Chronic Illness

IMPACT AND INTERVENTIONS

Chronic Illness

IMPACT AND INTERVENTIONS

Ilene Morof Lubkin, R.N., M.S., C.G.N.P.
California State University, Hayward

Jones and Bartlett Publishers, Inc.
Boston/Monterey

Editorial offices: Jones and Bartlett Publishers, Inc., 23720 Spectacular Bid, Monterey, CA 93940.
Sales and customer service offices: Jones and Bartlett Publishers, Inc., 20 Park Plaza, Boston, MA 02116.

Printed in the United States of America
10 9 8 7 6 5 4

Library of Congress Cataloging-in-Publication Data

Lubkin, Ilene, [date]
  Chronic illness.

  Includes bibliographies and index.
    1. Chronic diseases—Psychological aspects.
2. Chronically ill—Family relationships. 3. Nurse
and patient. I. Title. [DNLM: 1. Chronic Disease—
psychology. 2. Professional-Family Relations.
3. Professional-Patient Relations. W 62 L929c]
RC108.L83 1986   616   85-26468

ISBN 0-86720-354-4

Sponsoring Editor: Jim Keating
Project Coordinator: David Hoyt
Production: Cece Munson, The Cooper Company
Manuscript Editors: Susan Thornton and Meredy Amyx
Interior and Cover Design: Lois Stanfield
Illustrations: John Foster
Typesetting: Omegatype Typography, Champaign, Illinois
Printing and Binding: Malloy Lithographing, Ann Arbor, Michigan
Cover Art: Paul Jenkins, *Phenomena Reverse Spell.* Reproduced with permission of the Hirshhorn Museum and Sculpture Garden, Smithsonian Institution, Washington, D.C.

The selection and dosage of drugs presented in this book are in accord with standards accepted at the time of publication. The authors and publisher have made every effort to provide accurate information. However, research, clinical practice, and government regulations often change the accepted standard in this field. Before administering any drug, the reader is advised to check the manufacturer's product information sheet for the most up-to-date recommendations on dosage, precautions, and contraindications. This is especially important in the case of drugs that are new or seldom used.

Foreword

Ilene Lubkin's book marks a new phase in the growing recognition of chronic illness as a major policy area. Awareness of the prevalence of chronic illness has increased during the past forty years, but its full implications for training, care, insurance, and health institutions are not yet clear to health professionals or the general public. As the publication of this book attests, we are now entering a period when the study and management of chronic illness are given the attention they have long deserved.

No country has yet made the adjustment that will be necessary to manage chronic illnesses effectively, either inside or outside of health institutions. Modern medical technology has been termed a "half-way technology," because the equipment, drugs and procedures, no matter how wonderful they seem, do not cure chronic illnesses. Rather, they allow people to live longer with their diseases and experience a better quality of life. Today's technology, while greatly refined, derives its medical perspective from the days when acute diseases were rampant. This perspective is not at all adequate for thinking about the many issues related to chronicity—social, psychological, ethical, legal, organizational, and financial.

This is true not only in the hospitals, but to an even greater extent when the ill return home to cope with medical equipment, drugs, and other features of their regimens. Home management is complex and often requires considerable skill and resources, including the help of family, friends, and agencies. Some diseases engender a great deal of stress for the spouse and other family members, especially children. The impact of extended illness on family income can be disastrous, even in nations where health insurance is adequate to defray strictly medical costs. Ilene Lubkin's book treats these problems with admirable thoroughness.

The pages of this book contain a wealth of information, impressive even to well-informed specialists in the fields it covers. The writing is clear, the format effective, the bibliographies useful. Professor Lubkin addresses policy issues and avoids the inappropriate disease-oriented approach to chronic illness. Her emphasis is not simply physiological, procedural, or medical/technical; chronic illness is put into perspective. The table of contents suggests the areas in which the study of chronicity must continue to develop if we are to have an effective system of care and support for the ill and their families.

In sum, I believe that you, your colleagues, your students if you have them, and your relatives and friends can gain measurably from reading *Chronic Illness*.

Anselm Strauss, Ph.D.
Professor of Sociology
University of California, San Francisco

$\Diamond$

Preface

$\Diamond$

This text focuses on the many factors and issues that influence the ways individuals and families deal with chronic illnesses. The emphasis is not on disease process or specific disease management, since this material is well covered by numerous other sources. Although physiological or psychological alterations initiate the illness process, the sum of other factors has more impact on an individual's life than does the disease process itself. Chronic illnesses have a broad spectrum of social, economic, and behavioral aspects. One individual's illness affects members of the family and others, sometimes disrupting the functioning of the individual or family. Chronic illness often becomes a family illness.

Although primarily intended for a nursing audience, the concepts discussed are applicable to all health care providers. As more and more individuals survive the ravages of diseases, their need for long-term self-management grows. To help these clients adapt successfully, the health professional must be aware of the individual's premorbid personality, past experiences, coping mechanisms, life-style preferences, and other past and current influences. Professional support and intervention can enhance the quality of clients' lives in addition to maintaining their health regimens.

The experiences and themes that proved meaningful to nursing students over several years have guided the selection of the text's content. In integrating the concept of chronicity into my courses, I sought and adapted material that would help students become more effective and sensitive health care providers. The reader will find many familiar topics presented from a different perspective: their application to chronicity. Only by understanding this perspective can one attain a thorough understanding of the long-term impact of chronic diseases.

The book is organized into four parts, reflecting the primary author's perspective. Part One, The Impact of Disease, first explores what chronicity is and then discusses illness perception, major illness roles, stigma, and mobility problems. These topics apply to most chronic disease processes. Part Two, Impact on Client and Family, examines more closely the individual and family unit and discusses quality of life, compliance, family caregivers, body image, and sexuality. Part Three, Impact of the Health Professional, covers the roles of change agent, teaching, advocacy, and research and explores ways of applying each to assist the chronically ill client. Unique to this section is a discussion of some alternative modalities used by clients and families who seek assistance beyond the medical model. Part Four, Impact of the System, examines some components of the system that influence client, family, and professional, focusing on ways of dealing with agencies, finances, and rehabilitation. Interventions that are appropriate to the specific topics discussed are introduced throughout the text.

The text presents a cohesive whole by developing the interrelationships of topics throughout. However, each chapter can stand alone, providing information and help in the area discussed. The goal is to expand health professionals' knowledge of chronicity, so they can better help their clients take on the responsibilities of self-care management while maintaining a high quality of life.

Someday, we may be able to prevent or cure diseases that are now considered irreversible. Until that time, health professionals need to help their clients accept the fact that their lives are still meaningful, though different. It is important that the affected individuals retain their intrinsic dignity and sense of self-worth.

ACKNOWLEDGMENTS

No book comes into being without the assistance of numerous people. I wish to acknowledge the many individuals who supported and encouraged me in the creation of this text. My teaching colleagues deserve credit for the ongoing work involved in putting together and modifying content we covered in our classes, much of which is reflected in the text. A special thanks to Adrian Perenon, now Marketing Director at Brooks/Cole Publishing Company, who had faith in me and my idea and provided much support and encouragement early on. I am also grateful to the publisher's editors and editorial assistants, who have been extraordinarily patient with my slow process of writing and rewriting, and to Patricia Watters and Joanne Whitmore, who typed so many pages of manuscript onto computer disks so that I could better utilize my time in editing.

I am grateful to the following professors, whose insightful reviews contributed greatly to the development of the manuscript: Dr. H. Terri Brower of the School of Nursing, Auburn University; Dr. Joyce Colling of the School of Nursing, Oregon Health Sciences University; Dr. Harriet A. Fields, now of New York City; Professor Kathleen Meyn of the School of Nursing, University of Miami, Coral Gables, Florida; Dr. Moira D. Shannon of the Department of Nursing, George Mason University; Assistant Professor Ann Stoewer of the School of Nursing, Wright State University; and Professor Nancy C. Wilson of the Valley View Medical Center, Plymouth, Wisconsin.

I offer special thanks to special people: to Anselm Strauss, Ph.D., who was always available to discuss my ideas and provided valuable input in several areas; to Arlene Kahn, both friend and colleague, who unstintingly reviewed manuscript in spite of her busy teaching schedule and graduate work; to my many other friends, who have seen to it that I remained involved in other activities when I was driven to isolate myself to work on the book; to my children, who were always encouraging with their pride in my achievements; and to my husband, who deserves a very special thanks for putting up with me, keeping our home functioning, and keeping things from getting too chaotic during the three years I invested in this book. Finally, I am grateful to my trusty computer, which now seems a part of myself. How did anyone ever write without one?

Ilene Lubkin

Contents

Part Three Impact of the Health Professional 209

Chapter 11 Change Agent 210
Brenda Bailey

Chapter 12 Teaching 227
Audrey Bopp & Ilene Lubkin

Chapter 13 Advocacy 248
Eileen Jackson & Ilene Lubkin

List of Contributors

Ilene Lubkin, R.N., C.G.N.P., M.S.
Professor
Department of Nursing
California State University
Hayward, California

Brenda Bailey, R.N., M.S.
Assistant Professor
Department of Nursing
California State University
Hayward, California

Dorothy Blevins, R.N., M.S.N.
Associate Professor
School of Nursing
Kent State University
Kent, Ohio

Audrey Bopp, R.N., M.S.N.
Instructor
School of Nursing
University of Northern Colorado
Greeley, Colorado

Karna Bramble, R.N., M.S., C.G.N.P.
Lecturer
School of Nursing
California State University
Long Beach, California

Sheila Charlson, R.N., M.S.,
    C.G.N.P.
Nurse Practitioner
Veterans Administration Medical
    Center
Palo Alto, California

Mary Curtin, R.N., M.S. candidate
Coalinga, California

Marie-Luise Friedemann,
    R.N., Ph.D.
School of Nursing
Eastern Michigan University
Ypsilanti, Michigan

Eileen Jackson, R.N., M.S.
Assistant Professor
School of Nursing
University of Missouri
Columbus, Missouri

Katheliene Kohler, R.N., B.S.,
    C.A.N.P.
Nurse Practitioner
Kaiser Permanente Hospital
Martinez, California

Karen Thornbury La Buhn,
    R.N., Ph.D.
Cincinnati, Ohio

Terri Neifing, L.C.S.W.
Golden, Colorado

Geri Neuberger, R.N., Ed.D.
School of Nursing
College of Health Sciences
University of Kansas
Kansas City, Kansas

Margene Nordstrom, R.N., M.S.
D.N.S. candidate at University of
    California
San Francisco, California

Katheliene Kohler, R.N., B.S.,
  C.A.N.P.
Nurse Practitioner
Kaiser Permanente Hospital
Martinez, California
Altered Mobility, with M.T.
  Schweikert-Stary and I. Lubkin

Karen Thornbury Labuhn, R.N.,
  Ph.D.
Assistant Professor
School of Nursing
University of Virginia
Charlottesville, Virginia
Research

Terry Neifing, M.S.W., L.C.S.W.
Social Worker, Oncology and
  Burn Units
Alta Bates Hospital
Berkeley, California
Financial Impact

Geri Budesheim Neuberger, R.N.,
  Ed.D.
Associate Professor
School of Nursing
College of Health Sciences
University of Kansas
Kansas City, Kansas
Alternative Modalities, with
  C. Woods

Margene Nordstrom, R.N.,
  D.S.N.c
Manager of Clinical Training
Care Enterprises West
Anaheim, California
Quality of Life, with I. Lubkin

Coleen Saylor, R.N., Ph.D.c
Assistant Professor
Department of Nursing
San Jose State University
San Jose, California
Stigma

Barbara Scheffer, R.N., M.S.
Assistant Professor
Department of Nursing Education
Eastern Michigan University
Ypsilanti, Michigan
Agency Maze, with M.
  Friedemann

Mary Therese Schweikert-Stary,
  M.S.
Disability Management Counselor
Disabled Student Center
California State University
Hayward, California
Altered Mobility, with K.
  Kohler and I. Lubkin

Ann Shanck, R.N., M.S., M.A.
Professor
Department of Nursing
California State University
Hayward, California
Rehabilitation, with I. Lubkin

Cynthia Thorne Woods, R.N.,
  M.S.
Assistant Professor
School of Nursing
College of Health Sciences
University of Kansas
Kansas City, Kansas
Alternative Modalities, with
  G. Neuberger

Chronic Illness

IMPACT AND INTERVENTIONS

PART ONE

The Impact of Disease

◇

CHAPTER ONE

What Is Chronicity?

◇

Introduction

Chronic illness constitutes a major challenge for health workers now and in the future. Growing awareness of the increased incidence of chronicity has led to recent legislation that has helped some people with long-term illnesses. For example, the availability of home care funding allows some individuals to carry out their complex care so that they can remain within the community rather than residing in institutions. Provisions for wheelchair ramps and toileting facilities in public areas allow the disabled to be involved in community life. Chronic illness presents a further challenge to society to expand efforts that will permit clients more self-determination; such efforts require that health care workers redefine their roles, activities, and goals.

Historical Perspective

Human beings throughout history have recognized the presence of illness and attempted to repair or minimize disease. Evidence of early healing attempts is shown in a Sumerian tablet (approximately 2100 B.C.) that deals primarily with poultices. The "Treatise of Medical Diagnosis and Prognosis" (Mesopotamian tablets possibly of 1600 B.C.) lists diseases and outcomes based on a variety of signs (Majno 1975). Interventions that combined medical means and mysticism were often used to treat the tangible and intangible aspects of disease.

Beginning in the 19th century, after discoveries in disease causation and process, people began to apply scientific methodologies to health care. Health fields such as medicine and nursing now deal with an increasing variety of health events that move from acute to chronic, as well as dealing with the iatrogenic effects of successful and wide-ranging interventions. Current health workers face the prospect that by the end of this century there will be clients with health conditions as yet unknown that will require health care by means not yet comprehensible. Health planners and legislators have the complicated task of defining future environments and responsibilities for health and health care, while dealing with the present implications of chronic disease on society.

The Shape of Chronicity

Chronic illnesses take many forms. They can occur suddenly or through an insidious process; they can have episodic flare-ups or exacerbations or remain in remission with an absence of symptoms for long periods of time. Maintaining a degree of wellness or keeping symptoms in remission can be a juggling act of balancing treatment and regimens. For example, heart failure makes one person a bedridden invalid, although another with a similar degree of failure attains a satisfactory social life simply by manipulating the time at which Lasix is taken.

The course of any disease follows some kind of general trend or trajectory (see Chapter 2), depend-

---

◇ CASE STUDY ◇
Mr. W.: A Case of Progressive Dermatitis

While looking after his small herd of cattle, Mr. W., aged 52, wore boots that were higher than his sock length, producing chafing in both calves. One area became increasingly inflamed and then infected. He self-medicated for a week with veterinary penicillin ointment on hand for use with cattle. By the time he went to his physician, the formerly reddened area had progressed into cellulitis with draining lesions from foot to midthigh. Two medications were tried without improvement.

After 2 weeks, a dermatology consultation led to hos-pitalization and orders for bedrest, daily leg soaks, diet restrictions, and further medication changes. Several months later he had still not healed. Social contacts were reduced; he sold the cattle herd because he was unable to work regularly. Reemployment as a yard foreman required job modification due to exacerbation of the leg lesions with activity. When not at work, Mr. W. kept his legs elevated and wrapped with ace bandages. At age 58 he retired because of chronic leg debility and osteoporosis.

---

ing on the specific entity diagnosed, severity, rate of progression, and psychological makeup and expectations of the person. In the past, trajectories were thought to be fairly predictable, but the advent of new technology such as donor and mechanical organ transplants has dramatically altered such courses. The presence of multiple disease entities further changes the trajectory, making projecting outcomes difficult for physicians and other health professionals as well as making future planning uncertain for client and family.

Factors Influencing Increasing Chronicity

Developments in the fields of bacteriology, immunology, public health, and pharmacology have resulted in a precipitate drop in mortality from communicable and other acute diseases. For example, smallpox, once the scourge of thousands, is controlled and, for all practical purposes, eliminated. Decreased mortality from acute illnesses has led to lengthened life spans and, incidentally, greater vulnerability to accident and disease events that can accumulate in chronic conditions. Medical success has also contributed, in part, to the unprecedented growth of chronic illnesses. For instance, biotechnology and nuclear medicine bring about lifesaving and life-sustaining interrelationships with machines.

Given these factors, it becomes apparent that the prevalence of chronic disease is increasing dramati-cally. This growth is especially apparent in cohort populations as they age. Nearly half of all noninstitutionalized persons over 65 are limited by at least one chronic condition. Additionally, 24% of those aged 45 to 64 and 7% of those 45 or younger are so limited (U.S. Dept. of Commerce 1980).

Chronic illness can begin with a seemingly insignificant acute condition that is only partially resolved. Although the outcome may be free of profound disability or death, the accumulation of events can lead to a drastically altered life-style. The case history of Mr. W. demonstrates such an occurrence.

Perceptions of Chronic Illness

Health professionals can view chronicity positively, as a state that can continue to contribute to potential growth of an individual, family, or society, or negatively, as a state of failure to recover completely. Some of this negativity flows from the fact that a majority of health workers participate in the client's care only at the worst times, since most health care settings provide episodic care based on worsening or exacerbation of symptoms. With this piecemeal exposure, the disease entity reinforces the attitude that the extended life indeed may offer only increasing disability, pain, and deterioration. To counteract negativity of this kind, the health professional must strive to keep the client's entire life pattern in focus.

Statistics, which are an invaluable aid for appreciating the scope of a particular disease condition through analysis of characteristics, impact, prevalence, costs, and so on, also influence attitudes about chronic conditions. From a positive dimension, statistics provide information that allows projection of outcomes. For example, data on heart disease in the United States indicate that there has been a decrease in the number of deaths since 1965: mortality among adults 22 to 64 years of age has fallen by about a third (compared to figures from 1950) and for the elderly population by about 25%. On the basis of findings on associated risk factors of cardiovascular diseases, James Schoenberger, president of the American Heart Association, predicted in 1981 that heart disease and stroke could be preventable conditions if healthy lifestyle habits to decrease risk factors for atherosclerotic disease began in childhood (Pater and Pater 1982). These factors include cigarette smoking, poor eating habits, and lack of exercise (Williams et al. 1979). Statistics also point out that cardiovascular disease in adults could be slowed by controlling serum cholesterol, weight, hypertension, and perceived psychosocial stress (Theorell 1980).

In spite of these findings, statistics tend to reinforce negative attitudes about chronic diseases. For example, information about the decline of heart disease in the United States describes the disease's characteristics in terms of physical disability, economic costs, and death rates. Seldom are reemployment rates provided for comparison to rates demonstrating individuals' dependency on society. Health workers must recognize the often one-sided presentation of statistics and the way they influence issues and attitudes surrounding chronicity and professional practice.

Acute illnesses generally have a sudden, dynamic onset, with signs and symptoms usually related to the disease process itself. Acute illness ends shortly with either complete recovery and resumption of prior activities or with death. Acute illness may be compared with an unexpected visitor who leaves one's house after a short-term stay.

Chronic illness, on the other hand, announces plans to visit for an indefinite stay and gradually becomes part of the household. Although this "guest"

is a welcomed alternative to death, the illness provides a mixed blessing to the host household and to society at large. In addition, the illness frequently becomes the person's identity. For example, an individual having leukemia, even in remission after chemotherapy, acquires the label "that person with leukemia" (see Chapter 4).

Difficulty of Defining Chronicity

Answering the question of what chronicity is becomes very complex. Many individuals have attempted to present an all-encompassing yet clear definition of chronic illness (see Table 1–1). It is interesting to note that there are no nursing definitions. The characteristics of chronic diseases were identified by the Commission on Chronic Illness as all impairments or deviations from normal that include one or more of the following: permanency, residual disability, nonreversible pathological alteration, required rehabilitation, or a long period of supervision, observation, and care (Roberts 1954). The National Conference on Care of the Long-Term Patient added a further time dimension to these characteristics: chronic disease or impairment necessitating acute hospitalization exceeding 30 days or medical supervision and rehabilitation of 3 months or longer in another caretaking setting (Roberts 1954). Many conditions, such as birth defects and postinjury and postsurgical states, are included within the umbrellalike classification of chronic illness under the terms these two agencies present.

Determining a definition for chronic disease is more difficult when one attempts to establish the origin of a specific condition. Many chronic diseases have multiple factors that can take many years to accumulate sufficiently to produce frank symptoms. Do we say that bowel cancer that manifests itself at the age of 50 originated when the first mutant cell divided 30 years earlier? Or was it the result of a particular diet or life-style? Or can we say it started at the time of biopsy? Like life itself, the time of origin is debatable. For chronic disease, origin is highly critical in seeking those measures that may prevent or ameliorate the eventual disease.

TABLE 1-1. Multiplicity of Definitions of Chronic Illness

Author	Definitions	Advantages	Disadvantages
Verbrugge (1982)	a degenerative illness	—	Too simplistic
Commission of Chronic Diseases (1949)	all impairments or deviations from normal which have the following characteristics: permanency, residual disability, caused by nonreversible pathological alteration, require rehabilitation, and may require a long period of supervision, observation, or care	Concise Generally applicable	Patriarchal Medicine-based interventions Not flexible Unilateral approach
National Conference on Care of the Long-Term Patient	requires a continuous or prolonged period of care, at least 30 acute hospital days, or 3 months of medical supervision and/or rehabilitation in a different setting [summarized]	Gives definite time dimension	Primarily based on hospital settings Now much intervention emphasizes shortening hospital stay and preventing exacerbations
Feldman (1974)	ongoing medical condition with spectrum of social, economic, and behavioral complications that require meaningful and continuous personal and professional involvement [summarized]	Directs attention to context of all human involvement Provides sound basis for intervention by all disciplines	Complex More cognizant of caretaker's than client's role
Cluff (1981)	A condition not cured by medical intervention requiring periodic monitoring and supportive care to reduce the degree of illness, maximize the person's functioning and responsibility for self-care [summarized]	Puts person with chronic illness into a major self-care role Flexible Includes other disciplines subtly Defines role of medical intervention	Somewhat medically oriented
Abram (1972)	Any impairment of bodily function over a period of time requiring general adaptation [summarized]	Behaviorally oriented Concise	Too brief
Mazzuca (1982)	A condition requiring a high level of self-responsibility for successful day-to-day management [summarized]	Acknowledges role of self-help Futuristic	Too brief
Buergin et al. (1979)	Symptoms and signs caused by a disease within a variable period of time that runs a long course and from which recovery is only partial	Concise Traditional	Disease-oriented

The extent and direction of chronic illness further complicate attempts to provide a firm definition. A measurable quantity of disability from chronic illness depends not only on the kind of condition and its severity but on the implications it holds for the person. A teenager may require greater adjustment to the restrictions necessitated by a bone cancer than an individual who is past 60. The degree of disability and altered life-styles, part of a traditional definition, may relate as much to the client's views of the impact of the disease on self as to the specific disease.

Long-term and iatrogenic effects of some treatment methods may constitute chronic conditions eligible for definition as chronic illness. This situation is well represented by the necessary changes in life patterns required of clients on hemodialysis. Lifesaving procedures can create other problems. Abdominal radiation that arrested metastatic intestinal cancer when an individual was age 30 can contribute to a malabsorption problem several years later, so that almost continuous diarrhea may force the now cachectic and exhausted person to stay close to toilet facilities. Fortunately, these are extreme examples of life-style changes provoked by treatment procedures.

Chronic illness, by its very nature, is never completely cured or prevented. The inevitable breakdowns of cultural, economic, emotional, and social factors all affect body integrity. Biologically, the human body continues to wear out unevenly. Medical advances cause older persons to need a progressively wider variety of specialized services for increasingly complicated bodily conditions. In the words of Emanuel (1982), "Life is the accumulation of chronic illness beneath the load of which we eventually succumb."

So we are left with the problem of defining chronicity. All of us, depending upon our own state and perspective, may well define it differently, but a more comprehensive and flexible definition is needed. This author offers the following in hopes of meeting these conditions:

Chronic illness is the irreversible presence, accumulation, or latency of disease states or impairments that involve the total human environment for supportive care and self-care, maintenance of function, and prevention of further disability.

Impact of Chronic Illness

Confirmation of a chronic condition tends to affect social, psychological, physical, and economic aspects of the person's life, often in a cyclic manner. The impact of physical disability changes the psychological status, which impinges on economic capability, and so on. Each area acts as its own stressor. Problems inevitably faced include intrafamily and sexual stresses, social isolation, independence versus dependence conflicts, enforced self-image insults and modifications, economic pressures, and threat of death (Levy 1979). The case history of J.O. illustrates the impact of progressive disability on the individual, the family, and the community.

The way an individual responds to diagnosis and then copes with chronicity usually relates to prior experiences with crises and accumulated strengths and weaknesses (Feldman 1974). The case study of J.O. demonstrates the interrelatedness of aspects of this illness on one individual client's life. J.O. initially denied the presence of a physical problem. When confronted by the diagnosis, he heard threats to his marriage and the prediction of his pending death. He responded by sequestering himself and family as he grappled with his newly acquired sick role and changed image. For the first time as an adult he became dependent on others to fulfill his needs.

Self-imposed isolation led to jealousy, perceived loss, hopelessness, powerlessness, and finally depression. Family and friends were then unable to maintain the degree of support sufficient to confirm his own esteem and worthiness. The threat of suicide led to potent crisis intervention and interruption of that overwhelming cycle. He grieved for his lost premorbid potential and independence and finally concluded "I'll live with it." In Feldman's terms, he has accepted being "different" rather than sick (1974). This successful accommodation to different levels of

◇ C A S E   S T U D Y ◇
J.O.: Interrelated Problems of Chronic Illness

Seven years ago, J.O., then a 30-year-old, was surprised by a sudden inability to control his hand grip. Tools fell unaccountably, and he noticed a numbness of his hands and a gradual inability to identify hand-held objects. For several months he attributed the lack of sensation to other causes until intermittent double vision led him to a family physician, who diagnosed multiple sclerosis. The doctor provided J.O. with what he saw as a dismal description of progressive deterioration. He also alarmed J.O. with the statement that "90 percent of marriages end in divorce by the fifth year." Recurrent, progressive symptoms led to J.O.'s decision to remain at home.

Friends and associates who visited were confused and apprehensive when looking at this robust-appearing man who had been so physically strong. They often talked all around the subject of his health, preferring to keep communication light. He did not benefit from these visits. He felt tired, defeated, and resentful and experienced pain from muscle spasms. He also was suspicious of his associates' intentions toward his wife. He rebuffed offers of activities that once were pleasurable and maintained an uncivil attitude toward all. Rarely did he leave the house for fear of being trapped in a situation in which his awkward ambulation or appearance in a wheelchair would cause him to seem foolish or pitiable.

J.O.'s marriage was under stress. He felt that his wife deserved a more sexually capable mate and their young children a more involved parent. The children knew

their father was ill and that his legs wouldn't work, but they did not understand his frequent irritability. They seemed to take particular delight in adapting or mimicking his dysfunctional mannerisms. He considered suicide to hasten the ultimate outcome. This threatened action necessitated a psychiatric consult and treatment and later referral to vocational rehabilitation.

He has adapted. Presently, he is employed at home as a telephone research surveyor for a political party. His wife has taken a full-time position in a nearby town. Monthly visits to a neurologist provide a consistent medical regimen and support, some pain relief, and increased optimism about the disease progression and remissions. Family and friends continue to visit occasionally and some invite J.O. out to their homes or to various community events. He now feels more relaxed in public places that afford accessibility to him, and he looks upon his wheelchair as a good friend that provides comfort and safety. Conversation frequently turns to hopeful talk about a new medication or cure, or at least to lengthy remission. General plans include events several years in the future.

J.O. says, "This is not a pleasant thing to have but I've got it and I'm going to live with it." The couple seem to agree that life will be a struggle. Communication is more open than ever before. However, the subjects of their most frequent arguments, including finances, sexual inequalities, and child management, are not brought to resolution.

---

normality allows J.O. to face and participate in day-to-day problem solving. He finds that life holds value (Strauss 1975).

Issues of Quality and Quantity of Life

Adapting successfully to chronic illness includes a conception that the quality and quantity of life are worth the struggle. Illness is only one of a myriad of factors that influence the totality of a perceived life scheme that impacts a person's quality of life. The same medical condition may be tolerable to one person and overwhelmingly intolerable to another. Qual-

ity of life is also assessed by the individual's community. The characteristics of the illness, age of individual, degree of collective disability, and extent of medical intervention required to maintain a condition all have implications for individual and community decision making (see Chapter 6).

Professional caregivers face changing dilemmas as medical technology creates new methods to preserve and prolong life. The medical community has long confronted the question of who receives which life-giving measure and who should finance treatment. With the advent of multiple complex treatment modalities and mechanical organ transplants, broad-based planning must establish the guidelines for designating recipients. Even the process of dying and the moment of death itself can be controlled by machinery that dictates bodily functioning. Physicians daily face the challenge of determining when maintaining life is inhumane or ceasing to maintain it is murder. Medical/legal decisions entail a collected summary of ethics, legal guidelines, individual caregivers' consciences, and wishes of the individual and the community (Bohle 1979).

Self-autonomy is one quality of life a healthy person takes for granted. Chronic illness may make individuals feel victimized by their altered body. Outsiders expend efforts to increase treatment compliance and effectiveness, including shifting greater responsibility for self-management and control to the client. Inherent in control of one's life may be the ideal of control of one's death. Presently, "Living Wills" that provide more autonomy over the way of death are being tested in hospitals for practicality and in courtrooms for legality. Of crucial importance to society is seeking an answer to the question, When is a client's request for cessation of treatment or procedure death with dignity, and when is it suicide?

Impact on the Client

An individual is destined to age, progressing toward senescence. Age and life stages influence the types of problems and consequences impacting the person having a chronic condition. In spite of the disability, the individual must also accomplish developmental tasks allowing psychological and cognitive transition from one stage to the next. Each age group—child, adolescent, middle aged, and old—demonstrates particular characteristics.

Infancy through Adolescence. Chronic illness has replaced acute illness as the leading health concern for children. In her article on children in long-term care, Cullinane (1983) reports that 10% to 15% of all children under 18 years have some type of chronic condition, with 1 to 2.8 million limited in daily activities. The degree of disability or potential for independence has far-reaching implications. A

newborn with spina bifida faces outcomes that range from a life of institutionalization and custodial care to one of productivity with only residual disability. If the child is at home, parents face the role of long-term caregivers, requiring medical and nonmedical support. Categories of services most parents need include acute illness care, health care maintenance, education, general advice, future planning, emotional support, genetic counseling, and coordination of services (Stein et al. 1983). Stein also points out that although seriously ill children generally receive most of these services, studies have found gaps in effective delivery of services to all children with chronic illness.

Women are now able to carry pregnancies to full term; babies who would not have survived full gestation with lesser technology are born. Diagnosis and treatment of fetal defects in utero can preserve function and life. Surgery corrects some tissue defects, but infants born with congenital disorders often depend upon caretakers for a lengthened life span. This dependency creates a situation that can be destructive for some families; to others such a child brings unlimited loving unity and an increased value system.

Maintaining a medical regimen can conflict with a child's growth and development needs. Important parental contact and response during infancy affect the baby's mental and physical progress. Separations due to hospitalizations, testing, or treatments can influence the early establishment of trust and security. Later, the child looks outward, seeking interaction with peers and other adults. Awareness of the way one appears to others and self-value develop during these early relationships. Treatment procedures and regimen scheduling can interfere with a normal lifestyle. Siblings experience a gamut of emotional reactions to having a "different" brother or sister (Cullinane 1983).

The adolescent who has a chronic illness faces a dual role of normal adult development and acceptance of a life with limitation. A major task confronting an adolescent is the necessity to grow into a life of what is and can be, rather than one of what might have been. Dunlop (1982) identified six major prob-

◇ CASE STUDY ◇
Impact on the Client and Family

M.T. was the second-born and seemed normal until repeated upper respiratory infections and consistent lack of weight gain necessitated a referral to a regional medical center when M.T. was 14 months. Cystic fibrosis was diagnosed through a positive sweat test. The diagnosis could not have come at a worse time! The mother was in her second trimester of pregnancy, and the family's finances already were not covering assorted medical expenses.

M.T.'s parents learned to perform the postural drainage and percussion exercises required several times daily to keep M.T.'s lungs functioning. With urging, they attended group meetings at the center. Inherent in these meetings were shared experiences and emotional support. After two meetings the father stopped attending: "I wasn't getting anything from them. My wife became the expert and ran the meeting. Even the therapists had a hard time talking."

As M.T. grew older, the mother became obsessed with the home regimen and perceived need to keep M.T. away from disease-causing people or things. People were not invited to the home, and M.T. did not go into crowds. The father gradually assumed a background role in family decision making in regard to M.T.'s illness. His concern for his wife's preoccupation led him to suggest that she consult a psychiatrist. She of course refused. When the public health nurse, visiting for Crippled Children's Services, suggested mental health counseling to the mother, she was told to mind her own business: "I'm not crazy."

The older sibling, a girl five years M.T.'s senior, had always been expected to conform to the demands her sister's illness placed on the household. She was a serious child, close to her father, and until she was 16 was the major caregiver to the youngest girl. She eloped at that time. The youngest girl, who proved to be free of cystic fibrosis after delivery, varied between overdependence and stubborn independence. Although close to M.T. in age, she generally kept an emotional distance. The siblings chose not to entertain their friends around M.T. and centered their activities out of the home.

By the time M.T. reached school age she needed to rise an hour and a half earlier than her sisters to allow for the first pulmonary exercise program. Dietary requirements and occasional added postural drainage at noontime necessitated that the mother transport M.T. home and back to school daily. After school, a pulmonary session was followed by homework, a rest period, and dinner. M.T. had an early bedtime. She slept nightly in a mist tent.

Regardless of the restrictive circumstances, M.T. developed into a bright, energetic child who was outgoing and well-liked. Friends did not visit often, because of the home routine and the unpleasant but necessary production of sputum. Until she was 10 years of age, M.T. followed her mother's directions without argument.

During the fifth grade, illness forced M.T. to miss a lot of school. All her spare time had to be spent studying. One day she told her mother she was joining the Girl Scouts "to have some fun with my friends." The mother pointed out that group activities would expose her to fatigue, germs, and a change of routine, but the child was adamant. From that time on, regardless of her mother's wishes, M.T. continued to direct her own life.

---

lem areas specific to young adults who have cancer that also pertain to all young people whose futures are less than certain as the result of a chronic condition:

1. The uncertainty of the future
2. Identification with the illness and the sick role
3. Taking negative risks
4. Illness and death as unexpected life events
5. Dependence/independence conflicts with parents
6. Being different

Cystic fibrosis, presented in the case study of M.T., is a disease that typifies the impact made on family life. The very fact that individuals are now surviving into young adulthood is a tribute to devoted family members, cooperation with complicated therapeutic regimens, and advances in medical technology.

Young to Middle-Aged Adults. The young to middle years are typically a time of high activity and productivity. Individuals launch careers and marriages, begin and raise families, experience changes

---

◇ CASE STUDY ◇
Cancer and the Middle-Years Family

S.W.'s attitude during the crisis of discovery, diagnosis, and treatment of lung cancer largely determined the way she and her family dealt with the experience. She is a 38-year-old secretary whose complaint of continued coughing and weight loss took her to a private physician. X-rays demonstrated an infiltrate with pleural effusion. Further testing resulted in a diagnosis of small-cell carcinoma, stage III, with limited survival expectation (Golomb & DeMeester 1979). A one-pack-a-day cigarette smoker for 20 years, she suddenly became one of the statistics showing a sharp increase of females with lung cancer and mortality approaching that of breast cancer (Rosenow & Carr 1979).

S.W. and her family had to work through the turmoil of diagnosis, treatment, and role changes. She began chemotherapy and radiation hopeful of effects, but fearful of reactions, disability, and expense. During this pe-

riod, her husband took over the family and household tasks. He admitted fearing present and future losses and being angry that his wife should fall victim to a smoker's disease. After a period of flight from usual and required responsibilities, the two teenaged children began taking on some of the work at home.

Gradually, S.W. and her family entered the *coping phase*, a time of rebuilding life. S.W. lived day to day, spending quality time with family and friends. Although some conversation centered on the future and possible absence of S.W., she and her family shared what was really important to them. S.W. returned to work part-time, as symptoms allowed. For the rest of her life, she established a balance between what had to be changed and maintained and what could be resisted or challenged.

---

in status, and prepare for retirement. According to 1979 statistics, this age group shows a three- to four-fold increase of diabetes, heart conditions, arthritis and rheumatism, and hypertension without heart involvement. The presence of a chronic condition can complicate the conception and completion of goals and dreams. At a time when creative energy generally goes outward, the individual may need to utilize most inner resources to cope with the condition.

The case study discussing cancer in the middle years demonstrates the impact that chronic disease, cancer in this situation, can have at this time of life. A diagnosis of cancer engenders great fear regardless of the type of cancer or age of the individual affected. That fear and allied overwhelming emotions are described as the *cancer mystique* (Dagrosa 1980). Accordingly, remission of the cancer depends on gaining control over one's body, allowing reduction of anxiety and stress concerning the disease. At such a time, the body's healing potential can be optimally activated.

Older Adults. The greatest proportion of chronic illness affects the older population. Diagnoses of

chronic illness are frequently multiple. To the older chronically ill person, longer life expectancy means periods of disability, vulnerability to other health problems, financial expense, and increasing care concerns.

Combined with the normal aging processes, management of ailments can be formidable. A body weakened by neurological pathology may become more fragile through bony calcium loss. An elderly person having hypertension may eat canned soups, high in sodium, because of lack of easy access to fresh foods or because canned products are an easy meal for one person. And if mental faculties are affected, he or she may be unable to follow a complex medical regimen.

Demographics from 1979 show a preponderance of older women over men in North America. From the ages of 75 to 79, there are 1000 women to every 673 men. Over age 80, the proportion increases to 1000 women to 558 men (Grundy 1983). The older woman who is alone must meet the normal challenges of financing and running a household. Her support system often depends on the presence of children and friends and their ability to help. This

---

◇ CASE STUDY ◇

Losing Independence

A.C., a 72-year-old retired businesswoman and widow of six years, was healthy except for a history of peptic ulcer and cataract of the left eye. She stumbled and fell, sustaining a fractured femur that was pinned without complication. She was transferred from the acute care facility to a convalescent hospital for continued physical therapy and recovery. During a transfer from her wheelchair to the toilet, she fell without sustaining injury. However, her self-confidence was shattered. Subsequently, two nursing assistants helped her with ambulation and transfers. Her daughter, who lived out of town, noted this increase in aid and advised her mother to stay at the hospital until she could take care of herself as before.

A bladder infection caused problems with urinary continence. A.C. began to exhibit confusion and made several attempts to get out of bed at night without alerting the staff. After retrieving her from the floor twice, they applied restraints at night to prevent further falls. A representative from a home health agency attempted to arrange discharge and visitation schedules. A.C. expressed fear about being at home alone. Family and staff now assumed most of her daily living tasks and business transactions. Alternative living situations were considered. Her wish to return to her own home is very uncertain.

---

woman tends to be less assertive and less well educated than the younger single woman. Cohort differences in the changing role of women and their dependence exist.

In general, society views both the aged and chronically ill negatively. There is a tendency to look at age and disability in terms of their effect on the national pocketbook. Services needed for both populations are on the increase. Unlike that for children, the investment for older adults brings limited promise of return. The old who are chronically ill also carry a double yoke of undesirability when they become inpatients. Circumstances often cause them to be less rewarding to care for in terms of recovery, reduction of disease states, and economics.

Even though an older person may have been independent just before a crisis, other persons' caution and reluctance to relinquish the helping role may negate return to an independent state. The case study on loss of independence demonstrates just such a situation.

Sociocultural Impact

To date, society defines illness and debility largely with a disease-specific focus. This acute illness model places chronically ill individuals at a disadvantage. Rather than seeking cure of disease, the chronically ill person needs to be considered not as incurable, but as modified. Such a perspective leads to maximization of well-being, creativity, and productivity. However, society often sees the disabled as nonproductive.

Hamera and Shontz (1978) studied clients', families', and nurses' attitudes toward positive and negative aspects of chronic illness. Those subjects who had closest contact to the illness had a more positive perspective than those who were less close. One may take some liberty with the conclusion by casting society in the role of an outsider who emphasizes negative aspects of chronic illness because of perceived dismal outcomes.

Recently, nationally recognized political figures have stepped forward to make statements as active persons who coincidentally have disabling or terminal illnesses. These conditions include alcoholism, cancer, and neurological and coronary diseases. These persons' courage and far-sightedness encourage a more objective and closer appraisal of legislation and funding by lawmakers.

Use of Health Services. Traditionally, chronic disease has been that condition left after incomplete resolution of acute disease. As a result of the gradual evolution of chronic disease in this manner, acute modalities have been the management approaches used. The physical design of hospitals well defines this mode, since they are planned for efficient disposition of diagnosis, treatment, and care.

The great uncertainty clouding the future of an individual's life may not be caused by the demands of his or her condition, but by the intricacies of the medical system. Dealing with various service or provider elements can be difficult for those people who lack knowledge or energy. Physicians' offices tend to reflect efforts to maintain efficiency and control of the clients' behaviors. Health personnel often do not recognize that a general conversation can elicit the extent to which a person is affected and the adaptation required for lengthy disability. The need for professionals to see chronic illness as more than pathology is essential for providing optimal support and interventions.

Utilization of services varies by sex and age. Both the elderly (65 years and older) and women in general use health services more than younger populations or men (Verbrugge 1982). Not only do 39% of all persons 65 and older have major activity limitations due to a medical condition (Metropolitan Life Foundation 1982), but they often require closer medical supervision and therefore more frequent physician visits. Women who attend prenatal and well-baby care programs are more exposed to the importance of prevention and health promotion, which may partly account for their increased utilization of these services. Stein's study demonstrated that although children with chronic illness received acute illness care, needs for general advice or future planning, support, genetic counseling, and coordination of services often remained unmet (1983).

Society's laws have supported illness and disability as acute processes that shape and dominate the environment of the client's life. The nursing home industry well illustrates this perspective. Although striving to make the most of remaining health and ability, these facilities offer a pervasive illness model with stark walls and white uniforms of caretakers serving as a daily reminder of the need for intensive care. Health workers need to appreciate how the en-

vironments they work in may influence attitudes toward chronic illness and the chronically ill.

Recent inroads in chronic care management are redefining environments. Traditional or shopping-mall offices are often decorated to encourage relaxation and comfort. Many nursing homes have decor that stimulates and helps orient their residents. Also for the residents, increased accessibility to the community encourages fuller life experiences and expectations.

Rehabilitation.   Rehabilitation for the chronically ill can play a major role in restoring or maintaining function. As with acute illness, planning and implementation of restorative methods must soon follow diagnosis. Critical functions, such as hand flexibility and bladder continence, must be assessed for competency. Efforts should address those areas that potentially lessen independence. In response to heavy financial burdens, public policy and health planning tend to deny the accessibility of physical and socio-psychological rehabilitation to the chronically ill (see Chapter 18).

Cultural View of Illness.   Illness belief systems form the cultural milieu that defines caregivers' and individuals' attitudes toward illnesses. Conceptions about the source of illness and required treatment affect the types of therapy the caregiver offers as well as the outcome the client expects. A recent study of White and Chinese families revealed striking contrasts in attitudes toward ill children. Whites expected children to integrate normalization strategies so as to reduce deviance. Chinese families emphasized the comfort and contentment of the child, often to the exclusion of treatment priorities (Anderson & Chung 1982).

Language Differences.   Blumhagen (1980) found that 72% of a studied population having biomedically defined hypertension defined their illness as "Hyper-Tension," a problem of excessive nervousness caused by untoward social stress. A lack of basic agreement on diagnosis affects compliance to a treatment regimen. It is vital that professional caregiver, client, and family share a common language, which should include agreement on terminology for disease etiology, treatment, prognosis, and experiences symbolic to the person.

Political Impact

In 1954, Dean Roberts, director of The Commission on Chronic Illness, proposed that the result of improved medical technology would not be that fewer people would need long-term care, but that progressively older people would need care (Roberts 1954). Population structure changes, numbers, and varying requirements of health service needs all pose complex problems for health planners and social policy leaders. Institutional provision of long-term care has been customary for clients with highly debilitating conditions. Currently, legislators are looking at ways to increase home health benefits to clients and families.

Financial Cost

Illness is expensive. On a national scale, private health expenditures in 1981 came to $159 billion. Public health expenditures, including Medicare and public assistance, totaled $114.5 billion. Nursing home care leaped from $10 billion in 1975 to $24 billion in 1981 (Metropolitan Life Foundation 1982). Economic effects of chronic illness cause legislative turmoil on a national level and community impact and family desperation on a local level. Families are characterized by reduction of income and benefits, change to poorer housing, marital instability, and decreased opportunities to educate their children. Generally, chronically ill persons are not eligible for individual insurance coverage, unless they were previously covered by a group policy (see Chapter 17).

Interventions

Illness behavior can be defined as a total expression of meanings held by the individual and is attributed to interplay between the nature of the illness and the nature of the person (Byrne 1982). The goal of com-

ing to terms with chronic illness necessitates an acceptance of being permanently different. Harris and associates (1982) compared the acute sick role to the chronic impaired role in a study about survival rates and coping styles of maintenance hemodialysis clients. In the sick role, the person is exempted from normal role expectations. In the impaired role, the person is expected to maintain normal activities and care responsibility for the chronic illness. Although this new identity allows for maximum independence and freedom of choice, it also may involve varying amounts of inward stress to fulfill role expectations. Ideally, the involved individual will set a goal of achieving the highest level of wellness through focusing on strengths, following the medical regimen, and preventing further disability (see Chapter 3).

Coming to Terms with Chronicity

Successful management of chronic illness requires a high level of client or family responsibility. The individual's attitudes toward a specific therapy can have profound effects on outcome. A very personal problem the client must confront is determining the treatment that offers the chances of wished-for benefit at an acceptable level of risk (Pearlman and Speer 1983).

Although professionals hold positions in which they judge the client's life situation and potentials, in the final analysis, clients maintain the responsibility for determining the quality of their own lives. The ability to "get on with life" is one of these inherent qualities. Johnson recommends methods to achieve acceptance of cancer, a chronic illness, including word desensitization, self-belief, education, and acknowledgment of potential disease outcome (1982). She lists patterns of resistance such as being oneself, guarding against depression, refusing limitations, and resisting isolation. These suggestions apply to other chronic illnesses as well.

Support from Providers

Long-term care responsibility requires varying types of expertise provided by a variety of professionals.

Learning to deal with the system is an ongoing accomplishment. Individuals and their families are entitled to information and counseling about the mechanisms for obtaining care. They need access to opportunities to provide feedback on care received and to report problems with the system.

The professional community and society at large have joint responsibility to assist the chronically ill person and family to achieve maximal function and to slow or prevent functional impairment. This responsibility may require that novice practitioners learn how to enter and negotiate the system (see Chapter 16). Constructive attitudes and new models of health care should be considered.

A disease-specific focus or cure-oriented model is not practical for long-term care. The dominant issue in chronic illness is management, rather than a search for remedial results. Functional improvement and well-being can usually be achieved without curing the underlying disease. Health professionals must examine their reactions to chronically ill persons and recognize feelings of frustration and previous disappointments caused by the impossibility of effecting a total cure. Disease management can be viewed more positively and objectively by emphasizing success in modifying discomfort and disability. The satisfaction of crisis prevention can replace the drama of crisis intervention.

Professional and Community Responsibility

Committed professionals must be advocates for commonsense prevention planning. Such planning is useful in preventing congenital and early life illnesses that can necessitate a lifetime of care. Mother/child services include prenatal care, nutrition supervision, and well-baby care. Since it is known that low-birth-weight infants are more likely to suffer permanent disabilities (California Department of Consumer Affairs 1982), preventive services may have a greater impact than state-of-the-art monitoring equipment for high-risk deliveries and neonatal intensive care equipment for low-birth-weight and premature infants.

The older individual benefits from community preventive programs that offer nutritional supplementation, blood pressure monitoring, social and intellectual stimulation, daily telephone contact services, and so on. In spite of governmental funding for many such programs, they remain limited in number and often have long waiting lists. Low-cost preventive interventions could resolve the increasing demand for higher forms of technology that becomes necessary when physical status deteriorates.

Client Education. Client education has been considered one of the basic components of ensuring self-determined care. Educational programs include preventive health measures to retain function and prevent further disability from other health problems. Since education can pave the way for the individual to assume a greater role in management of chronic illness, the individual and family must be included as participants in the therapeutic decision-making process. A position of mutual trust and respect diminishes the undesirable connotation of long-term illness and care.

In a review of experimental effects of client education, Mazzuca (1982) found that behaviorally oriented programs were most successful at improving the clinical course. Interventions to integrate regimens into daily routines included regular contact with the same professional caregiver and daily self-care rituals designed to carry out the individualized self-management plan.

Preventive Education: The Client. Scientific validation of relationships between psychosocial factors and disease etiology has given rise to numerous life-style change workshops. Community college and hospital-based curricula offer free health promotion programs. Program content ranges from direct bodily change, weight reduction, smoking cessation, and so on, to knowledge expansion and attitudinal control, first aid, cardiopulmonary resuscitation, and stress reduction. In addition to decreasing the incidence of primary disease, the workshops are designed to prevent deterioration of current chronic conditions.

In 1982, the Department of Health and Human Services strategy on health promotion emphasized the promotion of behavioral and life-style changes for healthier Americans. Component activities included those relating to life-style, as well as those pertaining to prevention of disease and disability through appropriate use of preventive health services (Brandt 1982).

Preventive Education: The Professional. Increasingly, medicine relies on advanced technology to treat health care problems that may be preventable. From the *Nei Ching*, a Chinese medical book compiled around 350 B.C., comes this observation on preventive medicine (Majno 1975):

> The superior physician helps before the early budding of the disease.... The inferior physician begins to help when [the disease] has already developed; he helps when destruction has already set in.

Hence, prevention of disease has been long recognized as a noble endeavor of medicine. A cure-focused orientation, however, does not emphasize prevention but cure.

New models for prevention-oriented education of the professional are mandatory. According to Jonas (1982), preventive medicine must be the preeminent discipline. He advocates that disease-oriented physician education (DOPE) change to health-oriented physician education (HOPE). Computer-assisted instruction will lead comfortably to a computer-assisted practice, freeing physicians from the overwhelming amount of random memory work and allowing them to provide client education and communication necessary in a prevention-oriented practice.

Educating the Health Professional Student. Health educators cite the lack of comprehensive programs for students in medical and nursing schools and propose that classes on chronic illness be a major part of the curriculum. Clinical experiences should relate to the care of long-term illness and disability for all ages. The curriculum must integrate techniques to improve communication between caregivers and clients, families, and allied personnel. Professional caregivers must learn ways to increase individual self-assertiveness and self-care skills. The partnership of client and caregiver can then focus on self-determination.

Attitudinal Change. Changing attitudes toward chronicity is a slow process. Television documentaries, newspaper articles, and community hospital and college courses are laying a solid foundation of knowledge about the implications of living with chronic illness. Society's lack of empathy and concern may have been the result of lack of interaction with those affected. Because of degree of illness and debility, an unfriendly physical environment, and absence from the workplace, the chronically ill were not integrated into the mainstream. At present, the chronically ill still are identified frequently by debility rather than ability.

Among the highest rewards of self-determined care are societal recognition and respect of individuals' knowledge of their conditions. These individuals, who also are survivors and equalizers between positive and negative aspects of life, could be valuable resources at all levels of education and legislation to reverse bias and ignorance.

Research: A Key to Change

Research in chronic illness is a key to unlocking evidence that clarifies etiology, treatment, and prevention. Technology is allowing studies that are multifactorial in design and interdisciplinary in conception and execution. Resulting data may lead to more complicated questions. Professionals are at the horizon of chronic illness research. A large body of knowledge exists, yet what is still to come may change entirely the perception of chronicity. Research questions about chronicity, its cause and effects, have to be an integral part of medical practice (see Chapter 14).

◇ CASE STUDY ◇
The Client and the Computer

T.R., 36, became a paraplegic through a traffic accident. Because he is a type I diabetic, his brittle control and probable insulin reaction contributed to the accident. Following stabilization of the paraplegia and a program of rehabilitation, professionals and T.R. felt he was ready for home care. In collaboration with T.R., the physician facilitated a computer analysis using educational level, culture, other life-style preferences, medical history, and laboratory and treatment information. The following care program was listed in the computer: basic instructions for the medical regimen, information on expected or adverse reactions of treatment and medications, appropriate diet program, and all resources pertinent to the client's care.

T.R.'s prior employment as a telephone lineman was no longer possible. A telecommuter schedule with a terminal in his home enabled him to contact a vocational economist, have an employment assessment, and receive retraining. He was also able to schedule his infrequent in-office visits through the computer. Utilizing the terminal tied into an outpatient diabetic program, T.R. made daily adjustments of insulin dosage based on serum and urine glucose levels until his condition was stable. He has referred himself to a listed nutritionist and podiatrist. All referrals and their reports are printed out for the monthly meeting with his health team.

New Models of Care

Models of care that vary from the prevalent acute illness model give a new perspective to chronicity; rather than picturing the omnipresent disease or condition centrally, they focus on the function of one's entire life. Feldman (1974) stressed objectives interrelating a person's psychosocioeconomic function with readaptation and maximal social function. These objectives would channel components of medical care toward realistic and socially meaningful goals.

Tasks that could accomplish these objectives include the following broad categories, which give attention to all aspects of life (Strauss 1975). The individual would be assisted with funding and money management; revamping of the physical environment; and provision of access to a wide assortment of medical, educational, counseling, daily maintenance, and client representative services and programs. Professionals from medical and social fields would redesign support networks, work toward supplying the most functional technical equipment and aid, and educate those persons who encounter the chronically ill to increase understanding. Other models of care stress the development and utilization of

particular services. As one example, Levy (1979) describes the treatment of stress, a consequence of chronic illness, by a liaison psychiatrist.

Different models change the relationships between those who are afflicted by chronic illnesses and conditions and those who encounter them professionally. Rather than one or two persons directing modifications in life-style that are warranted, a number of individuals would share the required interventions. A collaboration of client with professional caregivers defines health service needs and methods for meeting them.

Effects of Computerization. Computerization of administration, research, education, and practice is affecting all aspects of medical care. Automated processing is capable of dealing with the complex and detailed recordkeeping and health planning that advanced medical technology necessitates. The presence of computer-based client care data systems will improve accuracy, so that the chronically ill person will receive enhanced care and individualization of health planning and promotion. The case study of the client and the computer illustrates the application of computer technology.

Social scientists are concerned about whether computers are tools of great promise or dehumanizing machines. More than any other modern implement, computers allow for creativity, networking, and ongoing evaluation of traditional methods of health management not previously possible. Current professional roles will evolve or be intensified. *The Post-Physician Era* (Maxmen 1976) projects a 21st century with a medic-computer model of client care in which the physician's traditional role would be greatly diminished. Other health care roles, including those of medics, professional nurses, physician assistants, and alternative care providers, would be extended. Computers would supply most of the technical, diagnostic, and treatment "decisions." Health workers would provide most supportive and technical tasks.

Nursing leaders question whether clients and caregivers will become appendages to computers (Happ 1983). Policies are being formulated to ensure humane, ethical client care. As computers change client treatment and the basic premises for these policies, constant updating of ethical concerns will be necessary. Professional caregivers must work to keep a healthy interdependence with machines to maximize human uniqueness while reaping the benefits of machine capabilities. The human being must be affirmed as the master of the designed technology, rather than the servant (Bohle 1979).

Value of Alternate Models. At-home care, regardless of complexity of condition, is becoming increasingly important to client and family and attractive to health care cost payers. Nonprofessionals now carry out parenteral nutrition, renal dialysis, ventilator-dependent care, maintenance of aseptic living quarters, and a myriad of other complicated procedures. A well-coordinated system of support services facilitates these at-home procedures, and efforts to increase feasibility of home care are increasing. The landmark Surgeon General's Workshop on Children with Handicaps and Their Families was held in December 1982. A cross section of all persons and agencies involved with the welfare of severely handicapped children focused on the requirements for at-home quality care, and recommendations for meeting the needs of all disabled children were disseminated through official channels (Koop 1983).

Nursing interventions to develop a child's self-care skills and family caregiving skills are the primary goal of Rural Efforts to Assist Children at Home (REACH), a Florida demonstration project (Pierce & Giovinco 1983). This project provides community-based nursing services to chronically ill children. Nurse managers supplement health care to improve treatment compliance, lessen need for medical services, and reduce exacerbation of the primary illness.

Meeting Individuals' Needs. Through involvement in health planning at local and regional levels, professional caregivers and chronically ill persons can work to meet the social and personal needs of individuals. The deficiencies and inefficiencies of health services can be brought to the attention of those persons who make policy and legislation.

Changing Focus of Legislation

Professional caregivers must act as advocates to change the focus of legislation from cure orientation to care orientation. Improvement of impaired function must receive equal attention in order to preserve the independence of the chronically ill. Medicare and Medicaid were designed primarily for short-term, acute illness; this focus must change. More funding for home health services and hospice care must be available.

Methods for reversing escalating medical costs are being tried. Nationally, policymakers are emphasizing competition and cost containment in the health industry to control prices. Replacing the fee-for-service system, rate of payment will be determined by categories called diagnosis-related groups (DRGs). On a state level, pilot projects organize new public agencies to negotiate rates with doctors and hospitals for medical services. The state pays the agency a predetermined flat fee for all medical services provided that year. Public assistance funding will change, as the client increasingly participates in cost sharing of expenses.

Summary and Conclusions

Chronicity is a state of unwellness produced by disease or disability requiring medicosocial intervention over an extended interval and affecting many aspects of an individual's life. Human beings may be chronically ill to some extent at all times. The chronically ill exert efforts to survive with self-determination and quality of life in what is often an unaware society. One of the most pressing obligations professional caregivers have toward chronically ill persons is to make society recognize that this struggle is being waged.

The degree of an individual's health may be determined by interventions of caregivers made at the most primary levels. Accident and disease prevention lowers the incidence of future chronic conditions. Changes in life-style with reduction of stress and smoking seem to play a major role in lowered heart disease incidence, for instance. The recommendation to change ways of eating may lessen bodily destruction and ultimately redesign health roles and concerns of professional caregivers. The world of prevention contains great power and potential for eliminating some disease and reducing the degree of others.

A challenge to all levels of health service workers is an increase of empathy for the chronically ill through direct involvement with them. The tendency may be to stand back and diagram chronically ill individuals and their needs as students once diagrammed sentences. However, people and their environment are not that elemental. To be effective, we, as professional caregivers, must be part of that diagram. A partnership of care requires information exchange and mutual decision making and offers an opportunity to share a part of courageous, creative lives.

Because of tumultuous effects of technology, constant change in disease and disability states, and efforts to meet resulting needs, a partnership with computers has been made necessary and desirable. Computers release caregivers from mundane and highly complex work to concentrate on heightening the unique human qualities in the care of the ill.

A partnership in health care also changes societal focus from the chronically ill as dependent victims to persons inconvenienced, but responsible. Chronically ill or disabled persons benefit from expanded rehabilitation, education, employment, and recreation opportunities. Caregivers promote full partnership in society of individuals with chronic illness through support of research, continued efforts to make the physical environment accessible, application of technology, and networking communication.

STUDY QUESTIONS

1. How do the many factors and conditions (technological, historical, and so on) lead to the increase in chronicity that exists today?
2. In what ways do statistics influence our perspective of chronic illness positively and negatively?
3. What factors should be considered in defining chronicity?
4. How do age and developmental level influence an individual's response to being chronically ill?
5. From a sociocultural and political perspective, how does society in general react to and treat the person who is chronically ill? How does this approach differ from treatment of acutely ill people?
6. How can the person come to terms with his or her chronicity?
7. What roles and actions can professional health care workers take to prevent, support, or improve care given to the chronically ill person?
8. In the future, how can computers or new models of care enhance or improve the care of the chronically ill?
9. What is the role of research in answering questions about chronicity?
10. In what way can the professional serve as an advocate to secure changes in the focus of legislation?

References

Abram, H., (1972) The psychology of chronic illness, editorial, *Journal of Chronic Diseases*, 25:659–664

Anderson, J., and Chung, J., (1982) Culture and illness: Parents' perceptions of their child's long term illness, *Nursing Papers*, 14:4:40–50

Blumhagen, D., (1980) Hyper-tension: A folk illness with a medical name, *Culture, Medicine, & Psychiatry*, 4:197–227

Bohle, B. (ed.), (1979) *Human Life: Controversies and Concerns*, The Reference Shelf, 51:5, New York: Wilson Co.

Brandt, E., (1982) A national health promotion strategy, editorial, *Public Health Reports*, 97:5

Buergin, P., (1979) Chap. 29 in Phipps, W., Long, B., and Woods, N., *Medical-Surgical Nursing*, St. Louis: C.V. Mosby Company

Byrne, D. G., (1982) Psychological responses to illness and outcome after survived myocardial infarction: A long term follow-up, *Journal of Psychosomatic Research*, 26:105–112

California Department of Consumer Affairs, (1982) Pregnant women and newborn infants in California: A deepening crisis in health care, California State Dept. of Consumer Affairs, Division of Consumer Services, Sacramento, California

Cluff, L., (1981) Chronic disease, function and the quality of care, editorial, *Journal of Chronic Disease*, 34:299–304

Cullinane, M., (1983) Children in long-term care, *Nursing Times*, March 9, 79:10:30–32

Dagrosa, T., (1980) Cancer in America: The socialization and promulgation of the mystique, *Nursing Forum*, 19:4

Dunlop, J., (1982) Critical problems facing young adults with cancer, *Oncology Nursing Forum*, 9:3:33–38

Emanuel, E., (1982) We are all chronic patients, *Journal of Chronic Diseases*, 35:7:501–502

Feldman, D., (1974) Chronic disabling illness: A holistic view, *Journal of Chronic Disease*, 27:287–291

Golomb, H., and DeMeester, T., (1979) Lung cancer: A combined modality approach to staging and therapy, *CA—A Cancer Journal for Clinicians*, 29:6:258–275, as reprinted in the American Cancer Society, Inc., booklet, *Lung Cancer*, 1979

Gordon, R., (1983) An operational classification of disease prevention, editorial, *Public Health Reports*, 98:2:107–109

Grundy, E., (1983) Demography and old age, *Journal of the American Geriatrics Society*, 32:6:325–332

Hamera, E., and Shontz, F., (1978) Perceived positive and negative effects of life-threatening illness, *Journal of Psychosomatic Research*, 22:419–424

Happ, B., (1983) Should computers be used in the nursing care of patients? *Nursing Management*, 14:7:31–34

Harris, R., Hyman, R., and Woog, P., (1982) Survival rates and coping styles of maintenance hemodialysis patients, *Nephrology Nurse*, Nov./Dec., 30–39

Johnson, J., (1982) Call me healthy, *Oncology Nursing Forum*, 9:3:73–76

Jonas, S., (1982) A perspective on educating physicians for prevention, *Public Health Reports*, 97:3

Koop, C. E., (1983) Meeting the health care needs of children with disabilities, editorial, *Public Health Reports*, 98:2:105–107

Levy, N., (1979) The chronically ill patient, *Psychiatric Quarterly*, 51:3:189–197

Majno, G., (1975) *The Healing Hand*, Cambridge, Mass.: Harvard University Press

Maxmen, J., (1976) *The Post-Physician Era, Medicine in the 21st Century*, New York: John Wiley and Sons

Mazzuca, S., (1982) Does patient education in chronic disease have therapeutic value? *Journal of Chronic Diseases*, 35:521–529

Metropolitan Life Foundation, (1982) *Statistical Bulletin* (US-ISSN-0026-1513), One Madison Ave., New York, N.Y. 10010, Jan.–Mar.

Pater, A., and Pater, J. (eds.), (1982) What they said in 1981. *The Yearbook of Spoken Opinion*, Beverly Hills, Calif.: Monitor Book Co., Inc.

Pearlman, R., and Speer, J., (1983) Clinical conferences: Quality-of-life considerations in geriatric care, *Journal of the American Geriatrics Society*, 31:2:113–120

Pierce, P., and Giovinco, G., (1983) REACH: Self-care for the chronically ill child, *Pediatric Nursing*, Jan./Feb., 37–39

Roberts, D., (1954) The over-all picture of long-term illness. Address given at *A Conference on Problems of Aging*, School of Public Health, Harvard University, Massachusetts, June, 1954. Subsequently published in *Journal of Chronic Diseases*, February 1955, 149–159

Rosenow, E. II, and Carr, D., (1979) Bronchogenic carcinoma, *CA—A Cancer Journal for Clinicians*, 29:4:233–245, as reprinted in the American Cancer Society, Inc., booklet, *Lung Cancer*

Sandrick, K., (1983) *What Every Hospital Employee Should Know About DRG's*, Care Communications, Inc., 200 E. Ontario, Chicago, Ill. 60611

Stein, R., Jessop, D., and Riessman, C., (1983) Health care services received by children with chronic illness,

American Journal of Disabled Children, *137*: March:225–230

Strauss, A., (1975) *Chronic Illness and the Quality of Life*, St. Louis: C.V. Mosby Company

Theorell, T., (1980) Life events and manifestations of ischemic heart disease: Epidemiological and psychophysiological aspects, *Psychotherapy and Psychosomatics*, *34*:2–3

U.S. (1977) *The Global 2000 Report to the President—Entering the 21st Century*, A report prepared by the Council of Environmental Quality and the Department of State. (Superint. of Doc., U.S. Govt. Printing Office, Wash., D.C., 20402)

U.S. Dept. of Commerce (1980) Statistical Abstract of the United States, 101st Edition, Series P-25, Nos. 802,888

Verbrugge, L., (1982) Sex differentials in health, *Public Health Reports*, *97*:5:417–437

Williams, C. L., Carter, B. J., Arnold, C. B., and Wynder, E. L., (1979) Chronic disease risk factors among children. The "Know Your Body" study, *Journal of Chronic Diseases*, *32*:505–513

C H A P T E R   T W O

Illness Trajectory

Trajectory. *1. The curved path of a projectile, comet, planet, etc.   2. (geometry) A curve or surface that passes through a given set of points or intersects a given series of curves or surfaces at a constant angle.*

(World Book Dictionary, 1967)

Introduction

Implicit in the preceding definition of *trajectory* are the ideas of direction, movement, shape, and predictability. These four characteristics are apparent when one thinks of some object, such as a missile hurtling toward a landing site determined by calculating physical properties involved in movement over time and through space. The concept, however, is less obvious in relation to illness.

Yet the course of an illness can be seen as a trajectory if one thinks of a process that begins with some physiological change and ends with either a positive or negative resolution. By taking into account a disease's characteristic symptoms, phases, and treatment over time, one can predict potential or probable outcomes. Physicians use knowledge of these potential outcomes to plan appropriate therapy to correct, reverse, or slow disease progression. Nurses use this same knowledge to determine staffing needs and plan and perform work necessary to care for and provide support for clients.

Glaser and Strauss (1968) introduced trajectory, as a concept applicable to illness, in a study of the dying client in a hospital setting. Their efforts to increase understanding of the distancing that sometimes occurred between staff and the terminally ill

client (without placing blame for that unfortunate situation) created an awareness that dying was an event that different people perceived differently. The concept served to provide a sociological perspective on the phenomenon and the way it was being managed.

For the health professional, trajectory is a relatively new psychosocial concept. First, the concept focuses on the difference in perception, over time, of those involved in the situation (for example, the health professional, client, and family). Second, it considers the impact on these people and their responses. Finally, this perspective takes into account the resultant identification, organization, and performance of tasks involved in management over the entire course of the illness (Strauss et al. 1985). Different diseases have different trajectories, much as they differ in symptomatology; like symptoms, these trajectories are influenced by many factors: the medical plan, each person's background, problems or complications, cooperation among those involved, and so on.

To date, studies related to this concept have looked at dying trajectories, pain trajectories, technology and the intensive care nursery, and aspects of task work done by staff or family and client. Once understood, trajectory can allow analytical ordering of a variety of events that are present and can lead to distancing and perspective on why some problems occur between health professionals, between professional and client and family, or between client and family (Strauss et al. 1985).

Considering both the definition and the inherent characteristics of any disease, one might feel that *illness trajectory* should be synonymous with the unfolding of the physiological course of that illness. Such a conclusion tends to be true with acute, noncomplicated diseases because there may be no discernible distinction between projected and actual outcome. As an example, several clients undergoing uncomplicated cholecystectomies vary slightly from one another in their expected rate of recovery, generally within tolerable or acceptable limits. However, in many diseases the actual course of an illness often can and does differ from the perceived course. In the preceding example, the client who is not progressing as expected behaviorally or physiologically illustrates the divergence between the perceived and actual courses.

Perceptions depend on people's knowledge, experiences, and capabilities (Strauss et al. 1984). Just as several witnesses report varying versions of one accident, so professionals see a disease's progression somewhat differently from each other and from the client. Once a diagnosis is made, the physician, nurse, or other health professional knows the physiological basis of what is happening, what could happen with treatment, what probably might happen without treatment, the range of possible complications, and procedures necessary to achieve a positive resolution. Each health professional then develops an image of the disease and predicts what can or will happen. If each health team member's perception of a trajectory was graphed onto a transparency, the differences and similarities would become apparent even though they might be minimal. Subtle differences seen in trajectory generally do not adversely impact on necessary work.

The client may have a markedly different perception, focusing not on physiology but on the effects of symptoms, on anxiety and concern over long-term effects, or on a sense of uncertainty secondary to limited understanding of what is happening. With acute illnesses, clients tend to move into the sick role,

in which the responsibility of managing the illness rests on the staff (see Chapter 3). For the chronically ill with multiple hospital experiences, and often multiple trajectories, this situation is vastly different. Chronically ill individuals have a fuller sense of their disease, its progression and management, and are aware of what works and does not work for them. Unlike hospital personnel, who tend to base their perception on the episodic nature of disease, chronically ill clients may be focusing not only on the primary condition but on managing secondary, but currently quiescent, illnesses (Fagerhaugh & Strauss 1977).

Reif's study (1975) implied that individual perceptions lead to responses that are appropriate to those perceptions. The man who is recovering from a myocardial infarction can respond with too much or too little activity based on his perception of his cardiac status. If he considers his heart highly damaged rather than healing, he may see himself as a cardiac cripple and markedly limit activity. His wife may believe that he is now well and his heart healed and urge him to return to work. The physician, if conservative in approach, may be concerned about recurrence and encourage the client to take things easy, reinforcing the cardiac cripple status. If, however, the physician feels that activity maximizes recovery, conflict about how much is enough activity can arise between this client and doctor.

And what about a situation in which the physician, client, and family agree that returning to work is a reasonable choice sometime in the near future, but other individuals involved in the situation disagree? For instance, an employer may consider the person permanently disabled or be concerned about the possibility of another heart attack, which would affect productivity, safety, and disability insurance rates. In either case, a forced early retirement may be in store for this individual, despite his and others' wishes.

Trajectory Terminology

An adequate understanding of trajectory requires that health professionals clearly understand the terms, concepts, and distinct characteristics involved (see Table 2-1). The concept of trajectory has been introduced and the difference between actual and perceived course, as well as the importance of predictability in relation to outcome, covered briefly.

All trajectories occur over time and move in some direction. These characteristics can be perceived differently because they are influenced by actions taken by participants or by the contingencies of a given situation. Trajectories can range from swift, like those following a fatal accident, to slow and progressively downhill, with a full gamut of variations between these two extremes (Glaser & Strauss 1968).

Shape of a trajectory results from changes that occur. It may go straight down, vacillate slowly, plateau for periods of time, and then move quickly or slowly in one direction or another (Glaser & Strauss 1968). A trajectory's shape can be accurately graphed retrospectively. However, once a diagnosis is made, professionals tend mentally to graph what they feel probably will occur.

The word *shaping* is used rather than *management* because the latter does not adequately cover the complexity of trajectory work, medical outcome, or consequences for the workers. Although health professionals are more comfortable using the word *management*, *shaping* more accurately reflects the conscientious, but not always effective, efforts to deal with complex trajectories or the iatrogenic effects of new technologies. One can say that shaping the trajectory helps give shape to the course of an illness. Only when illness courses are routine and trajectories are nonproblematic is the term *managing* appropriate.

Work involved in shaping trajectories has temporal relationships (timing, pacing, sequencing), occurs spatially, is diverse, and has complexities in relation to the tasks involved. In the hospital setting, when people are being worked on, over, or through, they can react and affect or participate in the work (Strauss et al. 1982, 1985). In the home, client/family work includes not only necessary procedures to control the illness, symptoms, or complications but management of the household and family (Corbin & Strauss 1982).

Phases, like trajectories, can have predictable or unpredictable sequences or unknown timing. When there is certainty, chronically ill individuals and their families can plan for changes, for example, moving to a new home prior to an individual's loss of mobility or making financial arrangements before an expected death. When there is uncertainty, planning becomes difficult, and social arrangements lack stability (Strauss et al. 1984).

Biographies are like other trajectories in that they are perceived; have duration, shape, and predictability; and involve work. Client biographies include previous hospital experiences, usual ways of dealing with symptomatology, feeling tones, and other factors. Staff also have biographies that impact the situation; each staff member's personal biography includes "a host of individual attitudes, impressions, conceptions, mood changes" that influence much of what happens (Wiener et al. 1979).

Biographies should be considered *perceptions* rather than *actualities* of personal history since each individual includes certain components of events and excludes others. As in the case of the varying eyewitness accounts of an accident, others who know us may recall events in our lives much differently from the way we do. As an example, family members and clients recall differing information when providing social history on admission.

The ideal of *predictability* also applies to biographies, although it seems unlikely that one can determine future personal social events in a way similar to predicting illnesses with known expected changes. Yet the tendency to plan activities to reach hoped-for goals can be considered a way of predicting future events in our lives. For example, adequate grades in school are a prerequisite to advanced educational opportunities needed to reach employment objectives. The high school student predicts that his athletic prowess, coupled with an adequate grade point average, will gain him an athletic scholarship to the college of his choice. If he should suffer an injury that leads to a cervical spine fracture and paralysis, the course of his biography will change radically, negating his predictions about his future.

Balancing can be a necessary process to keep

TABLE 2-1. Definitions of Trajectory Terminology

TRAJECTORY: a concept that deals with the way disease progression is perceived over time by those involved in the situation, the responses resulting from this perception, and the relationship of these factors to the organization and performance of necessary work.

PARTICIPANT: anyone involved in the illness situation. Participants include client, family member, nurses, physicians, even friends, neighbors, and employers if they influence the trajectory.

DURATION: the time span involved in the trajectory, which may range from swift (as following a fatal accident) to slow and progressively downhill. Duration is not an objective physiological property since it varies in each situation and is perceived differently by each person.

DIRECTION AND MOVEMENT: the progression of a disease from point *A* to *B* to *C,* and so on. Direction and movement occur over time and are influenced by actions taken to manage the trajectory.

PERCEPTION: what participants define as occurring or expect to occur, given their knowledge and experience. Participants' perceptions of events vary, even when their knowledge and experience are similar. "Perception" of what is occurring differs from the "actual" unfolding of a disease.

PREDICTABILITY: the ability to anticipate the way the trajectory will progress, including the rate at which changes will occur. Some diseases are highly predictable; others are not.

SHAPE: the mental image that the course of an illness is expected to take. Since shape has direction and movement that occur over time, it can be graphed. Like duration, shape is a perceived property, with each participant having a somewhat different image.

SHAPING: actions that influence the outcome of a disease (different from shape, but similar in meaning to management). Management implies successful outcomes, whereas shaping implies that unexpected problems are handled in the best way possible, even when the trajectory is not in full control. Shaping covers the complexity of trajectory work, medical outcome, and consequences to the workers.

WORK: effort directed to accomplishing an objective. Work occurs over time, is diverse, and has complexities related to the tasks involved. Trajectory work includes performing technical chores and providing comfort and clinical safety, managing or supervising machines, coordinating efforts, and so on. Hospital work is done by patients and family, as well as staff. At home, the client and family do the work.

PHASES: major divisions of trajectory consisting of stages that contain clusters of necessary interrelated tasks; phases include diagnosis, various therapeutic steps, and recovery. Each phase has points of decision concerning the cluster, sequence, and organization of tasks necessary for that phase. Like trajectories, phases can be certain or uncertain. When phase tasks go awry or conflict with tasks for another trajectory arises, problems that result may affect the shape of the trajectory.

BIOGRAPHIES: the background or life history that makes each individual unique from others (social identity, family and social relationships, work history, life-styles, and so on); also called *social trajectories.* Like all trajectories, biographies are perceived; have duration, shape, and predictability; and involve work. All participants (staff, client, and others) bring with them aspects of their biographies (such as attitudes, impressions, and moods) that influence interpretation and reaction to events.

CONTINGENCY: problems of a medical, interactional, organizational, or biographical nature. Contingencies can be expected (such as side effects of drugs) or unexpected (such as effects of technology whose outcomes are unknown). The former allows for advanced preparation to manage the problem; the latter cannot. Contingencies influence the shape of the trajectory; the interplay between contingencies and efforts at illness control creates the specific details of trajectories.

BALANCING: the process of making choices. Often a matter of determining priorities, balancing generally entails giving up some considerations in exchange for others. Families do much balancing at home to avoid adverse physiological aftermaths or to retain some acceptable degree of life-style. Hospital staff also performs balancing tasks.

---

symptoms and disease under control, especially in multiple chronic illnesses with regimens that have conflicting task requirements (Strauss et al. 1985). Balancing at home also helps clients and families deal with illness in relation to other needs by determining adjustments that must be made in regimens so they fit into life-style or the timing of other activities. Often balancing occurs without the knowledge or consent of the primary health care provider—for example, the individual who omits occasional doses of a diuretic prior to planned outings.

During hospitalization, clients and family continue to do what they see as necessary balancing. The client and family and the health professional may have different perspectives of what should be balanced; that is, clients may weight options differently from professionals (Strauss et al. 1985), leading to contests over control (Fagerhaugh et al. 1977).

Staff also balances situations in the hospital setting. For example, the precarious condition of premature infants in an intensive care nursery (ICN) requires balancing provision of sufficient oxygen to keep fragile lungs functioning with ensuring that quantity is insufficient to cause blindness. Balancing in these situations can be adversely influenced by such factors as (1) lack of knowledge, for example, of side effects of new drugs or other innovative treatment modalities; (2) staff's tendency to focus on the primary trajectory to the exclusion of other, currently stabilized disorders; and (3) personnel's actual lack of knowledge of other diagnoses or illnesses (Strauss et al. 1985).

Problems from a Trajectory Perspective

The ranks of the chronically ill grow not only because there are more chronically ill elderly people but because of an ever-increasing number of middle-aged and young adults as well as children who are surviving formerly fatal diseases and trauma. Wiener and associates (1979) point out that the ranks of the chronically ill are even being increased by premature infants, now graduates of ICNs, many of whom

need long-term care and treatment. Many illnesses progress in an expected manner, with treatment handled routinely and work patterns anticipated and planned—all without untoward difficulty or problems. Other illnesses, in growing numbers, have multiple problems, which adversely influence perception, increase the number of possible outcomes, and in turn influence the trajectory.

Technology as a Contingency

A major factor affecting the chronically ill is modern medical technology (Strauss et al. 1985). The avant-garde nature of technology causes *contingencies* that often are unexpected and difficult to evaluate and decrease the ability to predict outcomes. Lack of predictability creates uncertainty for the staff as to how to respond, in turn affecting the organization and work that are necessary (Strauss et al. 1985). In other words, each *participant* in the situation may be unsure of what is happening or what to do.

Advancing technology has also expanded the range of alternative lines of action that are available, meaning that choices must often be made to shape the trajectory most effectively (Strauss et al. 1985). In medical centers, where new and often innovative diagnostic and treatment modalities (equipment, medication, and techniques) are devised and tested, uncertainty is anticipated and built into medical and nursing management. Participants accept that details of a disease or treatment may not be within their realm of knowledge or experience. Take, for example, the first artificial heart transplant, in which shaping was difficult, contingencies were both expected and unexpected, and predictability was often impossible.

Furthermore, the impact of technology no longer resides exclusively in major medical centers but has been extended into community-based hospitals and even into the home as the result of the availability of more and more sophisticated equipment and advanced skills (Morris 1984). Community-based hospitals now have computed axial tomography (CAT) scans and other sophisticated diagnostic tools. Specialty units such as intensive care and coronary care units are commonplace. High-risk intensive care nurseries and dialysis centers (or their satellite units) are within relatively easy reach of most of the population in this country.

Technology and New Trajectories

Technological advances have prolonged existing trajectories or created new ones, through which lives are maintained by machines, procedures, or drugs. Clients who would have died in the past face uncertain futures, often stemming from iatrogenic effects of treatment that impacts not only on the originally diseased body system but also on other body systems. For some of these people, long-term complications or contingencies remain unknown; the impact on life-styles and on the organization of in-hospital or at-home work is often enormous (Strauss et al. 1985).

End stage renal disease (ESRD) is an example of an iatrogenic condition created by technologic developments; ESRD has radically altered the social and illness trajectories of kidney failure (Plough 1981). Before federal funding, renal dialysis and transplantation were marginal experimental treatments. Once funding became available, these expensive treatments were accessible to all individuals in renal failure (Plough 1981). Because dialysis and transplants keep people alive but do not cure them, the ESRD client faces the difficult choice of dialysis versus transplant versus dying.

Treatment focuses on the pathophysiology of the kidney and physiological complications. Figure 2-1 is a graph reflecting the health professional's view of the ESRD trajectory. Physicians differ in their opinions of optimal intervention. Surgeons advocate transplants, arguing that they free clients from the dialysis machines; nephrologists argue for dialysis by pointing out the high failure rate of transplants, the complications from immunosuppressant therapy, and the development of advanced forms of dialysis (Plough 1981; Calland 1972).

Psychological Impact.   Quality of life and clients' perceptions of their renal diseases receive limited consideration (Plough 1981). The literature dealing with psychosocial aspects of ESRD does not focus on social and emotional needs; rather, it tends to label the client who finds coping difficult as deviant, deficient in emotional responses (Plough 1981), wrapped up in nonuseful coping mechanisms, showing depressive or paranoid ideation, or exhibiting the organic brain syndrome that accompanies uremia (Calland 1972). Uncooperative behavior by clients is considered inappropriate, rather than a result of the stress of therapy.

Calland (1972), who was both physician and ESRD client, raised a number of questions that evolve from reality-based client problems. How does one deal with fluid and electrolyte restrictions that make meals unpalatable? Should marriage be considered, or is it even possible? Can or should the individual start a family? Is it worth struggling for the rest of one's life with the problems that dialysis creates? Plough (1981) points out that most clients are unable to work because they cannot deal with additional stresses beyond dialysis and because the time spent on the machines and in commuting blocks many job opportunities. Role changes and role reversal can occur. Expression of problems is not reinforced by physician or nurse. Clients therefore conceal these problems, and the staff remains unaware of the difficulties they experience (Calland 1972). Figure 2-2 is a graph reflecting the way that an individual who has ESRD might view the trajectory of this condition.

Families also undergo tremendous stress, as evidenced by the increase in the divorce rate that occurs shortly after treatment begins (Plough 1981). Even nurses who are more attuned to the psychosocial needs of clients are often critical of families who have difficulty retaining supportive stances. Often the staff becomes so involved in the technological management of the disease that they tend to assume that current problems are the result of prior problems and that dialysis is just another event in the client's life (Plough 1981).

Physiological Impact.   Clients and staff perceive physiological responses to ESRD differently. Physicians and nurses use laboratory values to evaluate

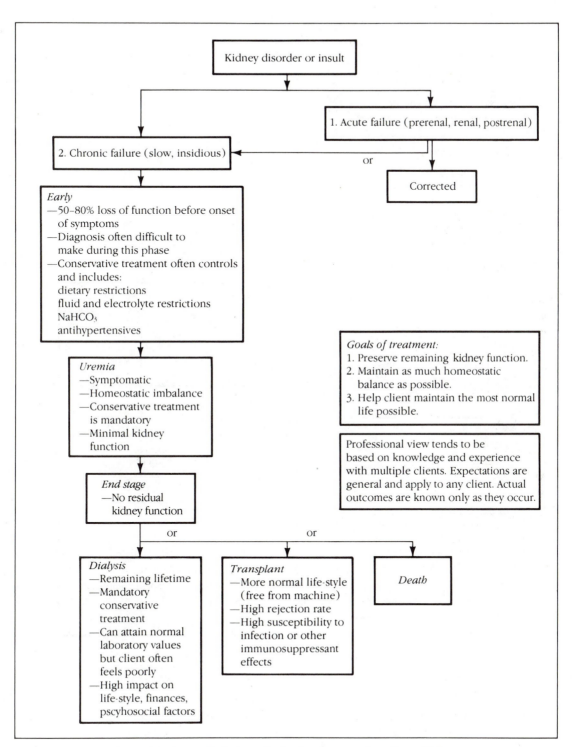

FIGURE 2-1. Trajectory: Professional perception of renal failure

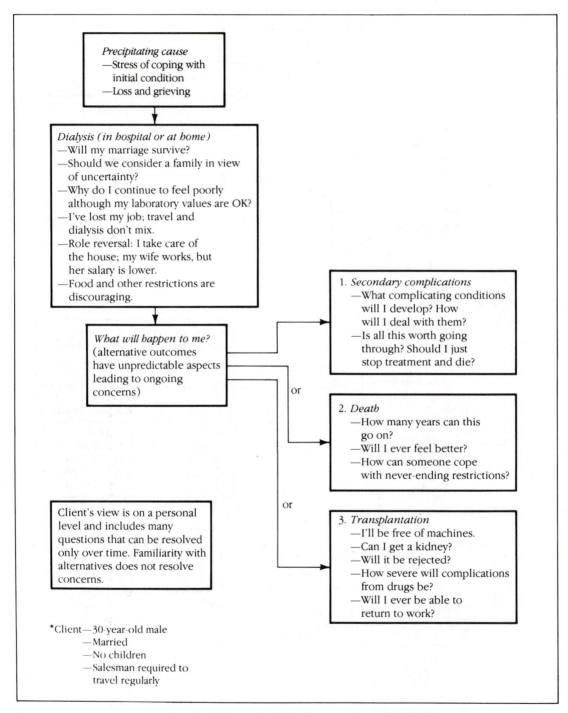

FIGURE 2-2. Trajectory: A client's perception of renal failure

homeostasis. Clients do not always find laboratory reports in line with the way they feel or are able to function (Calland 1972) since accumulated fluids, metabolites, and waste products create unpleasant symptoms (Plough 1981). In addition, dialysis causes secondary illness trajectories, such as cardiac disorders, neuropathies, or atherosclerosis, that nephrologists consider "nonrenal complications." Once the impact of complicating trajectories is removed from the realm of the disease model, the health professional can continue feeling successful at shaping the disease (Plough 1981).

Many clients see transplantation as a valid alternative to dialysis. Yet, when it is possible, the client is not necessarily freed from anxiety or contingencies. The possibility of rejection or of complications from immunosuppressant therapy remains. In addition, there may be no improvement in social or financial problems because knowledge about life expectancy after transplantation is still limited (Calland 1972). The trajectory continues to show uncertainty. Problems may become so severe that the client loses the desire or will to live and refuses continued treatment.

Work Problems

Trajectory work consists of organizing and performing necessary tasks and actions that shape trajectories. With chronic illness, this work moves from home to hospital and back to home, depending on the phases or contingencies that are currently present in the situation. Such movement makes it obvious that work is shared by clients and families as well as staff in shaping trajectories (Strauss et al. 1982).

Staff Work. The diagnostic phase marks the beginning of trajectory work for the health professional. The multitude of tests and procedures require time, organization, preparation, and follow-through of staff. Once the disease is identified, the image of the illness's potential course helps the physician map out interventions and allows the nurse to plan appropri-

ate care. The occurrence of new symptoms signifies change in the disease trajectory that may require that diagnosis and mapping recur at intervals (Strauss et al. 1985).

In the hospital, the staff often sees clients in relation to the amount of work they create for the expected trajectory. "Good" clients are those without problems or complaints, or those who have multiple problems but are cooperative. "Problem" clients are individuals who are uncooperative, complaining, or overly emotional, as well as those who respond poorly to treatment and therefore need a great deal of staff time (Lorber 1981).

Advancing technology has led to an increased number of hospital tasks that relate to machines, drugs, and procedures. When situations are highly unpredictable, unanticipated tasks occur, organization of work may become confused, and a great many ad hoc approaches may be needed to get things done. Some trajectories are unclear, making a search for different options necessary; additional medical specialists are involved to help make decisions. The increased complexity of who is managing what complicates the entire picture and adds to the work that is involved (Strauss et al. 1985). A situation in which authority and responsibility are not clear-cut evolves.

Client Work in the Hospital. In their home environment, the chronically ill carry out all work involved in trajectory shaping by balancing the interplay of technology and their own bodily reactions (Strauss et al. 1982). When they require hospitalization, this experiential knowledge goes with them even though the staff does not always try to gain such information. In the hospital setting, clients are expected to delegate responsibility of care to the staff and to conform to the medical model in the traditional sick role (see Chapter 3). Such conformity (especially when other nonacute conditions need management) may be inappropriate except when the individual is helpless during acute phases. Conflicts between client and staff may arise.

Work required of clients changes as trajectory or phases change. When diagnosis is in process, client work includes cooperation with procedures. During the treatment phase(s), other clusters of work are performed: minimizing pain, following regimens, learning what needs to be learned (Strauss et al. 1984). When trajectories are problematic, client involvement in decision making is often necessary, especially when the chronically ill person is highly knowledgeable about the condition (Strauss et al. 1982). For example, an individual having chronic obstructive pulmonary disease can provide information on timing of medications to maximize effectiveness.

Visibility. Client work in the hospital can be visible or invisible to the staff. Decision work and cooperation are highly visible; other work sometimes is invisible. Invisibility may be deliberate if the client feels the staff would disapprove of the client's actions or interpret them as criticism. Some work, such as getting up when ordered on bedrest, occurs when the client deems it necessary for trajectories related to secondary illnesses. Invisibility can also occur when staff focuses completely on the main trajectory and does not notice the client's work or realize that it is part of another trajectory (Strauss et al. 1982).

Explicit or Implicit Work. Explicit work is recognized or supplements staff work; it includes such tasks as monitoring machines, carrying out painful rehabilitation procedures, and providing feedback to teaching done for home management. Staff generally realizes that the client is involved, often regarding that participation as cooperation rather than work. Sometimes clients do not identify their own activities as work because they differ from the official work that the staff does (Strauss et al. 1982).

Implicit work tends to be unrecognized; that is, it includes activities not seen as work. Implicit work includes the many activities of daily living performed by the client: providing information in relation to admission, responding to treatment, and so on. It includes giving cooperation and maximum performance required by tests, procedures, or interventions. Being uncooperative with such tasks is considered a noncompliant or recalcitrant behavior when

the staff deems such cooperation important (Strauss et al. 1982).

Family Work in the Hospital.   Families also do various kinds of work in the hospital: helping clients deal with reactions and maintain the necessary composure required for technical, sometimes painful tasks; providing comfort (positioning, requesting medications); helping with safety (raising bed rails, checking on procedures); and doing much of the necessary legal/administrative work, including filling out forms, signing documents, making financial arrangements, and so on (Strauss et al. 1984).

Families are often responsible for crucial decision-making work that may require choices among less-than-perfect options. Intelligent decisions are often difficult, since obtaining information may be difficult. Doctors may be hard to reach, or specialists and primary physicians may each feel that the other is responsible for providing information. Moreover, specialists may not agree among themselves about the medical consequences of actions. When all this uncertainty is coupled with new or little-tried interventions, as in large medical centers, it is not surprising that the family is impeded in its decision making (Strauss et al. 1984).

Client and Family Work at Home.   Once a client returns home, someone must take responsibility for all trajectory management, as well as the home management that is necessary despite the presence of an illness. The trajectory work includes many of the tasks performed in hospitals but also involves other tasks, such as crisis work (preventing and handling), symptom and regimen management, time management, and providing psychological support (Strauss et al. 1984).

In chronic illness, work of considerable range and complexity goes on 24 hours a day, 7 days a week, often in a setting not designed for such work (Corbin & Strauss 1982). Families usually have minimal equipment, no shift relief, and little training, which is eventually supplemented by what they learn over time. The way family members share medically related tasks depends on the degree and kind of physical impairment, financial resources, and interpersonal relationships and communication patterns. With each change in the trajectory, the family must reassess social arrangements, daily life, and future development. Changes can lead to increased physical labor, altered financial status, changed family mood, and altered identities (Strauss et al. 1984; Corbin & Strauss 1982).

The Child as Client. When children are ill, physical and psychological problems generally impact on the parents, with most of the work load falling unequally on one parent, usually the mother. Parents may also be tortured by guilt (as with genetic illnesses) or feel that they are at fault (as with an accident). When a disease, such as cystic fibrosis, is known to be eventually fatal, uncertainty about the way to raise the child may exist. Should the emphasis be on helping the child go through normal developmental stages that might adversely impinge on the medical condition, or should the child be protected to limit medical hazards, even at the risk of causing psychological problems? Such difficulties cause tension; as tension rises, an increasing marital gap may result, sometimes leading to divorce (Strauss et al. 1984).

Life cycle phases of the parents and child have a great deal of influence on the success of shaping. A young couple with limited income and a sick baby is affected quite differently from a more established family in which a chronically ill teenager is creating other kinds of problems. Siblings are impacted by expectations that they will assume responsibility for helping with symptom control, as well as by feelings of guilt, a sense of loneliness during illness crisis, resentment, and adverse responses to death (Strauss et al. 1984).

The Adult as Client. For adult clients, the burden of work usually falls on the spouse, especially when children are too young to help or have left home. Work consists of all the responsibilities and activities that the ill person cannot manage but that are necessitated by the illness and by the household's requirements.

Biographical diversity among couples can cause problems. Young married persons may find illness destabilizing to their relationship, while an elderly couple may lack the physical or mental abilities to cope effectively with ongoing illness. In addition, partners may have different perspectives, and problems that arise from the strain of dealing with the disease may adversely affect the relationship. The arithmetic of time and energy for all tasks can total up to quite an exhausting, even crushing burden. Even when the ill individual is able to manage the regimen and monitor symptoms, crisis work may be enormously stressful, producing a devastating cumulative impact on the spouse (Strauss et al. 1984; Corbin & Strauss 1982).

Work Overload. The amount of work that must be done is often unbalanced, depending on factors such as illness status, availability of outside resources, and presence of contingencies that may increase the work load. The key to balancing is not the actual amount of work being done but the perception of this load and the conditions under which one is working. With adequate support or help, positive change in status, and so on, the amount of work can seem to contract (Corbin & Strauss 1982).

Managing both illness and home can overwhelm caregivers, causing a sense of being stretched to the limits of energy and tolerance (Strauss et al. 1984) and leading to resentment, anger, or other negative responses. Should the caregiver find no relief, the impact on the family may be devastating; decisions to end the marriage or to place the client in a nursing home may seem to be the only viable alternatives (Corbin & Strauss 1982; Strauss et al. 1984).

Respite from continuous responsibilities can make the difference in a caregiver's ability to continue. Respite takes various forms and lasts for variable periods of time. The caregiver can try to get a friend or family member to take over responsibility for a short while, to get assistance from outside resources, or to go away temporarily or for several days. This latter alternative can sometimes be accomplished by placing the client in a care facility for a few days (Corbin et al. 1982; Strauss et al. 1984) (see Chapter 8).

Specific Trajectories

As noted in the introduction to this chapter, several areas have been studied: various pain trajectories, dying trajectories, biographies as applied to intensive care nurseries, and problems of work involved in shaping the illness. Variations in perceptions of trajectories are apparent in some of these studies, especially those dealing with pain and dying.

Pain Trajectories

In the hospital setting, clients may experience acute or chronic pain, which may be disease-related or iatrogenic, resulting from procedures or treatment. Most staff feel that they manage nonproblematic pain well in the hospital setting and that chronic pain is managed adequately. However, investigation of pain trajectories indicates that they may not be entirely right.

Surgical Pain. Not all surgical procedures are performed for acute conditions. Many chronically ill individuals need surgical interventions: joint replacement for arthritic conditions, cancer-related procedures, and so on. Clients who enter the hospital for surgery anticipate that pain will accompany these treatment modalities.

Hospital personnel believe that pain accompanying nonproblematic surgery is adequately managed. Incisional pain has a known physiological basis and usually necessitates injectable narcotics for 24 to 72 hours, followed by a decreasing need for pain medication over a relatively short period. Pain work performed by the staff includes assessing, preventing,

minimizing, relieving, and avoiding complications that could increase the pain. The client's pain-related tasks include informing the staff about the pain and its characteristics (where, when, and so forth), maintaining reasonable limits for expression of pain (no screaming or carrying on), and cooperating and enduring painful but necessary procedures such as turning and coughing (Fagerhaugh & Strauss 1977).

On surgical units, high client turnover and busy work schedules create competition between pain management and other work priorities. The staff relies heavily on medications to manage pain trajectories, rather than on more time-consuming minimization techniques (splinting, positioning, distracting, and so on). Because pain tends to be relatively short-lived and since the client usually improves rapidly, hospital staff generally feel that pain is satisfactorily controlled (Fagerhaugh et al. 1977).

Yet interviews with clients indicate less satisfaction with pain management than the staff realize (Fagerhaugh et al. 1977). Clients reported inconsistencies in staff philosophy about pain management. Some staff encouraged waiting for medication and others supplied it on request; some administered maximum doses of ordered pain medications, others minimum. Some gave clients more control over when medications should be given, others less. Because most of these clients were aware of the limited duration of the acute pain phase and tended to compare themselves with others who were more critically ill, there was a greater willingness to endure pain. The lack of overt complaining reinforced the staff's perception that pain trajectories were being fully managed.

The case study of Mrs. J. demonstrates the differences in the way the staff and one surgical patient regarded pain management.

Obviously Mrs. J. did not see her trajectory in the same way that the staff did. Biographical data that were obtained focused on information related to usual surgical responses. Had more psychosocial data been obtained, staff work would have included a consistent approach to giving medication and greater personal support to assuage her fear. Mrs. J.'s pain was not well managed.

◇ CASE STUDY ◇
Postsurgical Pain

Mrs. J., age 50, was admitted for a hysterectomy. The frozen section showed some precancerous involvement. Her doctor assured her that surgery had been successful and that she need not feel concerned. This was her first hospital admission. Her history (medical and nursing) showed that she was widowed 2 years earlier, had no children, had mild osteoarthritis but no other disease conditions, and was slightly overweight and moderately active. No difficulties that should adversely affect her recovery were identified. Mrs. J. was seen as quiet but slightly anxious.

She was now 5 days postoperative and continued to complain of postsurgical pain severe enough to require intramuscular (IM) narcotics. She was also reluctant to get out of bed. Her wound was healing well, with no signs of infection; bowel sounds were present; and she was tolerating a soft diet. The staff thought that she should be taking oral pain medications, ambulating readily, and be ready for discharge. Instead she was improving slowly. There was frequent disagreement about why she was still having so much pain and was so dependent.

The staff had not obtained some pertinent biographical material about this woman. She was a very dependent person, and being in the hospital allowed her to nurture this dependency. No one had asked her how she would manage at home, but she was very apprehensive about leaving the hospital since she had always relied upon her husband to do things for her. She also tolerated pain poorly and was fearful that her incision would "open up," something she had heard about. When the staff summarily ordered her out of bed on her second postoperative day, she was having severe abdominal cramps and became convinced that the staff was uncaring and unconcerned.

To compound her hesitancy and distrust, the differences in the ways the staff administered her pain medications made her feel that they did not know how to manage pain. Why else would the nurses tell her different things? She was not even sure that the doctor was telling her the truth: that she didn't have cancer. Her mother had died of uterine cancer.

Clients with multiple illnesses who need surgery have trajectories with greater probability for complicated, unpredictable outcomes (Fagerhaugh et al. 1977). Staff and client may have discrepant pain priorities. Staff concern may emphasize balancing risk of addiction with pain care. Clients may try to gain control because they may feel the need for more management of stable, sometimes painful, chronic conditions. Increased pain work and client/staff problems may result (Fagerhaugh et al. 1977).

Chronic Illness and Pain. People who have recurrent or long-term pain states find that hospitals are settings geared to managing acute, short-term pain. These people have extensive illness biographies that include experiences with hospitals, personnel, pain, conflict with staff, and so on. This background influences reactions to personnel and new pain experiences. Any attempts to retain some control of their pain management can lead to personnel's

stereotyping or labeling these clients as uncooperative or difficult (Fagerhaugh et al. 1977).

Skilled nursing facilities (SNFs) handle chronic pain differently; they are primarily custodial, with social and illness trajectories generally on a downward course. Care focuses primarily on physical maintenance and stabilization of the medical condition to the extent possible. Even when efforts are made to increase humane factors, care tends to be bureaucratic because of limited numbers of staff. Routines serve as a basis of care since they are a more efficient way to accomplish tasks and to manage pain within the constraints of the work routine (Fagerhaugh et al. 1977). In these settings, pain management relies less on medications than on the use of minimizing techniques (positioning, distraction, and so on). The exception, of course, is the terminally ill individual.

Interviews demonstrated that client-residents of SNFs had come to terms with living with their chronic pain. The major priority residents expressed was the social contact provided primarily by staff. Social contact therefore becomes a means of social control (Fagerhaugh et al. 1977). Although many residents had voiced many pain complaints for a period of time after admission, they soon learned that excessive pain expression can lead to possible isolation.

Clients also balanced priorities in relation to their pain. Relief provided by narcotics was balanced against possible addiction, decreased sociability, and side effects. Tolerating some pain became the better alternative. Eventually client and staff grew somewhat insensitive to ongoing pain (Fagerhaugh et al. 1977).

Dying Trajectories

Many chronic illnesses are on some kind of downward spiral: death is a known outcome. Repeated hospitalizations are not uncommon during the course of these illnesses. Often death comes while an individual is hospitalized. Planning care for the dying patient was found to be dependent on the perceived course of the dying, rather than its actual course (Glaser & Strauss 1968). Participants had varying degrees of awareness and acceptance of the client's dying and expectations of the way the process would progress. Shaping of the dying trajectory tended to focus on the medical aspects of dying: managing the physical dying, since caregivers demonstrated less ability to fulfill psychological than physical needs (Strauss & Glaser 1970).

Types of Dying Trajectories. Dying trajectories can be divided into *quick* and *lingering* categories (Glaser & Strauss 1968). Quick dying trajectories that occur over relatively short periods of time may be expected or unexpected. Sometimes it is apparent that death will occur quickly and expectedly within hours or at most a few days (the head trauma client kept alive by life-support systems). Or quick death can come when someone who was expected to die eventually dies unexpectedly as a result of a sudden deterioration (the terminal cancer client who has a massive myocardial infarction). The quick dying tra-

jectory that is most traumatic for the staff occurs unexpectedly to someone who was not expected to die at all (recovery is expected after surgery and death results from massive pulmonary emboli).

Lingering trajectories have two major features: long duration and slow but steady downward movement. Lingering trajectories have a greater potential for biological, human, or psychological unpredictability than do quick trajectories. If lingering is relatively short (days to weeks), with little pain and a reasonably high level of family acceptance, it is not greatly upsetting (Glaser & Strauss 1968). When the lingering exceeds perceived reasonable limits, much stress for family and staff results.

Dying in the Hospital. Quick deaths in the hospital may sadden the staff, but the sadness passes rather quickly and work resumes. Lingering deaths are different since dying is a process constantly undergoing change, requiring staff to redefine the trajectory continually to assure appropriate medical and nursing care for each phase (Strauss & Glaser 1970; Glaser & Strauss 1968). Although some degree of certainty is often present, the total length of time involved in the dying may not always be clear to personnel. Time miscalculations can lead to crises on the unit that necessitate changes in work load (Strauss & Glaser 1970). For example, the individual who suffers a major cerebral vascular accident may linger for weeks, rather than days.

Difference in perception of the dying process can also lead to inconsistencies in care. The nurse who senses that the client is now terminally ill may be more generous with pain medications than the nurse who feels that death is a long way off and is worried about addicting the client. Staff often become more involved in the dying of young clients than of the elderly, especially if they themselves are young (Strauss & Glaser 1970).

Dying trajectories are handled differently on various units. Because the emergency room is geared for a constant shift to new emergencies rather than routine kinds of care, relatively few deaths occur in that setting: transfer to other units occurs within hours. Intensive care units handle dying clients for longer periods of time if these people might survive through heroic efforts or are on machines that need constant monitoring. Medical wards are units structured to deal with lingering trajectories (Glaser & Strauss 1968).

Time as a Factor.   Dying takes time, and staff work is organized around the amount of time it is expected to take. Routine work (physical care, tests, procedures, and so on) is scheduled to avoid conflict with other activities involved in terminal care. Because staff time is finite, care of the dying competes with care of clients who are recovering (Glaser & Strauss 1968).

Work Changes.   Accurate expectations make possible arrangements that provide adequate personnel to perform necessary tasks. As dying moves into the terminal phase, tasks and relationships change (Glaser & Strauss 1968). Evaluative tests or therapy may stop and comfort care increase. When family provide some of the care, the staff is relieved of these aspects of physical work, even when the presence of family is disruptive because of their responses to the situation (Glaser & Strauss 1968).

The dying client may also have a concurrent pain trajectory, so that the significance of pain must be considered (Fagerhaugh et al. 1977). Balancing questions arise: Should pain medications be temporarily withheld because they might obscure diagnostic symptoms? Should opiates be given, knowing their administration may hasten death? Should milder medications be given rather than stronger ones to avoid grogginess or respiratory depression? Is it more important to keep the client pain-free or alert but in some pain? And what are the client's wishes or preferences?

Dying at Home.   Clients may prefer to die at home, where time and work involved in providing care and support allow the family and client to shape the trajectory and gain a sense of control over events (Glaser & Strauss 1968). Dying at home provides the family

the satisfaction of knowing that they were able to maintain solidarity and to fulfill proper social obligations to the dying individual. The most obvious problems of management in these situations relate to physical needs: giving enemas, preventing or treating bed sores, managing pain, and so forth. The case study of D.M. shows the way one individual handled his dying in the environment that met his needs.

Interventions that Consider the Trajectory Concept

The trajectory concept furnishes the professional with an alternative perspective to problems or conflicts: a way of highlighting the entire environment and the participants within. The concept can lead to a greater depth of understanding of disease processes in relation to both client and work done to manage the disease regardless of setting. This perspective can promote greater accountability and development of interventions that are more humane and improve the client's quality of life. In addition, professionals might well find themselves in a better and more effective work environment. Strauss and others (1984) also feel that a greater awareness of the influence of illness perception on actions could lead to a broader-based national social policy: a policy that relieves individual providers of sole responsibility for components of health care, such as maintaining the terminally ill with machines, by establishing national guidelines for consistency of care and sharing of responsibility.

Accountability

In addition to health professionals' sense of responsibility, which guides their actions, hospital policy requires professional accountability, especially in relation to proper diagnosis and treatment by the physician and nurse (Strauss & Glaser 1970). The major

◇ CASE STUDY ◇

Dying at Home

D.M. knew that he was dying long before anyone else did. In spite of having non–insulin-dependent diabetes, mild hypertension, and chronic constipation, he saw himself as well until he passed his 75th birthday. Each year after that, he developed another medical problem. One year he had problems with his ear, the next year, a prostatectomy, and the following year, cataract surgery. Then came the painless hematuria, but no definitive diagnosis was made. At age 79 he began to feel "poorly" and was diagnosed as having pancytopenia, cause unknown.

When his condition deteriorated to the point that death would have ensued within a matter of weeks, he finally agreed to have a splenectomy. D.M. realized that he might well die on the operating room table but decided that it was worth the risk for the probable 18 months of relatively comfortable living the doctor told him was the alternative. He survived the surgery without any complications but never fully recovered. Over the next 6 months he lost weight slowly but continuously.

Shortly after his 81st birthday he developed severe low back pain, which the doctor diagnosed over the phone as a lumbar strain.

But he knew he was dying. He finally persuaded his physician and wife that a trip to visit his daughter would be beneficial. His real goal was to die in his daughter's home rather than in a hospital. He threw a pulmonary embolus shortly after arriving and had to enter the hospital again. There a diagnostic workup revealed pathological fractures of the lumbar spine and other bony involvement secondary to metastatic prostatic cancer. His request to die at his daughter's home was honored, and he was subsequently discharged. The visiting nurse and hospice program in that area made it possible for his wish to be fulfilled. Pain control was the greatest problem his family faced. Surrounded by his wife, his daughter, and her family, D.M. died 3 weeks later. Even though his dying lingered over several months, awareness of the process for family and health providers involved only a few weeks.

emphasis of this accountability is on following medical orders and performing medically supported tasks. There is little required accountability for ensuring that knowledge about the client's biography or experiential history with disease and pain is gathered or reported (Strauss et al. 1984).

The acute illness orientation of most hospital settings, plus the multitude of tasks and procedures that are intrinsic to hospital work, serves to block accountability in issues other than those of a medical nature (Fagerhaugh et al. 1977). But the chronically ill individual often enters the hospital with multiple kinds of trajectories related to illness state(s) that should be considered. Yet only limited amounts of social and psychological information are collected systematically, primarily by nurses and social workers.

The complexity involved in a client's long-term management and hospital experiences can lead to a great variation in the client's responses to the staff's handling of the acute problem. When there are diffi-

cult clients, the staff tends to organize efforts to collect data that will help them solve the immediate problem(s). This course is usually effective in resolution of the present difficulty. However, since the same problems arise repeatedly, staff would find permanent solutions or interventions more beneficial than repeatedly gaining and analyzing information and selecting appropriate solutions. The repeated need to resolve the same kind of problem indicates little accountability for nonmedical aspects of care (Strauss et al. 1984).

Personnel tend to focus on the reason for the admission and not on other existing illnesses that may impinge on trajectory management (Strauss et al. 1985; Fagerhaugh et al. 1977). With the advent of recent changes in government regulations (Medicare and Medicaid payment based on disease classification rather than length of stay), accountability in relation to the primary illness has increased. Ironically, if quiescent illnesses flare up or complicate the situation, their importance grows and the primary illness can even become secondary. For example, the older person admitted with a fractured hip whose chronic pulmonary problems become acute presents two trajectories that the staff must consider.

Biography: Seeing the Whole Client

Chronically ill individuals who manage their own care at home frequently find delegating full responsibility to hospital personnel difficult. Concerns arise over personnel's lack of knowledge about the intricacies of disease regimens carried out at home. To ease this transitional phase, a rational approach would be to allow the client greater participation in decisions while in health care facilities or to extend the health care system so that personnel could play more of a role in helping the chronically ill and their families inside and outside the hospital setting (Strauss et al. 1984). Such approaches require inclusion of a more extensive client biographical history than is usually obtained.

Importance of Biography. Ordinarily, biographical material collected by hospital personnel pertains to current work, an emphasis that distorts the total identity of the client. For instance, the client who has long managed chronic pain can have difficulty trusting the staff when they change the frequency, amount, or even the medication itself without gaining information about prior experiences with medication effectiveness, sensitivity, or alternative methods for minimizing pain. Having such knowledge would help the staff control the distressful symptom without the complex, time-consuming process of trying out different medications to determine which works best. Prior hospital experiences have conditioned chronic pain sufferers to expect that the staff will not attend to their long-term needs and that requests for medication will periodically be delayed or unanswered. This mismanagement contributes to the creation of somewhat difficult clients (Strauss et al. 1984).

Obtaining Biographical Data. Interviewing is a very effective way of obtaining biographical information. Interviews need not be time-consuming: in-

formation can be collected while care is given or during multiple short sessions, which would also be less tiring for the client. Once obtained, such information should be added to a master form specifically provided for this purpose, a form that should be used with each subsequent admission. Family members should also be interviewed, since they often have additional information or a different perspective that may provide insight into family dynamics as well as confirming the client's information (Strauss et al. 1984).

Biographical information can be used in several ways. First, it can help shape work and responses in terms of specific information about the client. Second, information gathered over time from multiple clients can be useful for planning care for the types of individuals who generally enter that specific unit. Finally, this information can help determine the proportion of responsibility the client should retain and the proportion the staff must assume. These actions lead to more individualized care and provide support for the client in dealing with disease and contingencies. In addition, biographical information would also ease some of the staff's work by providing long-term solutions to dealing with "difficult" individuals (Strauss et al. 1984).

Improving Care for the Dying

Currently, accountability required in relation to the dying client includes maintaining a reasonably pain-free environment, notifying the family of the impending death, pronouncing the individual dead, and informing the family of the death. Many of these tasks are performed in a perfunctory manner. Personnel are held less accountable for such factors as information the client can be given and the way work is done around the dying person. Accountability is also affected by the distancing between staff and the terminal client that results from the stress of providing care sometimes triggered by awareness of one's own mortality (Strauss & Glaser 1970).

When hospital staff face unexpected client or family responses, their discussions recalling similar situations can lead to problem solving. Organization of work improves for the betterment of client, family, and staff. Unfortunately, after the death and post-mortem care, this learning does not evolve into a set of permanent approaches but seems to disappear until another crisis or negative situation occurs (Strauss & Glaser 1970).

Terminal care should be directed to ease inconsistency of interactions and to improve accountability to the dying client on a personal level. This goal could be accomplished by increased sensitivity to the process of dying and by an increased awareness of one's own perceptions and feelings about dying. Within the hospital setting all staff members need training in terminal care to enhance their understanding of the social relationships associated with lingering deaths. This training should not be limited to hospitals but should be integrated into medical and nursing schools' educational programs (Glaser & Strauss 1968; Strauss & Glaser 1970).

Accountability requires familiarity with the social and psychological needs of the client and family and the organization of ward work to include these needs. Hospitals could increase accountability to the dying by explicitly reviewing social, psychological, and organizational aspects of terminal care as well as focusing on nursing and medical matters (Strauss & Glaser 1970). Increased accountability would require that the hospital take responsibility for such actions, which are currently left to personal discretion and therefore are unreported.

For most people having some kind of lingering trajectory, the dying process often requires multiple admissions to the hospital between stays at home. These individuals and their families need some kind of reasonable plan to provide adequate medical and nursing care without financial ruin. Home hospice care is not uniformly available throughout the country, and governmental policy toward financial support limits the availability of hospice care for prolonged time periods. Advocacy by the health care provider could help assure a national policy that would provide moneys to train personnel and to make hospice care available throughout the country. The entire cost in money, time, and energy would be lower in the home environment, and the presence of support would decrease the anguish for those involved (Strauss & Glaser 1970).

Also needed in the public domain is a policy governing issues that transcend professional responsibilities for terminal care, for example, on withholding addicting drugs or prolonging life when it results in increased agony or financial ruin (Strauss & Glaser 1970). Medical and nursing personnel should encourage public discussion of these issues.

Applying Trajectory to Nursing Practice

To date, no studies have specifically related trajectory to direct nursing care. However, its value becomes apparent when an understanding of the concept is combined with the nursing process and a dose of imagination. Fewer conflicts, improved care, and greater efficiency at work can result.

Gathering and utilizing more complete information on client biographies and illness trajectories and respecting the client's and family's knowledge about management of disease will help the medical staff determine what care is appropriate and how it should be implemented. Involving the client and family in this way can help resolve many current and recurrent problems. The use of biographical data enhances quality care by increasing awareness of the whole person.

Work improves when medical personnel see beyond pathophysiology and become aware of differences in perception based on psychological and sociological needs. Increased sensitivity to the perceptions of others improves communication with the client and family as well as with other health professionals (physicians, nurses, therapists, and social workers). Staff/staff and staff/client disputes become more amenable to resolution when the need to place blame is eliminated.

Trajectory phases can provide a basis for determining the work the staff and client need to do. During the diagnostic phase staff work includes instructing the client about procedures or tests, preparing the client, obtaining needed supplies or equipment, providing postprocedural follow-up care, and supporting the client in areas of concern. Clients are expected to cooperate with procedures, save specimens, and so forth. During the acute treatment phase the staff observes, assesses, implements medical and nursing orders, and records information, and the client follows restrictions, reports symptoms, and so on. During recovery the staff teaches, evaluates, and provides feedback; the client takes increasing responsibility for the regimen and eventually for full at-home responsibility. Teaching can focus on areas of learning need rather than following a general teaching care plan, to promote greater continuity of care between hospital and home setting.

The health professional can apply the trajectory concept in other ways. There is an interplay between growth and development and trajectory, with each impacting on the other. Roles and self-identity can be influenced by participants' understanding of the trajectory. Contingencies and the importance of ultimate responsibility become apparent. Imagination will identify many other applications.

One Application of Trajectory in a Hospital Setting

Given that growing numbers of clients have chronic illnesses that require long-term management, involvement of clients in planning care could increase their responsibility toward maximizing functioning in the hospital and at home. Usually in the hospital only limited time and work are devoted to furthering such personalized rehabilitation goals. To increase effective posthospital management, clients should help set goals and determine interventions while still hospitalized. Plans developed with client input lead to greater integration of client and staff work and allow the client an opportunity to influence outcomes and effect continuity of care.

Davis (1980) studied a setting in which the staff philosophy encourages client involvement. Clients participate in developing their own goals and care plans and help identify activities necessary to carry out these plans, all with the staff's blessing. Because the medical chief of service accepts and supports this philosophy and program, nonphysician members of the staff are treated in an egalitarian rather than a subordinate manner. Each person's expertise is accepted as the basis of work done, and all personnel are accountable for appropriate decision making. Consequently, the unit's physician can focus on acute care, while the staff can focus on social, biographical, and other matters.

Examination of this program reveals that the staff has become more sensitive to the clients' biographical background, perspectives, and needs. Helping clients master necessary skills and knowledge and take greater responsibility when appropriate creates individuals who cope more effectively and function more efficiently when they return home. The staff gains work satisfaction when their expertise is utilized and they are accountable for more than medically centered tasks.

Summary and Conclusions

Trajectory is a sociological concept that broadens understanding of client problems and needs beyond the acute medical model. Trajectory deals with individuals' perceptions of situations, their responses to those perceptions, and the organization of work that is involved. The various kinds of trajectories—illness, biographical, dying, pain, and so on—all have the qualities of duration, movement, predictability, and shape. Work that is necessary to shape or manage the trajectory is performed not only by staff but by clients and their families.

Management problems, especially with chronic illnesses, have increased as trajectories have become more complex. Increased complexity leads to decreased predictability and changes in work and organization. Technological advances have become a major factor impacting on trajectory because they create new illnesses and phases of illnesses and add to the numbers and kinds of chronically ill individuals. Individuals who have end stage renal disease illustrate the iatrogenic impact of technology.

The episodic nature of admissions and the acute illness orientation of hospital personnel often lead to conflict with chronically ill individuals who are experienced managers of their own illnesses. When the staff manages illness without adequate awareness of the biographies and experiences of the client, care that is less than satisfactory may result. Both staff and clients contribute to the work at hand, but goals and tasks may differ. Staff tend to focus on acute illness, and clients on maintaining their chronic conditions in a stable state. Families also participate in work, both in the hospital and at home.

Involving clients in the work of managing their own care can promote better continuity of care. Accountability must increase in the hospital setting, and there needs to be a more comprehensive social policy directed at integrated management of long-term illnesses, not just the acute phases that occur.

Clients and family must cope not only with physiology but with a host of health-related social problems that affect roles, relationships, and adjustments. Chronic illness must be integrated into the lives and needs of the client and family, not the reverse. The business of the chronically ill is to live as normally as possible despite the symptoms and the disease. The problems of managing and the perspective of each individual influence this living (Strauss 1981).

The professional has a role in this drama. Focus must extend beyond the medicophysiological perspective to take into account the lives and expectations of the client and family; compassion and medical or nursing competence are not sufficient. Through an awareness of such concepts as trajectory, professionals can expand their knowledge and sensitivity to the social aspects of symptom control, regimen management, and crisis prevention, as well as to management of pain and dying. To accomplish these objectives, illnesses must be viewed from a social as well as a medical perspective (Strauss 1981). Integrating social concepts into their work will allow professionals to develop strategies or tactics and to influence public policy that would provide a more humane approach to all who are afflicted with chronic diseases.

STUDY QUESTIONS

1. How would you define trajectory as it relates to illness?
2. What is the difference between the actual course of chronic illness and its perceived course? How does the latter relate to trajectory?
3. Define the following terms in relation to trajectory: *participants, duration, perception, predictability, shape, shaping, work, phases, biographies, contingency, balancing.*
4. How does technology influence trajectory? How does this influence affect staff and client?
5. In the hospital, how does the work of staff and client differ? What work does a family do in the hospital? What influences staff's awareness of client work?
6. What kinds of work do the client and family do at home when they have a regimen that must be followed?
7. What are the contingencies that impact on the effectiveness with which client and family manage at home? How do they lead to work overload?

8. In the hospital, how do staff and client differ in their perceptions of pain management? How does this difference influence pain management? Discuss the difference from the perspective of both acute and chronic pain.
9. What two categories of dying trajectories have Glaser and Strauss identified? What are their characteristics?
10. Why are lingering dying trajectories more prone to contingencies? What are these contingencies?
11. How could health professionals increase their accountability to clients in the hospital setting? How do biographical data influence this accountability?
12. How could care for the dying client improve in the hospital setting?
13. What reasons that would encourage health professionals to serve more readily as client advocates can you identify? What issues deserve emphasis?
14. If you could set up a unit to increase clients' involvement in their own care, how would you go about doing this?

References

Calland, C. H., (1972) Iatrogenic problems in end-stage renal failure, *New England Journal of Medicine, 287*: 334–336, August 17

Corbin, J., and Strauss, A., (1982) Trajectory and Work and Biography, paper presented: International Sociological Meeting, Mexico City

Davis, M. Z., (1980) The organizational interactional and care oriented conditions for patient participation in continuity of care: A framework for staff intervention, *Social Science and Medicine, 14A*: 39–47

Fagerhaugh, S. Y., and Strauss, A. L., (1977) *Politics of Pain Management: Staff-Patient Interaction*, Menlo Park, Calif.: Addison-Wesley

Glaser, B., and Strauss, A., (1968) *Time for Dying*, Chicago: Aldine

Lorber, J., (1981) Good patients and problem patients: Conformity and deviance in a general hospital, in Conrad, P., and Kern, R. (eds.), *The Sociology of Health and Illness: Critical Perspectives*, New York: St. Martin's Press

Morris, E. M., (1984) Home care today, *American Journal of Nursing, 84*: 3: 340–347

Plough, A., (1981) Medical technology and the crisis of experience: The costs of clinical legitimation, *Social Science and Medicine, 15F*: 89–101

Reif, L., (1975) *Cardiacs and Normals: The Social Construction of a Disability*, (unpublished), Abstracts, UCSF

Strauss, A., (1980) Editorial comment, *Social Science and Medicine, 14D*: 351–353

Strauss, A., (1981) Chronic illness, in Conrad, P., and Kern, R. (eds.), *The Sociology of Health and Illness: Critical Perspectives*, New York: St. Martin's Press

Strauss, A., Corbin, J., Fagerhaugh, S., Glaser, B., Maines, D., Suczek, B., and Wiener, C., (1984) *Chronic Illness and the Quality of Life*, St. Louis: C.V. Mosby

Strauss, A., Fagerhaugh, S., Suczek, B., and Wiener, C., (1985) Illness trajectories (Chap. 2), *Social Organization of Medical Work*, Chicago: University of Chicago Press

Strauss, A., Fagerhaugh, S., Suczek, B., and Wiener, C., (1982) The work of hospitalized patients, *Social Science and Medicine, 16*: 977–986

Strauss, A., and Glaser, B. (1970) *Anguish: A Case History of a Dying Trajectory*, Mill Valley: The Sociology Press

Wiener, C., Strauss, A., Fagerhaugh, S., and Suczek, B., (1979) Trajectories, biographies and the evolving medical technology scene: Labor and delivery and the intensive care nursery, *Sociology of Health and Illness, 1*: 3: 263–283

$\diamondsuit$

CHAPTER THREE

Illness Roles

$\diamondsuit$

Introduction

Living together in social groups, as most of us do, requires guidance so that interactions do not lead to chaos. Society establishes guidelines, which in turn influence the responses and behaviors of group members. *Role theory*, based on the premise that most of the time, most people define most important situations in approximately the same way (Berger 1963), provides a vehicle for understanding these guidelines. According to role theory, society defines every recognized position and assigns roles that contain a set of *norms*, or behavioral rules, that are socially accepted (Wu 1973; Berger 1963).

Roles not only include norms for behaviors, actions, emotions, and attitudes but lead to the emergence of identities that others recognize and that help one maintain an individual self-image (Berger 1963). The mechanism by which socially assigned identities are learned is called *socialization*, which Mead (1934) explains as a process in which the individual discovers self and society at the same time. Interactions with and direction from significant others (parents, teachers, friends, and others) reflect the expectations and recognition of society at large. Children play at different roles, practicing behaviors inherent in these roles. Over time, the person becomes a repertoire of multiple roles, much as an actor in the theater does, with the ability to focus on behaviors that are part of the individual role appropriate to a given situation. For example, the young mother who

is also a nursing student utilizes appropriate but different role behaviors in each of her life situations.

During periods of illness, role expectations must change so that affected individuals can move from daily responsibilities to behaviors deemed appropriate to their changing health status. The individual who fully recovers returns to prior behavior and roles. However, when there is only partial recovery or residual pathology, the individual has to modify or adapt prior wellness behavior to accommodate both social expectations and the illness. The nurse who is aware of the roles that occur during illness, the behavior appropriate to these roles, and interventions that can support the client during and after transition into these roles is in a position to help the client and family.

Illness Behavior

The onset of symptoms leads to a response, called *illness behavior*, which helps individuals determine their own state of health and need for treatment (Wu 1973). Illness behavior has been defined as "the way in which given symptoms may be differentially perceived, evaluated and acted (or not acted) upon by different kinds of persons" (Mechanic 1961).

Viewed from this perspective, illness behavior is limited to help-seeking behavior that either identifies and assesses changes that are occurring or searches for solutions. Because it is health-seeking, it can be triggered whenever an individual feels that a symptom demands explanation, desires a means of managing the underlying disorder, or disagrees with current treatment. For example, the client with recurring, nonspecific neurological symptoms may consult many physicians and receive several diagnostic opinions and treatment plans before multiple sclerosis is finally confirmed. Or a family who finds that current medical treatment is not helping their dying child may move to Mexico to try laetrile treatments.

Influences on Illness Behavior

In 1966 Rosenstock formulated a *health belief model* (HBM) to explain the way one's beliefs about health and illness can predict health service consumption. The HBM showed that attitudes, personal values, beliefs, previous life experiences, and present life stresses may alter actions, choices, and responses to illness (Rankin & Duffy 1983). Although the HBM is more useful in evaluating preventive health teaching and in assessing compliance to treatment regimens, it also clarifies illness behavior (see Chapters 7 and 12). According to Rosenstock's model, people hold four basic beliefs: (1) one is susceptible to a disease, (2) the disease is harmful or serious, (3) preventive actions or health interventions can reduce the likelihood of contracting or the severity of the disease, and (4) these actions and interventions are worth any cost or barrier that exists (Rankin & Duffy 1983; Redman 1984).

Sociocultural factors also influence beliefs and illness behavior. People tend to be internally consistent with their own cultural system; that consistency can result in a gap between the values and beliefs of segments of the population and those of health practitioners (Redman 1984). As an example, those Mexican-Americans who believe that illness is a result of life-style and an imbalance in the body between "hot" and "cold" would carry out treatment at home, seeking outside advice only when such treatment proved ineffective (Gonzalez-Swafford 1983). An-

other factor influencing health behavior is economic status, which affects educational level, economic level, family structure, and so forth. The poor, who often have less knowledge of preventive measures and know of fewer resources to obtain services, tend to delay seeking medical help until symptoms interfere with daily independence or ability to function in usual daily roles (Redman 1984). Table 3-1 lists many determinants or influences that can affect illness behavior.

Actions and Responses to Symptoms

The occurrence of symptoms does not necessarily lead an individual to seek a definitive diagnosis or treatment. Rather, behavior can take several directions: action, inaction, remaining in flux, or counteraction (Lewis & Collier 1983; Wu 1973). The symptomatic person tends to go through a process encompassing several stages (see Table 3-2). Action taken to identify the basis of symptoms is illness behavior. When a diagnosis is made and the individual accepts a treatment plan, illness behavior gives way to the *sick role*.

Action. Possible actions include making self-diagnosis and using self-help–home remedies, seeking advice from others, consulting culturally acceptable healers, and finding professional medical help. One's sociocultural group or the kinds of symptoms being experienced often determine the kind of help sought. Individuals are more likely to choose self-help and self-management when symptoms are vague or do not seem serious. If symptoms, however, appear significant or life-threatening, individuals usually seek professional help. Whereas clients with colds usually self-treat, those who are bleeding or having chest pain generally go directly to the doctor without attempting home remedies.

Inaction. Involving a "wait and see" attitude, inaction can be influenced by fear of some diagnoses (for instance, of cancer), inadequate knowledge of resources, worry about costs of receiving help, or

TABLE 3-1. Determinants of Illness Behavior

Recurrence of the Aberrance: The more frequent a symptom, the more the individual feels that help is needed. If relief is obtained from home remedies, less outside help is sought.

Visibility and Consequences: Symptoms that are more apparent lead to more illness behavior. However, if the individual feels that the disorder will lead to stigma, there may be a lessened tendency to seek help. Community tolerance toward certain symptomatology will allow for less help being sought, whereas a prejudice against a symptom or disease forces help-seeking behavior. When a symptom is seen as life-threatening, help will usually be sought regardless of other factors. Also influencing a person's willingness to seek help are the consequences on other roles or significant others.

Perceived Seriousness or Severity: How overt or life-threatening are the symptoms? What influences do they have on social or work relationships? Are they associated with stigma or guilt? What organs are involved? What is the prognosis or rate of recovery? Disorders seen as serious lead to earlier illness behavior. However, how serious or severe a person considers an illness may differ by social class and by health belief system. In addition, when seriousness is viewed on a hierarchy of other needs and desires, symptoms may be considered to have lesser consequences.

Influences of Availability of Treatment and the Medical Care System: Distance, costs, convenience, time, effort, and fear of outcomes all influence a person's willingness to seek help. In addition, the health care system tends to subordinate the individual's needs, requires conformity, removes personal identity and privacy, and places the client in a situation similar to that of parent/child. Such subordination can influence willingness to begin illness behavior.

Knowledge of Significance of Symptoms: Lack of knowledge of the significance of symptoms can influence help seeking. For example, older, symptomatic individuals can interpret their symptoms as illness or as part of the aging process.

Cultural and Social Expectations: Cultural and ethnic variations of symptom interpretation and notions of what is acceptable health care all serve to guide individuals toward or away from seeking help from a physician. Socioeconomic class, age, and sex influence how symptoms are interpreted. Lower classes give more credence to symptoms that interfere with important roles; the aged utilize more health services; women seek more medical care than men.

Adapted from Alonzo (1980).

concern over the possibility of being labeled should symptoms not lead to diagnosis (Wu 1973). People tend to inaction when symptoms are vague or have previously occurred and have been alleviated within a relatively short period of time. Abdominal cramps, colds, and so on, fall into this latter category.

Remaining in Flux. The client who is in flux vacillates between wanting to take action and remaining inactive. Vacillation implies an ambivalence about various concerns: wanting treatment versus feeling constraints of time and money; avoiding discomfort versus regaining health; getting help but not both-

ering others; and so on. Such conflicts can lead to a delay in treatment that can have an adverse impact on disease outcome.

Counteraction. Considered anti-illness behavior, counteraction often reflects a denial of symptoms and is sometimes considered a form of deviant illness behavior (Wu 1973). Some individuals tend to seek help in an effort to negate or minimize the significance of symptoms—that is, to disprove the seriousness of symptoms or to avoid "giving in" to them. For example, the man who, in spite of recurrent mild chest pain after activity, insists that daily jogging is

TABLE 3-2. Stages of Acute Illness

Stage	Behavior
1. Symptom experience	Identifies symptoms as not compatible with own concept of health.
2. Assumption of the sick role	Relinquishes normal duties and activities. Seeks validation from nonprofessional individuals. Becomes preoccupied with signs, symptoms, and bodily functions. May take action, wait and see, vacillate, or take counteraction. Action taken may include self-help, help from significant others, or help from cultural healers. Desires to get well even when not contacting a health professional.
3. Contacting health professional	Seeks legitimization from professional. May be willing to undergo treatment and to work to return to normal role or may continue illness behavior and shop around for another diagnosis and treatment plan.
4. Dependent role	Accepts diagnosis and treatment plan and must want to get well. Becomes compliant and conforms to opinions or demands of health provider, acknowledges need for physical assistance and for emotional support. Increased dependence manifested by egocentrism, decreased interest in other activities, regression, and so on.
5. Recovery	Must relinquish the sick role and resume normal tasks. Often moves to a higher level of wellness through health teaching. If no improvement occurs, condition may be considered malingering or could be result of secondary gains (enjoying dependency to gain attention or wanting no pressures or responsibilities).

Adapted from Lewis and Collier (1983) and Wu (1973).

essential to maintaining health is taking counteraction. For the client ignorant of the significance or meaning of particular symptoms, inaction or counteraction may be a result of this ignorance, rather than a form of denial.

The Sick Role

The *sick role* concept was introduced in juxtaposition to the physician's role by Talcott Parsons (1951). These two roles were not seen as equal, since the physician retained leverage to influence client movement toward a positive health change (Cockerham 1978). In fact, the physician–client dyad presented by Parsons contains a quality of the parent–child relationship, despite the physician's more limited involvement with the client than the parent has with the child (Parsons & Fox 1952).

Parsons saw illness as a response to social pressures (for example, evading responsibilities), and therefore both biologic and sociologic in nature. Anyone could take on the role he identified; therefore it was *contingent*—that is, negatively achieved through failure to keep well. In addition, the role also carried with it the connotation that ill individuals were not competent to help themselves (Parsons 1951). Table 3-3 lists the four major components or characteristics of this role. Like all roles, the sick role is learned and is influenced by evaluation and legitimization from others (Alonzo 1980). One assumes the sick role when one has accepted being ill, initiated some form of action, and demonstrates a desire to be well again. Should the individual continue to seek another, more acceptable diagnosis or treatment, then illness behavior continues.

TABLE 3-3. Characteristics of the Sick Role

Component of the role	Associated expectations and behaviors
Rights	
Exemption from normal role responsibilities	Dependent on nature and severity of illness. Requires legitimization (validation) by others and by physician, thus discouraging the malingerer. Once legitimization is obtained, the individual is obligated to avoid responsibilities.
Right to be cared for	The individual is not expected to become well by an act of will or decision. Not responsible for becoming sick, the individual therefore has a right to be cared for. Physical dependency and the right to emotional support are therefore acceptable.
Obligations	
Obligation to want to become well	Being ill is seen as undesirable. Since privileges and exemptions of the sick role could become secondary gains, the motivation to recover assumes primary importance.
Obligation to seek and cooperate with technically competent help	The patient needs technical expertise that the physician and other health professionals have. Cooperation with these professionals for the common goal of getting well is mandatory.

Adapted from Parsons (1951).

The Impaired Role

It becomes evident that the sick role assumes major importance in medical sociology on the basis of its reasonableness in relation to acute illness and its focus on movement toward recovery; consequently, it has little applicability to chronic illness.

Gordon (1966) carried out the first study that identified behaviors applicable to chronically ill clients when he examined responses and expectations of several socioeconomic groups toward illnesses that differed in severity and duration. He found, among all groups, that prognosis was the major factor in defining someone as "sick"; that once someone was so defined, acceptable behaviors were consistent with Parsons's model. When prognosis worsened, all groups encouraged increased exemption from social responsibility. Socioeconomic groups varied in terms of *who* was defined as sick, with members of lower socioeconomic groups equating sickness with functional incapacity. In ad-

dition, Gordon found that individuals and their families made illness-related decisions primarily during either the early, nonhelpless stages or during the recuperative stage; they made few of these kinds of decisions during the highly dependent phase.

Gordon identified two illness role statuses. The first was the *sick role*, as presented by Parsons, which was seen as valid when the prognosis was grave and uncertain. When this role was deemed appropriate, all social groups felt that pressure should be applied to insulate the client from usual role responsibilities. The second role, which he called an *impaired role*, was considered appropriate for disorders in which the prognosis was known and was not grave. When individuals were seen in the impaired role, social expectations supported normal behavior and usual role involvement (Gordon 1966). In other words, the study showed that social pressure would discourage normal behavior if the individual were considered sick but would encourage an individual who was disabled and was not experiencing illness to maintain normal behavior, within the limitations of the condition.

The impaired role assumes the following characteristics:

1. The individual has an impairment that is permanent.
2. The individual does not give up normal role responsibilities but is expected to maintain normal behavior within the limits of the health condition. Modification of life situation may be necessitated by the disability.
3. The individual does not have to "want to get well" but rather is encouraged to make the most of remaining capabilities. The individual must realize potentialities while accepting the existence of the impairment and recognizing limitations and performance commensurate with the disability (Wu 1973).

Inherent in the impaired role is the attitude that retaining sick role behaviors prevents the disabled from taking over their own management of care. However, once the impaired role is accepted, any activity that helps maintain control of the condition, prevents complications, leads to resumption of role responsibilities, and results in full realization of potentialities is acceptable (Wu 1973). Since the impaired role incorporates both rehabilitation and maximization of wellness, assumption of this role indicates that illness is not defined as deviance. If the individual retains sick role behaviors at this time, such action is considered deviant and inconsistent with the medical condition (Wu 1973).

Problems and Issues Related to Illness Roles

Parsons's sick role model, which was presented as an ideal type (Segall 1976), was accepted on its reasonableness and logic (Cockerham 1978). Most research that has explored its various components in relation to the acutely ill tends to support Parsons's basic assumptions (Steward & Sullivan 1982). But the nature of some illnesses is such that there is no clear societal agreement over when the person should be admitted to the sick role (Segall 1976).

When originally presented, Parsons's model indicated that the ill person could be considered deviant since he or she was evading social responsibility (Parsons 1951). This hypothesis has not received widespread agreement among sociologists, who feel that using deviance as a model for illness negates the biological reality of the disease itself. Parsons, however, was not equating illness deviance with criminal deviance, despite some similarities between illness and crime: Both mobilize agencies of social control, initiate a social process to alter behavior, contain role changes that presume irresponsibility, require others to intervene to control behavior, and lead to a decrease in personal autonomy (Twaddle 1973).

Illness and crime differ in key ways. Society sees criminals as individuals who are responsible for their behavior and knowingly violate social norms. Consequently, society attempts to punish those individuals, seeks agents to control their behavior, and tries to force criminals to engage in normal activities (Twaddle 1973). The sick are not seen as being responsible for their behaviors or able to correct their deviance independently. Therefore, they are given exemptions from normal role responsibilities, along with encouragement to recover so they can willingly return to normal roles and accountability. Helping agents, in the form of health care providers, are designated to assist in the attainment of this goal (Twaddle 1973). In other words, society expects the criminal to alter and conform but is willing to alter conditions that prevent conformity in dealing with the sick.

The major deficiency of the sick role model is that it is based on acute episodic illness. Consequently, it overlooks chronic illness characteristics: the long-term rather than temporary nature of the illness, the reality that full recovery is not a reasonable expectation, and acknowledgment that management is often the responsibility of the client or family and, therefore, that the individual must adjust to a permanent change. Acute and chronic illnesses vary not only in biomedical aspects but in client responses: findings, symptom recognition, help-seeking behavior, and therapeutic encounters (Steward & Sullivan 1982). The chronically ill are often unable to resume prior roles fully and need to focus on retaining (not regaining) optimal role performance, restricted only in relationship to limitations imposed by the disease (Kassebaum & Baumann 1965). Yet society does not provide a clear and acceptable role for this group (Segall 1976).

Criticisms of Parsons's Model

Application of the sick role model has limitations among different sociocultural groups in relation to attitudes toward sickness. Many populations have distinct concepts of the way illness is defined and the sociocultural patterns of help-seeking behavior that are valid for themselves or others (Cockerham 1978; Twaddle 1969). The only universal agreement seems to be that the role is undesirable (Segall 1976). Behaviors described in the model have a middle-class orientation; the impact of poverty on people's responses is ignored. The poor, who have to work to survive, often deny sickness unless it entails functional incapacity (Cockerham 1978). In spite of symptoms, people who are poor may not move into the sick role. Few studies have actually explored sociocultural differences toward the sick role itself or the relationship of role expectations regarding appropriate behavior for sick persons and those with whom they interact.

Seeking and Cooperating with Competent Help

The four components of the sick role have been studied quite extensively, especially the component that deals with seeking out and cooperating with technically competent helpers. Yet little research has addressed the influence of social groups on these health care decisions (Hover & Juelsgaard 1978) and the roles of nonphysician health care providers. Also missing from the model is a "healthy stage" when individuals may seek contact with the health care system for purposes other than treatment of illness (Hover & Juelsgaard 1978). Other criticisms concern the oversimplification of behaviors and the model's

not taking into account the personality and orientation of the individual, aspects that influence dependence, knowledge, psychological needs, and so forth. Many people are less dependent than Parsons's model would indicate (Hover & Juelsgaard 1978).

Exemption from Role Responsibilities

Studies dealing with role responsibilities and performance assume that the person who is willing to consult the doctor is ready to adopt the sick role. The relationship of taking on this role to the individual's willingness to give up normal work responsibilities or to become dependent on others (Segall 1976) has not been studied.

Exemption from role responsibilities also requires legitimization, or validation, from others to prevent malingering by those who are not truly ill (Cockerham 1978). Studies have not analyzed legitimization when a social question of personal responsibility for causing the health conditions is involved.

Alcoholism and mental illness are both disorders in which obtaining release from role responsibilities can be difficult (Segall 1976). Although alcoholism is now considered a disease needing treatment, most people, including most health professionals, still feel that legitimizing this disorder removes the responsibility that society believes alcoholics should take for their behavior. Consequently, alcoholics are frequently denied the legitimacy that allows them to take on the sick role.

Mental illness presents a somewhat different perspective of social role exemption. The literature shows that the mentally ill are not exempt from performance of normal roles and responsibilities while they are trying to get well (Segall 1976). Hospital treatment programs include work incentives and activities that are similar to those found in the community. The mentally ill are expected to be active, independent, and self-directed in their interaction with the physician and other health care providers. They are not expected to be helpless, passive, submissive, or dependent. When mental illnesses, such as depression, are treated in community settings, these individuals maintain their normal roles while undergoing outpatient treatment. Once recovered, the mentally ill, especially those who have been hospitalized, must prepare for the stigma and rejection associated with being labeled as "formerly mentally ill" (see Chapter 4).

Who Should Legitimize Illness? Parsons's model emphasized primarily the physician's role in legitimizing illness; he did not deal with the roles of nurses, social workers, and other health care providers in the process. Legitimizing actions by family and others was also considered less significant. Although the physician may give the final validation with acute illnesses, one must question whether this prerogative applies to situations involving the chronically ill or permanently handicapped. Since most health care management of chronic illnesses occurs in the home, dependency on nonprofessional sources for evaluating client status increases. One study found that a "more crucial role in their treatment was assigned [by patients] to the lay significant others than to professionals" (Honig-Parnass 1981). In other words, care and support by lay caregivers were felt to be more important legitimizing criteria for the chronically ill than was medical care in relation to managing their daily activities.

Obtaining Legitimization of Illness. With some chronic illnesses, especially when early symptoms are not well defined, receiving legitimization from the physician, other health professionals, or nonprofessionals can be difficult and frustrating. Denial of opportunity to move into the sick role forces continued illness behavior, including "doctor hopping," placing the client in a problematic relationship in which the individual must "work out" a solution alone (Steward & Sullivan 1982). As a result symptomatic persons may be left to question the truth of their own perceptions.

Multiple sclerosis (MS) is a good case in point since it averages about 5 years from onset of symptoms to diagnosis. This period of time has three phases: (1) the nonserious phase, (2) the serious phase, and (3) the diagnostic phase (Steward & Sul-

livan 1982). During the nonserious phase, symptoms are so vague that they receive only minimal action. The individual tends to respond as if they constituted a minor ailment.

The serious phase begins when the client moves into illness behavior and starts to define symptoms as illness needing a diagnosis. The lack of definitive tests makes obtaining such a diagnosis difficult; visits to doctors result in a multitude of incorrect diagnoses, with symptom relief being elusive. Confusion and uncertainty result; illness behavior must be continued. Should significant others accept these diagnoses, the still-complaining client is viewed as a hypochondriac or malingerer. Because the individual is not socially defined as sick, he or she finds that stress symptoms increase, becoming more troublesome than the MS. An ambiguous situation with unclear role definitions results: there are increasing symptoms and increasing need for the sick role, but the lack of diagnosis and legitimization prevents the individual from adopting the role. The individual then feels forced to take a more active role and "shops around" for a physician who can correctly identify what is wrong.

When diagnosis is finally made, the client frequently shows an initial somewhat joyous response to having a name for the recurrent and troublesome symptoms. As the case study of J.A. illustrates, this initial reaction results from the decrease in stress. In addition, now professional legitimization and greater social support from significant others follow. This initial response carries with it optimism and hope that the illness will have long remissions, mild or no progression, and a potential future cure.

Delay in Seeking Help

Symptomatic people are sometimes reluctant to seek medical care. Such delay can prove detrimental when illnesses that require early consultation and diagnosis are not identified so that effective, and sometimes lifesaving, treatment can be instituted. Delay can also have an adverse economic effect if it results in treatment that is prolonged or less efficient or if correcting or minimizing the condition consequently

◇ CASE STUDY ◇

Trying to Obtain Legitimization

Because of their vague nature, 24-year-old J.A. paid little attention to her symptoms. When the weakness and numbness in her left leg continued for several weeks, abated, and then recurred, she decided to consult her physician. Her history and clinical manifestations were so vague that the physician felt that nothing was physiologically wrong with her, and she accepted the evaluation. Over the next year she developed two episodes of diplopia and some spasticity in the left leg, followed by scotomas and vertigo. Each time, although symptoms did not persist, they were more severe. Repeated visits to J.A.'s family physician did not result in a diagnosis. In fact, the physician believed that J.A. had a "pseudoillness" and recommended that she talk to a psychiatrist because she had recently undergone a traumatic breakup with her boyfriend of several years. Because her initial symptoms predated this breakup and because each recurrence of symptoms was slightly more pronounced, she interpreted her findings as more significant than the physician did. She went to another physician, who treated her for a low-grade infection. Treatment seemed to help at first, but when symptoms

again recurred, J.A. rejected the diagnosis and actions as ineffective.

J.A.'s parents, who had no reason to question the ability of their long-time family physician, supported his suggestion that she seek psychiatric help although her symptoms were growing worse with each exacerbation. This attitude was very upsetting to J.A. because she felt she was losing vital support in her efforts to find out what was wrong with her. She began keeping records of tests and findings and asking more and more questions. Her goal was to assist, not to impede, the physician.

In addition to being time-consuming, the uncertainty caused her to doubt her own mental state. Her distress continued as her search proved fruitless. She eventually was referred to a medical center, where a diagnosis of multiple sclerosis was made. Her initial response was a sense of relief, although she soon found out that treatment would not lead to cure but only to some symptomatic relief. J.A. was 28 when diagnosis was finally made.

requires more time. At times, delay can even affect the total community's health. For example, should active tuberculosis remain untreated, others might contract the disease (Blackwell 1963).

Many factors influence individuals' timing in seeking medical help. When symptomatic, individuals reach a point when they decide that now is the time to see the doctor. Psychological stress can serve as the trigger to action, or the decision may be based on an individual's pattern of illness behavior. Crisis, as the capacity to adapt is lessened, can cause enough disequilibrium to make the individual seek help (Stoeckle et al. 1963). Care seeking is also associated with family's or friends' evaluation of a situation, when they decide that symptoms represent an illness requiring expedient medical intervention (Alonzo 1980).

In spite of factors that move clients to seek health care, delays having potential adverse effects on outcome of the disease process occur. Choosing to be-

come a patient or to remain a nonpatient does not necessarily depend on the nature or quality of the distress, the seriousness of the complaint, or the ability to treat the disorder. Some sociocultural groups allow delay until symptoms interfere with relationships, others when physical or functional activity is prevented, and still others until after approval or decisions of the family or group (Stoeckle et al. 1963).

Blackwell (1963), analyzing studies dealing with delays involving cancer patients, points out that these studies primarily indicate that delay does exist and that many people are not saved because they postpone seeking diagnosis and treatment. Individuals with mental problems often remain at home and do not seek treatment. Once their families feel they have reached the limits of tolerance, their demand that the individual seek medical care often moves the client into therapy.

Three features seem to influence help seeking (Stoeckle et al. 1963). These are the client's

TABLE 3-4. Influences: Delay in Seeking Help

Symptoms are a normal part of life: The presence of symptoms of one kind or another is so widespread that it is considered a norm in most populations. In fact, total absence of any complaints even among the "healthy" over long periods of time may be the exception. Respiratory, abdominal, and muscular skeletal symptoms occur on a regular basis and are generally treated by the individual or family with home remedies or over-the-counter medications. What the individual identifies as "sickness" requiring medical intervention may differ from what the health professional defines as illness in relation to signs and symptoms alone. It is a fact of life that a large percentage of those people with illnesses do not seek medical assistance.

Type of onset: Concern about symptoms often depends upon whether onset is acute or slow and insidious, or on the individual's perspective of the significance of the symptom(s). Rapidly developing, acute symptoms such as bleeding, crushing chest pain, or severe trauma lead people to seek medical care. Care may not be sought with slow insidious symptoms.

Significance of "chief complaint": Medical significance of a symptom is not the criterion used by individuals in seeking help. Health care is sought if the client's *chief complaint* or concern about a symptom is distressing to that individual. Take, for instance, the individual who focuses on edema that causes leg discomfort rather than other nephrotic signs and symptoms. The symptomatic individual may be more concerned about impairment of his or her social roles than about the meaning of physical symptoms. When symptoms are seen as indicative of possibly incurable disorders, the individual might choose to avoid the "truth" about what the illness is, especially if there is a feeling that the health care providers cannot help.

Differences in symptom perception: Different cultural, ethnic, or social groups perceive and respond to symptoms differently. What may be operating is a difference in the very definition of what constitutes a symptom. The same symptom can lead to different courses of action. Some cultural groups may see the onset of pain as requiring immediate attention and be concerned about physical and social effects of the illness; others may be more concerned with the functional impact of the disease. Social class also influences whether the individual will seek medical care. For example, the upper classes will seek treatment for "nervousness," but this problem might be ignored by the lower classes as of little significance.

Attitudes toward and expectations of the health care provider: The acceptance and use of a particular caregiver are frequently determined by the client's reason for seeking health care or the client's perspective and attitude toward health providers. People who only want to be reassured about the disease and symptoms or who rate "personal interest in the patient" as more important than technical competence delay seeking help from health providers who emphasize technical competence. Primary providers may be seen as less influential than caregivers who seem more helpful. The advice of the physical therapist who helps in the rehabilitation of the stroke patient may carry more weight than that of the physician.

Definitions and beliefs regarding health care: The stages that people go through in the process of health care, from deciding something is wrong to doing something about it, may depend on their definitions of and beliefs about health and illness. Individuals who see avoidance of disease as an achievement undergo more health checkups to assure such attainment; others who show more apathy regarding health may make fewer visits. People who are concerned about anything that interferes with their usual activities will seek care when they develop ailments that impede such activities.

Content based on Stoeckle et al. (1963).

(1) perception, knowledge, beliefs, and attitudes about the objective clinical disorder or symptom; (2) attitudes toward and expectations of the physician and medical services; and (3) personal definitions of health and sickness and beliefs about when medical care is necessary (see Table 3-4).

Who Seeks the Sick Role?

Individuals gauge sickness more by the disruption of their ability to function than by organic parameters. Emotional stress, which occurs with many disorders, has been identified as an important cause of illness

(Mann 1982). For example, stress was found to frequently predate coronary problems (Weidner 1980). Perception of the significance of symptoms influences whether an individual seeks medical care. One study found that individuals who as children received rewards (toys, food, and so on) when they were sick tended to move into the sick role more readily, voiced more somatic complaints, made more doctor visits, had more acute and chronic illnesses, and missed a greater number of work days (Whitehead et al. 1982).

Other factors that influence moving into the sick role include economic ability to pay for medical care, sense of responsibility to one's own health, and personal views of medicine, professionals, surgery, and the body itself (Redman 1984). As an example, the elderly often see bodily changes as a "natural" part of aging rather than as symptoms, and this attitude adds to their reluctance to seek care, especially when it is coupled with economic concerns. Psychological factors such as anxiety and fear play a role. Individuals may have to experience a crisis or realize that symptoms interfere with important activities to seek help (Redman 1984).

Mechanic (1972) points out seven important variables that influence moving into the sick role; some of them tie into an individual's health beliefs:

1. Number and persistence of symptoms
2. Individual's ability to recognize symptoms
3. Perceived seriousness of symptoms
4. Available information and medical knowledge
5. Cultural background of the defining person, group, or agency in terms of emphasis placed on qualities such as tolerance or stoicism
6. Extent of social and physical disability resulting from the symptoms
7. Available sources of help and their social and physical accessibility

Role Insufficiency and Role Conflict

Transition into the sick role, sudden or gradual, is not always easy. Such movement, which includes loss of some current roles during the acquisition of new roles, requires the person to incorporate new knowledge, to alter behavior, and to define self in a new social context (Meleis 1975). Any difficulty that arises in making the transition between role behavior and expectations can cause *role insufficiency* or *role conflict* (Meleis 1975). Insufficiency denotes some disparity in meeting role obligations and indicates that one's role performance is seen as inadequate by oneself or others (Meleis 1975). Role conflict, on the other hand, indicates that contradictory expectations cannot be met simultaneously (Stuart & Sundeen 1983). This incongruence can make acceptance of a necessary role change difficult. In either case, the client is faced with stresses that can be manifested as anxiety, depression, apathy, frustration, grief, powerlessness, unhappiness, or aggression and hostility (Meleis 1975).

Secondary Gains

Wanting to get well is an essential aspect of Parsons's model, but at times clients choose to remain in the sick role; many of their reactions and responses to illness are influenced by premorbid personality, lifestyle, and level of psychosocial competence (Feldman 1974). When clients remain in the sick role overly long, the role becomes a form of deviant behavior (Wu 1973), with secondary gains serving to meet unconscious needs (Feldman 1974). Some individuals use the sick role to withdraw from normal responsibilities or routines or to meet dependency needs (Mann 1982). Some have used the sick role to gain power over others through aggressive or demanding behavior or through appearing pitiful. In any case, people who interact with these clients feel they must provide more time, more attention, and a willingness to accede to demands (Wu 1973).

Byrne, Whyte, and Butler (1981) found that 85% of patients who had been working prior to their myocardial infarction (MI) returned to work. The objective severity of the infarct showed no relation to their resumption of employment. Those who had not returned to work 8 months after their MI were more likely to have remained in the sick role. Anxiety also influenced movement back to prior activities. Those individuals whose anxiety predated the MI and persisted over time showed reluctance to engage in social activities (Byrne 1982). This group tended to show greater concern for aspects of bodily functioning and well-being, which reflected affective responses rather than recognition of physical symptoms.

Life Cycle Differences

Responses to illness differ, depending on people's developmental stages, tasks, and roles. The ill child can develop behavioral problems or poor resolution to developmental tasks. Siblings can be adversely affected and undergo change, with which they may require assistance. Families face much stress, which impacts each member. Each age group deals with illness roles, especially the impaired role, differently; individuals in each cohort group can feel a need for secondary gains. The aged, who are involved in many role changes—often in a negative way—will be discussed here to illustrate the interaction of illness and life cycle roles.

Although our society purports to value each individual, many societal actions do not support this contention. Our society values youth, productivity, and independence, and many of these values no longer exist for the elderly as they face more and more role and responsibility losses. The loss of esteemed roles forces the elderly into dependent positions in which they receive little of the positive feedback that allows individuals to consider themselves valued (Kiesel & Beninger 1979). Being old is sometimes similar to being ill, even for a person who is physically and mentally able (Gillis 1972). In fact, some social attitudes toward aging and retirement are more appropriate with respect to the soon-to-be-terminally-ill than to those who have many long years ahead (Clark & Anderson 1967).

These role losses impact on physical and emotional well-being (Robinson 1971). In addition, the resultant role vacuum needs filling. Given the greater number of illnesses found among the aged, and given that the sick role is a socially acceptable role, albeit of lower status than others, the aged sometimes find focusing on symptoms easy.

In the elderly, illness can be precipitated by many factors aside from physical and mental deterioration. Limited finances, poor housing and nutrition, social devaluation, and multiple losses all contribute to social isolation and illness (Robinson 1971). Despite acute onset, most of these illnesses are chronic in nature. Being ill, which allows dependency without obligation, contains many features already present in their lives. For those older persons who are alone even when they have families, the onset of symptoms can bring more attention from family members, attention that is unwarranted by the illness but that is considered culturally appropriate behavior (Hyman 1971). This preferential treatment may become symbolic to the elderly client in two ways: (1) it indicates that some change in status has occurred and (2) it reinforces the sense of the sick role. The coupling of a socially acceptable role with the lack of other positive roles for the aged leads to a cycle in which the person adopts the sick role as normal and ongoing, as the case study of A.B. illustrates.

Professional Responses to Illness Roles

Health providers generally expect those entering the acute hospital setting to conform to sick role behaviors. Most people entering the hospital for the first time are quickly socialized and expect to cooperate with treatment, to recover, and to return to their normal roles. Provider expectations and client responses are in line with social expectations and fit with the traditional medical model of illness as acute and curable.

When clients are compliant and cooperative, health providers communicate to them that they are "good" (Lorber 1981). When clients are less cooperative, the staff may consider them problematic. In line with the acute illness model, discharge is frequently equated with cure.

But the percentage of chronically ill individuals entering hospitals increases. Such admissions occur when symptoms flare or acute illnesses are superimposed. Many of these people have had their chronic illnesses for indefinite periods of time and have had prior hospital experiences. Being in the impaired role is integral to their daily lives. Although willing to delegate some responsibility for care to

---

◇ C A S E S T U D Y ◇
The Elderly and the Sick Role

A.B. had passed most of her adult life without serious health problems. At 68 she was widowed, 3 years after retirement from her job as a candy maker. Her children had long since married and left home, and only one daughter lived in the same community. Her former activities as wife and mother and her involvement with her work had ended. In spite of adequate income to meet her needs and occasional phone contact from her children, A.B. felt lonely and deprived of a meaningful role.

A.B. had some long-standing but mild symptomatology that her physician had evaluated and treated: dysphagia (never diagnosed), mild coronary artery disease, and occasional low back pain. She had also been overweight most of her adult life. Within months of her widowhood, A.B. began making more frequent visits to her physician for evaluation of any symptom, regardless of how minimal. This illness behavior brought forth concerned responses from her family and provided her

with a topic of conversation and a socially acceptable behavior: waiting in the doctor's office. She also enjoyed striking up conversations with others who were waiting as a change from her daily routine of cleaning house and watching television. No suggestions by her family that she would feel better if she would lose weight and increase her activity were effective. She insisted that the doctor would help her "get well." Visits to the doctor every month or two went on for several years.

By the time A.B. developed a terminal illness, her physician had become insensitive to her ongoing complaints of weakness, pain, fatigue, and so on. At age 74, A.B. consulted another physician, who became concerned by her insistence that she had been growing more fatigued over the last several months. A diagnostic workup revealed acute leukemia, and she entered a true sick role. She died two weeks later while undergoing chemotherapy.

---

personnel, they prefer to retain some control of their regimens when possible (see Chapter 2).

Those clients who have multiple chronic disorders may focus concern on maintaining stability of quiescent conditions to prevent unnecessary symptomatology, whereas staff most likely focuses on managing the current acute disorder (Strauss 1981). Clients who have had multiple prior admissions more likely will use their hospital savvy to gain what they want or need from the system (Glaser & Strauss 1968). During hospitalization, these individuals may demand certain treatment, specific times for treatment, or specific routines. They may keep track of times various routines occur or complain about or report actions of the staff as a means to an end they consider important. All these demands increase staff work and stress, and frequently the client is labeled a "problem patient" (Lorber 1981). Table 3-5 compares acute and chronic illness behaviors seen in hospitals.

Staff also receive secondary gains from their work, manifested in the form of a sense of accomplishment and the personal satisfaction in the drama of witnessing a recovery. The goals of acute care

(cure and full restoration of all faculties) provide a subconscious motivation or reward for many nurses, making them feel that they are healers (Wesson 1965) and generating a sense of omnipotence and self-fulfillment (see Table 3-6). The grateful client who recovers makes hospital work worthwhile for those who provide this care.

But cure is not possible for the chronically ill; only stabilization is. Frequent readmissions, often for recurrence of the same problems, can create a sense of frustration for the staff and require repetitive, tiresome care that may become boring. Long-term goals focus on maximizing remaining functional potential and minimizing further deterioration (see Chapter 18). These tasks do not provide those dramatic secondary gains that acute care does. Often caregiver attitudes demonstrate a lack of sensitivity to the meaning of illness to the long-term client (Abrams 1972).

Lack of Role Norms for the Chronically Ill

The chronically ill require that a variety of tasks be performed to fulfill the requirements of both the

TABLE 3-5. Comparing Acute and Chronic Illness Behavior in Hospitals

Acute	Chronic
1. Passive, dependent, regressive	1. Positive dependency*
2. Predictable symptoms and outcome	2. Symptoms variable, progressive, difficult to assess
3. Illness temporary	3. Illness permanent or long-term
4. Return to normal responsibilities	4. Modified responsibilities
5. Desire to get well	5. Accepts inability to get well
6. Role less desirable but acceptable since temporary	6. Role inferior, some nonperson status
7. Limited experience with this role in this setting	7. Knowledgeable about patient role since illness is full-time
8. Decision making by staff	8. Retains much decision-making power; wants familiar patterns followed
9. Sick role behavior reinforced by staff	9. Often seen as "problem" patients

*Recognizes and accepts help to achieve maximum function.

TABLE 3-6. Professional Role: Relationship to the Acute and Chronically Ill

Acute	Chronic
Responsibility	
Responsibility for patient health management	Directs care plan but not responsible for it
Accountability	
Held accountable for care by patient (i.e., lawsuits)	Holds patient accountable for managing own care Sees patient as problem; easily irritated at patient's use of manipulation or demands
Secondary gains	
Many for the staff:	Limited for the staff:
1. Patients' gratitude satisfying to staff	1. No available cures; only ability to stabilize condition
2. Feeling of omnipotence when helping to "save" others	2. Repetitive recurrences may become tiresome to caregivers
3. Seeing results of efforts through relatively rapid recovery	3. Long-term interactions lead to valuable relationships

medical regimen and personal life-style. In spite of residual disability that limits activity, society does not identify the chronically ill as individuals who are experiencing illness. Assuming sick role behaviors is discouraged. These individuals enter and remain in the impaired role, but implicit behaviors for this role are not well defined by society. Given this lack of norms, influences on the client include the degree of disability (with different attributes of disability producing different consequences), visibility of the disability (the lower the visibility, the more normal the response), self-acceptance of the disability (resulting in others' reciprocating), and societal views of the disabled as either economically dependent or as pro-

TABLE 3-7. Tasks Required of the
Chronically Ill

1. **Carrying out the medical regimen:** Learning
   the regimen includes the amount of time, energy,
   and often discomfort required to carry it out.
   Following the regimen is influenced by its visibility
   and its effectiveness in preventing symptoms

2. **Controlling symptoms:** Learning to plan ahead,
   to modify the environment, and to plan activities
   when symptom-free

3. **Preventing and managing crisis:** Learning what
   a crisis is, recognizing signs and symptoms,
   preventing its occurrence, and evolving a plan for
   handling it

4. **Reordering time:** Adjusting schedules to cope
   with too much or too little time that occurs with
   trying to manage health regimens along with other
   life experiences

5. **Adjusting to changes in course of the disease:**
   Learning to deal with predictable and
   unpredictable situations or symptoms and adapting
   to deterioration

6. **Preventing social isolation:** Preventing self-
   withdrawal or withdrawal by others

7. **Normalizing:** Learning to hide disabilities,
   manage symptoms, find ways to be treated as
   normal

Adapted from Strauss et al. (1984).

ductive (Wu 1973). Without role definition, whether
disability is present or not, the individual is unable
to achieve maximum levels of functioning. Table 3-7
outlines tasks chronically ill individuals must
perform.

Interventions Based on Illness Role Theory

The sick role and impaired role are sociological explanations of behavioral responses of individuals;
they are states of being, not problems requiring interventions per se. Through knowledge of these
roles, health providers can help their clients cope
more effectively with appropriate dependency and

can gain a better understanding of the relationship
that exists between client and health professional, as
well as between those roles and social expectations.
Because the application of illness role theory to clinical practice has not been fully explored, it provides
fertile ground for research. As with the sick role
model, which was accepted on its "reasonableness
and logic," rather than on empirical validation, this
section considers actions in terms of personal experience and is not all-inclusive. Where it exists, research supporting the validity of proposed courses
of action is noted. It is hoped that readers will find
many applications of illness role theory to their own
clinical practice.

Allowing Dependency

As noted, dependency is an inherent part of the sick
role. But health professionals are not always comfortable about the client's remaining in this dependent role without making some effort for movement
back to independence. Take, for instance, the practice
of beginning discharge planning soon after admission, even for the critically ill. Such action is based
on several factors: first, the societal expectations that
the sick should want to get well, and second, wariness
of the malingerer or the patient who might want to
stay ill for various secondary gains. For the client
whose disease improves as expected, malingering is
generally not a problem, but at times individuals,
whether suffering from acute or chronic illnesses,
remain in acute illness states longer than expected.
An additional incentive for planning for discharge is
the "cost-effectiveness" criteria imposed on acute
hospitals by diagnostic related group (DRG) regulations. When dependency continues longer than expected, one tends to forget that the majority of our
clients are also socialized to want to become well
and to make the effort to improve as their conditions
warrant.

Severely ill patients are more concerned with
physical than psychosocial aspects of care (Hover et
al. 1978) and are incapable of making many decisions
(Gordon 1966). Emphasis on the physical aspects of
care with these individuals is compatible with Mas-
low's *Hierarchy of Needs model*, which emphasizes

that meeting physiological and then safety needs precedes the emergence and fulfillment of higher, psychosocial needs. One client noted that during her hospitalization she did not have energy even to want to survive and was incapable of extending any efforts to improve her condition. Given these factors, the health professional must recognize and accept even total dependency. Awareness of behavioral responses and times when they occur can help the professional avoid premature emphasis on independence until the client can collaborate in working toward return to normal roles.

Utilizing illness roles in planning interventions allows the health professional to maximize time spent with the client. One such intervention that could benefit from integrating knowledge of illness roles is teaching (see Chapter 12), since the client still in the highly dependent phase cannot benefit from teaching. As improvement in physical status occurs, emphasis on the desire to return to normal roles creates motivation to learn about the condition and necessary procedures for maximizing health. As the client moves into the impaired role and becomes aware of the necessity to maximize remaining potential, teaching provides a highly successful tool both in the hospital and at home.

The nurse can also be instrumental in helping the client deal with role insufficiency or conflict in both preventive and therapeutic ways, through role clarification and role taking (Meleis 1975). *Role clarification* is the integration of the knowledge and cues necessary for performance of a given role. *Role taking* is the process of assuming the position or point of view of another person by imagining the position or viewpoint. The nurse or other health professional can help the client gain mastery of illness roles through intentional role instruction ("We expect you to . . ."), role modeling (letting the client observe the behavior of others in order to rehearse and emulate their behavior), or provision of opportunities for interacting with relevant others (Meleis 1975).

Learning to Deal with Personal Biases

Professionals who have limited awareness of illness roles are often insensitive to these roles, their mean-

ing, and the ways their own responses are affected by and affect the client. The health professional in the hospital setting deals with clients on an episodic basis and often has little knowledge of the entire situation that these people must live with on a daily basis. This limited perspective may hamper recovery or rehabilitation, especially for the chronically ill. The problem is compounded because individuals who are experienced with hospital settings are not always compliant and, in fact, are often considered "difficult" patients. Since these people are responsible for self-management at home, they are often unwilling to delegate control over all their care and have acquired ways of continuing aspects of their regimens that they consider important even though they are in the hospital for other reasons. They never fully move into the sick role, except during the most acute phases of illness.

Caring for individuals who have frequent recurrences of the same problems can block health providers from feeling that they are contributing to recovery. They may blame the client for their consequent frustration, since negative feelings about people influence interactions with them. To be truly helpful, health professionals must focus on the personal feelings and responses that are triggered by the client's needs to retain autonomy. Only through being aware of the impact of those feelings on patient care can the provider achieve objectivity. Objectivity leads to greater realization that such persons are trying to manage their symptoms and lives and to maximize their remaining potential. This knowledge makes joint goal setting and planning possible. Staff must see that demands for autonomy indicate that the client is adapting to the necessity to deal with the illness role while striving to achieve holistic wellness. This awareness also tempers the frustration that results from an increased work load or modifications in work necessitated by client actions.

Assisting the Client in the Impaired Role

Studies of the relationship of illness response, personality, and stress indicate different responses to different diseases, as well as variations in affective behavior and cognitive meaning of specific illness

(Byrne & Whyte 1978; Pilowsky & Spence 1975). These studies, using the same tool, found that individuals who had myocardial infarctions (MIs) had different patterns of concerns regarding their bodily functioning, recognition of the gravity of their illness, and responses to stress from those of individuals experiencing intractable pain. In fact, patients having MIs initially had difficulty accepting the sick role (Byrne et al. 1978). Such information could be useful in planning care and in devising programs of rehabilitation and prevention. The practicing professional could also consider utilizing such tools to identify characteristics of other chronically ill people in order to plan their short- and long-term care.

Not only is ongoing treatment necessary, but individuals in the impaired role are "continually threatened by a decrease in function related to the chronic illness" (Monohan 1982). This characteristic has led to the evolution of a modification of the impaired role described as the *at risk role*. Clients who perceive themselves as being at risk of having complications are more highly motivated to greater compliance with regimens (see Chapter 7). To encourage movement into this modified role, the health provider should persuade the client that compliance is valuable in maximizing health and wellness when developing symptoms or complications without such adherence is a possibility. The goal should be retaining, not regaining, optimal physical functioning. Helping the client decrease the risks of complications requires that the professional assess the following factors: health beliefs, environmental factors (family setting, role, and composition; medical and social supports; sociocultural factors), and present functioning level and symptoms.

haviors, accepting some congruence between old and new behaviors, and being motivated to take on new roles (Wu 1973).

The need to adapt has led the chronically ill to evolve several unique roles (Wu 1973). The *handicapped performer* develops a different and more limited repertoire than that of a well person. Goal achievement may require innovative approaches, and other role needs may require modified activities. The individual who has an *instrumental dependency* required to complete tasks needs to learn to be an object of aid, despite negative feelings about accepting such aid. The *co-manager* becomes actively involved in care by making decisions and assuming responsibility for controlling, maintaining, or improving current status. Finally, the role of *public relations* person includes the necessity of explaining one's health condition at times. Maintaining good public relations enables the person to receive aid and to satisfy the curiosity of others. It also helps to resolve inconsistencies between self and others who are not impaired, to focus on abilities relevant to employment or admission to college, to lessen social prejudice through education, and to maximize individual potential (Wu 1973).

But self-definition of roles is not adequate for meeting the challenges of our society. We all need to know the behaviors that society expects and accepts. The political activism of disabled, handicapped, and elderly advocacy groups is creating new norms. These groups are demanding a greater voice in society and more meaningful lives. Each professional can also help promote the development of norms that would lead to greater productivity of a growing segment of the population.

The Need for Role Definition

As mentioned earlier, chronically ill individuals do not have clear role norms to help them define themselves socially, especially since the impaired role, which continues as long as residual pathology or disability does, limits activity in many ways. For the chronically ill, adaptation requires learning new be-

The Need for Research

Although the body of research related to chronic illness is increasing (see Chapter 14), studies focus on the relation of illness to clinical practice. Most research on the sick role has emphasized the theoretical perspective. More research on clinical application of the sick role needs to be carried out by clinical practitioners. Two instances of the application of role theory research to clinical practice are noteworthy.

Theoretical research can have clinical application even when it was not specifically designed for that purpose. As an example, extensive worldwide research has analyzed the relationship of the Type A personality and illness behavior to the person who has a myocardial infarction (Byrne et al. 1978; Byrne et al. 1981; Heller 1979; Hackett 1982; Byrne 1982; Appels, Jenkins, & Rosenman 1982). These studies were intended to verify the role of personality factors in this condition and to determine whether the tool that was developed had international application. Outgrowths of this research led to development of preventive programs for Type A personalities, application of this information in post-MI teaching, and the integration of knowledge about personality with patient care and rehabilitation programs.

One qualitative study that considered the dialysis patient's ability to assume or reject the sick role identified several subroles (Artinian 1983). The *undecided role* is usually assumed by the newly diagnosed individual who is still questioning the necessity of dialysis; eventually the individual moves to one of the other roles. The *worker role* fits the individual who rejects the sick role, continues to define self as normal, and finds ways to fit dialysis into other life activities. The patient does so by cooperating with dialysis and selecting the type of dialysis most suitable to lifestyle. The *waiter role* is adopted by the person who does not accept the sick role but finds dialysis unacceptable as a way of life. This individual waits for a transplant or death, is least informed about the process, is least compliant, and feels trapped and deprived of a future. The *true dialysis patient* accepts the sick role and centers life around dialysis, which becomes his or her "job." This person is knowledgeable about the disease and its management, arrives early for treatment, and stays late to socialize. The *emancipated role* is not a dialysis role since an individual assumes it only after being freed from dialysis through transplantation.

The nurse can use these four identified dialysis roles in several ways in planning and implementing care (Artinian 1983). Doing so necessitates changing the power relationship to that of a partnership between nurse and client, with the nurse realizing that patients are responsible for their own lives and accepting the role that they adopt. Without this acceptance, the nurse will experience anger and guilt for failing to "help," and meaningful dialogue will decrease. Artinian also feels that individualization of care is essential to fulfilling the physical and self-esteem needs of each role group. The *undecided* need time without pressure to accept dialysis. Expeditious service allows the *worker* to feel in control. The *waiter* needs to have a nonhostile environment even when being noncompliant. The *true dialysis patient* needs praise for successfully managing the dialysis regimen, as well as opportunities for companionship.

Summary and Conclusions

When symptoms strike, the affected individual generally takes action to identify and correct the cause. This *illness behavior* is influenced by many variables, including the client's health beliefs. At some point along the illness behavior continuum, the acutely ill individual enters the *sick role*, in which it is acceptable to be dependent on others while being relieved of social responsibilities. In exchange, one is obligated to want to become well and to seek and cooperate with technically competent professionals. This role is more applicable to acute, rather than chronic, disorders. According to the *impaired role* model, chronically ill or disabled persons must be responsible for their own health management and can meet normal role expectations within the limits of their health condition. In other words, the impaired role entails adapted wellness.

The sick role was postulated on the basis of reasonableness and logic, rather than on research. Studies have investigated its four major components, and results indicate that although some weaknesses in the model have been noted, the model is validated in relation to acute illness. The lack of usefulness of this role to chronic illness is a major drawback, especially in light of increasing numbers of chronically ill people. The impaired role is problematic in that society has yet to define role norms clearly that maximize social integration of impaired individuals. The nurse can promote such integration by supporting individualized strategies for each affected person.

Health professionals must also come to terms with the differences in behavior of acutely ill and chronically ill clients in the hospital setting by recognizing the internal aspects of their relationship to the client. Using illness roles as a basis for clinical practice currently has a strong experiential component, since research data are limited. In the meantime, knowledge of illness roles can provide some direction for the health professional.

All theorists agree that illness is not only an individual matter but a biological and sociological event. Since social systems depend on individuals, the health status of all members is a matter of group concern. Society's responses to illness depend on many sociocultural factors, which are not always logical or scientifically based (Cockerham 1978). The health professional needs to be aware of the many factors that influence the chronically ill, including the roles assumed during acute illness and when residual disorders remain.

STUDY QUESTIONS

1. What is illness behavior, and what factors influence the symptomatic individual to adopt illness behavior?
2. How do illness behavior and the sick role fit into the process a symptomatic individual follows in regaining health? Discuss the stages that are involved and directions the client may take.
3. What are the characteristics of the sick role? When do symptomatic individuals take on this role?
4. How does the impaired role differ from the sick role? What are the characteristics of the impaired role?
5. What problems have been identified in relation to the sick role and its characteristics? Discuss them.
6. What other problems affect movement into or out of the sick role? How do they influence assuming, adapting to, or relinquishing this role? What roles do growth and developmental level play?

7. In what ways do professionals' expectations influence their response to clients?
8. In what way does the lack of clarity regarding role norms for the impaired role influence clients' behavior?
9. Consider a client you have cared for in the hospital setting. What criteria could you use in determining whether the individual is in a dependent role? ready to move toward greater independence?
10. How can you use knowledge about illness roles in planning your time and work? in helping the client adapt to the sick role? the impaired role?
11. Why is it important that nurses understand themselves and their personal biases?
12. What problems arise from an inadequate societal role for chronically ill or impaired people?
13. What value does research have for relating the sick role to clinical practice? Identify areas in which such research would be beneficial.

References

Abrams, H. S., (1972) The psychology of chronic illness, editorial, *Journal of Chronic Diseases*, 25:659–664

Alonzo, A. A., (1980) Acute illness behavior: A conceptual exploration and specification, *Social Science and Medicine*, 14A:515–526

Appels, A., Jenkins, C. D., and Rosenman, R. H., (1982) Coronary-prone behavior in the Netherlands: A cross-cultural validation study, *Journal of Behavioral Medicine*, 5(1):83–88

Artinian, B. M., (1983) Role identities of the dialysis patient, *Nephrology Nurse*, May–June, 5:30:10–14

Berger, P. L., (1963) *Invitation to Sociology: A Humanistic Perspective*, Garden City, N.Y.: Anchor Books

Blackwell, B., (1963) The literature of delay in seeking medical care for chronic illness, *Health Education Monographs*, 16:3–31

Byrne, D. G., (1982) Illness behavior and psychosocial outcomes after a heart attack, *British Journal of Clinical Psychology*, 21:145–146

Byrne, D. G., and Whyte, H. M., (1978) Dimensions of illness behavior in survivors of myocardial infarction, *Journal of Psychosomatic Research*, 22:485–491

Byrne, D. G., Whyte, H. M., and Butler, K. L., (1981) Illness behavior and outcome following survived M.I.: A prospective study, *Journal of Psychosomatic Research*, 25(2):97–107

Clark, M., and Anderson, B. G., (1967) *Culture and Aging*, Springfield, Ill.: Charles C Thomas

Cockerham, W. C., (1978) The sick role, in *Medical Sociology*, Englewood Cliffs, N.J.: Prentice-Hall

Feldman, D. J., (1974) Chronic disabling illness: A holistic view, *Journal of Chronic Diseases*, 27:287–291

Gillis, L., (1972) *Human Behavior in Illness*, London: Faber & Faber

Glaser, B., and Strauss, A. L., (1968) *Time for Dying*, Chicago: Aldine

Gonzalez-Swafford, M. J., (1983) Ethno-medical beliefs and practices of Mexican-Americans, *Nurse Practitioner*, 8(10):29–30,32,34

Gordon, G., (1966) *Role Theory and Illness: A Sociological Perspective*, New Haven, Conn.: College and University Press

Hackett, T. P., (1982) Sociocultural influences, the response to illness: Editorial comments, *Cardiology*, 69:301–302

Heller, R. F., (1979) Type A behavior and coronary heart disease, *British Medical Journal*, 280:365

Honig-Parnass, T., (1981) Lay concepts of the sick role: An examination of the professional bias in Parsons' model, *Social Science and Medicine*, 15A:615–623

Hover, J., and Juelsgaard, N., (1978) The sick role reconceptualized, *Nursing Forum*, XVII(4):406–415

Hyman, M. D., (1971) Disability and patient's perceptions of preferential treatment: Some preliminary findings, *Journal of Chronic Diseases*, 24:329–342

Kassebaum, G. G., and Baumann, B. O., (1965) Dimensions of the sick role in chronic illness, *Journal of Health and Human Behavior*, 6(1):16–27

Kiesel, M., Sr., and Beninger, C., (1979) An application of psycho-social role theory to the aging, *Nursing Forum*, XVIII(1):80–91

Lewis, S. M., and Collier, I. C., (1983) *Medical-Surgical Nursing: Assessment & Management of Clinical Problems*, New York: McGraw-Hill

Lorber, J., (1981) Good patients and problem patients: Conformity and deviance in a general hospital, in Conrad, P., and Kern, R. (eds.), *The Sociology of Health and Illness: Critical Perspectives*, New York: St. Martin's Press

Mann, S. B., (1982) *Being Ill: Personal & Social Meanings*, New York: Irvington

Mead, G. H., (1934) *Mind, Self & Society*, Chicago: University Press

Mechanic, D., (1961) The concept of illness behavior, *Journal of Chronic Diseases*, 15:189–194

Mechanic, D., (1972) *Public Expectations and Health Care*, New York: John Wiley & Sons

Meleis, A. I., (1975) Role insufficiency and role supplementation: A conceptual framework, *Nursing Research*, 24:4:264–271

Monohan, R. S., (1982) The "at-risk" role, *Nurse Practitioner*, May, pp. 42–44, 52

Parsons, T., (1951) *Social System*, Glencoe, Ill.: The Free Press

Parsons, T., and Fox, R., (1952) Illness, therapy and the modern urban American family, *Journal of Social Issues*, VIII:31–44

Pilowsky, I., and Spence, N. D., (1975) Patterns of illness behaviour in patients with intractable pain, *Journal of Psychosomatic Research*, 19:279–287

Rankin, S. H., and Duffy, K. L., (1983) A model for patient decision making and mutual goal setting, in *Patient Education: Issues, Principles, and Guidelines*, New York: J.B. Lippincott

Redman, B. K., (1984) Readiness for health education, in *The Process of Patient Teaching in Nursing* (4th ed.), St. Louis: C.V. Mosby

Robinson, D., (1971) *The Process of Becoming Ill*, London: Routledge and Kegan Paul

Segall, A., (1976) The sick role concept: Understanding illness behavior, *Journal of Health and Social Behavior*, 17:163–170

Steward, D. C., and Sullivan, T. J., (1982) Illness behavior and the sick role in chronic disease: The case of multiple sclerosis, *Social Science and Medicine*, 16:1397–1404

Stoeckle, J. D., Zola, I. K., and Davidson, G. E., (1963) On going to see the doctor, the contributions of the patient to the decision to seek medical aid: A selective review, *Journal of Chronic Diseases*, 16:975–989

Strauss, A., (1981) Chronic illness, in Conrad, P., and Kern, R. (eds.), *The Sociology of Health and Illness: Critical Perspectives,* New York: St. Martin's Press

Strauss, A., Corbin, J., Fagerhaugh, S., Glaser, B., Maines, D.,

Suczek, B., and Wiener, C., (1984) *Chronic Illness and the Quality of Life* (2d ed.), St. Louis: C.V. Mosby

Strauss, A., and Glaser, B., (1975) *Chronic Illness and the Quality of Life*, St. Louis: C.V. Mosby

Stuart, G. W., and Sundeen, S. J., (1983) *Principles and Practice of Psychiatric Nursing*, St. Louis: C.V. Mosby

Twaddle, A. C., (1969) Health decisions and sick role variations: An exploration, *Journal of Health and Social Behavior*, *10*:105

Twaddle, A. C., (1973) Illness and deviance, *Social Science and Medicine*, 7:751–762

Weidner, G., (1980) Self-handicapping following learned helplessness treatment and the type A coronary-prone behavior pattern, *Journal of Psychosomatic Research*, 24(6):319–325

Wesson, A. F., (1965) Long-term care: The forces that have shaped it and the evidence for needed change, *Meeting the Social Needs of Long-Term Patients*, Chicago: American Hospital Association

Whitehead, W. E., Winget, C., Federacivius, A. S., Wooley, S., and Blackwell, B., (1982) Learned illness behavior in patients with irritable bowel syndrome and peptic ulcer, *Digestive Diseases and Sciences*, 27(3):202–208

Wu, R., (1973) *Behavior and Illness*, Englewood Cliffs, N.J.: Prentice-Hall

Bibliography

Bauwens, E. E., Anderson, D. V., and Buergin, P., (1983) Chronic illness, in Phipps, W. J., Long, B. C., and Woods, N.F. (eds.), *Medical Surgical Nursing: Concepts and Clinical Practice* (2d ed.), St. Louis: C.V. Mosby

Blackwell, B., (1967) Upper middle class adult expectations about entering the sick role for physical and psychiatric dysfunctions, *Journal of Health & Social Behavior*, 8:83–95

Carasso, R., Yehuda, S., and Ben-uriah, Y., (1981) Personality type, life events, and sudden CVA, *International Journal of Neuroscience*, 14:223–225

Dery, G. K., (1983) Concepts of health and illness, in Phipps, W. J., Long, B. C., and Woods, N. F. (eds.), *Medical-Sur-gical Nursing: Concepts and Clinical Practice* (2d ed.), St. Louis: C.V. Mosby

Erikson, K. T., (1957) Patient role and social uncertainty: A dilemma of the mentally ill, *Psychiatry*, 20:262–272

Fross, K. H., Dirks, J., Kinsman, R. A., and Jones, N. F., (1980) Functionally determined invalidism in chronic asthma, *Journal of Chronic Diseases*, 33:485–490

Jelnick, L. J., (1977) The special needs of the adolescent with chronic illness, *Maternal Child Nursing*, January–February, pp. 57–61

Johnson, D., (1967) Powerlessness: A significant determinant in patient behavior? *Journal of Nursing Education*, April, pp. 39–44

Jourard, S., (1968) *The Transparent Self* (2d ed.), New York: Van Nostrand, pp. 3–18

Kawash, G., Woolcott, D. M., and Sabry, J. H., (1980) Personality correlates of selected elements of the Health Belief Model, *Journal of Social Psychology*, 112:219–227

Lawson, B. A., (1977) Chronic illness in the school-aged child: Effects on the total family, *Maternal Child Nursing*, January–February, pp. 49–56

Lewis, B. L., and Khaw, K.-T., (1982) Family functioning as a mediating variable affecting psychosocial adjustment of children with cystic fibrosis, *The Journal of Pediatrics*, *101*(4):636–639

Linn, M. W., Linn, B. S., Skylar, J. S., and Harris, R., (1980) The importance of self-assessed health in patients with diabetes, *Diabetic Care*, 3:599–606

Papper, S., (1970) The undesirable patient, *Journal of Chronic Diseases*, 22:777–779

Petroni, F. A., (1971) Preferred right to the sick role and illness behavior, *Social Science and Medicine*, 5:645–653

Pilowsky, I., and Spence, N. D., (1976) Illness behaviour syndromes associated with intractable pain, *Pain*, *2*:61–71

Pond, H., (1979) Parental attitudes toward children with a chronic medical disorder: Special reference to diabetes mellitus, *Diabetic Care*, Sept/Oct, *2*(5):425–430

Pritchard, M., (1977) Further studies of illness behaviour in long term haemodialysis, *Journal of Psychosomatic Research*, *21*:41–48

CHAPTER FOUR

Stigma

My car came to a stop at the intersection. I looked around me at all the people in the other cars. People of all shapes and ages, but no one there was like me. They were apart from me, distant, different. If they looked at me, they couldn't see my defect. But if they knew, they would turn away. I am separate and different from everybody that I can see in every direction as far as I can see. And it will never be the same again.

Anonymous cancer patient

Introduction: The Significance of Stigma

This chapter demonstrates how the concept of stigma has evolved and acts as a significant factor in many chronic diseases and disabilities. It also explores the relation of stigma to the more common concepts of prejudice, stereotyping, and labeling. Since stigma is socially constructed, it varies from setting to setting. In addition, individuals and groups react differently to the stigmatizing process. Those reactions must be taken into consideration when planning strategies to improve the quality of life of individuals with chronic diseases.

To date, the nursing literature has not discussed this subject prominently. Most of the nursing articles on psychosocial aspects of chronic disease are located in clinical journals. These journals are available in rehabilitation centers and university settings; but they are often inaccessible to many health care providers. This chapter attempts to bring many of the relevant problems associated with stigma to a larger nursing audience.

The word *normals* is used in this chapter to designate people without the stigmatizing characteristic under discussion. If one person has been diagnosed as arthritic and another has not, the designation of "normal" simply refers to the one without arthritis. The normal person may have other characteristics that could be stigmatized, such as being hypertensive, grossly obese, or abnormally tall. One should not infer that normal is "better" or "physically perfect"; the tendency to attach value judgments is evident in the historical beginnings of the concept of stigma.

Not all persons attach a stigma to disease or deformity, even though the stigmatizing process is very common. This chapter does not assume that all who come into contact with those who deviate from normal devalue them; rather, it does insist that each of us look penetratingly and honestly at our thoughts and actions.

Webster (1974) defines stigma as a "mark of shame or discredit." Roget (1977) lists synonyms such as *blemish* and *disrepute*. Goffman (1963) traces the historic use of the word to the Greeks, who referred to "bodily signs designed to expose something unusual and bad about the moral status of the signifier" (p. 1). These signs were cut or burned into a person's body as an indication of being a slave, a criminal, or a traitor. Notice the moral and judgmental nature of these stigmata. The disgrace and shame of the stigma became more important than the bodily evidence of it.

To illustrate the way a concept used by the Greeks relates to chronic disease, let us consider Goffman's view of stigma as a spoiled identity. We must first explore what constitutes social identity to develop a better understanding of the discrepancies that exist between expectations and actuality.

Social Identity

Society teaches its members to categorize persons and defines the attributes and characteristics that are ordinary for persons in those categories (Goffman 1963). Daily routines establish the usual and the expected. When we meet strangers, certain appearances help us to anticipate what Goffman calls "social identity." This identity includes personal attributes, such as competence, as well as structural ones, such as occupation. For example, university students usually tolerate some eccentricities in their professors; but stuttering, physical handicaps, or diseases may bestow a social identity of incompetency. Not based on occupational status, this identity of incompetence, once established, bestows a stigma.

Hooper (1981) does not use the term *social identity*, although she does describe similar important characteristics that make up a person's identity: (1) physical activities, (2) social roles, and (3) the concept of self. Anything that changes one of these, such as a disability, changes the person's identity and therefore creates a stigma.

Goffman's study (1963) used the idea of social identity to expand previous work done on stigma. His theory defines stigma as something that disqualifies an individual from full social acceptance. Goffman argues that social identity is a primary force in the development of stigma because the identity that an individual conveys categorizes that person. Social settings and routines tell us which categories to anticipate. Therefore, when individuals fail to meet expectations because of attributes that are different and/or undesirable, they are reduced from accepted people to discounted ones—that is, stigmatized.

Discrepancies

Society defines the attributes expected of ordinary people, such as personal accomplishments, health, and attractiveness. When these structural expectations are met, we evaluate those individuals as "good," "valuable," or "worthwhile." If these expectations are not met, our judgments are negative. These judgments, as well as the probable attributes, are an essential part of one's social identity.

We are often unaware of our expectations until the situation arises in which those expectations are not fulfilled (Goffman 1963). If our professor stutters or arrives in a wheelchair, we realize that we held unmet expectations. People expect others to be healthy and free from a debilitating condition. When deviations from this expected norm occur in any situation, the discrepancy between actual and expected is highlighted.

From Spoiled Identity to Stigma

Expected character attributes are called *virtual social identity* (Goffman 1963). There is a distinction made between the expected attributes and the attributes that the individual actually possesses. The latter are an individual's *actual social identity* (p. 2).

Stigma is defined as the discrepancy, or difference, between virtual and actual social identity; that is, there is some evidence of an attribute that makes an individual both different from and less desirable than others in his category (Goffman 1963). More specifically, stigma can "be considered the negative perceptions and behaviors of so-called normal people to individuals who are different from themselves" (English 1977b). Goffman (1963) states it in a slightly different way: stigma is "undesirable attributes incongruous with our stereotype of what a given individual should be" (p. 3). Both authors see stigma as a discrepancy between what is desired and what is actual by noting a special relationship between an attribute and a stereotype. This discrepancy "spoils" the social identity, isolating the person from self-acceptance and societal acceptance (Goffman 1963).

In the past, the words *shame* and *guilt* were used to describe a concept similar to stigma: a perceived difference between behavior or attribute and an ideal standard (Lynd 1958). From this perspective, guilt is defined as self-criticism, and shame results from the disapproval of others. Guilt is similar to seeing oneself as discredited. Shame is a painful feeling caused by the scorn or contempt of others (Lynd 1958). For example, an alcoholic may feel guilty about drinking and also feel ashamed that others perceive his or her behavior as less than desirable.

Most stigmata are considered threatening to others. We stigmatize criminals and social deviants because they create a sense of anxiety by threatening our values and safety. Encounters with sick and disabled individuals also cause us anxiety and apprehension, but in a different way: the encounter destroys the dream that life is fair. Sick people remind us of our mortality and vulnerability; consequently normal people avoid contact with individuals with chronic diseases (Katz 1981). Normals often make negative value judgments about persons who are ill or disabled. For example, some may regard blind people as being very dependent or unwilling to take care of themselves, an assumption that is not based on what the blind person is willing or able to do. As a result the blind have to contend with more than the loss of sight; some people perceive them as less worthy or valuable: they possess a stigma.

The attribute that provides the stigma need not be undesirable in itself. If everyone in town had diabetes, it would be expected and no discrepancy would exist. There would be no stigma; the disease would be normal. Only when expectations differ from actual experiences is a stigma possible. Discredit is caused by the relation of the expected and the actual. The difference between expected attributes and actual attributes provides the deficit.

Furthermore, the concept of *deviance* versus *normality* is a social construct. Individuals are de-

valued less because they display attributes that violate accepted standards than because some communities have chosen to call certain attributes deviant (Katz 1981). Since stigma is socially constructed, it can differ from setting to setting. Although many culturally constant values are extremely influential, others may vary from group to group. Use of recreational drugs, for instance, may be normal in one group and taboo in another.

Whenever a stigma is present, the devaluing characteristic is so powerful that it overshadows other traits and becomes the focus of personal evaluations (Volinn 1983). This trait, or differentness, is powerful enough to break the claim of all of the other attributes (Goffman 1963). The fact that a nurse is a brittle diabetic may cancel the remaining identity as a competent health provider. A professor's stutter may negate academic brilliance.

Although a stigma can be overpowering, the extent of stigma resulting from any particular condition cannot be predicted. Individuals having a certain disease do not universally feel the same degree of stigma. In one study of epileptics, their perception of stigma varied greatly depending on seizure severity, perceived job discrimination, perceived limitations due to epilepsy, as well as age, sex, and level of education (Ryan, Kempner, & Emlem 1980).

On the other hand, very different handicaps may possess the same stigma. In writing about individuals who are mentally handicapped, Dudley (1983) describes great variations in intellectual ability among these individuals; however, normals did not take the variation into account. All those who were handicapped shared the same stigma—mental retardation—regardless of their capabilities. People responded to the Down's syndrome stereotype rather than to actual physical changes (Dudley 1983). This is further evidence that the actual physical capability, or lack of capability, is not solely responsible for the social reaction. The diagnosis and associated stigma of mental retardation exclude individuals from social interaction; their intellectual or physical handicaps may or may not. This example of a spoiled identity that leads to stigma has excluded the individual from the societal interaction that could have otherwise been expected.

Discredited versus Discreditable

Two classifications of stigma must be clarified: discredited and discreditable (Goffman 1963). Some discrepancies between actual and virtual social identities are obvious; others are not. A discredited condition is one with visible cues. Limping, shortness of breath, physical deformity, and wheelchairs are immediately apparent. These and other kinds of clues identify an individual who is different from the expected norm. As soon as these clues are seen, the individual may be discredited in the eyes of others.

In other circumstances, the discrepancy may be hidden. An individual without obvious clues to a defect is known as discreditable. Diabetes, early stages of cancer, or a hearing impairment is not readily apparent; the differentness is not visible. If others knew about the hidden condition, stigmatization would occur. As long as the condition is hidden, the individual is not discredited.

A discreditable condition creates the problem of whether or not to reveal the defect. The issue becomes one of managing information about the failing. One must decide whether the defect should be displayed or not: should others be told or not? Is it worth lying about? To whom should the defect be displayed or discussed? How? When? Where? (Goffman 1963). The dilemma of managing this information will be discussed later in the chapter.

Types of Stigma

Stigma is a universal phenomenon. Every society stigmatizes certain conditions (Becker 1981). Goffman (1963) distinguishes among three types of stigma. The first is the stigma of physical deformity. The actual stigma is the deficit between the expected norm of perfect physical condition and the actual physical condition. Many chronic conditions create changes in physical appearance or function. These changes frequently create a difference in self-perception (see Chapter 9). Changes of this kind also occur with aging. The normal aging process creates a body far from the television commercial "norm" of youth, physical beauty, and leanness, although this "norm" is changing to include mature and elderly individuals.

The second type of stigma is that of character blemishes such as rigid beliefs, unnatural passions, or dishonesty. This type of stigma occurs in individuals who have a history of alcoholism or hospitalization for mental illness. Many obese individuals carry this type of stigma because others assume they could lose weight if they only had "will power."

The third type of stigma is tribal in origin and is known more commonly as *prejudice*. This type originates when features of race, religion, or nationality are seen as a deficiency of one group when measured against a socially constructed norm of another group. There is growing awareness of job discrimination against women and Blacks; but we may be less sensitive to discrimination against handicapped persons or former mental patients (Katz 1981).

Health professionals feel that prejudice, the third type of stigma, has no place in the health care delivery system. Although many professionals display both subtle and overt intolerance, most strive to treat persons of every age, race, and nationality with individual sensitivity. However, we may be surprised to find that prejudice against chronically ill persons does exist; it prevents humane and effective health care delivery as surely as racial or religious prejudice.

The three types of stigma may overlap and reinforce each other (Volinn 1983). Individuals who are already socially isolated because of race, age, or poverty will be doubly hurt by the isolation resulting from another stigma. Individuals who are financially disadvantaged or culturally distinct (that is, stigmatized by the majority society) will suffer even more should they become disabled or handicapped.

Furthermore, not only is stigma ever present, once it occurs, it is irreversible. If the cause of stigma is removed, the effects remain (Ablon 1981). Social identity is influenced by a history of a stigmatizing attribute. The alcoholic as well as the former cancer or mental patient continues to carry a stigma in the same way that a former prison inmate does. One's identity is not only spoiled, it is spoiled permanently.

Chronic Disease as Stigma

Persons with chronic diseases present daily examples of deviations from what we normally expect in our daily social interchanges. Most people do not expect to meet a person in a wheelchair or one with an insulin pump in ordinary personal or business encounters. Persons with speech or visual handicaps are not expected at most social functions. Some people consider any evidence of physical or mental deviation from the "normal" a stigmatizing trait; others have learned to regard deviation differently.

American values contribute greatly to the perception of chronic disease as a stigmatizing condition. The dominant culture emphasizes qualities of youth, attractiveness, and personal accomplishment. The Protestant work ethic and heritage of the western frontier provide heroes for us who are strong, productive, and healthy. Television and magazines demonstrate, on a daily basis, that physical perfection is the standard against which all are measured. These societal values collide with the reality of chronic conditions. A great discrepancy exists between the realities of chronic conditions, like arthritis, and the values of physical perfection that our society tells us constitute a worthwhile person.

A chronic condition such as deafness can be stigmatizing when hearing people become aware of the alteration and freeze or withdraw from contact (Becker 1981). Ironically, some hearing parents say to their deaf child who socializes with other deaf friends such things as, "You're not going out with those deaf, are you?" (p. 22). Even signing, that effective way that the deaf communicate with one another, has much stigma attached to it. Obviously signing is a continuous reminder that an individual deviates from the norm; it may even serve as a stigma.

Characteristics such as an unclear etiology can contribute to the stigma of many chronic diseases. In fact, any disease having an unclear cause or ineffectual treatment is suspect (Sontag 1977). Diseases that are somewhat mysterious and at the same time feared are often felt to be morally contagious (Ablon 1981). It is not surprising that cancer patients sometimes find themselves shunned by relatives and friends.

So far we have come to understand stigma as a perceived deficiency between expected and actual characteristics. What is the result of stigma on chronically ill people who possess less-than-desired characteristics—physical deformity, shortened life span, reduced energy level, medical and dietary requirements, and so on? All types of stigma share a common tie: In every case an individual who might have interacted easily in a particular social situation may be prevented from doing so by the trait that is seen as different from what had been expected. The trait may become the focus of attention and can actually turn others away. The following section describes the way many individuals respond to stigma.

Impact of Stigma

A stigmatizing condition has a profound impact on both the affected individual and on normals; the effects must be confronted when these people encounter each other. The stigmatized individual is often unsure about the attitudes of others and therefore may feel a constant need to make a good impression. At the same time, normal individuals may worry about whether to acknowledge the deficiency; they may be concerned about making unrealistic demands (Goffman 1963). One response of a person with a chronic condition is "People don't know how to act toward me so they don't include me in their groups" (Saylor 1984). Responses to stigmatized individuals vary. These responses will be discussed from the perspective of the stigmatized individual, the normal individual, and the professional.

Response of Stigmatized Individuals to Others

The way an individual deals with the reactions caused by a stigma varies depending on the length and nature of the condition, as well as that individual's personal characteristics. Previously used responses may be altered or abandoned as individuals live with their conditions for a period of time and learn what is effective and how to protect themselves. Dudley (1983) eloquently identifies how the stigmatized often feel when he states:

> A depreciating remark, cold stare, willful disregard of a person's viewpoint hurts in unimaginable ways. The pain derives not only from each stigma-producing incident, but also from the cumulative effect of numerous previous incidents, with the latest one serving as a further reminder of their inferior status. (p. 64)

Stigmatized individuals respond to this pain in a variety of ways.

Disregard.   A person's first response to a stigmatizing reaction may be disregard. Individuals may choose not to reflect on or discuss the painful incidents. At other times, individuals may lack an appropriate approach to dealing with the incident even when they realize the discomfort that has been caused. Well-adjusted individuals who feel comfortable with their identity, have dealt with stigma for a long time, and choose not to invest much effort in responding to the reaction may disregard it (Dudley 1983). For example, many proud and confident members of minority groups disregard demeaning comments directed toward their particular group.

Isolation.   Human beings have a proclivity for separating themselves into small subgroups. This tendency may not necessarily signify prejudice. Staying with one's own group is easier and requires less effort, and, for some individuals, is more congenial. However, this separation into groups tends to emphasize differences rather than similarities. Furthermore, communication among groups is impeded by this separation (Allport 1954).

Once a group has been set apart, a strategy of social interaction called *normalization* may occur (Becker 1981). In this process an ingroup seldom invites outsiders to participate and interaction is contained within the group itself. Closed interaction

from within enhances one's feelings of normality and validates one's worth because the individual is surrounded by others who are similar. Chronically ill or disabled persons often display this process, but it can occur any time outsiders are seen as threatening or anxiety producing. Outsiders are reminders that the world is different from the ingroup.

Trying to function as normal requires a lot of energy for an impaired person. Individuals may decide to save much of the energy used in frustrating interactions with normals for more self-actualizing relationships with similar others. Becker (1981) describes a group of hearing impaired individuals who were talkative, confident, and outgoing until they interacted with others who could hear normally, and then they became quiet and hesitant. This behavioral dichotomy not only reflects ways in which these hearing impaired individuals adapted, but softened the effects of stigmatizing situations.

Staying with others who are similar is a source of support; but *similar* does not always mean disabled or ill. Individuals who have a sense of normality, even though disabled or ill, may feel more comfortable when they are surrounded by normals. One young woman who was handicapped from a birth defect stated, "I always felt normal so I feel better around normal people. Other handicapped people sometimes make me feel uncomfortable" (Saylor 1984). Her statement reminds us to use caution when making assumptions about the perceptions of others.

During the process of normalization, the symbols of stigma sometimes undergo a transformation in such a way that they become a means of self-affirmation. The sign for "I love you," originally banned in a school for the deaf in order to promote an oral method of expression, has become a powerful symbol of unity among hearing impaired people (Becker 1981). This process is analogous to that reflected in the slogan "Black is beautiful," in which a stigmatizing attribute, skin color, reflects attractiveness and pride.

Secondary Gains.   Another possible response is to seek secondary benefits (Dudley 1983). If the deviance and its stigma are great enough, the individual may try to derive maximum benefit from the situation (Lemert 1972). For instance, the mentally retarded sometimes promote themselves as objects of pity. Dudley describes a docile, dependent mentally retarded individual who behaved in this way to gain favors. Health professionals are familiar with individuals who capitalize on their conditions in order to achieve special favors. Health professionals rarely value this behavior. It is, however, one real alternative for a stigmatized individual, perhaps the person's best one.

Actually, promoting the positive side of a negative identity is not necessarily bad (Dudley 1983). Some secondary gains from a chronic condition may be desirable. For example, sheltered workshops are places to foster social relationships, an important secondary benefit. Most individuals benefit greatly from these sheltered environments; but the rewards can deter a person from progressing beyond the sheltered environment itself. Caution must be applied if the benefits discourage growth.

Resistance. Another response to a stigmatizing situation is resistance (Dudley 1983). Individuals may speak out and challenge rules and protocol if their needs are not met. How many years were wheelchair-bound individuals unable to reach pay telephones? But the wheelchair-bound and others united in voicing their protests of the situation, and now, lower pay telephones are a much more common sight, as are ramps on stairs and curbs. Anger often serves as a catalyst for those seeking change. Dudley sees this resistance, at least in the case of mentally retarded individuals, as an important step toward autonomy.

Passing. An important potential response is *passing*: pretending to have a less stigmatic identity, or even a normal one (Dudley 1983; Goffman 1963). If the attribute is discreditable (not readily visible), such as being a type II diabetic or having hypertension, passing is a viable option. It may begin accidentally and be strongly reinforced. As time goes on, individuals become proficient at performing activities as though they were normal. Consider, for example, the illiterate individual who bought and carried a newspaper on the bus in order to appear normal (Dudley 1983), or the person with a hearing impairment who pretends to be daydreaming in order to pass (Goffman 1963). This process may also include the concealment of any signs of the stigma. Some individuals refuse to use physical equipment, such as hearing aids, because this will notify others of their defect.

In addition to visibility, obtrusiveness determines the ability to pass. In other words, how much does the condition interfere with normal functioning? For the individual in a wheelchair whose defect is very visible, being behind a desk or conference table makes this differentness easier to ignore (Goffman 1963). A person with a speech impediment has no visible symbol of stigma, but whenever he or she speaks, others are reminded of the defect.

Discreditable persons often divide the world into a large group to whom they tell nothing and a small group who are aware of the stigmatizing condition. Medical practitioners often recommend this type of information management (Goffman 1963). For example, the diagnosis for leprosy is often listed as Hansen's disease or mycobacterial neurodermatitis. The client then has the option of revealing only to certain persons the alternate name of *leprosy*, with its accompanying historical stigma (Volinn 1983). Intimates who know of the condition often protect and help the stigmatized individual. The classic case is that of the alcoholic's mate who provides necessary explanations for periods of absence from work or social occasions.

The final step in passing is for the stigmatized individual to move completely into the normal world (Goffman 1963). An epileptic or mildly retarded individual may live, work, and function completely in normal social activities. Only selected people may be aware of the stigmatized condition and offer assistance in helping the person pass.

Learning to pass is one phase of a stigmatized person's career. However, acceptance and self-respect will mitigate the need to hide the defect. Voluntary disclosure is a sign of a well-adjusted phase, "a state of grace" (Goffman 1963). The woman who voluntarily tells a casual acquaintance about her co-lostomy has achieved this phase.

Covering. Due to the potential threat and anxiety-provoking nature of disclosure of a stigmatizing defect, most people deemphasize their differentness. This response, called *covering*, is an attempt to make the defect seem smaller or less significant than it really is (Goffman 1963). Like passing, this process involves understanding the difference between visibility and obtrusiveness; that is, the condition is openly acknowledged but its consequences are minimized. The object is to reduce tension. We have all observed persons with special dietary requirements who, in a social situation, deny the importance of maintaining the restriction even though they follow the restriction: "I can eat almost anything I want." Minimizing the importance diverts attention from the stigma or defect and creates a more comfortable situation for all. This process is also illustrated by people in minority groups who change their names or have plastic surgery to change a facial feature, making the visible attribute less obtrusive.

Another way in which visible stigma becomes less anxiety-producing is the skillful and often light-hearted manner in which the stigmatized individual handles it. Although the defect is not deemphasized, as in covering, the person may joke about it, thereby reducing the anxiety of normals during the encounter. "I make a joke about my wheelchair and that lets others know it's OK to talk about it" (Saylor 1984). The anxiety-producing subject is therefore no longer taboo and can more easily be managed.

Responses toward Self: Changes in Attitudes

Societal norms and values are a major determinant of an individual's standards for self-esteem and self-worth. Children are socialized to adopt the attributes of their particular sociocultural group (Geis 1977). Most of our standards of what is normal or expected from our particular society are derived from this socialization. To use Goffman's terms, we expect of ourselves what is expected of those in our particular social category. Specifically, in the United States,

strength, achievement, and attractiveness are commonly held values.

The person who does not possess the expected attribute is quite aware of this nonacceptableness as an equal and desired individual in the society. In addition, individuals with chronic diseases or conditions may find that their own deformities or failings decrease their self-respect. Not only does the stigmatized individual have to deal with the responses of others but some individuals find their own attributes undesirable. Awareness of the handicapped individuals' possible rejection by others should not overshadow awareness of self-approval versus disapproval. This heavy, self-imposed cloak of being unsatisfactory is more numbing than any illness or handicap.

Some individuals can accept deviations from expected norms and feel relatively untouched. A strong sense of identity protects them and they are able to feel acceptable in the face of the stigma (Goffman 1963). This is true in groups of culturally distinct individuals such as Jews and Mennonites who have pride in the group identity of their members. Strong extended families and cultural pride also reinforce this acceptable identity for other groups such as Blacks and Chicanos.

This identity belief system, also called *cognitive belief patterns*, refers to a person's perspective. It includes one's perceptions, mental attitudes, beliefs, and interpretations of experiences (Burns 1980). Individuals who are stigmatized by the major society may believe and perceive that their groups are actually superior, or at least preferable. These belief patterns offer protection from the stigmatized reactions of racist societies.

In chronic disease, cognitive belief patterns help individuals achieve identity acceptance and protection in the face of stigmatizing defects. For example, after mutilating cancer surgery, patients may consciously tell themselves that they are full human beings since the missing part was diseased and useless. The body, although disfigured, is now healthy, whole, and totally acceptable. (See Chapters 5, 9, and 10.) One's perception of self-worth influences personal reactions to disease or disability. An individual's question "Am I worthwhile?" is answered by determining that person's own definition of what one is and the way one ought to be (Geis 1977). Clients' definitions of themselves are crucial factors in self-satisfaction.

In describing studies of cerebral palsy, cancer, facial deformity, arthritis, and multiple sclerosis clients, Shontz (1977) noted that what was uniformly regarded as crucial was the personal meaning of the disability to each individual client. For example, individuals who feel valuable *because* they are healthy and physically fit suffer feelings of worthlessness if they contract a chronic condition. The diabetic will never be without a regimen and the necessary paraphernalia; visually impaired individuals will never see normally again. Individuals' reactions and ability to accommodate these discrepancies from normal determine their own attitudes of worth and value.

Responses of Normals to Stigmatized Individuals

Responses of normals to a stigmatized individual vary with the particular stigma and the "normal" person's past conditioning. Since society specifies the characteristics that are stigmatized, it also teaches its members the way to react to that stigma. Children learn to interact with others who are culturally different by watching and listening to those around them. In the same way, we learn how to treat chronically ill or disabled individuals by incorporating societal judgments. Unfortunately, these reactions are usually negative, since the stigma usually identifies an individual as discredited.

Devaluing. Normals often believe that the person with the stigma is less valuable, less human, less desired. Many of us exercise more than one kind of discrimination, and by so doing, effectively reduce the life chances of the stigmatized individual (Goffman 1963). Many tend to stigmatize persons as inferior or even dangerous and use such words as *cripple* or *moron*. Those who accept the devaluing effect of the physical changes see the stigmatized person as having a spoiled, or contaminated, social identity.

This concept has been previously discussed, but bears repeating for emphasis.

Stereotyping. Categories simplify our lives. Instead of having to decide what to do in every single situation, we can respond to categories of situations. Most of our life's events fall into general categories and the responses are, therefore, simplified (Allport 1954). "The professor is always on time." "Church occasions require appropriate dress." Sometimes, however, the inclination to categorize leads to restricted and inaccurate thinking, such as assuming that men are better at mathematics than women, or that swarthy white people are untrustworthy. Many normals believe that the handicapped are incompetent. Not only do categories lead to dangerous thinking but they are difficult to change. Much less effort is required to sustain a bias than is required to reconsider or alter it.

Stereotypes are a negative type of category. Stereotypes are a social reaction to ambiguous situations and allow us to react to group expectations rather than to individuals. When normal people meet impaired people, expectations are not clear (Katz 1981). Normal people are often at a loss as to how to react. Placing the chronically ill individual into a stereotyped category reduces the ambiguousness toward that person and makes the situation more comfortable for those doing the stereotyping.

Using categories and stereotypes to understand people decreases our attention to other characteristics (Lynd 1958). If we are unaware of a person's positive attributes or capabilities, the negative characteristics become the major social identity. When people are put into categories, normal others are blinded and look no further.

Categorizing tends to make one see the world as a dichotomy. This is true of both normals and impaired people. The hearing-impaired tend to see the world as made up of two kinds of people: those who can hear and those who cannot (Becker 1981). Likewise, people are categorized as either mentally retarded or normal even though mental handicaps exist on a continuum, with all of us falling somewhere along the line. Often stigmatized people may see themselves as more similar to normals than different from them. Regardless of categories, individuals from different groups are similar in some ways, dissimilar in other ways.

Labeling. The label attached to a condition is extremely crucial and influences the way we think about that individual. For example, public drunkenness is a criminal offense and results in a jail term. The drunk is, therefore, seen as possessing a negative label. Yet alcoholism is a disease properly treated in an alcoholism treatment center (Volinn 1983). Mentally handicapped individuals sometimes do not mind being called *slow learners* but are startled by being called *mentally retarded* (Dudley 1983). Their response indicates that they see this term as if it were a taboo. Mentally handicapped individuals go to great lengths to explain why they are not retarded when they note that they work, fix their own dinners, clean up afterward, and so on. Their definition of this state is that it is less than human: "Mentally retarded, that's for very low people" (p. 38). The inability to perform certain functions was not nearly as traumatizing to these individuals as the connotations inherent in the dreaded label.

Professional Responses: Attitudes toward Stigma

Health care professionals share the values and expectations of their society. Most nurses, physical therapists, and allied health workers share the American dream of achievement, attractiveness, and a cohesive, healthy family. These values influence perceptions of individuals who are disabled, impaired, or otherwise less than "normal."

Expression of negative reactions by medical students and faculty when encountering clients with severe disabilities of uncertain prognosis have been documented (Ford, Liske, & Ort 1962). One young woman with Hodgkin's disease perceived that she had fewer voluntary interactions initiated by the staff after her diagnosis had been confirmed: "The nurses didn't come into my room as often after the diagnosis" (Saylor 1984). Medical personnel have been known to withhold care from those whose problems result from drunkenness, carelessness, or neglect (Ablon 1981). This behavior represents a moralistic blaming in response to the spoiled identity of the individual.

Society's values and definitions of stigma affect professionals' attitudes. These attitudes are also influenced by professional education; students in health professional schools are enormously affected by their faculty and staff (Cohen et al. 1982). These authors describe how faculty influenced medical students in developing attitudes toward cancer clients; students assimilated the attitudes they saw around them. That is, if faculty treated clients with intolerance or a demeaning attitude, the students often adopted that behavior. On the other hand, if humane acceptance of all kinds of clients was observed, that behavior was more likely to be copied.

In addition to the influences of faculty and staff, attitudes were also changed by interactions with clients and chronically ill acquaintances (Cohen et al. 1982). Students' confidence in clients' ability to cope with the disease increased with professional experience. In a similar manner, personally knowing someone with a chronic condition increased positive attitudes.

Health professionals display all the reactions that any unstigmatized person has toward those with discrepancies of some sort. Caregivers need a thorough understanding of potential responses toward individuals with stigma if they are to overcome the effects of this stigmatizing behavior. The responsibility to react with sensitivity, understanding, and wisdom is incumbent upon those who deliver care.

Interventions: Dealing with Stigmatized Individuals

A handicap imposes various kinds and degrees of constraints on a person's life. The stigma of that disorder adds additional burdens, often far greater than those caused by the disorder itself (Dudley 1983). Individuals with chronic conditions usually receive only medical treatment; little, if any, sensitivity and few interventions are directed at reducing the effects of the associated stigma.

Helping others to manage the effects of stigma is not simple and should be approached with caution. Individuals and their families react to stigma-producing situations in ways that society has long dictated. This statement applies to both normal and stigmatized people. We must question our ability to make significant changes in society's attitudes since "ever present social stigma can be seen as a symptom of a diseased society" (English 1977a). At best, change will be slow and uneven. Individuals are more likely to "comply" than to criticize staff for stigma-producing behavior (Dudley 1983). However, sensitive health care providers cannot afford to assume that the situation is overwhelming and therefore unsolvable. Consistent and knowledgeable interventions aimed specifically at reducing the impact of stigma are as crucial as those that reduce blood pressure or chronic pain. The following section discusses appropriate strategies for managing stigma.

Developing a Support Group of One's Own

Those who share the same stigma can provide the "tricks of the trade," acceptance, and moral support to a stigmatized person. Goffman (1963) used the term *the own* for those who share a stigma. Groups of like-afflicted individuals enable the stigmatized person to feel like any normal person. Self-help groups are examples of persons who are *the own*. Alcoholics Anonymous, for instance, provides a community of *own* as well as a way of life for its members. Members speak publicly, demonstrating that alcoholics are treatable, not terrible, people. They act as *heroes of adjustment*, to use Goffman's term.

Groups comprising people with similar conditions can be formal or informal and are enormously helpful. First, peer groups can be used to explore all the potential response options previously discussed, such as resisting and passing. Second, problem-solving sessions in the groups explore possible solutions to common situations (Dudley 1983). Finally, others who share the stigma provide a source of acceptance

and support for both the individuals with the disease or disability and their families.

One word of caution is appropriate. Sometimes stigmatized individuals feel more comfortable with normals than with like others, when there is a closer identity with normals that allows for a sense of not being different. For example, not all women respond positively to Reach to Recovery groups; some may feel more anxiety and depression than a sense of support. The "best" solution varies from individual to individual.

Developing Supportive Others

Supportive others are persons who do not carry the stigmatizing trait but who are knowledgeable and offer sensitive understanding to individuals who do carry the trait. These people were called *the wise* by Goffman (1963) and are accorded acceptance and courtesy within the group of stigmatized individuals. The wise, who see the stigmatized as normal others and do not make affected individuals feel shame, treat such individuals in a normal fashion. One handicapped college student, asked what behaviors she liked from others, indicated a preference for knowledgeable acceptance:

> I like to look people in the eye, but that means they need to sit down and come close. I like to be touched. Other students slap each other on the back, why not me? I really feel accepted when they ask to ride with me in my chair up and down the halls. Some people see *me*, not my wheelchair. (Saylor 1984)

Short of riding in wheelchairs with clients, these desired behaviors are simply the same ones two friends or acquaintances would use. The stigmatized person must be seen and treated as normal, viewed as more than body changes or orthopedic equipment, seen as a person who is more than a stigmatized condition.

The process of becoming wise is not simple; it may mean offering oneself and waiting for validation of acceptance. Health care professionals who encounter chronically ill individuals cannot prove themselves as wise immediately. Validation requires consistent behavior by the professional that is sensitive, knowledgeable, and accepting. For example, hypertensive clients typically have problems of adherence to long-term diet and medication regimens (Saylor 1980). Professionals who are informed and helpful regarding the real-life problems of implementing diet and medication changes over a long period of time will be seen as supportive.

One way an individual can become wise is by asking straightforward, sensitive questions such as inquiring about the disabled person's condition. Many disabled individuals would be delighted to have the opportunity to disclose as much or as little as they wish since that would mean that the defect no longer was taboo.

Wiseness can come from working around individuals with a particular stigma. Health professionals can acquire real-life knowledge about problems, effective strategies, and concerns of a particular illness. This knowledge can enable them to offer the sensitive understanding and practical suggestions of "the wise" to chronically ill individuals. Nurses who work with cancer clients, for instance, have the opportunity to find out which behavior is really effective and can learn about outcomes and clients' reactions. This information is extremely valuable to similar clients and their families.

Caring, close friends or relatives are another type of wise. Siblings, spouses, and parents have the opportunity to be powerfully wise since they see beneath the disorder to the human being and show that they see ill persons as persons first. A word of caution: not all relatives and friends become wise. Many cannot deal with the stigmatizing condition and tend to separate themselves from the ill individual.

Neither are all health care providers wise. Many people who work with chronically ill or handicapped compound the stigmatization of clients by their lack of acceptance and insensitivity.

Being wise is not a new role for nurses or other caring health professionals. Nurses have traditionally worked in medically underserved areas with discredited persons because they are knowing and caring persons who are accustomed to treating clients as people, not as conditions. In fact, poor urban and rural areas often depend on nurses for health care delivery, especially in expanded roles such as nurse practitioners (Backup & Molinaro 1984). Regardless, in both their traditional roles or expanding roles, nurses often assume the predominant role of gatekeepers to the health care delivery system for many devalued individuals. Often, clients with chronic diseases receive effective and efficient care from these and other health professionals, who have great opportunities to perform the role of the wise.

Advocacy

Others who demonstrate the concept of the wise are client advocates: persons who support the right of clients to make informed decisions and to determine the treatment they will accept (see Chapter 13). The client advocate supports that right by speaking in behalf of someone in need, combining professional expertise with a sensitive understanding of an individual or group of individuals. Advocacy is a demonstration of wiseness because both processes require treating the individual as valuable and worthwhile.

Such an act of advocacy becomes obvious when medical missionaries, working with leprosy clients, emphasize that this disease is so mildly contagious that none of those who lived in the leprosarium contracted the disease (Volinn 1983). The same is true when nurses, working in a Skid Row area, act as advocates of alcoholics by being protective of clients and seeing them as individual enough to know each of them by name (Volinn 1983). These and other acts of advocacy effectively reduce stigmatization and the resulting impact and are the expression and proof of mutual trust between client and professional (Volinn 1983).

Changing Definitions of Disability

One way to change stigmatized persons' perceptions of self-worth is to reassess the criteria by which they determine what is normal. This is also applicable to normals. For example, people with healthy minds and bodies can be crippled by an inability to enjoy happiness (Goffman 1963). Other people, such as those who have had life-threatening accidents or diseases, often reorder life's priorities. These individuals have learned to recognize that life is precious and that they should savor simple pleasures. This creates a feeling of being more fortunate and healthier than those who waste time complaining. In other words, such people receive strength from the knowledge that they are successfully coping and know what is important to them. Absence of disease or disability no longer is their sole criterion for self-worth. Rather, an alternate ideology develops to counter the ones that discredit them.

Saying that stigmatized individuals and their caregivers should simply "change definitions of disability" is condescending, trite, and ineffective. The type of individual one encounters and the type of social setting influence the salience of disability as a stigma. One's definition and projection of self as worthy or demeaned and one's ability to manage others also serve as an influence (Cogswell 1977). Each person, normal or chronically ill, can learn to judge what each individual is and what that individual can do, rather than what that person cannot be or cannot do. In other words, all people have a right to be seen as valid.

Family, friends, and health care providers who interact with the stigmatized person are powerful influences in the self-perception of value and worth (Becker 1981). Being treated as valuable and acceptable by significant persons enhances one's self-esteem. Stigmatized persons may find that this healthy perception of self counteracts negative reactions of others. A person who has been handicapped since birth stated that her family had always treated her as if she were normal, so she thought she was, until she encountered "prejudice and bigotry" as a teenager (Saylor 1984).

Changes in one's health, ability to function, or body image cause the individual to create new answers to the question "Who am I?" to counteract stigmatizing effects of disease or disability (Cogswell 1977). Individuals whose self-esteem or identity was dependent on an occupation or hobby may lose these attributes as a result of a stigmatizing condition. Just as a parent whose children are grown finds many

previously undeveloped personal attributes to fill the lost sense of identity, so many individuals with chronic conditions find new sources of identity to replace lost functions. Others may wish to establish a new activity that is consistent with individual limitations to enhance or restore their sense of intrinsic worth (Geis 1977). A person should be able to feel worthwhile without fulfilling any conditions. For instance, a nurse who can no longer work because of a chronic condition should be able to enjoy leisure time with professional friends and former colleagues without suffering a complete loss of self-identity. In the same way, changes of body image should not be catastrophic for those who answer "Who am I?" with intrinsic values rather than physical attributes.

Nonacceptance versus Nonparticipation

The distinction between nonacceptance and nonparticipation is important in caring for stigmatized individuals. *Nonparticipation* is a reasonable abstinence from social activities based on limitations caused by the handicap or illness. *Nonacceptance*, on the other hand, is a negative attitude; that is, a resistance or reluctance to admit the handicapped person to various kinds and degrees of social relationships (Ladieu-Leviton, Adler, & Dembo 1977). A disabled person who chooses not to join a rock-climbing outing is a nonparticipant. The physical disability serves as the basis for that person's decision not to participate. Deciding not to invite that person to join the group, whether or not participation seems possible, is nonacceptance, preempting the person from choosing to participate.

Commonly, normal people cannot correctly estimate the limits of potential participation by those having a disease or disability (Ladieu-Leviton et al. 1977). Usually, the physical limitations imposed by a disability are overestimated. If normals incorrectly assume that an individual is not able to participate, that is a form of nonacceptance. Such nonacceptance is created by the difference between the degree of participation that is actually possible and the degree assumed possible by normals. If the difference can be resolved, nonacceptance ceases to be a problem.

The remedy can be simple. Normals can simply indicate that they want the individual to participate, leaving the decision of whether or not to become involved to the person. Perhaps the disabled individual would like to participate in a different way. The young adult who has juvenile arthritis may not regret being unable to go fishing if he or she can elect to go along and spend time socializing with friends (Ladieu-Leviton et al. 1977). People who have been changed by a disease are often able to restructure situations to include them. Under these circumstances, even though disabled, persons may feel that others behave insensitively about whether participation is possible or not (Ladieu-Leviton et al. 1977). However, this feeling is preferable to one of nonacceptance.

Professional Attitudes: Care versus Cure

Traditionally, the goal of health care has been to cure the client. Even today health care providers tend to measure success in this way. Since chronic disease is now more prevalent than infectious disease or acute illness, this criterion of success must be changed. Cure is neither essential nor necessary in order that the client benefit (Kübler-Ross 1969). Rather, caring should be the criterion. With the increased number of people having chronic diseases, providers must learn to accept the characteristics of chronic disease: indeterminate course of morbidity, relapses, and multiple treatment modes (Volinn 1983).

Selecting an Appropriate Model for Health Care Delivery. The manner in which health care is delivered may increase or decrease the effects of stigma. Encouraging a client's participation in health care decision making is an outward demonstration of respect and regard for that person. Treating a client as a partner in establishing goals demonstrates one's acceptance of that individual as valuable. On the other hand, when health providers make decisions regarding treatment or goals without consulting a client, they reinforce the feeling of being discredited.

Therefore, any mode of delivery that increases client participation enhances that person's perception of self-worth and, therefore, reduces the effects of stigma.

All provider-client encounters fall into one of three basic health care delivery models (Szasz & Hollander 1956). Any relationship that exists implies participation of both client and provider, with varying amounts of activity. For reasons of stigma management as well as chronic disease management, it is wise to determine which model of health care delivery is most appropriate for chronic conditions.

Active-Passive. The *active-passive* encounter is not really an interaction, since the client is acted upon and makes no contribution to decision making. The provider is the only active participant. This model is analogous to the relationship between a helpless infant and parent. In emergency situations, this model may be the most appropriate one. However, this form of encounter essentially says the client is unworthy of inclusion in decision making.

Guidance-Cooperation. In the *guidance-cooperation* model, a client seeks help from a provider and is willing to cooperate. Implied here is that the client is expected to respect and obey the health provider. The power in this encounter is unequal because the client is not expected to question the provider's recommendations. This model of health care delivery comprises the majority of traditional client-provider encounters and is valuable with most acute illnesses. It allows little if any room for clients' expectations or goals, which may be different from those of the provider.

Mutual Participation. *Mutual participation* evenly divides power between provider and client and leads to a relationship that can be mutually satisfying. In other words, the client should be as satisfied with the recommendations and decisions as the provider is. In addition, each party depends on the other for information culminating in that satisfactory solution. The client needs the provider's experience and expertise; the provider needs not only the client's history and symptoms but priorities, expectations, and goals. Sometimes a choice between treatments with relatively equal mortality rates is necessary; for example, surgery or radiation for cancer treatment. The physician can offer expert knowledge regarding long-term effects of radiation and changes in body image due to surgery. The client must decide the relative value of side effects of the alternative proposed treatments. Some people are inordinately afraid of radiation or of surgery; others are not. Because the "right" decision depends on the individual, input from both client and health care provider is necessary to produce a course of action that is mutually acceptable.

An important tenet in combating stigma is to allow individuals who have limitations the opportunity to become "central participants in the battle" (Dudley 1983). This tenet applies to all stigmatized clients. If the provider dominates the interaction, fuller client involvement does not result. The traditional models of client-provider interaction that give power and the right to decision making to the provider must give way to one that allows increased client participation. Clients having chronic diseases not only acquire an ability to evaluate their own symptoms and treatment but know that health care providers do not base all their decisions on scientific, undisputed principles (Volinn 1983).

When providers become more comfortable with allowing clients a greater range of participation and decision making, the relationship loses some of the stigmatizing effect. Health professionals must create an atmosphere in which individuals with chronic conditions not only are expected to cooperate but are encouraged to express their concerns, observations, expectations, and limitations.

The mutual participation model is the model of choice in stigmatizing chronic diseases since it enhances the client's feelings of self-worth. The client is responsible for long-term disease management, and the health care provider's responsibility is helping the client help himself or herself (Szasz et al., 1956). Together, they explore alternative strategies and decide on one that is agreeable to both. Being treated as a valuable partner is incompatible with

being treated as discredited. When a client's priorities and goals are valued and incorporated into the regimen, an increased sense of being accepted and acceptable emerges. The respect and regard for clients demonstrated by this model are an effective tool to counteract stigmatizing effects of illness.

A model of mutual participation is not easily achieved. Such a model is impossible without informed clients. One study of doctors' communications with cancer clients found not only that 40% of physicians perceived that patients preferred not to know their diagnosis but that only 80% of the physicians in the study thought that clients should be told regardless of their wishes to know (Greenwald & Nevitt 1982). With the current concerns for client rights, it is intriguing that any providers would think that clients should not be informed. Providers should use caution in attempting to shelter or protect clients. These behaviors may well decrease participation and, therefore, perceptions of worth and value.

Another benefit of a mutual participation model is increased compliance with medical regimen. In chronic disease, the client carries out the regimen; therefore compliance becomes a particularly important issue (see Chapter 7). A review of many articles discussing compliance showed that (1) when professionals were highly authoritarian, clients were less compliant, and (2) when chronic illnesses or disabilities were more severe, clients were less compliant with the professional's recommendations (Anderson 1977). It is adequate to note here that the need for compliance provides further reinforcement for the use of a mutual participation model that increases the client's responsibility for health care. Then, instead of wondering why the client does not comply with recommendations, professionals would consider why the provider does not recommend an acceptable plan.

Inservice Training. Health care providers' attitudes are representative of general societal views and can, therefore, be expected to include prejudices. Since health professionals have prolonged relationships with chronically ill individuals, the impact of these prejudices can be great. Training programs to teach professional and nonprofessional staff to identify and correct preconceived and often unconscious notions of categories and stereotypes deserve high priority (Dudley 1983).

Health care professionals are usually caring, sensitive people who do not intentionally devalue or behave insensitively toward those in their care. However, culturally learned habits are ever-present and ever-stigmatizing. Nevertheless, learned behavior can be relearned; old habits can give way to new sensitivities and new standards for individual worth. Professionals and nonprofessionals who manage chronic disease with satisfaction and pride can to some degree counteract the source of discredit from these long-term diseases.

One study of stigma-promoting behaviors provides ideas for health care providers who wish to change their attitudes (Dudley 1983). The most frequent stigma-promoting behaviors included the following: inappropriate language in referring to clients, inappropriate restrictions of activities, violation of confidentiality, physical abuse, denial of opportunities for clients to present views, ignoring clients, and staring. Both staff and laypersons were guilty of such behavior. The first step necessary to decrease the deleterious promotion and impact of stigma is to develop awareness of one's own responses and behaviors.

One effective way to increase awareness is through planned contact with stigmatized individuals. This should be preceded by group work with a knowledgeable leader who can help identify and work through attitudes and reactions. For example, many nursing students do not like skilled nursing facilities (SNFs) because clients who are frail, old, and slow are seen as unappealing. A gerontological nurse specialist spent time with such a group of students before they began working in the facility. Her slides of faces etched with character, stories of interesting experiences, and sense of humor through mishaps helped the students see human beings inside aging bodies. A group discussion confronted myths and stereotypical thinking regarding the stigma of aging (Burnside, Saylor, & Taylor 1984). These students had a positive experience at the facility. Knowl-

edgeable preparation for contact with stigmatized individuals does not solve all problems; it is, however, one way to expose stigmatized reactions such as stereotypes, to examine them, and to provide information to caregivers.

The attitudes of nonprofessional staff also must not be overlooked, since they provide much of the care, especially in long-term facilities. The attitudes and behaviors of these caregivers can promote or decrease the process of stigmatization (Volinn 1983). Providing intensive staff education for the purpose of reducing stigma perception by all employees in any particular agency would be beneficial. The group sessions described earlier would be very appropriate for both nonprofessional and professional caregivers. In addition, professional staff are in a position to role model behavior and to give informal information to help nonprofessional staff treat clients in an accepting manner.

Community Education Programs

Educational programs that reduce the effects of stigma can be carried to the community at large. Many organizations such as the American Cancer Society and American Diabetic Association have educational programs and are active in supplying such information through speakers or literature in the community. Educational programs for young children, who are still being socialized, would be effective in preventing the formation of stigma-producing attitudes (Dudley 1983). Schools, scout troops, and church groups are ideal settings for sensitive introductions of human beings who have many positive values and characteristics but do not meet normal health expectations. For instance, individuals who are visually impaired or individuals with insulin pumps could be the focus of a group discussion in which children learn to see others as human beings.

In addition to formal community education programs, the following variety of interventions that can influence society's attitudes are recommended (English 1977a):

1. Increasing the amount of rewarding, mutual interaction between normal and chronically ill in-

◇ CASE STUDY ◇
Dealing with Stigma

As the result of an auto accident, Jo, a 44-year-old home-maker with two children, was left with residual neuro-logical damage. Ten days after the accident, she was in a rehabilitation hospital being trained to stand and to per-form activities of daily living. Her prognosis for a full recovery was guarded. Jo had been a jogger and had enjoyed backpacking with her family. She was now faced with a wheelchair, a walker, decreased sensation and movement, and an inability to care for herself, much less her family. Her sources of identity, self-worth, and satis-faction were obliterated to a large degree.

Her greatest help in overcoming this stigmatizing situation was redefining her disability. A strong religious faith strengthened the concept that her intrinsic worth was not tied to physical abilities. The rehabilitation cen-ter's counselor immediately began a series of therapy sessions and acted as one of "the wise." No subject was taboo and unfit for discussion as the two confronted sexual functioning, body image, self-esteem, and so on. The nursing staff did not reject her in any way, nor was she allowed any secondary gains at this institution. She was treated as a person who would take care of herself, to the maximum of her capabilities: a worthwhile indi-vidual, not a stigmatized one.

Her family was intimately involved in Jo's care. They participated in physical therapy so that they would know what to expect and would not be afraid or overprotec-tive; they were also involved with long-term planning, as was Jo. Exercise regimens and medications for muscle spasm, for instance, were planned *with* Jo, not *for* her, taking into account her desires and past experiences.

As time passed, Jo regained enough function to walk with a cane and special shoes, although she is slow and awkward. There are fewer stigmatizing orthopedic ap-pliances now, but she will never run again. She has been comforted by others who have gone through cata-strophic events of many sorts: "the own." Friends and family have become "wise" by learning to accept her with her limitations. Her husband and daughters per-form the heavy household tasks, but she has resumed most of the cooking. The family now spends more time attending musical performances and plays and eating at restaurants, all of which Jo can manage quite well. Jo has rejoined her church activities, as well as neighbor-hood social groups.

Her initial reactions of being physically unacceptable and unattractive have given way to new criteria of intrin-sic values. Some physical problems remain: muscle spasm, altered mobility, and decreased sexual sensitiv-ity—none of which is a minor problem. However, these problems would be compounded if they were coupled with the burden of stigma. Fortunately for Jo, reactions of health care professionals, family, and friends have greatly reduced the effects of stigma.

---

dividuals: For instance, encouraging service proj-ects, pen pals, and outings between groups of normals and the disabled such as the blind or deaf.

2. Providing individuals having chronic conditions with adequate information about stigma and its effects: Clients can be helped to avoid inviting the devaluing attitudes of others. Self-help groups could address the topic of stigma during their discussions.

3. Influencing the media to present a more positive portrayal of chronically ill people: Providers and others should write to commend television net-works that show disabled individuals functioning well.

4. Involving the client's family in the treatment pro-gram: Include family members in developing long-range goals.

5. Sharing knowledge and experiences about stigma with professionals and nonprofessionals: Invite a person with a stigmatized condition to speak frankly at an inservice meeting.

The case study of Jo illustrates ways of dealing with stigma.

Summary and Conclusions

This chapter has followed the evolution of the con-cept of stigma to its present meaning: a mark of discredit. Stigma is caused by a discrepancy between an expected, socially defined norm and an actual attribute. This discrepancy, or defect, attaches a value judgment to its owner: It becomes the stigma. The person is discredited and less valuable. The discrediting and socially isolating effects of stigma transcend any limitations imposed by the actual disease or disability.

Chronic diseases are an everyday example of stigmatized conditions. Shortened life span, physical deformities, medical and dietary requirements, and other limitations are not considered normal and cause anxiety among others who do not have these characteristics. This anxiety is met with the same kinds of prejudicial responses that have occurred throughout the ages: stereotyping, devaluing, and labeling. The affected individuals, in an effort to limit the impact of such responses, use techniques such as resisting and passing.

Several helpful interventions have been discussed. All individuals must redefine the criteria by which they value others and themselves, reexamining the definition of a person's worth. The stigmatized individual benefits by gaining support from like others and learning to cope with negative responses.

Health care providers are encouraged to become "the wise" and to act as knowledgeable and sensitive advocates for individuals bearing the stigma of chronic disease. In addition, a model of health care delivery characterized by a more equitable sharing of power and goals must be developed. Teaching becomes a valuable tool to create change. Inservice education for professionals and nonprofessionals can sensitize those who provide care to behaviors that create and enhance their own stigma-producing attitudes. Societal education is also necessary to make inroads into underlying causes of stigma.

The preceding are general ways of dealing with stigma. As mentioned earlier in this chapter, helping others to manage the effects of stigma is not simple. Stigma is a problem of overwhelming proportions in which realism and pessimism seem to merge and affected individuals may despair and lapse into a state of helplessness (English 1977a). The health care provider who tries to deal with this problem in toto may be wrestling with overpowering problems. However, choosing a single technique that reduces stigma's effects and devoting one's energy to improving or correcting that particular component can produce positive results.

STUDY QUESTIONS

1. How would you use Goffman's theory to identify diverse potential sources of stigma in a population of non-White, low-income individuals with high rates of hypertension, diabetes, and arthritis?
2. What strategies would you use to reduce the effects of stigma in a specific client family? Use the example of a child who has cerebral palsy and whose mother is responsible for his exercises and special care. Use strategies to reduce the effects of stigma for the mother and for the child.
3. What potential stigmatizing situations could arise for disabled individuals at a summer outing that involves food, games, and outdoor activities? What procedures could prevent or reduce the effects?
4. How do various client participation models of health care delivery differ in terms of the effect on potential or actual stigma?
5. What are the benefits and costs of increasing client participation in health care delivery? If a client chooses not to accept a typical diet or exercise regimen, how can this choice be managed so that stigma is not increased?
6. What reactions to personal and clinical experiences of stigma has a chronically ill person of your acquaintance had? What strategies does this person use to lessen the effects of the stigma?
7. What means of effective and sensitive health care delivery are available to clients who have chronic illnesses? How do such means prevent stigmatizing the client?

References

Ablon, J., (1981) Stigmatized health conditions, *Social Science and Medicine, 15B* (1): 5–9

Allport, G., (1954) *The Nature of Prejudice*, Reading, Mass.: Addison-Wesley

Anderson, T., (1977) An alternative frame of reference for rehabilitation: The helping process versus the medical model, in Marinelli, R., and Dell Orto, A. (eds.), *The Psychological and Social Impact of Physical Disability,* New York: Springer

Backup, M., and Molinaro, J., (1984) The new health professionals: Changing the hierarchy, in Sidel, V., and Sidel, R. (eds.), *Reforming Medicine: Lessons of the Last Quarter Century*, New York: Pantheon

Becker, G., (1981) Coping with stigma: Lifelong adaptation of deaf people, *Social Science and Medicine, 15B* (1): 21–24

Burns, D., (1980) *Feeling Good: The New Mood Therapy*, New York: William Morrow

Burnside, I., Saylor, C., and Taylor, T., (1984) A group activity for nursing students, San Jose State University, unpublished

Cogswell, B., (1977) Self-socialization: Readjustment of paraplegics in the community, in Marinelli, R., and Dell Orto, A. (eds.), *The Psychological and Social Impact of Physical Disability*, New York: Springer

Cohen, R., Ruckdeschel, J., Blanchard, C., Rohrbaugh, M., and Horton, J., (1982) Attitudes toward cancer, *Cancer, 50*: 1218–1223

Dudley, J., (1983) *Living with Stigma: The Plight of the People Who We Label Mentally Retarded*, Springfield, Ill.: Charles C Thomas

English, R. W., (1977a) Combatting stigma toward physically disabled persons, in Marinelli, R., and Dell Orto, A. (eds.), *The Psychological and Social Impact of Physical Disability*, New York: Springer

English, R. W., (1977b) Correlates of stigma toward physically disabled persons, in Marinelli, R., and Dell Orto, A. (eds.), *The Psychological and Social Impact of Physical Disability*, New York: Springer

Ford, A., Liske, R., and Ort, R., (1962) Reactions of physicians and medical students to chronic illness, *Journal of Chronic Disease, 15*: 785–787

Geis, H. J., (1977) The problem of personal worth in the physically disabled patient, in Marinelli, R., and Dell Orto, A. (eds.), *The Psychological and Social Impact of Physical Disability*, New York: Springer

Goffman, E., (1963) *Stigma: Notes on Management of Spoiled Identity*, Englewood Cliffs, N.J.: Prentice-Hall

Greenwald, H., and Nevitt, M., (1982) Physician attitudes toward communication with cancer patients, *Social Science and Medicine, 16* (5): 591–594

Hooper, S., (1981) Diabetes as a stigmatized condition: The case of low income clinic patients in the United States, *Social Science and Medicine, 15B* (1): 11–19

Katz, I., (1981) *Stigma: A Social Psychological Analysis*, Hillsdale, N.J.: Lawrence Erlbaum Associates

Kübler-Ross, E., (1969) *On Death and Dying*, New York: Macmillan

Ladieu-Leviton, G., Adler, D., and Dembo, T., (1977) Studies in adjustment to visible injuries: Social acceptance of the injured, in Marinelli, R., and Dell Orto, A. (eds.), *The Psychological and Social Impact of Physical Disability*, New York: Springer

Lemert, E., (1972) *Human Deviance, Social Problems, and Social Control* (2d ed.), Englewood Cliffs, N.J.: Prentice-Hall

Lynd, H. M., (1958) *On Shame and the Search for Identity*, New York: Harcourt Brace Jovanovich

Roget's International Thesaurus (4th ed.), (1977), New York: Thomas Y. Crowell

Ryan, R., Kempner, K., and Emlem, A., (1980) The stigma of epilepsy as a self-concept, *Epilepsia, 21*: 433–444

Saylor, C., (1980) *A Study of the Relationship of Hypertensive Clients' Beliefs and Their Degree of Compliance*, Master's thesis, San Jose State University, San Jose, Calif.

Saylor, S., (1984) Personal communication, July 8, 1984

Shontz, F., (1977) Physical disability and personality: Theory and recent research, in Marinelli, R., and Dell Orto, A. (eds.), *The Psychological and Social Impact of Physical Disability*, New York: Springer

Sontag, S., (1977) *Illness as Metaphor*, New York: Farrar, Strauss, & Giroux

Szasz, T., and Hollander, M., (1956) A contribution to the philosophy of medicine, *American Medical Association Archives of Internal Medicine, 97*: 585–592

Volinn, I., (1983) Health professionals as stigmatizers and destigmatizers of diseases: Alcoholism and leprosy as examples, *Social Science and Medicine, 17*: (7): 385–393

Webster's New Collegiate Dictionary, (1974) Springfield, Mass.: G. & C. Merriam

C H A P T E R   F I V E

Altered Mobility

Introduction

To observe people is often to observe people in motion: children running and jumping, adults walking and jogging. Being in motion is a natural state of the human body. Imagine not being able to move freely or pick up objects with your hands. Picture yourself bedridden or dependent on a wheelchair or a cane. Think of yourself as restricted because you are unable to see where you are going or hear the sound of danger. In all these situations some kind of mobility has been lost.

Without the ability to move, we lose independence, and our world shrinks. Mobility allows us to function independently and to enjoy leisure and recreational activities at will. Participation in formal education is enhanced and enriched by independent mobility; employment often requires the ability to get around, especially to and from the work setting. Access to medical services and health resources is limited for an individual who is unable to get to them freely (Welsh & Blasch 1980).

Mobility and activities tend to change throughout life. Children are usually active; adult years bring a more sedentary, but still mobile, existence. Most aged individuals are still active and involved, despite the common association of aging with lessened activity and often chronic illness.

Diseases, especially chronic ones, may affect mobility. How does the person who has undergone a change in mobility make necessary adjustments?

How does society treat such a person? What are the potentially ego-shattering psychological effects on a human being who has lost some degree of mobility? How do these changes affect family relationships, self-esteem, and self-motivation? And how can people deal with societal and environmental barriers that inhibit maximum independence?

Problems of Altered Mobility

Health professionals usually think of altered or impaired mobility in terms of bedrest, "confinement" to a wheelchair, or loss of use of lower body extremities. In other words, they see mobility changes as apparent musculoskeletal impairment.

But mobility alterations can involve other aspects of an individual's life. Mobility can be influenced by sensory loss, pain, or energy depletion, none of which directly involves the musculoskeletal system. In addition, mobility loss tends to occur in patterns: intermittent, progressive, or permanent, or combinations thereof. Regardless of pattern, alterations in mobility are associated with psychosocial problems that affect the client and significant others. This chapter touches on all these factors.

Bedrest

First we should look at the effects of bedrest. Although illness is often measured by the length of time spent in bed (Asher 1983), extended periods of bedrest may not always be efficacious because, beneath the comfort of the blanket, there lurks a host of formidable dangers. Studies reveal that even a few days of bedrest result in adverse physiologic and psychologic effects (Olson et al. 1967; Lentz 1981; Greenleaf & Kozlowski 1982). This observation has prompted physicians to insist that their bedridden patients sit up as soon as possible. Interestingly, altered physiologic responses associated with bedrest are not abnormal; they are the body's attempts to optimize its functions and to enhance its survival potential (Greenleaf & Kozlowski 1982) (see Table 5-1).

Bedrest is a restricted level of activity often necessitated by times of illness, either acute or chronic. In acute illness, for example, when surgery is necessary, periods of bedrest tend to be temporary, improvement is expected, and complications are uncommon. Recovery and rehabilitation are usually short in duration, with body functions quickly regained: the individual rapidly regains mobility, independence, and, by society's standards, productivity.

Unlike acute illnesses, many chronic disease states demand longer or more frequent periods of bedrest. Effects of long-term rest can be irreversible, but if homeostasis is maintained, the client can retain some functional capacity (Lentz 1981).

Cardiovascular Effects. Even three days of bedrest cause changes in the cardiovascular system. These changes include decreased venous flow with increased probability of thrombus formation and decreased orthostatic tolerance, resulting in dizziness or fainting upon resuming an upright position. Following prolonged periods of bedrest, fatigue or weakness results from limited periods of exertion (Olson et al. 1967; Lentz 1981). Goldman (1977) found that healthy young adult males, after three to six weeks of bedrest, required at least six weeks to regain full cardiac function.

Respiratory Effects. The respiratory system shows a decrease in oxygen transport capacity after short-term bedrest. In his study of healthy young adult males, Goldman found that respiratory deconditioning included an 18% decrease in maximum oxygen uptake. The increased oxygen debt led to lactic acidemia and symptomatic fatigue with exertion. Recovery of respiratory function required two to five weeks (Goldman 1977). Lack of oxygenation and fatigue, coupled with decreased coughing ability and increased hypostatic pooling, can lead to increased risk of atelectasis (Olson et al. 1967).

Musculoskeletal Effects. Musculoskeletal changes can significantly reduce the ability of a client, regardless of age, to resume normal activity. Demineralization of bone is thought to be secondary to the decreased stress on long bones in the upper and lower legs (Olson et al. 1967). Muscle mass and strength diminish without frequent stress and work demands on the muscle. An aged individual with decreased bone density and muscle mass has increased risk of fractures. A decreased ability to resume activities of daily living leads to slower recovery (Lentz 1981). Limited joint mobility results in decreased range of motion, lack of joint stability, and eventually to contractures (Olson et al. 1967). Prolonged pressure, inadequate nutrition, and other factors lead to decubitus ulcers; often slow to heal, such open wounds make the body susceptible to systematic infection (Olson et al. 1967).

Genitourinary Effects. Bladder emptying is incomplete in the supine position. An in-dwelling catheter aids in draining the bladder but may result in infection and perhaps bladder dysfunction such as incontinence. Urinary stasis in the renal pelvis due to dorsal recumbency fosters both infection and calculus formation (Goldman 1977). The kidneys must then filter larger amounts of minerals and salts, which are released into the blood plasma as a consequence of hemodynamic and metabolic changes. The passing of renal calculi, usually composed of calcium salts, may injure the mucosal lining and increase the urinary tract's susceptibility to infection (Olson et al. 1967).

TABLE 5-1. Effects of Bedrest

Cardiovascular
1. Orthostatic hypotension: neurovascular reflex control decreases, producing decreased muscle tone and decreased muscle action on veins.
2. Increased work load on heart: changes in resistance and pressures lead to redistribution of blood and increased circulation. The Valsalva maneuver increases intrathoracic pressure.
3. Thrombus formation: thrombi form secondary to venous stasis, hypercoagulability, and external pressure on legs.

Pulmonary
1. Decreased basal metabolism reflects a lessened cellular oxygen need; carbon dioxide production decreases.
2. Chest expansion is limited (compression), muscle power and coordination diminish, and compliance and elastic recoil decrease.
3. Increased secretions resulting from less effective coughing, pooling, and thickening lead to hypostatic pneumonia.
4. Poor ventilation and gas exchange result in carbon dioxide retention and hypoxemia with eventual respiratory acidosis.

Musculoskeletal
1. Contractures: disuse leads to atrophy and loss of muscle tone and mass. The integrity of muscle function (lengthening and shortening of muscle fibers) lessens, leading to an imbalance between opposing muscles (spasm) and decreased function of ligaments, tendons, and joint capsule (decreased range of motion).
2. Osteoporosis: the absence of weight-bearing stress on the skeleton causes a decrease in osteoblastic function; osteoclastic action continues.
3. Decubitus: increased pressure and decreased circulation lead to decreased nutrition and ischemia; necrosis and ulceration can develop, with eventual osteomyelitis or systemic infection.

Genitourinary
1. Calculi: stasis occurs when urine must move against gravity; infection can result. Urine becomes more alkaline. Stasis and alkalinity plus protein breakdown and bone demineralization increase minerals and salts that need to be excreted; any particle can become the nucleus for formation of a renal calculus.
2. Voiding: difficulty relaxing the pelvic muscles for micturation causes distention and overflow incontinence leading to skin breakdown and lowered self-esteem; voiding difficulties can lead to reflux and kidney damage. In-dwelling catheters help drain the bladder but invariably lead to infection.

Gastrointestinal
1. Negative nitrogen balance results from increased catabolic activity (protein breakdown) and anorexia (common with many illnesses). Stress (parasympathetic stimulation) can lead to dyspepsia, distention, anorexia, diarrhea, or constipation.
2. Constipation is secondary to several factors: malnutrition and decreased exercise cause muscle atrophy and loss of tone, decreased response to defecation reflux occurs secondary to unnatural position and disruption of familiar patterns, and withdrawal of water from fecal material in the bowel causes hard, dry stools.

Metabolism
1. Decreased metabolic rate, tissue atrophy, and protein catabolism occur. There is bone demineralization; anabolic processes are retarded, while catabolic activity accelerates.
2. Body temperature: heat conduction and radiation are lessened by bedclothing. Sweating increases wherever skin surfaces touch, contributing to fluid and electrolyte loss.
3. The supine position reduces the production of adrenocortical hormones, which affect the metabolism of carbohydrate, protein, and fat and affect electrolyte balance.

Psychological
1. Motivation and ability to learn and retain information decrease; ability to solve problems lessens.
2. Emotional behavior becomes exaggerated and manifests as apathy, withdrawal, anger, aggression, or regression; drives are diminished.
3. Body image is altered. There is a loss of feelings of self-esteem, self-worth, and pride.
4. Efficiency of sensory processes is reduced, leading to sensory deprivation, which in turn causes a decrease in perception. Time distortion occurs.
5. Role activities and drives change; roles are altered, reversed, or eliminated.

Summarized from Olson et al. (1967).

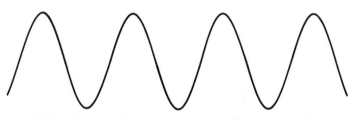

FIGURE 5-1. Intermittent pattern of altered mobility

Gastrointestinal Effects. Bedrest leads to psychological and mechanical effects on gastrointestinal functions, especially ingestion and elimination (Olson et al. 1967). The loss of appetite, perhaps initially from stress or pain, leads to anorexia, which in turn results in a negative nitrogen balance (Greenleaf & Kozlowski 1982). Bowel dysfunction, constipation, and fecal impactions, along with accompanying discomfort, may well undo many of the goals that necessitated bedrest.

Metabolic Effects. Immobility markedly reduces both the energy requirements of cells and their metabolic processes. Bedrest interferes with metabolic homeostasis, influencing the efficiency of homeostatic mechanisms. Functional changes include reduced metabolic rate, tissue atrophy, protein catabolism, bone demineralization, alterations in the exchange of nutrients and other substances between extracellular and intracellular fluids, fluid and electrolyte imbalance, and gastrointestinal hyper- or hypomotility (Olson et al. 1967).

Psychosocial Effects. Dependency, depression, and dissociation are common. Changes in body image also occur. The dependent person often overreacts to perceived threats to self-image. The anxious or depressed person interprets required bedrest as serious illness. Problem-solving ability decreases, motivation lessens, and discriminatory ability decreases (Olson et al. 1967). When bedrest is prescribed for aged individuals, hazards become much graver because of reduced reserve; death is frequently an outcome (Goldman 1977). Immobility often sets the stage for the expression of either exaggerated or inappropriate emotional reactions; for

example, individuals may voice expressions of loss of personal worth, fear, wounded pride, guilt, disgust, or anger.

Patterns of Mobility Alteration

In most chronic illnesses, bedrest is only a temporary phase. Most of the time people with chronic illnesses follow patterns of activity and altered mobility; some of these patterns are quite characteristic of certain diseases. Although each of these patterns is described here as if it were a separate entity, one must remember that affected individuals may fluctuate between patterns, depending on the activity of the disease or on the current situation. As an example, the Type I diabetic shows *intermittent* changes in mobility patterns when blood sugar levels vary radically, resulting in hyper- or hypoglycemia. Later, when chronic complications set in, the same individual either shows a *progressive* pattern or stabilizes at a *permanent* level. Such movement between patterns of mobility is demonstrated in most chronic illnesses.

Intermittent Changes in Mobility. Intermittent changes come and go, often at unpredictable times (see Figure 5-1). This unpredictability creates difficulty for client or family in planning activities of any kind because of the ambiguity of tomorrow. Holding a job, participating in social events, or planning other activities becomes uncertain.

Frequently, intermittent mobility patterns have a variety of recurrent physiological responses or effects. As an example, the client having arthritis may experience repeated episodes of weakness, pain, and swelling of joints. Classically, clients with intermittent

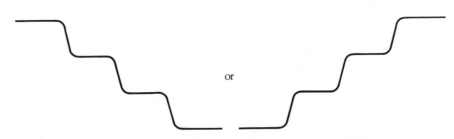

or

FIGURE 5-2. Progressive pattern of altered mobility

mobility have sporadic rises in energy and activity occurring during phases of remission or when they feel better. In other words, overactivity becomes an overcompensation for the function loss that occurs at other times. This behavior pattern tends to exhaust the individual and in turn leads to more episodes of bedrest than might otherwise be necessary.

Progressive Changes in Mobility. Progressive changes continue over time in a given steplike direction (see Figure 5-2). A negative progression has continuous downward steps; a positive direction demonstrates some kind of improvement. For example, an individual having multiple sclerosis (MS) may show steplike deterioration over time, whereas the person with myocardial infarction may progress to increased activity. Stabilization at a plateau sometimes occurs, providing opportunities for client and family to adjust before another change occurs. In some disease states, progressive immobility is associated with physical or functional decline, pain or fatigue.

Psychological responses are associated with the steplike quality of progressive changes. Downward progression often has physical and emotional components making client or family coping difficult. Should the strain become excessive, major disruption of family cohesiveness may result. Some families have greater adaptive ability than others and are less disrupted by these changes. Even positive progression can have adverse effects. Expectations for continued improvement can exceed the client's potential or ability; client and family may be greatly disappointed when their hopes are not realized.

MS is characterized by chronic progressive decline and is accompanied by problems of adjustment, especially since it is a disease of the young, with a mean age of 33 years (Booz, Allen, and Hamilton 1980). Adjustments include increased dependence and altered ability to meet the demands of employment and daily living, especially during stages of exacerbation. Marsh, Ellison, and Strite (1983) note that three of ten people having MS reported altered marital relationships or family plans, and 42% lost their jobs.

Permanent Change in Mobility. Permanence refers to mobility loss that does not vary, assuming that good maintenance care is provided (see Figure 5-3). Permanent change can occur after a period of intermittent or progressive change but frequently results from sudden trauma or injury, as with spinal cord injuries (SCIs) or cerebral vascular accidents (CVAs). Damage to the central nervous system, with its instantaneous effect of paralysis, results in major life-style disruption and thus places a heavy burden of financial, emotional, and psychosocial demands on the client and significant others, especially in the beginning. Adjustment may be slow and painful; however, if it is achieved, the family functions in a reasonably stable way.

The client having rheumatoid arthritis (RA) is representative of changes from one mobility level to another. Some forms of RA are chronic systemic disorders associated with restricted activity, deformity or disfigurement, expense, and physical and emotional pain (Mooney 1982).

Pam's case study, which illustrates the effects of changes in mobility, demonstrates movement from one level to another. (We will return to Pam's case frequently throughout this chapter.)

◇ CASE STUDY ◇
Pam: Changes in Mobility

Pam, now 28, was 13 years old at the onset of juvenile arthritis (JA), rheumatoid type. At age 25, she developed Sjogren's syndrome, manifesting as diminished glandular secretion, resulting in dryness of mucous membranes. During the early years of her illness, Pam had difficulty keeping up with her friends' activities because her levels of energy were lower than theirs. She often found herself bedridden after an active day. Recently, while vacationing in Japan, Pam enthusiastically decided to participate in mountain climbing during a "good" day. She spent the following two days in bed recuperating, rather than sightseeing.

As her arthritis progressed, Pam developed ulnar deviation of her hands and finger joints, necessitating extensive changes in the ways she used her hands. She needed a large ring on her keys to allow her to pick up and turn them, kitchen utensils adapted for her use, and so on. Initially, Pam's husband had difficulty understanding her need for these adaptations, but with time they both adjusted.

The permanent quality of changes she faced created problems for Pam, her husband, and her parents. With specialized counseling over several years, Pam eventually accepted her disease and has come to terms with these irreversible changes. Pam realizes that JA is a part of her identity, not a foreign element. Her adaptations are now integrated into everyday living.

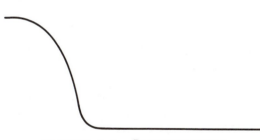

FIGURE 5-3. Permanent pattern of altered mobility

Sensory Loss

Generally, one does not associate mobility alteration with sensory problems, since loss of sensory function does not directly affect the musculoskeletal system. However, inability to see or to hear has a great impact on ability to move freely in one's environment.

Visual Loss. Visual loss alters mobility indirectly. Ease of travel decreases, since most cues for moving about are visual. Diminished cues prevent individuals with partial visual loss from full awareness of stairs, pathways, curbs, and obstacles. Loss of access to visual information is restricting because if one is unable to read signs, directions, and printed material, the ability to act on that information is lost.

Visual impairment adversely impacts independent living; loss of the ability to perceive the environment makes ambulating precarious. Eye changes can also result in light and glare sensitivity and reduced color perception (Genesky 1981). Visual impairment reduces grooming skills and confidence when in public surroundings.

The impact of visual loss depends on visually impaired people's development of spatial ability (Pick 1980). *Spatial ability* encompasses organizing information so that the individual senses how to get from one area to another by interpreting incoming nonvisual stimulation. Additionally, selection of travel aids (a cane, a guide dog, or a sighted guide) affects potential travel routes. For example, an individual who has a guide dog moves about comfortably in familiar territory but may experience difficulty in unfamiliar territory.

Hearing Impairment. Persons having hearing loss usually have few mobility problems in the physical environment (Welsh & Blasch 1980). However, they experience indirect obstacles to mobility. Many people do not realize that hearing-impaired persons frequently do not possess high oral or written language skills, so that communicating their mobility needs is difficult. Even those who are proficient in lip- or speech-reading are limited in their ability to communicate, since a person with good skills usually understands only about 30% of a conversation. As an example, sign language incorporates visual concepts rather than the verbal language structure familiar to those who can hear. The person with a hearing impairment may be reluctant to solicit needed help or information because of this difference in language skill.

Individuals who have hearing losses may be vulnerable to danger, unable to hear warning signals. In an emergency they may be immobilized, not knowing what is happening or the best way to move out of danger. Other hearing-impaired persons tend to have less experience in traveling independently if their family and friends are overprotective (Welsh & Blasch 1980) and therefore may lack confidence in their ability to travel on their own.

Pain and Loss of Energy

Pain can be an invisible handicap that becomes a disabling condition in itself. Fatigue or energy loss (for example, caused by multiple sclerosis or rheumatoid arthritis) can be so overwhelming that even being with other people becomes unbearable. Opening doors, driving, and carrying items are tasks that may intensify pain or, because they require energy and agility, become impossible.

Pain. A review of the literature indicates that the pain of chronic disease is both physical and psychological (Lewis 1984; Mooney 1982; McCaffery 1979). In addition, society has attached a stigma to complaints of pain, making people hesitant to talk about it. Instead, they tend to ignore or hide pain experiences (Jacox 1979).

The chronically ill client often experiences anticipatory pain (Mooney 1982) based on prior disease experiences or reactions. The anxiety associated with pain expectation may cause them to choose inactivity, ultimately creating isolation or limiting the quality of life.

> Pam: Pain is physically and emotionally draining. Even if you try to keep up with others to the point of total exhaustion and great physical pain, there is no one to confide in about your great emotional pain.

Loss of Energy. Many chronic conditions, such as myocardial infarctions or chronic obstructive pulmonary disease, cause fatigue that makes mobility more difficult. Although many of these energy-depleting conditions have no visible manifestations, they are nevertheless incapacitating. Even a simple act such as stepping up onto a curb can seem impossible to a person whose body is receiving inadequate oxygenation.

Energy loss can also develop directly from musculoskeletal problems. Small, simple movements may demand great effort when arthritis has reduced flexibility and range of motion. Painful joints and weak muscles cause an extra work load for normal joints and muscles so that unaffected areas must "take up the slack" and therefore tire more rapidly. The cyclic nature or intermittent pattern of some diseases increases fatigue because of the tendency to compensate by overexerting when one is feeling well (Gould 1982; *National Arthritis News* 1984).

Depression and frustration, which often accompany chronic diseases, can cause energy loss. The accompanying fatigue may heighten feelings of depression, for example, when the ill individual is unable to complete a favorite activity or to participate in events with friends as in the past. Thus, a vicious circle is created.

> Pam: It's hard to justify my fatigue to friends and relatives; my husband often asks, "Why are you so tired?" It took an article in the *National Arthritis News* to finally help me convince myself and him that my fatigue was real, physiologically as well as emotionally.

Psychosocial Aspects

Altered mobility affects the total person. Human beings do not experience life solely in physical terms, but also in psychological and social terms. Decreased mobility impedes one's sense of independence and productivity, and ultimately one's sense of worth and social value.

Psychological Effects. When physical ability to move changes, a psychological adjustment must occur. Adjustment is a process of redefining self that requires reconstruction of self-image. The mobile, ambulatory person who has difficulty accepting changes in locomotion or agility finds that adaptation rarely entails an agreeable, acceptable, or easy change.

Clients have compared times of adjustment to riding on a roller coaster: constantly challenged or angered by the uphill struggles, never knowing when another curve will come, and unable to stop the motion. They have a sense of instability during this period of mixed and conflicting emotions, of bewilderment, of a sense of helplessness. The process does not move easily or steadily from one stage to the next, but is usually characterized by inconsistency, questioning, and occasional hopelessness.

Loss. The emotional response to loss of mobility expresses itself as grieving, a process unique to each person, developing at an individual pace, that must be understood as such. Behavioral responses may seem irrational and inappropriate to both client and health provider; the health professional should be aware that this behavior accompanies psychological adaptation. In addition, somatic manifestations (pain, anger, loss of appetite, sleep disturbances, and slowed thinking and action) may be symptoms of the grieving and adjustment process.

Guilt, or a sense of being punished, is usually characteristic of this loss (Walker & Lattanzi 1982): "If only I had done (or had not done) this, then I would not be sick/paralyzed/bedridden." Of course, sorrow accompanies loss: loss of physical function, body image, social status, employment, familiar life-style, or previously stable emotions.

Chronic progressive diseases cause emotional readjustment each time the person must adapt to a new loss of mobility state, just as readjustment may become necessary at each new growth and development level. Recovery from loss (sometimes referred to as *acceptance*) is indicated when the person becomes more open to change, is able to use the experience for personal goals, and again welcomes life (Lattanzi 1983).

Self-Image. One's perspective of self has many components. Body image changes are common when mobility changes (see Chapter 9). When changes are visible, the client may deny the reality of the visible outer body, viewing it as perfect and totally functioning, or as ugly and deformed. Other people may perceive the client's outer body differently and interact on the basis of that perception. When these viewpoints of the body contradict, the client's concept of self may become confused.

Contradictions may also exist in cases of non-visible chronic illnesses, as with some cardiovascular or respiratory diseases. Although outwardly others may perceive the individual as actively mobile, the inward physique may be intensely altered by illness. The expectations of the client and others may exceed the client's ability to perform many functions.

Self-esteem is also affected. Earle and associates (1979) compared people having RA to those who did not have the disease and found that subjects with more severe joint disease showed more feelings of lower self-esteem and meaninglessness than those who had less active disease or who were disease-free. Such feelings can lead to difficulties in coping with the disease and can result in depression.

Isolation. A decreased ability to move may result, perforce, in the individual's becoming isolated. Inability to enter a facility or to gain access to transportation prevents social and professional development and interaction. Physical limitations may inhibit the individual's involvement in social activities, restricting social contacts and friendships. Fatigue or pain may preclude endurance for a prolonged endeavor, forcing the person to leave an activity early or not to attend it. Ironically, social isolation may reflect a loss of self-esteem rather than the ability to participate. Many people who can perform various activities choose not to do so.

Because of the emotional and physical stress associated with relating to others who have a negative or misinformed attitude, individuals may isolate themselves to avoid stigma (see Chapter 4). It may appear easier and healthier for a client to remain at home, where the social atmosphere is recognizable and the physical environment is constant and manageable.

> Pam: I had a poor self-image because I was so depressed about the chronic, painful JA and its disfigurement. It's hard when you're a teenager and can't keep up with your physically energetic friends. I spent much of my life in total isolation with no one to talk to about my disease. I consequently denied my JA to myself and to my friends, who couldn't or wouldn't understand.

Fear.   Fear emerges when the body is suddenly or gradually transformed from functioning in its usual expected manner to responding in an unexpected way to an unknown disease. Anger may erupt because of limited choice. Many individuals have the feeling "Why me?" Fear of rejection and abandonment is common. According to Marsh, Ellison, and Strite (1983), many individuals fear that other people consider them abnormal, deformed, or contagious. Themes include frustration at being handicapped and dependent on others for meeting some needs, frustration and anger concerning disabilities and insensitive treatment by others, reluctance to assert oneself, faulty communications with family members, and an unrealistic expectation that other people should "understand."

Travel.   The client's ability to move from one location to another is a complex interaction between independent travel and psychological factors (Welsh & Blasch 1980). Lack of independent travel may lead to increased dependency, isolation, hopelessness, and poor self-concept. The process becomes cyclic, with these factors serving as obstacles to independent movement. On the other hand, successful independent travel improves self-concept, gives a greater sense of independence, and improves motivation for other tasks. Overcoming fear of independent travel requires development of self-confidence and acquisition of new mobility skills.

Stress.   Stress can exacerbate disease activity or associated pain (as in systemic lupus erythematosis [SLE]) and in turn affect mobility. The client, consequently, is in a double-bind: trying to avoid stress because it intensifies the disease, yet experiencing stress by the very nature of the disease. Loss of control produces an attitude of helplessness and depression and may generate a setback in psychological and physical well-being. In the case of SLE, for example, depression may be magnified by emotional stress, normal life tensions, and steroid therapy. For this reason, emotional adjustment to the disease and its effects is very important (Lewis 1984).

Sociological Effects.   Disability frequently includes necessary dependence on relatives and professionals. In addition, architectural barriers impact on sociological well-being by preventing access. It is not only the pathology that affects the individual, as the medical model would suggest, but also the physical, social, political, and economic environment that limits choices (DeJong & Lifchez 1983).

Family.   Family members may face life-style changes necessitated by the immobilized member. Altered home life strains all family members by causing adjustments to accustomed routines. Financial concerns are common, and family members may feel frustrated by an inability to meet the special needs of the ill individual.

Family and client may be at odds in their assessments of the role of independent travel as a contributing factor to a healthy adjustment. Members of the family can be fearful, overprotective, or embarrassed to "expose" the client to the world (Welsh & Blasch 1980). Because such fears are real and understandable, health professionals must help the family to overcome their anxieties so they can understand the client's need for independence (see Chapter 8).

Role Changes.   Throughout all life stages, mobility allows individuals the opportunity to take on roles set out for them by society and in this way allows for needs satisfaction. Our American culture reflects its value orientation, social attitudes, and norms through role behaviors centering on wellness, work, individual independence, social justice, and social responsibility.

When mobility is altered, accustomed roles may change or appear to change from a familiar status to a perceived dependent role, creating anxiety and a sense of hopelessness. This change occurs through modified physical and occupational activity and through altered sensory and motor interaction (Olson et al. 1967). Concomitantly, leisure time for the recreational role increases, but with diminished physical ability and energy to expend on recreation. The roles of spouse, parent, sibling, sexual partner, and provider may be altered, reversed, or eliminated.

Altered mobility also influences social mobility since it has consequences of psychological and sociological deprivation that lead to downward movement. In a society that places prime value on the worker role, the nonworker role is generally interpreted as a lesser position, with consequent lowering of status in the societal hierarchy (Olson et al. 1967); the disabled person experiences diminished personal worth.

Sexual Functioning. Mobility changes influence sexual behavior. Depending upon the physiological impact of the chronic disease and its physical effects, the individual may be limited in sexual functioning (see Chapter 10). For example, a decreased range of motion, an inability to assume sexual positions or to shift to another position, or the presence of paralysis may cause the person to perceive his or her body as asexual or undesirable. The loss of visual or auditory acuity may impede the ability to see or hear sexual cues. Physical pain may accompany any movement, or chronic fatigue may hinder sexual interest or arousal. If movement changes greatly, the individual may feel unable to "perform" well sexually. Guilt or fear can result from inability to satisfy self or partner.

Altered mobility of one person has impact on the sexual partner as well. The partner may need a period to adjust to physical differences and may also be affected by psychological reactions the client experiences. The partner may be afraid of causing pain, hesitating to initiate sex or changes in position. A visible mobility aid (braces, wheelchair) may hinder the "sexual overtones" of sexual cues and arousal.

> Pam: It is difficult to express sensual pleasures—intercourse, touching, holding, hand-holding, hugging—when the body hurts. I often feel pain when trying new positions, which is also effected by my limited range of motion. Sjogren's syndrome causes dysfunction of saliva and mucous glands, leaving the vagina excessively dry and painful.
>
> Sexual expression was limited. My husband was afraid to try new things and positions sometimes because of fear he might physically hurt me. I was afraid of trying new things because I might hurt myself or cry out in pain and spoil the mood or feel embarrassed. I am now able to tell my husband, either verbally or through gestures, if I feel like assuming other positions—for I do worry about our sex life being boring.

Aging. The aging process also effects a decrease in mobility. This change in mobility is gradual, often coupled with psychological adjustment to the aging process itself. The aging client may have decreased vision or hearing or be "slowing down," unable to walk long distances, negotiate stairs or uphill grades, or drive an automobile. The possibility of injury from falling restricts mobility. The previously accessible environment may now contain barriers erected by their lessened agility or increased vulnerability to attacks. The elderly may be embarrassed in public situations, feeling that they look older, are less agile, and are not the people they used to be (Welsh & Blasch 1980).

Add a chronic disease to these elements, and the problem is multiplied. Since aging and illness often accompany each other, the elderly person may lose the ability, desire, or encouragement to maintain a previous state of mobility. For example, the fear of falling is a common deterrent to ambulation. Even though most falls do not cause injuries, one fall can be devastating to an individual's pride and confidence (Ham 1984). The case study of Grandpa illustrates the impact of aging and illness on mobility.

◇ C A S E S T U D Y ◇

Aging, Illness, and Mobility Changes

Grandpa's progressively decreasing mobility was first noticed at age 75 with a significant difference in his gait. He was diagnosed as having a partially occluded left femoral artery, diminishing his endurance and distance while walking, causing a discouraging change in his lifestyle.

Grandpa experienced a major stroke at age 84 that interfered with his sense of balance. Transient ischemial attacks (TIAs) occurred occasionally throughout the next nine years. At age 86, Grandpa fell, suffering a fractured hip. During his hospital stay, he progressed to the use of a walker, which he chose to place in the basement after he returned home. Grandpa learned to ambulate with a cane; his movements were cautious and hesitant, overcompensating so he would not fall forward. He progressively became slower and slower.

A few months later Grandpa fractured his pelvis, forcing him to use the walker he so disliked. His pride and confidence interfered with his acceptance of the wheelchair, except when necessary for mobility beyond a short distance; for example, to go to the doctor's office.

At age 92 Grandpa had a minor cerebral vascular accident (CVA), followed by bronchitis. He chose to remain bedridden except to use a commode or to make rare trips outdoors in the wheelchair. He lost strength and agility in his hands and upper body, further limiting him. Although he refused further physical therapy, he continued to maintain control of his personal life. During his remaining years, he felt secure in his environment at his daughter's home.

Barriers: Societal and Architectural. Barriers impede an individual's quality of life; in the broadest sense, they include physiological, psychological, and social difficulties that limit chronically ill persons whose mobility is altered. Depending on perspective, they may be environmental or architectural obstacles only, or they may encompass social attitudes as well. Even when societal and architectural barriers seem to be mutually exclusive, there is a tremendous overlap that affects employment, education, transportation, and social activities.

Attitudes. Of all the barriers that disabled or chronically ill people experience, the strongest and most difficult to eliminate is societal attitudes. One's feelings about oneself are often affected by the attitude of others; one's behavior is ruled by attitudes. Even more so, laws, rules, and even etiquette are governed by individual or group attitudes.

Family attitudes can prevent the client from improving to maximum potential. A study of attitudes of spouses of stroke patients found that the spouses responded primarily with overprotective and unrealistic attitudes, rather than expected feelings of rejection or guilt (Kinsella & Duffy 1980). This re-sponse was usually based on anxiety about the client's condition: sometimes overprotecting was the only way the worried spouse could cope with the situation without being overwhelmed. Although an expression of loving concern, overprotection can impede adjustment because it tends to hinder one's attempts to function independently.

Stigma. Stigma is a reflection of societal attitudes. Often changes in mobility are visible—a different gait, use of walking aids or wheelchair—to others. Since society expects perfection, youth, and beauty (note advertising messages), gaining social acceptance and approval is extremely difficult for an individual who is visibly different. A person who was previously perceived as "normal," "mobile," or "agile" may be avoided, even by acquaintances or friends. People are not always able to ignore external differences (see Chapter 4).

The individual tends to internalize society's stigma (Welsh & Blasch 1980). Even assistive devices may appear to the individual to reflect stigma, as do the ongoing problems associated with fear of falling or losing balance in public or crossing a street before the light changes. This attitude can be further complicated by the need for assistance in certain situations, such as entering inaccessible buildings, boarding a bus, or walking upstairs. When clients lack appropriate or effective communication skills to solicit needed assistance, the feelings of stigma intensify, causing difficulty in accepting offers of help or expressions of curiosity or sympathy.

> Pam: How I felt had a lot to do with social nonacceptance. It is difficult to be a young woman in this society and have a disfiguring but sometimes hidden disability—no one could believe the difficulties I have. They would say things like "you're too young to have arthritis," "you look like you're healthy," "why can't you keep up—all you have are minor aches and pains," and "why are your hands crooked?"

Language Use. The way that people use language reflects their attitudes and perceptions of other people (California Governor's Committee for Employment of the Handicapped 1984). Terms with negative connotations directed to chronically ill persons stigmatize them and influence others' attitudes toward them. When persons who have a chronic illness are described as a "victim" "suffering" with the "tragedy" of a disease or as having "agonizing" pain that "cripples" or "deforms" the body, "confining" them to a wheelchair, they become the object of a negative social stereotype of sorrow and pity (Brady 1984). Society, through its members, then judges and alienates. Self-image and self-esteem drop, and altered mobility becomes a greater handicap. One could even say that the health professional is a "victim" of this insensitivity, "suffering" from terminology that "confines" "cripples" to an "unfortunate affliction," dehumanizing them.

The use of inappropriate language or behavior reflects lack of sensitivity or ignorance. People often have difficulty speaking to someone with altered mobility. This difficulty becomes apparent when conversation is directed through a third person or through comments such as "How well you look" when the person looks and feels awful. Ignorance is apparent when one assumes that being in a wheelchair means paralysis without other physical problems (Gould 1982).

Environmental and Architectural Barriers. Stairs, narrow doorways, inclines, and lack of visual or auditory cues are architectural barriers. These barriers not only are safety hazards for people with altered mobility but are obstacles that limit their quality of life: restricting their opportunities, limiting their choices, and increasing their dependency.

Architectural barriers also compound the problems of gaining adequate housing. Choices are limited when apartments or houses have lengthy entrance stairways, when heavy security doors may be locked or impossible to pull open, or when tall cabinets are difficult to reach.

Van de Ven's study of lower limb amputees (1982) observed that individuals who used wheelchairs encountered many architectural barriers. Most subjects lived in homes with steps leading outdoors that restricted access to their external environment; several subjects lived in homes that had steps indoors. Indoor mobility was further impeded by narrow corridors and doorways. Of those who used prostheses, few were able to successfully negotiate the environment that included steps and other architectural barriers.

Social mobility is limited by architectural barriers. Travel can be difficult, requiring an accessible mode that is not overly fatiguing. When lodging is necessary or desired, it must be accommodating. Facilities that have stairs, limited bathroom space, or unmaneuverable water faucets prevent use. Attendance at many functions is difficult and therefore avoided by persons who do not own a car, do not live near a bus route or bus stop, or live where bus service stops too early. Seating arrangements might not allow for wheelchairs or provide room for storing a walker or crutches. Social life with friends is also impacted when the friend's home has many stairs or a bathroom lacking devices for allowing the person to sit down on or rise from the toilet or use the water faucet.

> Pam: Architecture is a real physical barrier; the wheelchair disabled aren't the only "cripples" who face architectural barriers. Doors, curbs, car doors, opening jars, turning keys, eating (holding utensils), cooking, dressing, driving—*everything* is difficult

when you have pain everywhere and arthritis makes it harder to do everything.

Transportation. For people accustomed to driving a car, being unable to drive can be very difficult to accept and limits their participation in activities, thus affecting their social esteem and self-concept (Welsh & Blasch 1980). The advent of hand controls, special mirrors, automatic shifts, and other devices, as well as necessary training, now makes automobile driving accessible to many (but not all) people with altered mobility.

Public transportation is a necessity for many, yet is not always accommodating. Limitations include lines that are not reachable, infrequent schedules, limited routes, early termination, and lengthy travel. Without wheelchair lifts, many buses have limited accessibility. Other people are restricted because they use devices that impede use of public transport or must depend on others for assistance.

> Pam: It is very difficult to handle money for public transportation like buses or the rapid transit system. The usual public routes are not very helpful for me. Standing is very tiring, and bus stops usually have no benches to sit on or shelter from the weather. When no seats are available on the bus or train, it is difficult for me to hold on to handles; I am embarrassed to ask for a handicapped seat because my disability is almost invisible. I'm able to get around only because I drive an automatic car.

Impact of Barriers. Employment and education are prime examples of the impact of barriers on individuals and their families. Employment is limited when a person cannot enter an employment site because of stairs or toilet stalls that are difficult to use. Because of altered mobility, an individual may not be able to accomplish a task as rapidly as coworkers or may need someone else to read work material. Since transportation to the workplace is necessary for most people, those persons who can no longer drive or use a bus because there is no lift are prevented from gaining self-esteem through being employed.

Also limiting are the attitudes of employers, many of whom still believe in the myths that discredit the abilities and skills of disabled persons to function in the workplace. Employers have been known to discriminate against a person who uses a wheelchair or guide dog. Employers often feel that accommodating altered mobility is expensive or that having a disabled person on the payroll will increase their insurance premiums.

On the positive side, the growing role of computerization has had a positive impact on creating home-based employment. Positive change will continue with ongoing input and involvement from physically disabled persons who help create avenues to reach into the business community.

Formal education is carried out at various schools, public and private. Getting an education has been a cherished expectation in America, one that is considered available to all citizens. Because of architectural barriers and social attitudes, many individuals with altered mobility have found the educational process barred to them. Current federal and state laws now mandate equal access to education, requiring accommodations for mobility differences and demanding high-quality teaching to allow disabled persons to learn and to progress. Nevertheless, many schools and campuses still have numerous architectural barriers that impede access to classes and facilities. And stigma that adversely impacts on the disabled person who wants to learn still prevails.

> Pam: Notetaking was hard, as was getting around campus and into classes. I was afraid to ask for help because I thought my disability was not bad enough. I was initially advised to major in business administration because I was told that this was something that could get me a job behind a desk, since I "would probably be in a wheelchair." These courses were easier for me but were not mentally challenging.

Much work has been done to improve these obstacles, through the national efforts of the disabled population and their fight for a barrier-free life (DeJong & Lifchez 1983). Some of that progress is reflected in federal and state legislation such as the Architectural Barriers Act of 1968 and the Rehabilitation Act of 1973. However, barriers still exist, and laws often are nonexistent or are not enforced.

Interventions for the Client with Altered Mobility

The major goal of the health care practitioner is to help the client gain maximum mobility. This requires initial and ongoing detailed assessment of physiological, psychosocial, and environmental factors that limit mobility. Assessment should also consider positive steps that can be integrated into any plans that are developed.

Coping with altered mobility depends on many elements that are not always considered in early stages of disability management: health, accommodations, family, outside support, finances, and individual motivation. For example, Van de Ven (1982) notes that it seems foolish to fit individuals with prostheses if they cannot put them on and live alone or are confronted with unmanageable stairs inside the home. The client who becomes exhausted by the effort to get to a physical therapy clinic finds the time spent there far from productive (Burnfield & Burnfield 1982). Assessment would indicate the need for a physical therapist who makes home visits so that therapy can be provided to a more energetic client.

Realistic treatment goals should be developed. Goal setting should take into account the client's objectives and set a series of successive goals on which success can be built. For example, the homebound client may wish to walk around the block. First, the professional needs to note the environment, as well as the client's stamina, agility, and self-confidence in walking. Properly fitted walking aids may need to be incorporated in the plan. The client may first need to increase stamina within living quarters, and furniture arrangements may have to be altered. Then compensation is made for stairs or other impeding barriers. Finally, the client will be able to focus attention on the energy necessary to walk around the block.

Interventions should focus on correcting or compensating for daily problems: physical limitations, barriers in the environment, and psychosocial components of living. Health professionals already have a large repertoire of interventions at their disposal or easily available in texts (medical-surgical, rehabil-

itation, psychology or psychiatry, and so forth) to assist the client and family. Although some specific interventions are discussed here, the major thrust of this section is to suggest ways in which the health professional can increase self-awareness in order to find creative ways of improving client mobility or quality of life.

Dealing with Physiological Aspects of Altered Mobility

As we have seen, the most complete form of altered mobility is long-term bedrest, which impacts on most body systems as well as on psychological well-being. Interventions for the problems of bedrest (Olson et al. 1967) are summarized in Table 5-2. Regardless of which body system is affected, adequate fluids and some kind of movement (range of motion, turning, sitting up, or ambulating) are essential to reverse adverse effects. Other interventions are more specific to the system involved.

Most chronically ill individuals, however, are relatively mobile except when their diseases require restrictions. Even those having permanent disabilities tend to use crutches or wheelchairs or to be ambulatory in a modified way. It is beyond the scope of one chapter to deal effectively with the many ways to compensate for musculoskeletal limitations. Here again, the health professional should consult the rehabilitation literature to address specific needs or should plan interventions with those specialists who have the expertise to maximize mobility.

Regardless of whether physical limitations manifest themselves during intermittent, progressive, or permanent levels of change, interventions should be geared to maintaining function and maximizing the home environment. The health professional should remember that most people are creative in meeting their own mobility needs; given time and opportunity, they develop satisfactory ways of managing obstacles. Teaching, resources, and equipment should be provided to meet physical and emotional needs, but their ultimate utilization depends on client and family interpretation, layout of the home, preferred life-styles, and coping and adaptation skills.

TABLE 5-2. Interventions to Avoid Complications from Bedrest

Cardiovascular
1. Position changes, including from horizontal to vertical, alter intravascular pressure and stimulate neural reflexes, which help prevent orthostatic hypotension.
2. *Progressive* activity and exercise, including active or passive range of motion, isometrics, and so on, prevent loss of muscle tone and improve flow of blood to the heart.
3. The Valsalva maneuver should be avoided when moving.
4. Adequate fluids prevent hypercoagulability.

Pulmonary
1. Accurate periodic observation of respiratory function (rate, depth, accessory muscles, neurological signs, hypoxia signs) is preventive.
2. Increased activity helps move secretions. Activity includes activities of daily living and position changes (including the upright position if possible).
3. Routine turning, coughing, and deep breathing benefit chest and lung expansion, move secretions, and facilitate gas exchange.
4. Increased fluids thin secretions.

Musculoskeletal
1. Weight bearing and muscle movement help increase osteoblastic activity and lessen decalcification. Increased calcium is not recommended since it ends up excreted in urine or deposited in muscles and joints.
2. A functional position should be maintained. Hip and knee flexion should be avoided (no pillows or gatch). A firm mattress, bed or foot board, shoes, padded splints help maintain body alignment.
3. Range of motion, position changes, and exercise prevent contractures.
4. Regular turning and skin care help prevent decubitus ulcers; alcohol (drying) or doughnuts (decreases circulation) should not be used. Toilet schedules help decrease incontinence, which contributes to skin breakdown. Maintaining healthy tissue or regeneration of damaged tissue requires adequate protein, carbohydrates, and fats in the diet.
5. If ulcers form, infections should be prevented and healing measures instituted promptly.
6. Teaching the client to shift body weight, perform range of motion, and so forth, assists in prevention.

Genitourinary
1. Activity (exercises, turning, ambulation, positioning) helps prevent urinary stasis.
2. If incontinence occurs, a check for bladder distention should be done; normal urination is facilitated if women sit and men stand to void.
3. Adequate fluid intake must be maintained to keep urine dilute, limit precipitates, and decrease stasis. Recording intake and output may be necessary.
4. An acid-ash diet will lower the urine pH. Cranberry juice also decreases the pH. Low calcium intake helps decrease stone formation.
5. If catheterization is necessary, in and out catheterizations every 6 to 8 hours leads to fewer infections than a Foley catheter. Scrupulous aseptic technique should be maintained for any catheterization.

Gastrointestinal
1. Sufficient nutrient intake maintains the basal metabolic rate and compensates for catabolism. Diet should have increased protein (overcomes protein breakdown) with adequate amounts of carbohydrates and fats.
2. Small frequent feedings that include liked foods compensate for anorexia.
3. Stress and tension reduction techniques help alleviate parasympathetic nerve stimulation.
4. Food with bulk and cellulose material (bran, prune juice) help elimination. Stool softeners or gentle digital stimulation may be necessary to maintain bowel habits or decrease straining at stool. Regular use of enemas and laxatives is not recommended.
5. Adequate fluids stimulate reflex activity and provide enough water in the feces.
6. Prior bowel habits should be incorporated into nursing care plan (most people defecate after meals). Adequate time should be allowed for defecation and if possible a position that promotes evacuation should be assumed; the environment should be modified to provide privacy.
7. Exercises can strengthen abdominal muscles.

TABLE 5-2. Continued.

Metabolism
1. Sitting up or having the head of the bed elevated helps alleviate many of the basal metabolic and hormonal level changes.
2. Minimal but adequate bedcovering enhances body heat loss.
3. Increased fluid intake and high protein nutrition hasten healing and help maintain electrolyte balance.
4. Range of motion, exercise, and weight bearing prevent atrophy and help limit elevated serum calcium levels.
5. Stress reduction helps maintain metabolic homeostasis.

Psychosocial
1. Reminders about reality, clocks, calendars, and so forth help maintain orientation.
2. Planning and participating in care promote independence and a sense of control.
3. Increased sensory stimulation and physical activity provide spatial mobility, help reconstruct body image and ego identity, and enhance roles.
4. Promoting independence stimulates physiologic and psychologic mobility.

Summarized from Olson et al. (1967).

People who have difficulty in walking frequently develop creative ways of ambulating. Unless another method is simpler or safer, the method used should not be discouraged. Ascending and descending stairs in the traditional fashion may not be possible in light of pain or hip and knee contractures. Some individuals can descend stairs only by grabbing the railing with two hands and going down backward.

Getting into and out of bed can also be difficult. A variety of home adaptations are usually devised by clients or their family, such as the use of an adjacent door or a strap attached to a radiator or headboard. If their own techniques for bed mobility are safe and satisfactory, a more traditional method (such as an overhead trapeze) need not be utilized. For example, an 85-year-old woman having bilaterally fused hips from previous inflammatory arthritis uses a belt attached to the headboard to pull herself onto her four-poster bed. She gets out of bed by wiggling on her back to the edge of the bed so that her knees extend over the side and then digging a cane into the mattress to thrust herself upright (Liang et al. 1983).

Since grooming can enhance one's self-esteem, professionals should intervene to encourage such self-care. This in turn creates a willingness to interact with others or be seen in public. A shower seat and a spray hose may facilitate bathing, and support in getting into and out of the tub or shower can be attained by use of a hand rail and a nonskid mat. The psychological benefits of dressing oneself each day should not be overlooked because it provides exercise and promotes a sense of independence and purpose.

Aids for Sensory Impairment. Professionals should become sensitive to the stigma of visual and auditory impairment. They should be informed about causative diseases and preventive measures and about services available to those who need them. The ability to interact effectively with those experiencing sensory loss is another essential quality for professionals in human service settings (Welsh & Blasch 1980). Teaching and modifying the environment are two ways in which the health care provider can best assist with sensory problems.

For people with visual impairment, many services to help in the performance of daily living skills are available, especially in major metropolitan areas. In fact, formalized instruction in independent mobility travel is more extensively developed for visually impaired people than for any other disability group (Welsh & Blasch 1980). Information about such services should be provided, and client and family should be encouraged to use them.

When an individual has partial vision, improved lighting, especially floor lighting, helps reduce falls or other home accidents. Steps with edging colors, vibrant contrasting colors to mark changes in height or location, or enlarged size of lettering can alert that person to surroundings and thus enhance mobility.

For general safety with any degree of visual impairment, it is necessary to reduce the hazards of loose rugs, telephone cords, and waxed or wet floors. Tactile or auditory interventions generally are useful. Tactile aids include raised lettering or braille to designate doorways, business locations, elevator floors, and so on. Auditory information can be provided by a sound system, such as bells to sound alarms.

Interventions to compensate for hearing loss increase willingness to initiate independent travel in public places, thereby increasing mobility. Effective interventions require attracting the attention of those with auditory impairments through visual cues (blinking lights and hand and facial gestures) and tactile cues (touching the individual to gain attention or creating vibratory contact through pounding on a table or floor). General measures include facing the auditorily impaired person to allow him or her to focus attention on the speaker's face and gestures. Speech should be natural but slow, although not too slow. Care providers should enunciate clearly but without exaggeration, using simple terms and short sentences. When writing any kind of notes, professionals must use simple language, since impaired individuals may have only limited understanding of written language.

Hearing aids, although helpful, can create problems. Although sounds are amplified, the ability to make sense of these sounds requires a new mode of concentration (Liang et al. 1983). The health professional and family should encourage the patience necessary to master the use of hearing aids.

Interventions for Pain and Loss of Energy. The client must learn that chronic pain may not be correctable and that depleted energy may never be regained. However, some interventions or actions can help decrease pain or increase energy sufficiently to enhance mobility.

Pain.   The health professional must learn to listen actively to the client's description of the type and quality of experienced pain in order to take effective action (McCaffery 1979), especially when analgesics (narcotic and nonnarcotic) are to be used. People are more receptive to suggested interventions when they feel that the health provider is genuinely interested in seeking joint solutions (Mooney 1982). For example, arthritic pain varies, as do individuals having arthritis. Pain management requires individualized interventions.

In research on endorphins and their action in relieving pain, West (1981) points out that many of the traditional nursing techniques of comfort may indeed have physiological as well as psychological effects. Specific comfort techniques, such as relaxation, positioning, massage, acupressure, and distraction stimulate endorphin release, providing pain relief (West 1981; Lewis 1984). Thus, these time-honored comfort techniques are now proved to be physiologically sound as well.

When pain is severe, the client tends to become less active in an effort for control. Inactivity increases fatigue, weakens muscles, stiffens joints, and decreases circulation (Lewis 1984). Unless bedrest is medically necessary, the client must be as mobile as possible. When pain is responsive to analgesics, they should be used appropriately to decrease the fear or anxiety that accompanies pain (McCaffery 1979). This should be done in conjunction with the comfort measures discussed previously. When specific medications, such as antiinflammatory drugs for arthritis, can ease pain, they should be used.

Some disorders, such as arthritis, are characterized by pain associated with even simple tasks such as using the toilet, turning in bed, or moving a hand. Except during exacerbations, a properly designed and implemented exercise program should be followed to help keep joints flexible, maintain muscle strength, and build overall stamina (Becker 1984). Such general conditioning and maintenance can be accomplished by frequent repetitions of normal activities within the energy and comfort limits of the person. This process can include walking or performing simple exercises such as raising the arms and straightening the legs (Liang et al. 1983). Exercise helps to develop a more positive mental attitude by improving self-image and reinforcing a sense of worth (Becker 1984).

When hospitalization becomes necessary, successful home medication routines that control pain should continue. Such regimens can differ from the hospital's scheduled medication times, but the staff should nevertheless integrate these proven methods into their plan of care for the client, with the physician's approval as necessary (Mooney 1982). Such actions do not release the nurses from their responsibilities to ensure that medications are taken properly and regularly.

Loss of Energy. Clients must understand that energy loss frequently accompanies many diseases and that different disease processes have different bases for energy loss. Fatigue usually demands an altered lifestyle, requires a conscious effort to assess one's own energy flow, and demands learning how to balance fatigue and needed rest with activities.

When energy is affected by long-term decreased cardiac output or oxygen intake, strategies should limit any decrease in functional capacity. When medically possible, energy should be rebuilt by progressive increments of activity. An initial program may involve walking slowly each day, gradually increasing the distance for improved exercise tolerance. Riding a tricycle is a form of exercise that also serves as a mode of transportation in accomplishing errands. Meals should be eaten at the table with the family, rather than in bed, and the client should dress each day. These techniques enhance self-esteem as well as increasing activity. In the home, walking should take precedence over using a wheelchair.

For energy that is decreased by inflammatory processes, rest and prescribed medications can reduce the inflammation. Complete bedrest is needed only during disease activity. After a flare-up, average daily activities should resume slowly, guided by attention to the body's response. Allow time to adjust: a few months may be necessary for resuming all previous activity levels. The client should be attentive to fatigue as a signal to rest and not overexert, maintaining a regular schedule to provide a structure for monitoring activity and rest. Even when an individual

is bedridden, some types of exercises should be maintained (Lewis 1984).

Various energy conservation techniques provide methods for coping with energy loss (*National Arthritis News* 1984). Physical therapists can serve as resources for teaching and implementing the following techniques:

1. Exercise program: for strengthening muscles and increasing range of motion.
2. Pacing: avoid overactivity when feeling good, since it can increase pain and fatigue.
3. Modifications: adapt the environment by various means such as constructing ramps, rearranging frequently used rooms, utilizing assistive devices.
4. Body awareness: be attentive to body and energy levels. Plan around times of high energy for tasks and low energy for rest periods.
5. Be realistic: since frustration results from not acknowledging limitations, develop activity alternatives.
6. Teaching others: educate support persons about fatigue and its effects.

Overcoming Barriers

The presence of barriers, both physical and social, impacts adversely on many individuals with mobility problems. These people want to interact with society, and barriers make such interactions difficult. The professional who is not a rehabilitation counselor or therapist can help these clients by developing a sensitivity to barriers. In this way, the professional can become an advocate by encouraging agencies to move toward greater accessibility and finding creative and workable alternatives for the client and other pertinent individuals.

The professional has a responsibility for advocacy. This requires a genuine empathy to the client's status, physically and psychosocially. Many disabled people have become politically active to obtain changes in relation to all barriers and to achieve recognition as valued citizens who can contribute to society constructively and meaningfully (DeJong & Lifchez 1983). The professional needs to initiate advocacy projects by becoming knowledgeable about their impact on clients (see Chapter 13) and supporting client self-help and advocacy groups.

Environmental Barriers. Many interventions specific to environmental or architectural barriers have already been addressed. There are many other possible interventions, but addressing them all is beyond the scope of this chapter.

Awareness of the multiple aspects of barriers is enhanced by the health professional's developing insight into the difficulties that barriers produce. Developing sensitivity to such barriers is best accomplished by personally experiencing mobility problems. One can simulate situations limiting one's mobility in several ways. Although a simulated experience provides a limited perspective on living with disabilities, it does give some insight into the emotional as well as the physical barriers that many individuals confront. Health professionals can try the activities suggested here during their normal daily routines.

Increasing awareness of sensory deprivation could be accomplished by wearing a blindfold or glasses that do not fit one's own prescription. Ear plugs that block out most auditory input are available. Finger movement and tactile input can be restricted by mittens or gloves that are oversize and bulky. Limiting upper-body mobility could be accomplished by handcuffs or a sling; the lower body can be restricted by crutch travel. Using a wheelchair in the work environment or a favorite restaurant enhances one's awareness of obstacles and the attitudes the user encounters.

Once health professionals have experienced these obstacles and the responses they engender in ill persons and those they encounter, sincere empathy and understanding in their interactions with affected individuals come more readily and meaningful alterations for the client follow. In the home this may mean access to other rooms or the outside: ramps, wider doors, reachable shelves, handrails on stairways, and so forth. For example, a woman with decreasing mobility from osteoarthritis and hypertension found herself forced to consider a move to a more functional apartment on the second floor of her building. This move would mean that she no longer could go outside, further reducing her incentive to remain active. Aware of difficulties that she would encounter in a second-floor unit, a health professional initiated efforts to adapt her current apartment to her needs by providing a raised toilet seat, bathroom hand bars, raised chair blocks, and so on.

Outside the home, barriers restrict access to the rest of the world. Effecting change in these areas often requires adopting the role of advocate for the client: lobbying for ramps where even one step prevents entrance, having doors widened, altering bathroom space to accommodate a wheelchair, or placing some water fountains at an accessible height. Continued advocacy by health professionals can further support and enforce such adaptations.

Social Barriers. The greatest degree of sensitization must be achieved in the area of social barriers. Sensitivity includes an awareness of the attitudes the professional projects to clients. Language reinforces our perceptions of people (California Governor's Committee for Employment of the Handicapped 1984), and words with negative connotations carry negative expectations and attitudes. Professionals should listen to what they are saying, hearing their words and tone of voice, being alert to subtle implications that stigmatize. Others, including nonmedical professionals, family, friends, and acquaintances, imitate the language used by health professionals, who are seen as role models. Words that contain negative inferences present a model of negative attitudes, subtly reinforcing stigma. Care in choosing words and developing techniques to alert and educate peers about their language use helps deter unhealthy attitudes.

Psychosocial Interventions

Any program of care should clearly address the psychosocial needs of clients and their significant others (Baum & Rothschild 1983), to make these needs more manageable and less overwhelming. The health professional already has, or can attain, a number of skills to assist the client with many of the adaptations necessary in chronic illness.

Dealing with Psychological Difficulties. People have different coping styles (Walker & Lattanzi 1982) and adjust at individual rates appropriate to them. The health professional should encourage clients to be responsible for their own courses of adjustment. Positive support includes acknowledging that adjustment is hard work. A willingness to listen to the client conveys that the professional recognizes feelings of depression and helplessness but is not trying to change these feelings. For example, it is not helpful to say "You just have to accept it" or "It will be all right," when the client is not feeling that way.

Since feelings of insecurity and worthlessness often surface when a person is coping with mobility alterations, the health professional should nurture the individual's self-confidence. A positive, realistic perception of abilities as well as limitations can support self-confidence. Focusing on physical limitations can become frustrating and overwhelming, yet it is part of the adjustment process.

Coping with Social Problems. Prior roles may no longer be possible or may be drastically altered. A change in employment, responsibilities, or home life may be necessary. Rehabilitation assists the client and family in establishing a new life-style (Lewis 1984) by providing information related to mobility accommodations and offering emotional support. A positive perspective of fulfilling certain role responsibilities may also enhance a feeling of self-worth and meaning.

Coping with social problems caused by mobility differences demands that clients clearly communicate their own needs and abilities (Apple, Apple, & Blasch 1980; Welsh 1980). Since social attitudes toward people with altered mobility tend to be negative and misinformed, assertive communication by the client provides accurate and useful information. The professional can encourage such "assertiveness training"; such self-advocacy becomes a needed role and influences the attitudes surrounding the individual.

Clients may need encouragement to be socially active. Perhaps their old social roles have been altered by their mobility changes; or they may be isolated and need to develop new relationships. It is important to be sensitive to their feelings of readiness; social interaction can be encouraged but not pushed. Being able to communicate mobility difficulties effectively facilitates social interaction. Such communication can sometimes be enhanced by dialogue with others in similar situations.

Family. The client's entire network of caring others requires support. Developing a realistic understanding of the client's limits, abilities, and goals assists these individuals in working together cohesively. A proper assessment of the family situation and the emotional status of significant others can facilitate meeting their needs as a unit.

Roles within the family may change as a result of the client's situation or new responsibilities may be necessary to ensure family harmony. Each individual within the family may have a unique style of adjusting; their various styles may not progress in a similar manner or time frame. Respite time may be advisable, providing family members a change from responsibilities that may seem overwhelming (see Chapter 8). The financial situation may be burdensome and may create tremendous anxiety; referral to assistance such as an appropriate agency might be helpful. Spiritual affiliations should not be overlooked; support from a minister, priest, or rabbi or a church community may accelerate psychological and social adjustment.

Aging Client. Caring for older clients requires sensitivity to meet their basic human needs as well as the needs produced by a chronic condition. Professionals must become aware of their own aging process, identifying and anticipating needs. This awareness is transferred to the aging client by increased empathy.

Research by Rosenbloom (1982) indicates that many individuals who are elderly tend to view the gradual loss of mobility functions as an expected part of aging. Accepting this loss as inevitable, they are less likely to seek assistance or communicate their needs effectively. Yet older clients merit the same sensitivity and advocacy interventions as are given to younger ones. Health professionals must not assume that aging people do not need rehabilitation or will not benefit from it and must not overlook appropriate interventions or treatment.

Other Interventions

Support Groups.   Health care providers should encourage clients to create and nurture their own support groups (*National Arthritis News* 1984). By talking about their problems, individuals who are physically disabled overcome fear of the unknown and find compatible life-styles, satisfaction, and an extension of their productive years (Marsh et al. 1983). Relationship mending occurs, and employment opportunities are extended. They learn to educate others as well as themselves about their chronic illnesses and ensuing mobility difficulties.

> Pam: Support groups showed me I was not alone in my pains—emotional and physical—by grouping me with others who had the same disease. Different people react differently to the same disease. I met a young woman my age who had JA as long as I, and I realized that we had different concerns as young women with arthritis: childbirth/rearing, dating, sexual relations, and so on.
>
> You learn a lot about yourself in a support group. I learned to take responsibility for my own health care, along with the health professional, and to live with daily activities more easily. Sharing showed that we are all individuals and have control over our lives and how we choose to cope with pain and disability.

Outside Resources.   One final suggestion to help those with mobility problems is to utilize the many helpful agencies that exist outside the health profession. These agencies offer advocacy and additional means of support that are beneficial. The informed professional can be the hub of a wheel of resources by eliciting the skills and expertise within their own community (see Chapter 16). The following is a partial list of agencies that work with mobility difficulties:

- Support organizations (American Cancer Society, American Heart Association, Arthritis Foundation, MS Society, United Cerebral Palsy, and others)
- Associations of the Physically Handicapped
- Independent Living Programs
- Deaf Advocacy Programs
- National Federation of the Blind
- Department of Vocational Rehabilitation
- Senior Services Centers
- City and County Social Services Departments

Summary and Conclusions

Activity is part of everyday life. Disease states alter mobility adversely. The professional thinks of these alterations as affecting primarily the musculoskeletal system and leading to bedrest. Bedrest is often effective for acute illness, but in chronic illness, bedrest usually is a temporary state; mobility tends to follow several patterns: intermittent, progressive, permanent, or a combination of these patterns. Mobility can also be lost by indirect alterations of the external structure of the body. Visual loss, hearing loss, pain, and depleted energy also hinder mobility.

Of greater concern, the individual with a mobility alteration has problems that transcend the disease state. A goodly number of psychological and sociological adjustments become necessary. Psychologically the individual must handle loss (sometimes again and again), face changes in self-image (body image and self-esteem), and overcome fear and stress. Sociologically, client and family face a myriad of problems. Families and clients may experience role and life-style changes and need to face and resolve differences in perspective. The aging members of our society encounter the double problems of mobility changes, those of aging overlaid with chronic illness.

Barriers, both social and environmental, impede the individual from gaining maximum mobility. Physical barriers include steps, inadequate facilities within buildings, and so forth. In overcoming these barriers, the disabled have led the way in gaining change through legislative action. But the greatest impediment continues to be the attitudes of others, including health care providers. Negative attitudes, often verbally expressed by choice of language, create stigma that handicaps the chronically ill.

Many available interventions are known to the health care provider or readily accessible through sources such as rehabilitation texts. Some of the specifics discussed relate to visual and hearing loss, pain, energy depletion, and ways of overcoming barriers.

The health professional needs to develop insight into problems created by loss of mobility, best accomplished by sensitizing oneself through experiencing, even for a short while, some of the difficulties caused by limited mobility. Health professionals also need to become sensitive to their own attitudes, which often manifest as stigmatizing behavior and language. Given that health care providers are often seen as role models, they must observe the stricture "Know thyself." In this way, they treat the *person*, not the disease!

STUDY QUESTIONS

1. What are the primary concerns of clients and significant others among the problems that result from altered mobility?
2. Which physiological systems are affected by bedrest? Describe these effects.
3. How would you describe the patterns that characterize mobility alterations? Select a chronic medical condition. How does this condition "fit" into these patterns?
4. What are the major psychological areas that impact on a person having altered mobility? Describe the way this individual is affected.
5. What are the major sociological barriers resulting from altered mobility? How many can you identify? What are the effects of these barriers?
6. How can the health care practitioner help the client having altered mobility meet some of the physiological, psychological, social, and environmental limi-

tations that are present? How can the health provider help clients meet their own mobility needs creatively?
7. What interventions are common to all the problems of bedrest? Which are specific to individual systems?
8. What interventions can help to satisfy the needs of the sensorily impaired? Discuss some.
9. How do pain and loss of energy affect mobility? What interventions help management of pain or energy loss?
10. In what ways can the health professional develop sensitivity to barriers the immobile person faces? In what way would such sensitivity help the individual? family? society?
11. What skills in the health professional's repertoire assist the client in adapting and adjusting to changes in life-style? in meeting psychosocial needs?

References

Apple, M. M., Apple, L. E., and Blasch, D., (1980) Low vision, in Welsh, R. L., and Blasch, B. B. (eds.), *Foundations of Orientation and Mobility*, New York: American Foundation for the Blind

Asher, R., (1983) The dangers of going to bed, *Critical Care Update*, 10(5):40–41

Baum, H. M., and Rothschild, B. B., (1983) Multiple sclerosis and mobility restriction, *Archives of Physical Medicine and Rehabilitation*, 64(12):591–596

Becker, M., (1984) Therapist tells arthritics to exercise regularly, *Physical Therapy Forum*, Sept. 12

Booz, Allen, and Hamilton, (1980) National Analysts Division, Executive Summary: *Prevailing Incidence and Costs of Multiple Sclerosis: A National Study*

Brackett, T. O., Condon, N., Kindelan, K. M., and Bassett, L., (1984) The emotional care of a person with a spinal cord injury, *Journal of American Medical Association*, 252(6):793–795

Brady, T. J., (1984) Arthritis has an image problem, *National Arthritis News*, 5(2):4

Brown, E. L., (1978) Psychosocial needs of the aged: What nurses can do, in Seymour, E. (ed.), *Psychosocial Need of the Aged: A Health Care Perspective*, Los Angeles: The University of Southern California Press

Burnfield, A., and Burnfield, P., (1982) Psychological aspects of multiple sclerosis, *Physiotherapy*, 68(5):149–150

California Governor's Committee for Employment of the Handicapped, (1984) *Language Guide on Disability*, CA. GCEH-3, Sacramento, Employment Development Department

Campbell, A. J., Reinken, J., Allan, B. C., and Martinez, G. S., (1981) Falls in old age: A study of frequency and related clinical factors, *Age and Aging*, 10:264

Convertino, V., Hung, J., Goldwater, D., and DeBusk, R., (1983) Cardiovascular responses to exercise in middle-aged men after ten days of bedrest, *Circulation*, 68(2):245–250

Counte, M. A., Bieliauskas, L. A., and Pavlou, M., (1983) Stress and personal attitudes in chronic illnesses, *Archives of Physical Medicine and Rehabilitation*, 64(6):272–275

DeJong, G., and Lifchez, R., (1983) Physical disability and public policy, *Scientific American*, 248(6):40–49

Dunlop, B. D., (1980) Expanded home-based care for the elderly: Solution or pipe dream? *American Journal of Public Health*, 70:514–519

Earle, J. R., Perricone, P. J., Maultsby, D. M., Perricone, N., Turner, R. A., and Davis, J., (1979) Psycho-social adjustment of rheumatoid arthritis patients from two alternative treatment settings, *Journal of Rheumatology*, 6(1):80–87

Emerson, D. L., (1981) Facing loss of vision: The response of adults to visual impairment, *Journal of Visual Impairment and Blindness*, 75(2):41–45

Fatigue: The hidden disability, (1984) *National Arthritis News*, 5(2):8

Genesky, S., (1981) Data concerning the partially sighted and the functionally blind, *Visual Impairment and Blindness*, 72:177

Goldman, R., (1977) Rest: Its use and abuse in the aged, *Journal of American Geriatrics Society*, 25(10):433–438

Gould, J., (1982) Disabilities and how to live with them: Multiple sclerosis, *Lancet*, November 27, pp. 1208–1210

Greenleaf, J., and Kozlowski, S., (1982) Physiological consequences of reduced physical activity during bed rest, *Exercise and Sport Sciences Review*, 10:84–119

Ham, R. J., (1984) Problems of rehabilitation: Many can be prevented, *Generations: Quarterly Journal of the Western Gerontological Society*, VIII(4):14–17

Hathaway, G., (1984) The child with sickle cell anemia: Implications and management, *Nurse Practitioner*, 9:16–20

Hughes, S. L., Cordray, D. S., and Spiker, V. A., (1982) Evaluation of a long term home care program, *Working Paper #62*, Evanston, Ill.: Northwestern University

Jacox, I. K., (1979) Assessing pain, *American Journal of Nursing*, 79(5):895–900

Kinsella, G. J., and Duffy, F. D., (1980) Attitudes towards disability expressed by spouses of stroke patients, *Scandinavian Journal of Rehabilitative Medicine*, 12(2):73–76

Lattanzi, M., (1983) Coping skills: Working with grief, a workshop, Oakland, Calif., December 6

Lentz, M., (1981) Selected aspects of deconditioning secondary to immobilization, *Nursing Clinics of North America*, 16(4):729–737

Lewis, K. S., (1984) Systemic lupus erythematosus: The great masquerader, *Nurse Practitioner*, 9(8):13–22

Liang, M. H., Partridge, A. J., Gall, V., and Eaton, H., (1983) Management of functional disability in homebound patients, *Journal of Family Practice*, 17(3):429–435

Liang, M. H., Partridge, A. J., Larson, M., and Gall, V., (1982) An evaluation of stepped-up rehabilitation for homebound elderly with musculoskeletal disability: A preliminary report, *Clinical Research*, 30:302A

Liang, M., Partridge, A. S., Larson, M. G., Gall, V., Taylor, J., Berkman, C., Master, R., Feltin, M., and Taylor, J. (1984) Evaluation of comprehensive rehabilitation services for elderly homebound patients with arthritis and orthopedic disability, *Arthritis and Rheumatism*, 27(3):258–266

Liang, M., Philips, E., Scamman, M., Lurye, C. A., Keith, A., Cohen, L., and Taylor, G., (1981) Evaluation of a pilot program for rheumatic disability in an urban community, *Arthritis and Rheumatism*, 24:937–943

Marsh, G. G., Ellison, G. W., and Strite, C., (1983) Psychosocial and vocational rehabilitation approaches to multiple sclerosis, *Annual Review of Rehabilitation*, 3:242–267

McCaffery, M., (1979) *Nursing Management of the Patient with Pain* (2d ed.), Philadelphia: Lippincott

McDonald, G., and Hudson, L., (1982) Important aspects of pulmonary rehabilitation, *Geriatrics*, 37(3):12

Mentzer, W. M., and Wang, W., (1980) Sickle cell disease: Pathophysiology and diagnosis, *Pediatric Annals*, 9:287

Mooney, N. G., (1982) Coping with chronic pain in rheumatoid arthritis: Patient behaviors and nursing interventions, *Orthopedic Nursing Journal*, 1(3):21–25

National Arthritis News, (1984) Arthritis Foundation, National Office, Atlanta, Ga.

Olson, E., et al. (1967) The hazards of immobility, *American Journal of Nursing*, 67(4):779–796

Pavlou, M., and Counte, M., (1982) Cognitive aspects of coping in multiple sclerosis, *Rehabilitation Counseling Bulletin*, 25(3):138–145

Pick, H. L., Jr., (1980) Perception, locomotion, and orientation, in Welsh, R. L., and Blasch, B. (eds.), *Foundations of Orientation and Mobility*, New York: American Foundation for the Blind

Report to the Chairman of the Committee on Labor and Human Resources, United States Senate, *The Elderly Should Benefit From Expanded Home Health Care But Increasing These Services Will Not Insure Cost Reduction*, (1982) *GAO/IPE-83-1*, Gaithersburg, Md.

Rieser, J. J., Guth, D. A., and Hill, E. W., (1982) Mental processes mediating independent travel: Implications for orientation and mobility, *Journal of Visual Impairment and Blindness*, 75(5):213–218

Rosenbloom, A. A., (1982) Care of elderly people with low vision, *Journal of Visual Impairment and Blindness*, 76(6):209–212

Van de Ven, C. M. C., (1982) Management of bi-lateral lower limb amputees: An investigation, *Physiotherapy*, 68(2): 45–46

Vinchinsky, E., and Lulen, B., (1980) Sickle cell anemia, *Pediatric Clinics of North America*, 27(2):429–445

Walker, J. R., and Lattanzi, M., (1982) *Understanding Loss and Grief*, Boulder, Colo.: Boulder County Hospice

Weissert, W., Wan, T., Livieratos, B., Katz, S., and Pellegrino, I., (1980) Cost-effectiveness of homemaker services for the chronically ill, *Inquiry*, 17:230–243

Welsh, R. L., (1980) Psychosocial dimensions, in Welsh, R. L., and Blasch, B. B. (eds.), *Foundations of Orientation and Mobility*, New York: American Foundation for the Blind

Welsh, R. L., and Blasch, B. B., (1980) Training for persons with mobility limitations, in Welsh, R. L., and Blasch, B. B. (eds.), *Foundations of Orientation and Mobility*, New York: American Foundation for the Blind

West, B. A., (1981) Understanding endorphins: Our natural pain relief system, *Nursing 81*, 11(2):50–53

Wild, D., Nayak, U. S. L., and Isaac, B., (1981) Prognosis of falls in old people at home, *Journal of Epidemiology and Community Health*, 35:200

P A R T   T W O

Impact on Client and Family

CHAPTER SIX
Quality of Life

◇ CASE STUDY ◇
Quality of Life

All who knew her perceived Ms. V. as a skillful nurse, a professional nurse educator, and an extraordinarily caring person. Her concern for others was a force behind all her actions and behavior. Ms. V. often expressed her concern for others, in both her personal and professional life, as "a precious charge" (Nordstrom 1976). It was a commitment she diligently pursued during her goal-directed living and replicated during her dying. Perhaps the words of Mayeroff (1970) best express her perceptions of herself and the world in which she found herself: "Caring enables me to be 'in-place' in the world. Gratitude for being in-place makes me experience people and things as more precious, and I become more responsive to them and their need for me; gratitude further activates me to care for my appropriate others."

In her midlife years, Ms. V. found herself dying of cancer after radical surgery and extensive radiation therapy. She chose to remain at home during the dying process, where she could be in control of her life. Further, remaining at home allowed for a comfortable and familiar environment where her wide circle of friends and colleagues could come and go freely and provide a supportive network. She found that a few friends lacked the necessary coping skills to continue to interact with her comfortably. These individuals thus withdrew. Because of her caring nature, Ms. V. pondered how she might help these individuals cope with what was happening to her in a way that would allow them to benefit and grow from the experience. Thus, three months prior to her death, she brought together a small, intimate group of friends for what she called a soiree.

Ms. V. had planned a living celebration in her home as a tacit design to supplement the grieving process after her death. This dying but still dynamic hostess greeted all her guests with the warm loving words, "You honored me by coming . . . " (Nordstrom 1976), followed by a short but warm tribute to each of her guests. The group was then guided through preselected hymns led by the tenor voice of her church minister and the sensitive words of the young assistant minister in relation to "celebrating the temporary." The structured part of the evening was culminated by sips of champagne, gourmet hors d'oeuvres, and a large serving of warm, spontaneous singing. The dying thus comforted and counseled the living through a happy commemoration.

Introduction

Ms. V.'s case study illustrates the way, even during the dying process, this woman was able to maintain the quality of her life; that is, her invasive disease had compromised her energy level and productive career, but on a smaller scale she was still in control. She maintained her independence, continued to demonstrate her caring and concern, and remained an intact friend and colleague.

The concept of quality of life, its relationship to chronic illness, and the barriers that chronically ill people may perceive in their effort to retain this quality are the focus of this chapter.

But the meaning of quality of life varies across the life span. For the teenager, struggling for independence from parental controls, quality of life may mean successfully cutting the dependency ties. The young adult, occupied with career seeking, may consider quality the achievement of a successful and meaningful occupation. The majority of older Americans may interpret quality of life to mean maintaining health, financial resources, social approval, self-esteem, and social status. The institutionalized elderly place a different emphasis on quality of life. These individuals often emphasize retaining a degree of preinstitutional life-style: freedom of choice, privacy, support of independence, safety and security measures, and the availability of continued relationships with family, friends, and community (Enquist 1979). For the chronically ill client whose living is compounded by chronic impairments, quality may mean any of these criteria plus need to control pain, pursue a therapeutic regimen, and maintain normalizing activities of daily life.

Defining the Concept

The quality of life is an ambiguous concept that defies definition. *Webster's Dictionary* (1976) in defining quality "refers to a characteristic (physical or nonphysical, individual or typical) that constitutes the basic nature of a thing or is one of its distinguishing features": property, character, attribute, trait. Miller (1983) points out that this concept contains no consistent or universal meaning other than a general construct: to maximize satisfaction by living life to its fullest and functioning to the optimum of one's capability in all stages of life.

Strauss (1975) refers to quality of life for the chronically ill at home. He states that such quality requires management of the symptomatic indicators of the disease, as well as the accompanying psychosocial and financial liabilities. There are times that quality of life for the long-term client means maximizing life in a health care setting. To retain real quality, the client must continue to control and manage the environment as it relates to the condition and the individual's life-style.

Personal Value Systems and Standards

For the chronically ill, the meaning and value of the quality of life are judged solely by the individual. Because it is a very subjective process, only the person making the judgment can give it meaning at any given time. Individual judgments may be influenced by personal value systems, selected perspectives, and self-imposed standards (Cluff 1981). Personal value systems are derived from one's overall belief system. Belief systems relating to illness may encompass a belief in God, or another deity, that provides inner strength to cope with illness and other adversity; a belief in health care professionals that results in support to the client; a belief in medical or nursing regimens that affects compliance patterns; or a belief in oneself or confidence in one's own capabilities (Miller 1983).

Chronic disease, by virtue of its having a long-term effect, requires continuous observation and attention to preserve optimal personal function. The degree of maximal personal function varies from client to client as a result of self-imposed standards. The degree of function an individual chooses to accept varies, depending on the disruption it creates in the individual's life-style and quality of life.

Multidimensional Aspects

Quality of life may be influenced by four theoretical components of the total human condition—the physical, the psychosocial, the spiritual, and the cultural—that embrace the multidimensional representation of the total person. No one component must be abandoned for another if life's quality is to be maintained. These four dimensional components are integrated within the whole person as interrelated or interdependent parts of the human condition. The more balance that is maintained, the more functional the system becomes. However, the parts may not always be in balance: When the total human system breaks down as a result of illness or injury, one or more parts are affected. During the repair process of care and rehabilitation, all four multidimensional variables require managing to maintain an intact, functional system (Murray & Kijek 1979). Thus, it is clear that therapeutic care demands not losing sight of interrelated parts by treating a disease entity and neglecting the psychosocial, spiritual, and cultural aspects. Therapeutic care should recognize the whole person when promoting and maintaining the quality of life.

Quality of Life Goal

The preceding discussion demonstrates that the quality of life goal for individuals having chronic disorders is to attain optimal functioning at the highest level of independence. *Functional level*, a term frequently used during the rehabilitation process, refers to an individual's ability to participate in society, to perform activities of daily living (ADLs), and to care for personal needs. Therefore, the quality of life may be directly related to the effectiveness with which the multidimensional components are considered during care and treatment of the chronically ill client, and the degree to which these promote and support independent behavior. In short, maximizing a person's functional level generally enhances life's quality. Realistically, such goal achievement has a greater probability of success when the client participates in decision making.

The client, however, cannot achieve a meaningful quality without recognition and support from outside sources. Such support must come from family or significant others, as well as from the nurse and other health professionals involved in care management. In Ms. V.'s case study, Ms. V. and her physician jointly agreed that her remaining at home during her illness would be beneficial. This decision was based on the reality that, although Ms. V. lived alone, she was surrounded by a constant and supportive network of significant others who would contribute to the quality of her remaining life.

Family and significant others help increase quality of life by providing a buffer during stressful life events. Social support, sometimes referred to as an individual's *human climate*, is not always well under-

stood. The literature contains meager reports about ways the family hinders or aids one of its members during long-term illness (Dimond & Jones 1983). Generally, it appears that the most significant effect that the family might have on an ill member may be of a psychosocial nature (DiMatteo & Hays 1981; Dimond & Jones 1983; Miller 1983). A stable, cohesive, empathetic family unit that displays care and concern and yet is able to maintain what Strauss (1975) describes as a "normalizing" environment at home may best contribute to quality of life.

Symbolic Interaction Theory

As stated previously, the quality of life is an elusive concept and has no universal definition. Rather, the concept has individualistic meaning—that is, a different meaning for different individuals; meaning derived from the particular social setting in which it occurs. For example, the chronically ill client may perceive medical care in the hospital as intended to improve function to a premorbid level, whereas the physician may perceive such care only as diagnosis and treatment of disease (Cluff 1981). Symbolic interaction provides a helpful framework for understanding the quality of life concept.

In the midthirties, George Herbert Mead laid the foundation for a theoretical framework of human conduct called *symbolic interactionism* (Mead 1934). He proposed three major concepts in this theory: mind, self, and society. According to Mead, symbolic interaction examines the interdependence of the human condition and its natural and social environment. The human being reacts to the environment subjectively, thus constructing a meaningful environment.

Mead conceptualized the mind as containing a process capable of thinking and having the capacity to assess, weigh, anticipate, and construct courses of action. Later, the concept was reformulated as the "definition of the situation" (Turner 1978), meaning that people perceive, make decisions, and take action based on their definition of their world. That is, one weighs and assesses a situation and then determines the appropriate conduct of action. Ms. V. illustrates this process: she found herself dying and sensed that her friends were also suffering. Their friendship was being overpowered by grief, discomfort, and distance. Ms. V. therefore provided a vehicle, the soiree, as an environment for purposeful and comfortable sharing.

The *self* was seen by Mead as developing while assuming roles or sharing the perspective of others; *others* was conceptualized as the *generalized other*, a composite of other people reflecting society within the individual. Thus, the generalized other implies defining one's behavior in terms of the expectations of others. A good example of the generalized other is illustrated by the case study of Mrs. A. in relation to the incontinence pad placed in bed by the nurse. Mrs. A. may interpret the presence of this pad as meaning that the nurse expects her to be incontinent or that it is acceptable to be incontinent. The outcome might, in fact, be incontinence, reinforcing the nurse's original behavior.

Mead also visualized the human being in a world of objects, which could be physical, social, or abstract ideas. Although most of these objects were considered physical, they could also include guiding ideals, such as independence or honesty, or the activities of others, such as commands or requests (Blumer 1969). Thus an object becomes an object, in Meadian theory, when it can be referred to. In addition, human beings were seen as unique since they could create gestures (facial expressions, voice tones, and body postures) and symbols (words and pictures) to communicate. The response to, or meaning given to, symbols is the basis of symbolic interaction theory.

The symbolic interaction characterization of society allows it to become a medium for the development of human beings and a process by which human beings associate. Thus, Mead conceptualized the self and society as developing together. Further, he theorized the emergence of the capacities of the mind and self to permit interactions that form the basis of society.

From a symbolic interactionist's perspective, then, individuals construct the quality of life by defining and classifying situations in their world and then acting toward and within these situations. Fur-

ther, those who face long-term illnesses interpret their situation by their perceptions of themselves and of the world around them in relation to their health and well-being. For example, Ms. V.'s inherent enthusiasm for life and her caring for others, even during her terminal illness, perceived her friends as needing "permission" to share feelings. The soiree served that purpose. Although her physical image communicated her terminal state, her zesty spirit and optimistic attitude conveyed to her guests that the situation was to be a happy celebration. Through her skillful symbolic interaction, Ms. V. enabled her guests to perceive the situation she contrived in terms meaningful to her. In addition, their response added quality to her life.

Problems and Issues of the Chronically Ill

Chronicity affects quality of life in a number of areas, including questions of choices relating to quality versus quantity and the myriad of ethical issues relating to the decisions involved in life and death, treatment, and other aspects of chronicity. Although an in-depth discussion of these issues is beyond the scope of this chapter, problems and barriers in the health system that may influence the quality of life of the chronically ill or elderly client are addressed.

Quality versus Quantity: Daily Choices

When do clients have a choice in the quality versus the quantity of health care? Is choice actually a viable option, or is it merely rhetoric? Many factors have an impact on this issue. The chronically afflicted client faces the day-to-day management of a disease, whereas the professional sees the client/family only episodically. Often client and family make adjustments in the regimen warranted by the life situation or quality. Given the difference between managing disease continuously and episodically, conflicts between the client/family and health professionals may arise.

Professional versus Client. The physician remains the gatekeeper to medical care and, traditionally, to health care. Clients who perceive physicians as having a prestigious role may find questioning or opposing them difficult regardless of their wishes. Physicians by training and inclination generally focus on cure, rather than care. Yet chronically ill individuals require an emphasis on symptom control and disease stability. Physicians and other health professionals tend to pursue their own goals for the client without mutual acceptance by the client, causing client resistance and noncompliance, especially in long-term chronic illness. If the medical regimen is considered inconvenient or excessively time-consuming, causes undue discomfort, is energy-depleting, stigmatizing, or financially overwhelming, or forces an unwanted life-style change, the client may resist (Strauss 1975). Not only must physicians and other health care decision makers throw off the "paternalistic cape" when treating the chronically ill, but sensitivity to both the client as a person and that client's world is paramount if quality of life is to be maintained.

Nurses and other health professionals are also often perceived as authority figures who emphasize a hierarchical system of providing health care. This aggregate of caregivers focuses on medical regimens through delegation of tasks and assumed client compliance. Compliance is considered a means to an end. If values, priorities, and active decision making are not shared with the client, compliance and successful treatment may not be achieved (Conway-Rutkowski 1982). Thus, caregivers must understand what the client considers important and incorporate such priorities into interactions with and management of the client.

Bureaucracies. Bureaucratic organizations such as hospitals are health care systems designed primarily to provide physical care. These institutions are not structured to revere life's quality as the central purpose of client services. This orientation may conflict with client goals. The traditional hospital model of medical diagnosis, treatment, and medication orders has extended to the long-term care facility (Greenberg & Moffatt 1980). Consequently, time and priority needed to nurture the psychosocial and ADL needs may be neglected, and the facility and staff may be perceived by the client as dehumanizing (Kayser-Jones 1981). This potential conflict between the client and caregivers subtracts from quality of life when institutionalization is necessary.

Loss of Control

At times the quality of life of the chronically ill may be affected by their inability to retain control of the circumstances in which they find themselves. Contributing factors to this decreased opportunity include the following: lack of knowledge about their illness and management, feelings of deference in communicating with health care providers, lack of opportunity to participate in their care planning and management, unexplained delays in waiting for health care providers (outpatient clinics and doctors' offices), identified boundaries within institutions (such as the nurses' station and health records), and chronicity leading to social isolation and lack of energy (Miller 1983). When these situations occur, the client can become powerless.

Powerlessness. The phenomenon of *powerlessness* is the clients' expectation that their behavior cannot produce the outcomes or reinforcements they seek. Miller (1983) defines powerlessness as "a perception that one's own actions will not affect an outcome." The American social structure tends to stereotype chronically ill or aged persons by establishing and perpetuating the powerlessness phenomenon. These individuals are sometimes considered incompetent to work gainfully and at times are cast aside from the mainstream of social life. When affected individuals accept society's values, they assume the role of powerlessness.

Acceptance of a sense of powerlessness established by social others can be related to Mead's symbolic interactionism: that is, persons gain meaning of

---

◇ CASE STUDY ◇

Stereotypic Thinking

Mrs. A., a 92-year-old Caucasian widow, was an occupant of a multilevel life-care complex comprising independent apartments, supervised living areas, and a skilled nursing unit for inpatient care. Mrs. A. functioned independently and maintained her own apartment in spite of her mild Parkinson's syndrome and occasional periods of confusion. One evening she was admitted to the emergency room of a local hospital with second-degree burns on her face, trunk area, and fingers. After initial treatment was carried out, she was ordered admitted to an inpatient unit. The only information telephoned ahead to the medical-surgical unit nurse was that there was to be an admission of a 92-year-old female with burns on the head, face, and trunk.

Mrs. A. was transported to a four-bed ward on a gurney, with an intravenous (IV) unit running. The bed had been prepared, and the linens were fan-folded down, revealing a large incontinence pad in the middle of the draw sheet. Without inquiring of Mrs. A. whether she was able to move, the staff began to discuss ways to move her from the gurney to the bed. While the nurses were considering this decision, some relatives who had accompanied Mrs. A. instructed her on the way to assist herself during the transfer, which she then executed with little problem.

After several weeks, Mrs. A. was transferred from the hospital to the skilled nursing facility (SNF) of her long-term health care complex to continue postburn treatments. She had hoped to receive such treatment as an outpatient. Going to the SNF made Mrs. A. depressed and contributed to some minimal increase in confusion related to the unfamiliar environment. Her attending physician, who knew that she normally had a predinner cocktail, ordered two ounces of her favorite alcoholic beverage in an effort to counter her depression and restore a semblance of her usual life-style. The licensed staff nurse felt that alcohol was inappropriate for a 92-year-old, and her stereotypic attitude led to her subtle undermining of the order. She quietly placed the prescribed cocktail in front of Mrs. A. in a medicine cup and exited without speaking. The increased confusion from the change in environment plus her reticence to take medications of any kind made Mrs. A. view the "medicine cup cocktail" as an unnecessary medication, which she immediately rejected.

---

the world around them by interacting with that world. Proponents of symbolic interaction state that behavior is not just a mechanical response to the external stimuli of the environment; rather, one acquires meaning about the self by interacting and interpreting symbols of others. Thus, becoming aware of societal attitudes and accepting and believing that they are correct make individuals feel powerless.

Stereotyping.   Stereotyping is "an unvarying form or pattern; a fixed or conventional notion or conception, as of a person, group, idea . . . held by a number of people, and allowing for no individuality" (*Webster* 1976). Stereotypic thinking can be destructive since it has the potential of inducing powerlessness and dependence. The person who retires because economic conditions require defining age as a criterion for leaving the work force may be considered less physically or mentally capable because of this enforced unemployment. This same retired person, no longer receiving salaried income, may undergo a severe decrease in financial resources and consequently may become dependent on society to meet some of his or her needs. Society then may stereotype the person as old, nonproductive, and devalued. The result is often lowered self-esteem and sense of powerlessness.

Powerlessness of the long-term care client may be derived from nurses who lack gerontological preparation and may perceive the elderly or chronically ill individual as an incompetent object. Such perceptions invoke dehumanizing attitudes and behavior toward that person. The way that stereotypical thinking can produce dehumanizing behavior is illustrated in the case study of Mrs. A., an elderly, chronically ill individual who is facing hospitalization.

◇ C A S E S T U D Y ◇
Internal versus External Locus of Control

Miss D. was a single, attractive female in her early thirties who was struggling against multiple sclerosis (MS). This invasive disease had stripped her of almost total strength and mobility. Although it was a monumental task, she moved herself between her second-floor hospital bedroom and the first-floor physical therapy (PT) department via an electric wheelchair. Her treatments in PT involved muscle strengthening on the parallel bars with the assistance of the male therapist. While at PT she always managed to use the toilet independently with only minor assistance. When she was in the nursing unit, however, Miss D. complained of total helplessness and demonstrated total dependence in toileting activities. The nursing staff therefore assisted her regularly and completely in performing this activity of daily living. The staff was unaware of Miss D.'s disparate behavior in PT and the nursing unit for several weeks until a team conference was called.

The case study of Mrs. A. illustrates the stereotypic behavior of many acute and long-term care nurses caring for the chronically ill elderly client. These stereotypic attitudes of nurse caregivers may be summarized as follows:

1. A 92-year-old will be incontinent.
2. All 92-year-olds are unable to communicate.
3. Decisions cannot be made by 92-year-olds.
4. Instructions cannot be followed by 92-year-olds.
5. Patients, especially 92-year-old patients, should not have alcoholic beverages.

Following physician orders, providing attentive bedside care to maintain skin integrity and fluid balance, and performing functional skills are futile and inhumane acts when interaction and other humanizing aspects of nursing care are neglected. The client feels powerless because of such naive behavior, and this powerlessness in turn can contribute to a sense that the quality of life is eroding.

Locus of Control. Chronically ill clients frequently are experienced in the impaired role (see Chapter 3) and are usually comfortable about retaining control (Dimond & Jones 1983). Often they make choices about many aspects of their health care management, such as deciding to keep appointments, adjust medications, or modify their regimen if they see fit.

In contrast to powerlessness, which is situation-ally determined (Miller 1983), the concept of *locus of control* relates to the perception that outcomes are within or outside oneself regardless of the situation (Rotter 1966). Rotter conceptualized person-centered control as having two dimensions: internal versus external locus of control. *Internal control* is perceived by the subject as an event that is contingent upon personal behavior. The subject perceives *external control* as involving reinforcement following the subject's actions, but not necessarily contingent on such action. External control is thus perceived as chance or controlled by powerful others.

Studies reported in the literature do not conclude that client behavior can be categorized according to internal and external control. Instead, if one considers these constructs on a continuum, client behavior tends toward one or the other or fluctuates between the two (Dimond & Jones 1983; Miller 1983). Miss D.'s case study illustrates this point.

According to potential behavioral indicators of locus of control (Miller 1983), compliance with health care regimens indicates that those who use internal control ("internals") tend to manipulate regimens, whereas those who see control as externalized ("externals") tend to complain. Motivation is an indicator of internals, whereas externals tend to feel helplessness or powerlessness (Miller 1983). From the information presented, it is difficult to determine the locus of control for Miss D. The very fact that she demonstrated compliance with her PT therapy but portrayed

◇ CASE STUDY ◇
Who Should Be in Control?

Mr. T. was a large-framed male in his midthirties. He was not well-educated, but his lack of schooling did not inhibit his ability to communicate or become a barrier to his constant flow of conversation during his dialysis treatments. Mr. T. was Hispanic, and for this cultural group time orientation is relative; that is, there are wide parameters such as day and night rather than discrete intervals such as minutes or hours (Ebersole & Hess 1981). Mr. T.'s primary nurse, who was Caucasian, was accustomed to working by hospital clocks and strict time schedules. The disparity between Mr. T.'s relative sense of time and his nurse's strict sense of punctuality may have triggered conflict between them.

Frequently, Mr. T. would appear late for his treatment appointment. One day his tardiness triggered a verbal attack by his primary nurse. She did not hesitate to demand punctuality in maintaining his treatment schedule and his dialysis regimen. Unshaken by the nurse's reprimand, Mr. T. made it clear that the decision to comply was his choice, his alone, and that he would accept no coercion for compliance purposes. Other portions of the nurse-client interaction revealed that treatment duration (three to four hours) as well as posttreatment effects were interfering with Mr. T.'s other daily activities. Obviously, dialysis treatments were interfering with his life quality!

---

complete dependency in the nursing unit suggests that her behavior may have been an attempt to control the quality of her life while enduring chronicity.

Locus of control can also influence situations involving other clients. When clients' decisions affect others, these actions can trigger hostile feelings in the health professional, who may seek to gain some control. Mr. T.'s case study illustrates responses of a health professional to a less than compliant client who insists on retaining control even when doing so causes other problems.

One is left with questions about who has the right to control in this situation. Mr. T., for whatever reasons, insisted on maintaining an internal locus of control so that he could perpetuate some semblance of quality in his life that was altered by his failing kidneys. Is treatment solely Mr. T.'s choice, assuming that he understands all the personal costs and benefits? And what of his primary nurse? She showed a need to force an external locus of control on this client. Was she acting as an advocate for the client (see Chapter 13), or was she feeling a lack of control over her client, as well as a lack of control in maintaining the dialysis unit's schedule? Were ethnic disparities the basis for conflict of control? Further, is there an ethical issue at work here?

Ethical Issues

The professional faces ethical decisions in a number of areas. Ethical decisions are spawned when a value conflict exists. One obvious conflict may be embodied in a clash between the health care provider and the client as to who has the right to make decisions. Professionals may disagree among themselves or they may be caught in a conflict between client and family that may have many ramifications, especially when the professional agrees with one or the other. Another source of value conflict may be grounded in the health care professional/caregiver who holds dichotomous values; that is, the disparity of values may reside within the health professional's own personal and professional value system. Value conflicts may also exist between society and the client and family or between society and the health professional (Davis & Aroskar 1983).

The Right to Make Decisions.   When individuals seek health care and become "clients" within a particular health care system, do they become victims of that system, or are they participating members of the interdisciplinary health care team? The impact on clients becomes a critical issue and raises questions because decisions must be made about therapeutic courses of action. Further, the professional must take prudent action to assist the client to understand the advantages and disadvantages of prescribed treatment so as to make informed decisions. In fact, the question or decision may be reduced to accepting or not accepting treatment or to clients' choice to remain autonomous until they find a professional who respects their individuality. Do such decisions fall into the domain of the health professionals, or do they remain the clients'?

With today's technological advances, some might say that the ethical dilemma rests with the quality of life potential. Again from the perspective of the symbolic interaction theorists, how does the client define and interpret the quality of life under life-threatening conditions? Miss D. illustrates that the normal emotional feelings of a young woman attracted by the opposite sex can be exhibited and tested even under conditions of disease and illness that eventually will be life threatening. Her behavior could well have reflected her desire to maintain normalizing behavior with the opposite sex. Such overt behaviors, which stemmed from high motivation and the mobilization of considerable strength and energy, were indicative of retaining life's quality for this client, according to this interpretation.

Clients' rights to health care decisions are embodied among the many rights claimed in today's society. "Rights, as entitlements, are claimed to privacy, to life, to die, to a healthy environment, and to health" (Davis & Aroskar 1983). Within the American Nurses Association's *Code for Nurses* is noted the client's moral right to decide about his or her own person (Davis & Aroskar 1983).

Clients' rights to relocation must be acknowledged. Relocation, or change in living environment, for the chronically ill may mean moving from home to hospital, hospital to nursing home, or even room to room within the same institution. Studies (Borup 1981) have suggested that relocation can be stress-provoking when the person being moved is not the decision maker. Intrafacility relocation often occurs for the convenience of staff. Clients who become behavior problems may be relocated away from public

thoroughfares. At other times, a client may complain about a roommate, forcing relocation of one or the other. Sometimes institutions maintain designated areas for recipients of specific programs. For example, a nursing home resident may be admitted as a private payer or as a Medicare recipient; however, over time when the client's funds or program benefits are consumed, the client may become a welfare or Medicaid recipient. As a result, relocation to a less prestigious area or less desirable room may be imposed by the facility. Quality of life, as symbolized by the new environment, may be denigrating for the resident through such involuntary moves.

Professional Disagreement. Physicians are primarily concerned with the physical aspects of curing disease. Nurses focus on the subjective aspects of care; that is, the health and well-being of the human condition (Benoliel 1982). These differences can involve decisions on many issues: following regimens, the right to die, or even the issue of withholding information from the client. Physicians desiring to withhold information can place the nurse in a precarious position.

Nurses have ethical obligations to their clients and to the physician and their employing institution (see Chapter 13). When there is incongruence, the nurse is in a dilemma of *multiple ethical obligations* (Davis & Aroskar 1983). Such a dilemma can occur when the physician bases a decision to withhold information about a client's diagnosis on clinical judgment, and the nurse's clinical judgment leads to the belief that the client should have the information to function autonomously and to preserve the quality of life. Multiple considerations arise from this situation, but essentially two basic questions are involved (Davis & Aroskar 1983):

1. What is the nurse's ethical obligation in those situations in which she confronts multiple ethical obligations?
2. What is the extent of this obligation?

Clinical decisions regarding clients such as the chronically impaired should rest with at least two or more persons, including the client and an attending health professional. As chronic conditions change over time, the decision makers must evaluate the facts and values involved for each member of the health team. Professional and client may differ markedly in factors they consider significant. Occasions arise when treatment and care decisions are separated by a fine line as a result of conflicting values. Then they become ethical dilemmas.

Conflicts between the Client/Family and Society. Does the state have the moral right to impose a paternalistic attitude over individual rights, values, and beliefs? Paternalism in health care has no clear-cut answers, particularly in emergency situations, in which too many variables are involved. Resorting to either weak or strong paternalism is a visible solution. Acts of paternalism in health care must confront liberty, a natural and inalienable right in democratic societies. For example, nurses who advocate client autonomy do not consider strong paternalism to be justified.

More conflicts on ethical issues between the individual and society are emerging as public awareness increases through the medium of television. As an example, the question of whether the state has the right to interfere with a family's decision to withhold medical treatment for a minor child if such treatment is contrary to the family's religious beliefs has been discussed widely. Which side of such issues of paternalism one takes depends on the personal values of the health provider.

Living or Dying. Terminally ill clients who are able to remain at home rather than in the hospital generally can maintain a more desirable quality of life. Usually, such individuals have the advantage of controlling their lives, maintaining their life-style, and resuming "normalizing" (Strauss 1975) activities. Electing to remain at home with family provides the dying person a supportive human climate as well as a place of personal possessions and personal choices. It should be everyone's right to choose, given the family's ability to deal with the situation, to continue living at home in a more familiar or accustomed style as long as possible. In this way, quality of life can be preserved.

With terminal illness as the intruder, both the client and family must be assured of professional support and assistance because of the uncertainty of the situation (Koff 1980). Koff also suggests that a family's fatigue from grief and physical exhaustion may require professional guidance (see Chapter 8). With the recognized need and advancement of the hospice concept, more clients have the option of remaining at home during the dying process. The caring community of hospice programs is increasing through government reimbursement. This inpatient and outpatient health care service can provide great comfort to the terminally ill. Through hospice programs, home care or supportive inpatient care is provided to allow the client to remain in a familiar environment.

Problems faced by chronically ill persons who wish to remain at home may necessitate some unexpected adaptations, such as moving an upstairs bed downstairs, renting or purchasing a hospital bed for more comfort or ease of transfers, acquiring a walker or wheelchair for mobility, getting mechanical devices to aid in shampooing hair, rearranging furniture, obtaining stools and grab bars for toileting and bathing, and arranging for medication injections.

Euthanasia. The word *euthanasia* is of Greek derivation and means "good or pleasant death." When euthanasia is discussed, the question of when death is preferred over life arises. The basic moral law that guides us is "Thou shalt not kill." Is there a moral difference between "letting die" and "hastening" death? If so, who decides? What criteria should be used? What degree of consent is expected from the potential subject? Does the decision belong to the client, the family, or the professional? What are the legal implications?

Euthanasia may be considered on a continuum from *antieuthanasia* (treatment with all means), strict sanctity of life, to *passive euthanasia* (withholding extraordinary or heroic means), to *active euthanasia* (helping or speeding death) (Davis & Aroskar 1983). "Mercy killing" is considered active euthanasia, whereas allowing people to die and giving only comfort care can be considered passive euthanasia.

Three different ethical stances supporting euthanasia are relevant to health professionals, clients, and society (Davis & Aroskar 1983):

1. *The new morality*, which separates the values of humanness and personal integrity from biologic life functions. This principle supports the quality of life ethic; that is, that death is not the worst event.
2. *The ethic of benemortasia* suggests an ethic of obligation. Benemortasia supports a good or kind death such as relieving pain and suffering and allowing the individual to die. It also honors the client's right to refuse treatment.
3. *Mercy killing* supports active euthanasia and makes a moral distinction between killing and allowing the individual to die.

Details of these arguments are analyzed in medicolegal texts. However, nurses and other health professionals should be aware that legislation is emerging in response to the need to deal with these issues. California, which is a forerunner in such legislation, passed *The Natural Death Act* in 1976. This act "recognizes the rights of adults to prepare written instructions authorizing their physicians to withhold or withdraw life-sustaining procedures in specified circumstances of terminal illness" (Davis & Aroskar 1983). Other states are following suit.

Nurses and other health professionals should explore the euthanasia issue carefully, in light of the nature of their practice. Practitioners should examine their own values about death, quality of life, respect for individual client dignity, advocacy to prevent client harm, and distributive justice (Davis & Aroskar 1983).

Decision Conflicts. In caring for the terminal or near-terminal client, professional nurses, particularly young graduates, must deal with an apparent caregiving conflict. Nurses and other health care providers, whether life can be preserved or whether life is beyond preservation, may have cause to question whether nursing intervention should be continued. Some nurses have difficulty handling this type of sit-

uation, and may express it in many ways, including avoiding the client except to give required care, and responding nonverbally in a negative way. Difficulty can arise from problems in dealing with one's own sense of mortality or aging, to those secondary gains that come from helping clients recover.

The decision to intervene can be problematic, depending on the condition and desires of the client. Nevertheless, the critical issue is that the nurse must never abandon care (Davis & Aroskar 1983). This may mean assuring the dying that they are not alone and that someone will be present at all times if they wish. Sincere caring as displayed by the nurse's attentive presence exemplifies high-quality care. In addition, such care advances the quality of life.

Focus on Cure, Not Care

There are times that, in spite of good intents, the professional actually contributes to poor care. This most often occurs in the hospital in caring for the chronically ill. Physicians focus most often on pathology: their primary objective is to cure or alter the disease. In this pursuit, they often lose sight of the fact that the disease dwells within the human condition. Overloaded nurses focus on assisting the short-stay client toward a speedy recovery and discharge. They may expect and demand compliance with medical and nursing orders. Nurturing becomes elusive. The chronically ill, who are not cured, who require frequent or repetitive care, who remain for long periods of time, or who are not compliant, consequently often receive less individual, humane, high-quality care. Furthermore, many of these chronically ill clients may be among the poor and elderly poor.

Individuals in today's fast-paced society who develop chronic health impairments may find themselves in the most frustrating of circumstances, especially if they develop an acute episode requiring hospitalization. The *chief* concern in a hospital is to save lives and cure disease, not to meet needs with psychosocial dimensions. Health professionals, in their concentration on machines that monitor and on curing of disease, may compromise the care or humanizing component of therapeutics. The imbalance that results from machine and equipment monitoring plus recurrent nursing staff shortages supersedes comfort and care measures.

The cost of medical and technical advances leads to short-term hospital treatment and limited length of stay (McClure & Nelson 1982). Escalating hospital costs, now being mediated through a diagnosis related group (DRG) system for Medicare reimbursement, leads to more rapid discharge (Clifford 1983; Davis 1983; Meiners & Coffey 1984; Coleman & Smith 1984; Beyers 1985). The effect that earlier discharges based on limited length of stay will have on providing high-quality care is not yet known (Hegyvary 1983). However, Hegyvary suggests that costs and quality must be considered simultaneously, not just within one discipline or one type of health care setting but within the total health care system.

Some suggest that "nursing personnel must be better prepared and more sophisticated . . ." (Feldman & Goldhaber 1984), but such improved knowledge and skills of nurses in practice should not be limited to hospital nursing but should extend to all areas of community nursing practice (Davis 1983; Coleman & Smith 1984). In addition, health care professionals working in acute settings must be prepared to care for the chronically ill during acute episodes of disease process, but such care requires time, patience, and repetition and does not correct the underlying health problems. In sum, emerging cost-containment and cost-effective health care systems will have an impact on the quality of care clients receive and, ultimately, on the quality of life.

Community, Society, and Policy Issues

Chronic disease is the major health problem in America today and is the largest contributor to morbidity, mortality, and physical impairment. Reif and Estes (1982) state that increasing evidence suggests that the impact of chronic disease is especially great among both the very poor and the very old populations. Those who are at greatest risk of becoming chronically ill and impaired are individuals with poor housing and nutrition, low income, and a limited or nonexistent support network. This same group is at greater risk of being institutionalized in a long-term facility (Reif & Estes 1982).

Financial and Policy Issues. Although the problems of reimbursement, coordination of services, and policy issues are discussed elsewhere in this text, they do influence quality of life. Persons requiring long-term care have been greatly affected by the decentralization of fiscal and policy responsibilities from federal to state levels (Reif & Estes 1982). Long-range solutions to problems of reimbursement, coordination of services, and policy issues have negligible impact on meeting the needs of the chronically ill and disabled. Long-term funding is determined by what is currently available through government programs such as Medicare, Medicaid, and Social Services (see Chapters 17 and 18).

Institutional care, which dominates long-term care funding policies and is reimbursable, overshadows the underdeveloped and inadequately covered noninstitutional services. Insurmountable barriers to accessible, appropriate, and acceptable services for long-term care clients are erected by the eligibility constraints of age and income, the continued escalation of nursing home care costs, the poor quality of nursing home care, and the lack of integrated services in any health care setting or across settings (Reif & Estes 1982). Individual values of independence, self-worth, self-esteem, and productivity for the chronically ill and disabled have low priority in our affluent society.

Shortage of Health Care Providers. It is projected that there will be a substantial increase in the need for long-term care health professionals (Reif & Estes 1982). Such a shortage affects quality of life through the lack of available and needed resources to maintain, support, and promote the health and well-being of those with chronicity problems. Several studies indicate that the nurse shortage in long-term care will not be self-correcting over the next decade or so (Reif & Estes 1982). Factors that contribute to such a limited supply of nurses in long-term care have been identified by Reif and Estes (1982):

1. The potential expansion of the role and functions of nurses in many diverse long-term care services.
2. An obvious growth of the elderly population.

3. Unattractive work situations and noncompetitive salaries and benefits for nurses.
4. The expansion of agencies and services to meet long-term care outpatient needs.
5. A limited number of educationally prepared nurses to work in and keep pace with the expanding long-term programs and services.

Interventions

Persons having chronic diseases who also suffer functional impairments and disability are increasing in numbers. As a result, the roles, functions, and practice settings of nurses will be affected. Increased emphasis on prevention, health education, primary care, and long-term services will result in greater demand for nurses in ambulatory clinics, home care agencies, and long-term care facilities (Reif & Estes 1982). Nursing interventions for chronically ill clients must take into account the quality of care and the quality of life. Suggested here are some broad generalizations to provide a basis for a focus on quality of life that is applicable to caring for any specific chronic disease.

First, the health care professional should provide support and encouragement of measures that would assist the client who wishes to remain at home, whether chronically ill or terminally ill. Provided the opportunity, a nurse prepared in long-term care can skillfully assess the home situation and recommend appropriate assistive devices, specialized equipment, rearrangement of the home environment, education of the client/family/significant other/neighbors about the health condition and situation, and means of contacting appropriate community resources. These actions can assist clients to extend their time at home.

In addition, the health provider should consider the client's life-style in decisions concerning appropriate care and treatment. Recognition and support of a client's pattern of dependence and independence, abilities, strengths, and likes and dislikes, as they relate to the chronic condition and possible life-style changes, may be critical to successful acceptance of care and treatment (Nield & Mahon 1981).

The health professional should also be knowledgeable about the client's personal value system in terms of ethical issues that relate to health care. It is also important to know clearly when the client's value system is congruent or in conflict with those of professionals (Davis & Aroskar 1983). Utilization of such knowledge should precede planning of appropriate and therapeutic care and should then be incorporated into such interventions.

Comprehensive interviews and health assessments should be designed to meet not only physical needs but also psychosocial, spiritual, and cultural needs. For the chronically ill client, because of the long-term and changing nature of the condition, both admission interview and assessment and ongoing assessment are necessary. Gathering information regarding a client's multidimensional components provides the data base for planning continued care (Anderson & Bauwens 1981; Miller 1983). Such information gathering is fundamental to nursing diagnosis and goal setting (Burnside 1981).

The client should also receive continued support and encouragement as a participant in care planning and goal setting, especially since the client is the major source of information needed to assess, plan, and evaluate the situation (Marrinier 1983). Further, a client who understands and is involved in the planning of a regimen is more likely to be cooperative during the care process.

Maintenance of the nurse advocacy role in client-nurse relationships can assure the client of better care. Since the nurse spends more time with the client and has a more caring relationship than do other health team professionals, a deeper awareness of the client's condition and situation is possible. As a result, the nurse is empowered to obtain the best possible care for the client (Murphy & Hunter 1983).

Long-Term Problem Solving

Clients who have chronic impairments have an enduring two-pronged problem: maintaining health and psychosocial well-being (Miller 1983). Regardless of the setting, nurses and other health professionals must not let the medically regulated system negate the client's chronicity vis-à-vis focus on physical care, which often steals the spotlight. Inadequate attention to the accompanying psychosocial needs of the client can lead to neglect that may undermine physical outcomes. The health professional must maintain keen eyes and ears to those issues important to the client and family. The degree of responsiveness to the client's needs and concerns has the potential for amplifying or diminishing quality of life. Interventions useful to health professionals, primarily nurses, often require time, planning, and patience. These approaches often require fitting the system to the client rather than the reverse, but their utilization can add meaning and quality to the lives of clients and their families.

Changing Policy: Advocacy. Nurses must remember that their relationship with the client is one of advocacy. As client advocates, nurses also support client autonomy. Although nurses and other health professionals often are socialized into paternalistic behavior, paternalism is not justified if it restricts the liberty of clients without their consent. We need to ask, Can we ever justify paternalism when it presents harm to our clients or others?

The purpose of this section is to identify suggested critical areas requiring significant changes with which nurses individually and collectively may educate legislators. All these efforts have the potential of contributing to an improved quality of life for those with chronic health problems (Reif & Estes 1982):

1. Ensuring appropriate and professional health care services for clients receiving inpatient and outpatient long-term care services
2. Supporting availability and accessibility of long-term care for populations in need
3. Supporting efforts to improve programs and policies and to focus on prevention and causes, rather than end-stage problems

The Interdisciplinary Team. The interdisciplinary health team theoretically works as a cohesive group to benefit the client. Three considerations of the team approach warrant examination here in re-lation to improving quality of life: involving the client and family as team members, improving communication, and setting goals.

Involving Client and Family in Planning Care. Clients entering the health care system usually do so as a result of a perceived health need. The severity and complexity of the health problem often determine the health team specialists that are required. In rehabilitation care for the chronically ill or disabled, a rehabilitation team comprising multiple disciplines may be appropriate (see Chapter 18). The central focus—that is, the client and family and their needs—must not be lost in all this expertise. Health team planning that excludes the client and family and ignores the individual's uniqueness is irrelevant, unrealistic, and nonproductive.

Improving Communication. The use of an interdisciplinary team is a viable approach in more than the rehabilitation setting. The team approach benefits both client and interdisciplinary staff members through improved communication. The benefits to the staff members include a broader scope for information sharing. Through team conferences, team members can make judgments based on multifaceted rather than isolated viewpoints, as indicated in Miss D.'s case study. The client benefits through access to diversified expertise plus the validation of efforts and responses to therapy.

Setting Goals. Mutual goal setting by the interdisciplinary team is complemented by the client, who ultimately decides whether team goals are acceptable. Client acceptance often hinges on the way the goals alter behavior or life-style. The ultimate goal is to enhance, not to hinder, the client's quality of life.

Other Professional Roles

The nurse assumes many roles in professional practice that can affect many of the components of clients' quality of life. These roles include educator, caregiver, and researcher.

The Professional as Educator. The teaching role is integral to nursing. However, it is essential to remember that change in the learner depends on what is meaningful to that learner (see Chapter 12). The chronically ill must deal with their health problems and the myriad of psychosocial problems on a day-to-day basis that accommodates their life-styles and that enhances quality of life. Teaching should be adapted to the client, should move at a pace appropriate for the client, and should be planned over time so that change that occurs can be integrated by the client.

Dealing with Powerlessness. Clients who are chronically ill need intact power resources to manage their own care and their own lives. As client educators, health professionals, especially nurses, should assess the client's power resources: belief system, hope, energy, knowledge, and self-esteem. The nurse educator can then facilitate alleviation of powerlessness through empowering strategies (Miller 1983). These strategies may include identifying options for the client; increasing the client's knowledge of care and treatment to enhance rational choices; identifying environmental modifications for increased function, comfort, and safety; and helping the client to set realistic goals.

Learning to Set Goals. Clients having chronic conditions may need assistance in setting realistic goals when they feel powerless. Unachievable goals hindered by feelings of depression, hopelessness, or incorrect or limited knowledge about their illness all reinforce powerlessness. Client participation and mutual goal planning validate coping and self-care skills. Such validation results in positive reinforcement and power to accept responsibility for setting desired and achievable goals: to shape and control the quality of life.

The Professional as Caregiver. A major role of nursing is that of caregiver: the laying on of hands. This is the role encompassing the caring and nurturing quality identified by most clients and their families as nursing. For the acutely ill, the care received contributes toward recovery. To the chronically ill or disabled and to the dying client and their family, nursing care can make the difference between a more comfortable and functional life and an empty, possibly despairing existence. Good nursing care provides support for families even after death of a member.

Enhancing Quality of Life for the Living. Clients who are institutionalized with long-term illness or who are dying require palliative (mitigating or alleviating), as opposed to curative, care. When the nurse caregiver can help modify or control symptoms, clients have more opportunity to gain control of their lives, environments, and situations and to make decisions. Quality of life remains in the hands of the client. However, the professional nurse, as caregiver, continues to provide humane support as nurturer, counselor, teacher, and advocate.

This is also applicable to individuals who are not institutionalized. These individuals and families often face tremendous odds that detract from the quality of their existence. Often they do not know how to deal with the health care system (see Chapter 16) or are impoverished by their illnesses (see Chapter 17). Families, impacted by presence of illnesses, often have difficulty in managing their loved ones at home (see Chapter 8). The nurse can provide the support and direction that help these individuals to remain in their home environment, where their needs can be best met by those who are personally involved with them. The dying client who wishes to remain at home rather than in the impersonal environment of the hospital needs support and often special equipment to achieve this goal. Again, the nurse can be the link connecting needed services to client and family.

Support for the Surviving Family. The death of a client often leaves a family behind in the throes of grief and mourning. Grief is an accepted response in our society and a necessary reaction to loss. The ritual of funerals assists in bringing support to the bereaved family. In addition, where the concept and reality of hospice exist, the hospice program can be most supportive to the bereaved. The hospice team comprises both professionals and volunteers who are committed to bereavement support. The professional nurse often is a vital member of this team and provides family support during the client's dying process, immediately after death, and months after the event of death. In this way, the nurse along with other professionals and volunteers may become part of the bereavement process, a process aimed at comforting and restoring quality of life to those who are left behind.

The Professional as Researcher. Nursing research designed to improve the quality of life of the chronically impaired client must define *quality* before attempting to measure it. Further, research requires identifying the environment in which the client's enduring struggle for improved quality of care and of life is occurring: home or institution.

Some clients and families faced with long-term health conditions are overcome with the uphill battle and withdraw; others grow (Lenihan 1981). Why the great disparity? Is it the chronic condition itself (disability, disfigurement, pain and discomfort, dependence on others)? Or could it be the lack of appropriate or accessible health care resources, financial capability or assistance, attitudes of society or health care professionals, the health care system, or the inner resources of the client and significant others? For the chronically ill who are also elderly, some argue that psychosocial needs are critical to gerontological nursing research (Gunter & Miller 1977).

These are a few of the questions that the professional nurse must address before nursing practice, through nursing research, can contribute to improving the quality of life of the client. As a practicing professional, the nurse can contribute to research through daily observations of clients and application of scientific inquiry to these observations. Until chronicity is prevented or controlled, we face an ever-increasing population that needs supportive approaches to maximize their potential and enhance the quality of their lives (see Chapter 14).

Summary and Conclusions

The quality of life is unique to each person, just as each person is unique. Questions about the way that life's quality will be determined for those who are chronically ill and impaired and the person who will make such determinations appear to be simple, since the ultimate choice maker must be the client. The goal of these choices should be enhancing quality of life for the health care recipient. Quality can be viewed from the perspective of Mead's symbolic interaction theory.

Maximizing quality of life can be a dilemma. To add to this dilemma, the general population is getting older, and accompanying this aging is an increase in chronic illness. Society's values will continue to play a central role in the allocation of health care services and in determining the recipients. Decisions regarding allocations often result in inadequate services for the chronically ill. To offset such limitations of services, nurses must not relinquish their advocacy role at any level: practice, education, research, or policy development.

Currently an estimated 9 million Americans suffer from functional impairments, a proportion that may increase significantly in the coming decades (Reif & Estes 1982), providing a tremendous challenge for the nursing profession. If numbers can have strength and mobilization is possible, the more than one million practicing nurses could have considerable clout in reshaping public policy in long-term care.

STUDY QUESTIONS

1. What is quality of life? How does one's belief or value system influence quality of life?
2. Why is a balance between the physical, psychosocial, spiritual, and cultural components important to enhancing quality of life? How do these components help the chronically ill attain optimal functioning to maximize independence?
3. How does symbolic interaction theory help explain quality of life?
4. How does the professional influence a client's

choices about quality versus quantity of life? How do bureaucracies influence such choices?

5. How does powerlessness or stereotyping adversely impact the client's ability to maintain control in relation to quality of life? How does locus of control affect quality?

6. From the perspective of ethical issues, what factors influence health care decisions? What are some of the areas in which client and professional might disagree about these decisions? What influence does disagreement between professionals have on such decisions?

7. From your own experience and knowledge, what is the basis of conflicts that arise between individuals and society? Do you feel that society or government has a right to such actions?

8. What are the ethical issues involved in care of the dying person? Who has the right to make decisions for these individuals? Explain your answer.

9. How does the professional contribute to poor quality of care? What is the impact of the acute health care setting?

10. Which groups are most affected by chronic disease? How do financial and policy issues influence quality of life for the institutionalized? What influence does the number of available health care providers have?

11. In what ways can nurses or other health professionals enhance a chronically ill client's quality of life? Discuss in relation to professionals, clients, and changing policy.

12. How could an interdisciplinary team improve quality of life for the client?

13. How can the professional improve quality of life from the perspective of health educator? caregiver? researcher?

References

Anderson, S. V., and Bauwens, E. E., (1981) *Chronic Health Problems: Concepts and Application*, St. Louis: C.V. Mosby

Benoliel, J. Q., (1982) Ethics in nursing practice and education, *Nursing Outlook, 31*:210–215

Beyers, M. (ed.), (1985) *Perspectives of Prospective Payment: Challenges and Opportunities for Nurses*, Rockville, Md.: Aspen Publications

Blumer, H., (1969) *Symbolic Interactionism*, Englewood Cliffs, N.J.: Prentice-Hall

Borup, J. H., (1981) Relocation: Attitudes, information network and problems encountered, *Gerontologist, 21*:5

Burnside, I. M., (1981) *Nursing and the Aged*, New York: McGraw-Hill

Clifford, J. C., (1983) Discussion, in *Nursing Research and Policy Formation: The Case of Prospective Payment*, American Nurses Association, Kansas City, Mo.: American Academy of Nursing

Cluff, L. E., (1981) Chronic disease: Function and quality of care, *Journal of Chronic Disease, 34*:305–311

Coleman, F. P., and Smith, D. S., (1984) DRGs and the growth of home health care, *Nursing Economics, 2*:391–395

Conway-Rutkowski, B., (1982) Patient participation in nursing process, *Nursing Clinics of North America, 17*:3

Davis, C., (1983) The federal role in changing health care financing, *Nursing Economics, 1*(1):10–17

Davis, C., (1983) The federal role in changing health care financing, *Nursing Economics, 1*(2):98–104

Davis, J., and Aroskar, M. A., (1983) *Ethical Dilemmas and Nursing Practice*, Norwalk, Conn.: Appleton-Century-Crofts

DiMatteo, M. R., and Hays, R., (1981) Social support and serious illness, in Gottlieb, B. H. (ed.), *Social Networks and Social Support*, Beverly Hills: Sage Publications

Dimond, M., and Jones, S. L., (1983) *Chronic Illness Across the Life Span*, Norwalk, Conn.: Appleton-Century-Crofts

Ebersole, P., and Hess, P., (1981) *Toward Healthy Aging*, St. Louis: C. V. Mosby

Enquist, C. L., (1979) Can quality of life be evaluated? *Hospitals*, November 16

Feldman, J., and Goldhaber, F. I., (1984) Living with DRGs, *Journal of Nursing Administration, 14*(5):19–22

Greenberg, B. M., and Moffatt, J. D., (1980) Medical model—nursing model, in Stillwell (ed.), *Readings in Gerontological Nursing*, Thorofare, N. J.: Charles B. Stack

Gunter, L. M., and Miller, J. C., (1977) Toward a nursing gerontology, *Nursing Research, 23*(3):209–221

Hegyvary, S. T., (1983) Prospective payment: Focus on quality of care, in *Nursing Research and Policy Formation: The Case of Prospective Payment*, American Nurses Association, Kansas City, Mo.: American Academy of Nursing

Kayser-Jones, J., (1981) *Old, Alone and Neglected: Care of the Institutionalized Elderly in Scotland and the United States*, Berkeley: University of California Press

Koff, T. H., (1980) *Hospice: A Caring Community*, Cambridge, Mass.: Winthrop

Lenihan, S., (1981) Quest for meaning in the face of chronic illness, in Perdue et al. (eds.), *Chronic Care Nursing*, New York: Springer

Marrinier, A., (1983) *The Nursing Process: A Scientific Approach to Nursing Care*, St. Louis: C. V. Mosby

Mayeroff, M., (1970) *On Caring*, New York: Harper & Row

McClure, M. L., and Nelson, M. J., (1982) Trends in hospital nursing, in Aiken, L. H. (ed.), *Nursing in the 1980s: Crises, Opportunities, Challenges*, Philadelphia: J. B. Lippincott, pp. 59–73

Mead, G. H., (1934) *Mind, Self, and Society*, Chicago: University Press

Meiners, M. R., and Coffey, R. M., (1984) *Hospital DRGs and the Need for Long Term Care Services: An Empirical Analysis*, National Center for Health Services Research, U.S. Department of Health and Human Services

Miller, J. F., (1983) *Coping with Chronic Illness: Overcoming Powerlessness*, Philadelphia: Lippincott

Murphy, C. P., and Hunter, H., (1983) *Ethical Problems in the Nurse-Patient Relationship*, Boston: Allyn & Bacon

Murray, R., and Kijek, J. C., (1979) *Current Perspectives in Rehabilitative Nursing*, St. Louis: C. V. Mosby

Nield, L. J., and Mahon, N. E., (1981) Barriers to health care, in Perdue et al. (eds.), *Chronic Care Nursing*, New York: Springer

Nordstrom, M. J., (1976) *Farewell, Friends—a Reflection*, Tacoma, Wash.: The Hillhaven Foundation

Reif, L., and Estes, C. L., (1982) Long-term care: New opportunities in professional nursing, in Aiken, L. H. (ed.), *Nursing in the 1980s: Crises, Opportunities, Challenges*, Philadelphia: Lippincott, pp. 149–182

Rotter, J. B., (1966) Generalized expectancies for internal versus external control reinforcement, *Psychological Monographs, 80*:1

Strauss, A. L., (1975) *Chronic Illness and the Quality of Life*, St. Louis: C. V. Mosby

Turner, J. H., (1978) *The Structure of Sociological Theory*, Homewood, Ill.: The Dorsey Press

Webster's New World Dictionary (1976) Gevralnik, D. B. (ed.), Cleveland: William Collins and World Publishing

Bibliography

Aiken, L. H., (1982) The impact of federal policy on nurses, in Aiken, L. H. (ed.), *Nursing in the 1980s: Crises, Opportunities, Challenges*, Philadelphia: Lippincott, pp. 3–21

Barnard, R. M., (1979) Research and rehabilitative nursing, in *Current Perspectives in Rehabilitation Nursing*, St. Louis: C. V. Mosby

Fasano, M. A., (1980) The long term care ombudsman, *Journal of Gerontological Nursing, 6*:717–720

Little, D. E., (1981) A formula for professional nursing care, *Rehabilitation Nursing, 6*:1

Murphy, C., (1983) Nurses' views important on ethical decision team, *The American Nurse*, November–December, p. 12

Perdue, B. J., Mahon, N. E., Harves, S. L., and Frik, S. M., (1981) *Chronic Care Nursing*, New York: Springer

Shields, F. M., and Kick, E., (1982) Nursing care in nursing homes, in Aiken, L. H. (ed.), *Nursing in the 1980s: Crises, Opportunities, Challenges*, Philadelphia: Lippincott, pp. 195–210

Compliance

Introduction

Tradition and scientific knowledge support the belief that clients' well-being increases when health care behavior is in accord with health care providers' recommendations. Such compliance is often the stated goal of client-provider interactions, whether health care delivery is preventive, curative, or restorative. This traditional perspective places the major responsibility for enhancing compliance on the provider and overlooks mutuality.

The lack of agreement between health care recommendations and client behavior has received extensive study. Several theories and models have been developed to guide further research. Health care providers can apply these theories, models, and research findings as they work with clients who have chronic illnesses, even though the current state of knowledge has not resolved the many issues and problems influencing compliance.

This chapter describes the phenomenon of compliance in chronic illness and explores noncompliance as an issue of concern to health care providers. It describes specific problems and issues of compliance and proposes some basic guidelines for assessment and interventions in situations involving potential, apparent, or actual noncompliance.

Compliance and Chronic Illness

The predominant pattern of illness has changed from acute illness to chronic illness as science and technology have advanced. Treatment regimens have become more complex and, at the same time, have frequently required unsupervised implementation by the client or family caregivers in the home. As an example, after the introduction of insulin in the twenties, diabetes mellitus (DM) was described for decades as a unique disease since it required that the client or family member take responsibility for managing the daily therapeutic regimen. The regimen usually included diet, one or more daily injections of insulin, exercise, and urine testing.

Client responsibility for managing diabetes has grown. Currently, an individual having insulin-dependent DM (IDDM) may have a computerized insulin pump and a computerized or manual blood testing device and may at some point be a candidate for hemodialysis or renal transplant. All these modalities of treatment require compliant behaviors to effect therapeutic outcomes that ensure maximal benefit and minimal harm to the client.

Needless to say, DM is no longer considered unique in its requirements for knowledgeable implementation of a therapeutic regimen. The increase in numbers of clients with chronic diseases whose optimal treatment requires nonsupervised implementation of regimens has focused attention on the study of compliance and the development of strategies to increase desired behaviors. The evaluation of new technological and therapeutic measures for chronic diseases must take into account compliance of the study population when determining efficiency of these measures in achieving therapeutic outcomes. Practitioners must also be concerned with the extent to which clients comply in designing plans of treatment or evaluating client responses to treatment measures.

Definition of Terms

Compliance is an umbrella term for all behavior consistent with health care recommendations. *Noncompliance* denotes behaviors that are not consistent with such recommendations. These two terms are used with an acknowledgment of concerns expressed about their appropriateness for describing client responses. These concerns have focused on the notions that compliance implies that the client is passive and lacks autonomy and that the health professional is coercive and paternalistic. This chapter attaches no such meaning to these words. We agree with Connelly (1984), who laments that concerns about these words are unfortunate since they arise from inaccurate and unfavorable connotations associated with the concept of compliance, whereas ethical issues really center in the ethics of strategies to promote effective self-care.

Adherence and *nonadherence* are generally used as synonyms for these terms. One notable exception in meaning of these words is presented by Barofsky (1978), who proposed a continuum of self-care with three levels of client responses to health care recommendations: compliance, adherence, and therapeutic alliance. In this model, compliance is linked to coercion, adherence to conformity, and self-care to a therapeutic alliance with the provider. Thus, Barofsky described differing levels of client autonomy with differing types of provider-client interactions.

Components of Compliance

The relevance of compliance to the total wellness-illness continuum was described by Marston in 1970. She defined compliance as self-care behaviors that individuals undertake to promote health, to prevent illness, or to follow recommendations for treatment and rehabilitation in diagnosed illnesses. When compliance is defined as self-care, the *agent* of compliance is the client.

However, defining compliance in terms of self-care behaviors may be too limiting for understanding the phenomenon of compliance in relation to chronic illness; it may be more helpful to consider that the *agency* of compliance is often shared, since many clients cannot implement their medical regimens without the participation of family members. Strauss and associates (1984) noted that family members often take on an assisting or controlling role in influencing clients to adhere to medical regimens. Further study of how couples managed chronic disease revealed that coordination and collaboration between the couple was necessary to carry out the work of the medical regimen (Corbin & Strauss 1984). Given this shared responsibility, it seems reasonable to conclude that compliance-increasing strategies should be directed toward all individuals who are involved in implementing medical regimens.

The act of compliance may be analyzed by examining the frequency, occurrence, and variation of behaviors undertaken in response to health care recommendations. Compliance behaviors are often categorized by type: *general* (commission, omission, or modification) and *specific* (keeping appointments, taking medications, abstaining from alcohol). Several role conceptions reflect differences in clients' perceptions of their health status and the purposes for which health-related behavior is undertaken. Dimond and Jones (1983) summarize these role behaviors:

- *Health behavior:* Any activity undertaken by a person believing himself to be healthy for the purpose of preventing disease or detecting it in an asymptomatic state (Kasl & Cobb 1966, 246).
- *Illness behavior:* Any activity undertaken by a person who feels ill to define the state of health and to discover a suitable remedy (Kasl 1974; Baric 1969).
- *Sick role behavior:* Any activity undertaken by a person who is considered ill by self and others for the purpose of getting well (Kasl 1974; Baric 1969).

These role conceptions are inadequate when the agent of compliance is managing chronic rather than acute illness (Baric 1969). With chronic illness, even though the illness continues, subjective feelings of being ill may not be present during asymptomatic periods. In addition, the chronically ill client no longer expects a cure or return to prior health. Parsons's original presentation of the sick role (1951) related only to illnesses that lasted for relatively short periods of time, identified the fact that the client was granted privileges and exemptions from responsibilities and duties during that time span, and noted that the health care practitioner was directed to take responsibility for cure-focused care (see Chapter 3).

Baric proposed that a more appropriate role for chronic illness is an *at-risk* role that has risk reduction and maintenance of health as primary goals. In the at-risk role, the individual desires control of symptoms, not to become well but to decrease interference with life activities. Privileges and exemptions from social duties are only partially granted, depending on limitations imposed by the illness. Features of chronic illness that make the at-risk role more appropriate than the sick role include time factors, the necessarily active role of the client in management of the regimen, the lack of institutionalized or clearly defined reinforcement of long-term behavior by others, and the frequent lack of symptom relief (Baric 1969; Kasl 1974; Dimond & Jones 1983).

Prevalence of Noncompliance

Several reviewers of the vast compliance literature concur that, on the average, one-third to one-half of clients in study populations are noncompliant in some way with health care recommendations (Marston 1970; Sackett & Snow 1979; Gillam & Barsky 1974). Marston noted the wide variation in published rates of compliance, ranging from 4% to 100%. She also emphasized the difficulties intrinsic to comparing compliance or noncompliance rates because of the variations in conceptual and methodological designs. For example, Marston cites two studies, both using urine tests to detect the presence of antituberculin medications, which show disparity in criteria used to distinguish compliance from noncompliance. One study, by Morrow and Rabin (1966), characterized as noncompliant those who had 50% or higher negative urine test result; the other, by Nynn-Williams and Arris (1958), characterized as noncompliant individuals who had one negative test result. It becomes readily apparent that a "compliant" subject in the former study might exhibit more noncom-

pliant behavior than did a "compliant" subject in the latter study.

Compliance studies are typically disease-specific; that is, the study population is defined by the presence of specific diseases. These studies show the high rates of noncompliance noted throughout the literature. For example, in their review of compliance studies related to diabetes mellitus, Becker and Janz (1985) describe the alarming rates of noncompliance in this client population:

- Dietary noncompliance was reported at 73% (Korhonen et al. 1983), 65% (Christensen et al. 1983), and 35% (Cerkoney & Hart 1980).
- Noncompliance rates for testing urine in an acceptable manner were reported as 67% (Watkins et al. 1967), 70% (Korhonen et al. 1983), and 43% (Cerkoney & Hart 1980).

The reviewers also noted that although Cerkoney and Hart reported comparatively low noncompliance rates for specific types of compliance behavior, only 4% of the study population were found to comply with *all* components of the diabetic treatment regimen.

Although ascertaining the true picture of noncompliance in chronic illness is very difficult, one is impressed by the consistency with which high noncompliance rates are reported and must conclude that noncompliance is a major problem in the delivery of health care.

Problems and Issues

For more than 30 years, numerous studies have demonstrated that large numbers of people having acute and chronic illnesses do not follow health care recommendations thoroughly. These findings indicate that noncompliance is an endemic phenomenon. Noncompliance may be partial and/or episodic, complete and/or persistent; the former is much more frequent than the latter (Blackwell 1976). Partial or incomplete noncompliance can interfere with treatment as significantly as complete or persistent noncompliance.

Although noncompliance is increasingly recognized as a problem in health care delivery, there is less consensus about appropriate or effective methods to decrease noncompliance. Some of the difficulty lies in the inadequacies of research on compliance, some in differing role expectations of clients and providers; some relates to motivation and some to conflict in values. These difficulties often underlie questions and concerns about compliance-increasing strategies. As health care providers prescribe, teach, and counsel clients about medical regimens, they must be cautious in making assumptions about compliance or noncompliance in a given situation before imposing any one strategy upon the client. Understanding phenomena that adversely affect compliance is a preliminary to efforts to achieve more positive outcomes.

Barriers to the Study of Compliance

Although a comprehensive discussion of research and compliance is not appropriate to this chapter, some of the barriers that plague investigators and limit the confidence with which researchers or practitioners can use reported findings of specific studies can be indicated. As we shall see, the methodological and conceptual problems in the study of compliance and the lack of consistent results lead one to the conclusion that there is no well-founded knowledge base for selecting and using compliance-increasing strategies.

Methodological Barriers. Numerous methodological problems characterize compliance research (Gordis 1979; Haynes 1979). Sackett and Snow (1979) highlight the inadequacies of research design in their review of 537 original articles on compliance, which revealed only 40 studies meeting the methodological standards established for the review. They noted deficiencies in study design, specification of the illness or condition, compliance measurement, description of the therapeutic regimen, and definition of compliance. On the basis of the findings of this same review, Haynes (1979) proposed four specific suggestions for priorities in future research on compliance:

1. Studies should use inception cohorts rather than cross-sectional samples. These samples would follow all clients who were started on a therapeutic regimen, and the study would encompass the least compliant individuals who "drop out."
2. Complete compliance distributions of all study patients would be published to reveal determinants of variance in distributions.
3. Description of the relationship between compliance levels and the achievement of the treatment goal should be included.
4. The study design should be precisely described.

Sampling errors can cause a distorted description of the extent and nature of noncompliance. For example, studies of compliance with antihypertensive medications that use a cross-sectional sample generate a population of the most compliant individuals (Sackett & Snow 1979). In contrast, a longitudinal study using an inception cohort as the study population would follow all clients who were prescribed medication and thus present a more representative sample. The advantage of inception cohorts is readily apparent when one considers that many clients having hypertension never begin treatment and that others discontinue treatment within the first year (Steckel & Swain 1981).

Research designs in compliance studies often focus on specific diseases or treatment modalities, such as those on hypertension mentioned previously. This focus allows researchers to consider the special characteristics of a given disease and its treatment. Although such designs avoid the potential of some confounding variables, they limit applicability of results to the general population of persons having chronic illnesses and to the many clients who have multiple diseases and receive many treatment measures (Hulka et al. 1976; Kasl 1978).

Measurement is another area presenting inherent methodological problems. Measurements may be either direct or indirect; direct measures of health-related behavior are more costly and difficult to implement but yield more reliable data. For example, direct measures used to evaluate medication taking include urine or blood samples. Indirect measures used for the same purpose include client reports, prescription-filling, pill counts, and interviews of client and physician. It is generally believed that these indirect measures, which are used more frequently, yield compliance rates that exceed the actual level of compliance (Marston 1970; Hulka et al. 1976).

Although direct measures are considered more reliable, differences in time spans of chronic illness make drawing accurate conclusions difficult when such measures are used. For example, when testing a single sample of blood or urine for drug presence is the method used to validate compliance, the test reveals only whether medication was taken during the preceding hours or days. Accurate inferences about medication use over months or years are obviously difficult to draw from measurement made on a single day. The development of the glycosated hemoglobin test in diabetes mellitus exemplifies technological advances that provide better measures of compliance in chronic illnesses. This test gives information about the level of blood glucose over a 6- to 12-week period and thus is superior to a single blood glucose test.

Accuracy of findings may be affected by the presence of an investigator or by the client's knowledge of planned compliance measures. Studies have shown that the introduction of an observer into the home can increase compliance behavior (Marston 1970). Contradictory findings have been reported in studies using unannounced visits at homes or schools to collect urine samples to test for the presence of prescribed drugs. One study showed higher rates of noncompliance during unannounced visits than during scheduled visits; two other studies did not show this inconsistency (Marston 1970). This writer has been impressed with the frequency with which individuals with DM have described more compliant behavior on days immediately preceding their check-up visits.

Single Variables of Noncompliance.   Investigators of compliance have focused primarily on the relation of compliance to single variables such as characteristics of clients, providers, disease, and regimen, or to client-provider interactions (Dracup & Meleis

1982). Although correlations are found, studies of single variables without attention to interrelatedness among variables have contributed to contradictory or inconclusive findings and to the scarcity of studies that can be generalized to other populations (Dracup & Meleis 1982; Becker & Maiman 1978). These authors conclude that one reason for this situation is the complexity of the phenomenon of compliance and the complexity of the relationships between compliance and the variables studied.

Compliance has been shown to be poorly related to severity of illness, pain, disability, or threat to life (Hingson et al. 1981). In 1979, Haynes noted that no single study showed that severity of symptoms encouraged compliance, whereas four studies reported that lower compliance is present when there are more symptoms. According to Haynes's review of research studies (1979), few client characteristics have been shown to be influential in studies on noncompliance. Those that are influential include the following, cited by Haynes:

1. extremes of age in medication-taking (Becker & Maiman 1975)
2. some mental illnesses, particularly schizophrenia, paranoia, and personality disorders (Haynes 1976)
3. denial in clients with coronary artery disease (Craig, Shapiro & Levine 1971).

Complexity of the medical regimen was the characteristic most often found to interfere with compliance (Marston 1970). In medication-taking, complexity has two components: frequency of dose and number of drugs prescribed (Blackwell 1979). The degree of behavioral change required by the regimen and the duration of the regimen have also been associated with noncompliance (Hellenbrandt 1983). Hellenbrandt also lists the following variables that significantly influence compliance:

1. Inefficient and inconvenient clinics
2. Client-physician interactions characterized by
   Inadequate supervision
   Client dissatisfaction
   No explanation of illness given

Physician disagreement with client

Formality toward or rejection of client

The relation of low socioeconomic status to non-compliance reported in a few studies can be explained by two other factors that have been shown to decrease compliance (Hellenbrandt 1983). First, persons of low economic status are likely to have long waiting periods before and during appointments in clinics; second, there is a lack of consistent and continuous client-physician relationships.

Conceptual Barriers. A central issue of compliance and chronic illness is the lack of clear-cut evidence supporting the relative value of any one compliance-increasing strategy. Not only do methodological problems serve as barriers because of contradictory or inconclusive findings (Marston 1970; Dracup & Meleis 1982), but some authors believe that inadequate conceptualization of the phenomenon of compliance has led to the lack of consistent findings. For example, Sackett and Snow (1979) note the failure of many investigators to define compliance and noncompliance carefully, an inadequacy limiting the use of replication studies.

Theories and Models. Theoretical frameworks can provide direction for health care providers by guiding the focus and dimensions of assessment and providing structure to the interaction of client and provider. A model or theory alerts the practitioner to attend to specific factors known to influence compliance.

Several authors point out the lack of a unifying theoretical framework in studies that address the phenomenon of compliance (Becker & Maiman 1978; Dracup & Meleis 1982; Connelly 1984). The most popular theories and models in compliance research do not take into account important variables, nor do they emphasize the interactive and communication processes considered increasingly important by many researchers (Dracup & Meleis 1983; Connelly 1984; Anderson 1985; Hulka et al. 1976).

At this point it would be helpful to distinguish briefly between theories and models (Fawcett 1984):

The primary distinction between a conceptual model and a theory is the level of abstraction. A conceptual model is a highly abstract system of global concepts and linking statements. A theory, in contrast, deals with one or more specific, concrete concepts and propositions. Conceptual models are only general guides, which must be specified further by relevant and logically congruent theories before action can occur. . . . A conceptual model cannot be tested directly because its concepts are not operationally defined, nor are the relationships among concepts observable. More specific concepts and propositions have to be derived from the conceptual model, that is, a theory must be formulated.

Dracup and Meleis (1982) analyzed the medical model, the health belief model, the locus of control construct, and social learning theory, which are frequently used in compliance research. They felt that all contained conceptual inadequacies.

Interactional Model. Dracup and Meleis propose an alternate theoretical approach drawn from role theory and based on the health transaction model (initially introduced by Stone in 1979) of mutual participation of clients and physicians. The advantages of role theory as an appropriate framework are that it emphasizes interaction and communication processes and addresses the multiple compliance-related variables that have been identified. A central notion of their interactional approach is that enactment of the sick role or the at-risk role must be supported and validated in compliance-increasing strategies. Using this model, one would expect that communication would focus on compliance expectations of the client and providers and that there would be attempts to resolve conflicts about different expectancies of behavior and outcomes. Essential propositions of this framework include the following:

1. To the extent a client demonstrates knowledge and competency in enacting a proposed role, a higher level of health regimen compliance is expected. The relationship is mediated through the level of complexity and duration of the medical regimen.
2. Compliance is maximized when there is evidence that the sick or at-risk roles have been incorporated into the self-concept of the client.

3. Compliance is enhanced when relevant other roles are congruent and/or complementary with client roles.
4. Compliance is enhanced if the compliance role is reinforced by significant others and other reference groups.
5. The level and extent of the client's compliance with a health care regimen depend on the degree to which behaviors of compliance are judged valuable by the client and are validated by significant others (Dracup & Meleis 1982).

Client-Provider Interactions

From a traditional medical perspective, the client is considered passive and poorly informed about the prevention and treatment of disease. In addition, since treatment is directed toward the disease, any noncompliance indicates that the client is a problem (Anderson 1985). Here, three specific aspects of client-provider interactions are examined: expectations about interactions, feelings about personal control, and perspectives of the client.

Differing Expectations. An issue of importance to providers and clients centers on the question of how much active client participation is appropriate to interactions with providers. The question is framed in such a way that one must acknowledge that both providers and clients have expectations about the appropriate level of participation. Both make judgments based on these expectations about suitable behavior in various roles. The expectations are formed in large part from previous socialization experiences.

Providers and clients have, by and large, been socialized to expect the client to exhibit sick role behaviors and the provider to use complementary role behaviors (Parsons 1951). In the sick role, clients are expected to try to get well by seeking help and cooperating with the prescribed regimen. The complementary role of the provider is that of dominance as the professional expert and manager of the condition. Holding expert power based on mastery of specialized knowledge allows the provider to make recommendations to the client as the culmination of diagnostic and therapeutic decisions and actions. Parsons's view of a "competency gap" served to under-

line the asymmetry in doctor-client relationships (Hingson et al. 1981) and described an authority-to-subordinate relationship.

But alternative interactional roles that are characterized by more mutuality of responsibility and decision making have been noted in the literature. Szasz and Hollander (1956) describe a mutual participation model that is more appropriate to chronic illness because of the management role clients have in implementing their treatment regimens. The following are features of this model: (1) the physician's role is to help clients help themselves; (2) clients are in partnership with the provider; and (3) clients are users of expert help. The complementary roles presented in this model are that of a provider who offers guidance to the client and a client who cooperates with the provider.

Anderson (1985) describes an educational approach that has a different basic assumption from the medical model, which uses teaching as a means of persuading clients to comply. In this model the problem is viewed from the client's perspective, and the practitioner must understand and work through the client's frame of reference. In other words, clients are accepted as capable and responsible for managing their own lives and are allowed to define and meet their own needs.

Vincent (1971) applied a basic premise of role theory to compliance: compliance is dependent on an interactional system based on complementary expectations and cannot be predicted or understood in terms of client characteristics alone. It seems apparent that if clients and providers hold congruent or disparate expectations about appropriate role behaviors, different kinds of interactions with potential for influence on outcomes are likely to develop. Agreement that the relationship should be that of authority-subordinate or that of mutuality represents compliant behavior. Disparate expectations between client and provider about the level of participation represent noncompliance.

Dracup and Meleis (1982) note three studies that validate the importance of complementary roles in influencing compliance:

1. Compliance failures were highly correlated with

tension in physician-client interactions (Davis 1968).

2. Noncompliance was more likely when there was less reciprocal interaction between client and physician (Gouldner 1973).

3. Noncompliance was linked with failure of the primary provider to communicate the purpose of the treatment (Wilson 1973).

Although further research is needed to test the relationship of complementary roles to compliance, it seems logical to assume that communication between provider and client might well include discussing the expectations each holds about the level and kind of participation of the client and the kind of assistance to be offered by the provider. Providers might become more effective in their communication and interaction with clients if they viewed clients as occupying different positions on a passivity-to-autonomy continuum, rather than focusing on a preconceived notion of expected client behavior. The result would be increased sensitivity to each client's requirements for autonomy, guidance, and direction. Rather than posing a question about the extent of participation clients should have in interactions, a more appropriate question would be, What is the optimal kind of participation for a particular client? The answer can only be evolved by the provider-client dyad as they communicate about expectations, goals, and perceived problems.

Feelings about Personal Control. The locus-of-control construct has been used to study client choices of self-care behavior; it focuses on individual expectancies about outcomes (rewards, reinforcements) and the perceived efficacy of behavior to modify outcomes. According to this construct, persons are at different positions on an internality-externality continuum of orientation to perceived control. *Internals* believe in personal influence on future events and *externals* attribute influence to others. The health locus-of-control construct modifies this generalized expectancy to specific ones of health and illness outcomes and health behaviors (Rotter 1966; Wallston et al. 1976).

Research findings have been contradictory about

the relationship of locus of control to compliance (Wallston, Wallston, & DeVellis 1978; Dimond & Jones 1983). Schroeder and Miller (1983) describe externals as more compliant with treatment and less active in seeking information, whereas internals actively seek knowledge and manipulate treatment regimens.

Some researchers have suggested that treatment programs should reflect the differing characteristics and learning styles of internals and externals (Wallston, Wallston, & DeVellis 1978). Schroeder and Miller (1983) suggest that approaches for externals would be most appropriate if they included an authority-to-subordinate interpersonal relationship, support of a positive self-concept, and structured teaching plans. Approaches for internals would be appropriately tailored if they included multiple options, participation in decision making, and emphasis on personal responsibility and accountability for treatment outcomes.

Internality may be increased through educational programs that emphasize personal responsibility. However, Dimond and Jones (1983) point out that the inculcation of personal responsibility is stressful and not without danger. These authors caution:

> It would be foolish if not dangerous to attempt to make the orientation of all clients internal. Personal control can be so stress-producing as to outweigh the benefits ... attempts to control uncontrollable conditions are likely to induce self-blame, depression, or despair.

Perspectives of the Client. Clients and providers are likely to hold different perspectives of chronic illness, its treatment, and the relative merits of compliant behavior. The client lives with the disease, and treatment is only one aspect of that individual's life. Living with treatment consequences is vastly different from offering advice, counsel, education, or exhortation about health care recommendations. Clients rarely, if ever, seek help from health care providers because they want to comply. Rather, they ask for help for a variety of reasons: they feel ill, they are worried, they are responding to others' recommendations, they need evidence to validate claims for entitlement benefits, and so forth. Providers, on the other hand, are very much concerned about compliance, which may be seen as the desired outcome of the interaction (Anderson 1985).

Anderson points out two important ways in which clients' perspectives of chronic illness, in this case diabetes mellitus, differ from those of providers. First, there is a relative difference in understanding of the treatment regimen, not just on the level of specificity, rationale, and consequences, but with respect to the sources of problems. Clients may see treatment as part of the problem of having diabetes, whereas providers see treatment as a solution. Second, clients are more concerned about the "here and now" experience, in contrast to providers' concern over a problem that places future health at risk. For example, Anderson reports that clients express more frequent concerns about preventing hypoglycemic reactions than about managing higher than normal blood glucose levels. Providers, on the other hand, express more concern about the importance of compliance in achieving close to normal blood glucose levels because of their perceptions of serious long-term consequences if control of blood glucose levels is not achieved.

The client's perspective on chronic illness, its treatment, and compliance is also influenced by the demands of living, of time and energy, and of the talents required by life conditions (Strauss et al. 1984). Other commitments and demands compete with those of the treatment regimen so that treatment benefits may be viewed as less valuable than the costs that are incurred. According to Strauss and associates, whether the client takes up and adheres to regimens of treatment depends on certain conditions, including these:

1. There is an initial or continuing trust in the physician or whoever else prescribes the regimen.
2. No rival supersedes the physician in his or her legitimating.
3. There is evidence that the regimen works to control either symptoms or the disease itself, or both.
4. No distressing, frightening side effects appear.
5. The side effects are outweighed by symptom relief or by sufficient fear of the disease itself.
6. There is a relative noninterference with impor-

tant daily activities, either of the client or of people around him or her.
7. The regimen's perceived good effects are not outweighed by a negative impact on the client's sense of identity.

Motivation

In the traditional medical model, noncompliance is often attributed to poor motivation. The provider attributes one client's mastery of and continuation with the prescribed regimen as the result of high motivation and identifies the lack of motivation as an obstacle to compliance in others. In this model noncompliance is not viewed as an inadequacy of communication between client and provider.

Client's Life Perspective. Differing levels of motivation for health care behaviors can be more understandable when the client's perspective of life is taken into account. A demand for a client to comply with a treatment regimen competes with other valued tasks, roles, or relationships that may impede complying with provider recommendations. Chronically ill clients must continue to manage their daily existences under specific sets of financial and social conditions (Strauss et al. 1984). Consequently the strength of motivation to carry out health care behaviors may vary with perceptions of current life demands.

The brief case study of Mrs. J. illustrates the necessity of learning the client's life perspective to understand apparent low-level motivation for assuming recommended health care behavior.

The case study demonstrates the need to consider the primary motivating forces in the client's life at a given time and to determine the way that they affect the strength of motivation for specific health care behavior.

Labeling a client as poorly motivated without considering that person's life perspective impedes the progress of the helping process. Labeling offers no suggestions as to how to intervene in an effective manner. However, taking the client's perspective into account can assist the health care provider to gain

---

◇ CASE STUDY ◇
Mrs. J.

Mrs. J., a 52-year-old matron of Eastern European descent, seemed not to listen to or understand the dietician's explanation of a 1,400 calorie diet prescribed for newly diagnosed non–insulin-dependent diabetes mellitus. Educational level and learning abilities were rated as above average. The nurse noted that Mrs. J.'s conversations concerned her daughter's wedding, which was to occur in 2 weeks and had been planned for 2 years. According to Mrs. J., this wedding was to be the "biggest event of my life," and one in which her status as a good

mother, future mother-in-law, and member of a newly extended family would be affirmed. It would be "unthinkable for me not to join in the festivities . . . in which eating and drinking would last hours and hours." It was not until the dietician offered to work with Mrs. J. to plan this day's food intake and to negotiate with her some compromise between the ideal of 1,400 calories/24 hours and Mrs. J.'s ideal of feasting that Mrs. J. showed some willingness to engage in learning to incorporate the diet into her usual daily life pattern.

---

clues about the barriers to compliance perceived by the client. It is true that effective intervention may need to include negotiation and compromise by both client and provider, particularly around specific or short-term time periods. It is also true that clients may be more motivated to learn when their perspective is considered and they are involved in planning and thereby achieve more complete compliance over longer time periods.

Health Belief Model.   Motivation is clearly related to beliefs and attitudes held by an individual. The health belief model (HBM), which contains a cluster of pertinent beliefs and attitudes, was developed by Hochman, Leventhal, Kegles, and Rosenstock to explain preventive health behavior (Becker & Maiman 1975) and was later modified to include a general health motivation (Becker 1976). Dimensions of the HBM can provide direction for assessment of an individual client's attitudes and beliefs that are relevant to compliance with a particular regimen. The HBM's major proposition is that two variables increase the likelihood of an individual taking recommended health actions: the value placed by an individual on a particular goal, and the individual's estimate of the likelihood that a specific action will achieve that goal (Becker & Janz 1985).

Figures 7–1 and 7–2 show the dimensions of the HBM in preventive health behavior and in sick-role behavior. The four dimensions or basic components

that are present in each of these applications are the individual's perception of susceptibility to a certain disease or disease outcome, perception of severity of that condition, perceived values of the health behavior, and identified barriers to action.

The HBM is less effective in explaining noncompliance and compliance in curative situations than in preventive situations (Kasl 1978), yet findings of many studies have generally supported the HBM as useful in discerning the relationship of client beliefs to compliance (Becker 1976). Research using the HBM shows that perceptions of susceptibility, severity, and benefits are positively correlated with a variety of desirable health behaviors: taking medications, following dietary restrictions, observing exercise prescriptions, and keeping clinic appointments (Hallel 1983; Becker & Janz 1985). Perceptions and beliefs can be altered by "corrective factual information, motive arousing appeals . . . recommendations from other sources of information that have greater credibility to the patient" (Becker & Janz 1985).

Ethical Issues in Compliance

Health care providers see compliance as a major factor influencing the extent to which optimal health care outcomes can be achieved; noncompliance in chronic illness can contribute to more costly hospitalizations and to the need for more extensive and

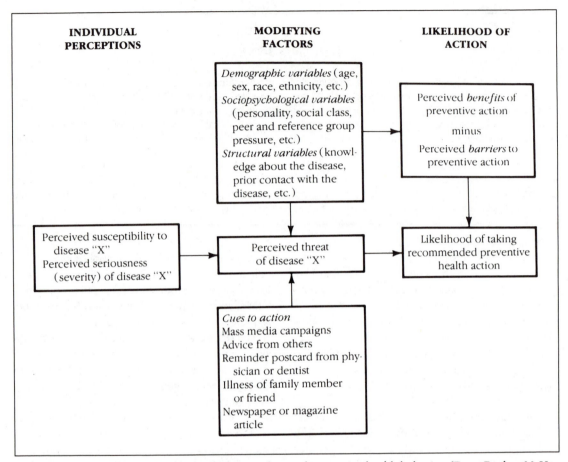

INDIVIDUAL PERCEPTIONS

MODIFYING FACTORS

LIKELIHOOD OF ACTION

Demographic variables (age, sex, race, ethnicity, etc.)
Sociopsychological variables (personality, social class, peer and reference group pressure, etc.)
Structural variables (knowledge about the disease, prior contact with the disease, etc.)

Perceived *benefits* of preventive action

minus

Perceived *barriers* to preventive action

Perceived susceptibility to disease "X"
Perceived seriousness (severity) of disease "X"

Perceived threat of disease "X"

Likelihood of taking recommended preventive health action

Cues to action
Mass media campaigns
Advice from others
Reminder postcard from physician or dentist
Illness of family member or friend
Newspaper or magazine article

FIGURE 7-1. The health belief model as predictor of preventive health behavior. (From Becker, M. H., and others: A new approach to explaining sick-role behavior in low-income populations, Am. J. Public Health 64:205-216, 1974.)

expensive treatments should severe illness result (Connelly 1984). Ethical issues that are raised center about reciprocal rights and responsibilities of caregivers and clients, use of paternalism and coercion by caregivers, autonomy of the client, relative risks and benefits of proposed regimens, and the costs to society of noncompliance.

Compliance or noncompliance with recommendations for health behavior is an increasingly important ethical issue in cost containment in health care since conflicts arise when health care resources are limited and decisions about the best use of time,

money, and the energy of providers must be made. However, economical and ethical issues differ. Whereas economic issues concern the most *efficient* distribution of resources, ethical issues concern the most *equitable* distribution (Barry 1982). Connelly (1984) believes that strategies that promote and improve clients' active and effective self-care are ethically and economically significant.

Sackett (1976) described three preconditions for ethical practice that must precede strategies to change client behavior toward increased compliance. These preconditions mandate the use of informed

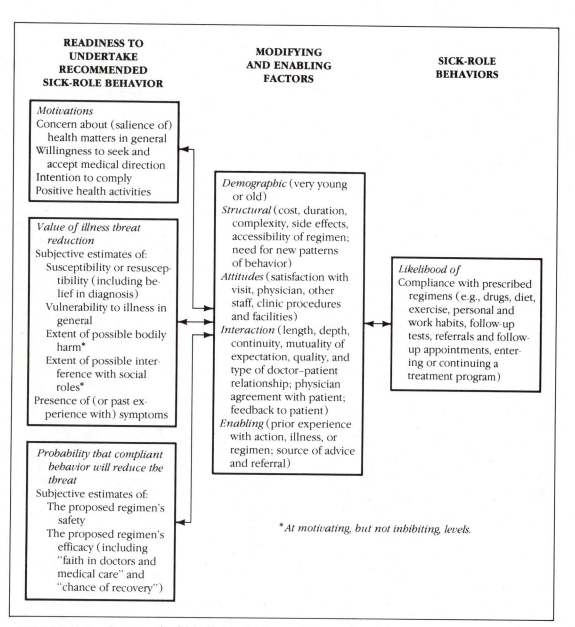

FIGURE 7-2. Summary health belief model for predicting and explaining sick-role behaviors. (From Becker, M. H.: The health belief model and sick-role behavior, Health Educ. Monogr. 2:409-419, 1974.)

consent and the development of a partnership with responsibility for compliance equally shared.

1. The diagnosis must be correct.
2. Therapy must provide more benefit than harm.
3. The client who accepts the treatment regimen must be a partner in strategies used to increase compliance.

Jonsen (1979) added a fourth condition, the importance of client consent to the regimen, and emphasized that the ethics of compliance are based on freedom, mutual understanding, and mutual responsibility. Connelly incorporated both Sackett's and Jonsen's conditions in an ethical approach to compliance that has three phases:

- Developing client competencies and reinforcing and supporting the client's self-care ability
- Evolving a consensual regimen and outcome goals through a client-provider interaction based on concepts of mutuality
- Focusing compliance-increasing strategies on joint exploration of problems and negotiation of conflicts in goals or implementation.

Threats, pressure, and inappropriate fear-arousal tactics are not ethical (Jonsen 1979; Connelly 1984). Punitive responses that can be implemented by the provider for revealed or suspected noncompliance include decreased time and attention from the provider, less availability for crisis management, and limitation of access to services, resources, or supplies. The high incidence of noncompliance and the provider's frequent inability to differentiate clients who comply from those who do not present an argument against the withdrawal or diminution of services to clients who disclose noncompliance. If others may be equally noncompliant, punitive responses to only those who are honest about noncompliance constitute inequality of care, an issue of social justice.

If the client has been informed and understands that the consequence of noncompliance is to be withdrawal by the provider, then termination of the relationship may be the right of the provider. Should economic or social conditions preclude access to other caregivers, this termination would raise serious questions about the ethical nature of withdrawing and abandoning the client. Assisting the client to find another caregiver is "ethically preferable to unilateral and abrupt termination" (Jonsen 1979).

Education

There is wide support for educational strategies in prevention and treatment of noncompliance among individuals interested in ethical implications of compliance behavior (Jonsen 1979) and researchers studying compliance (Green 1979). For example, the overwhelming suggestion offered by nurses in an opinion survey related to improving client compliance with medication taking was "teach, teach, teach" (Moree 1984). The relationships of client education to chronic illness and teaching are described in Chapter 12.

Sadly, knowledge about illness and treatment, in itself, does not ensure desired results. However, without knowledge, clearly compliance cannot occur (Sackett 1976; Becker & Janz 1985). For example, taking medication has been the focus of a large number of compliance studies. Reported results indicate that knowledge of drug function has been correlated with both decreased error rates and improved compliance (Hulka et al. 1976). In another study, using a sample of chronically ill elderly individuals, inaccurate knowledge about drugs was associated with a 20% error factor and occurred among 41% of clients (Schwartz et al. 1962).

Kasl (1978) described the complexity of the relationship of knowledge to compliance and cited the following studies as support:

Knowledge of the regimen is helpful (Kirscht & Rosenstock 1979) but may have dubious value when the regimen is relatively simple and not exceedingly demanding (Taylor et al. 1978).

Knowledge of disease seems to have little impact on compliance of those subjects who have a rich experience with their illness, treatment management, and the medical-care system (Tagliacozzo & Irma 1970).

There is contradictory evidence about the impact of information giving on compliance (Steckel & Swain 1981). One conceptual issue in the relation of education to compliance deals with the difference between information giving by the provider and a planned program of education designed to achieve specified cognitive, psychomotor, and affective health behaviors. This difference is not always appreciated in studies on compliance. To be effective, client education must include both an accurate assessment of learning needs and abilities, as well as barriers, and a plan designed and executed to maximize the potential for learning how to incorporate health care behavior into daily life.

Educational goals must be broader than the acquisition of knowledge alone if compliance is to result. Abilities beyond knowledge and comprehension are required. More complex domains of cognition include application, synthesis, and design, as described by Bloom (1971). It follows that the outcome of compliance depends on participation of the learner beyond that of listening, reading, or assimilating information.

In a review of compliance studies, Hogue (1979) observed that facilitating mutual participation of clients in their own care (including education) may be more effective than disseminating information in achieving compliance. In studies cited by Hogue, participation in learning included the following:

1. Using knowledge to increase one's level of wellness (Davis 1976)
2. Contracting with the nurse to change behavior (Sheridan & Smith 1975)
3. Discussing health, structure, and functioning of the family in relation to experience and abilities for health behavior (Fink 1969)
4. Receiving social support designed to increase competence and motivation to adhere (Caplan 1976; Hogue 1978)
5. Discussing ways to achieve congruence between the regimen and clients' life-styles (Hecht 1974).

Principles of adult education as defined by Knowles (1970) emphasize the necessity of involvement of adult patients in decisions about what to learn, when to learn, and how to learn. Adults learn best that which is clearly relevant and pertinent to them, not to the health care providers.

In summary, studies of compliance and education have led to the conclusion that transmitting information is not sufficient to overcome noncompliance, that engaging the client's participation in applying knowledge to his or her life holds more promise (Hogue 1979).

Interventions to Attain Compliance

The complexity of the problems involved in noncompliance should not deter the health practitioner from working with the client to achieve maximum possible integration of optimal health recommendations, given the client's needs, demands, and life-style. To accomplish maximum compliance, those who use compliance-increasing strategies have responsibilities to ensure the client's safety and comprehension. For the nurse, often working as liaison between client and physician, communicating with either or both is often necessary before matters are clear enough to select and begin specific compliance-increasing strategies.

Assessment Factors

Before any one intervention can be selected to assist a client in adhering to a proposed medical regimen, a careful assessment is necessary to distinguish those situational factors that can and will be modified from those that cannot or will not be modified. In addition, assessment will help determine the relative harm or benefit expected from a regimen implemented under the client's current conditions. The client and family should be included in the assessment process.

A systematic assessment of the client would include sociodemographic facts, knowledge level, beliefs, attitudes, and current understanding of the proposed regimen. There should be a determination of

◇ CASE STUDY ◇

An Appearance of Noncompliance

Mrs. Z., who was caregiver to her father, Mr. A., received from the pharmacist a vial of antibiotic medicine. The label on the vial was incorrect; instead of the prescribed "once a day" (q.d.), the label read "four times a day" (q.i.d.). Mrs. Z. remembered that six months previously the dosage of this antibiotic had been prescribed once a day. She decided that four times a day was too often and administered it twice a day. After a few days she decreased it to once a day and finally stopped giving it when her father became confused. Because her father attributed confusion to a prescribed vasodilator, she also stopped giving that.

She could not recall what she had been told about the dosage when she last saw the physician, nor did she recall receiving written directions. With her father's previous physician, Mrs. Z. had been comfortable about calling with questions about her father's care. That physician had stopped practicing because of his own sudden illness. The new physician seemed competent enough, but Mrs. Z. "did not know him well enough to call him." She readily accepted the home health care nurse's offer to call the physician to clarify the prescription, to report the onset of confusion, and to let him know about the omission of prescribed medications.

the "rightness" of the prescriptions for the particular client, including an estimation of relative harm or benefit that is expected. The outcome of assessment would allow the nurse to determine which aspects of the regimen management (1) are most unlikely to achieve compliant behavior, (2) are most important in attaining therapeutic goals, and (3) require most learning to attain desired behavioral change.

Hingson et al. (1981) suggest that the following questions be asked in a compliance-oriented history:

1. Have you been taking anything for this problem already?
2. Does anything worry you about the illness?
3. What can happen if the recommended regimen is not followed?
4. How likely is that to occur?
5. How effective do you feel the regimen will be in treating the disorder?
6. Can you think of any problems you might have in following the regimen?
7. Do you have any questions about the regimen or how to follow it?

Mrs. Z.'s case study illustrates many of the factors that interact and result in decisions and actions that lead to compliance or noncompliance. This case example also demonstrates the importance of properly

identifying the sources of noncompliance, as well as using guidelines for analysis of a situation involving apparent noncompliance.

First, we should recognize that health care providers are not infallible and that errors can occur in prescribing, in dispensing, in the process of communication with the client and family caregiver, or in maintaining updated written records, especially in clinics where health care is provided by different physicians and nurses. A second consideration is that the client/caregiver simply may not understand, or remember, instructions. Hulka and associates (1976) emphasize that lack of comprehension is different from volitional noncompliance and may be responsible for considerable errors in medication taking. In the Hulka and associates study, when clients were informed of the behavior expected of them and understood it, more than 85% of the time behavior conformed to that expectation.

Third, it is important to be aware of a tendency among care providers: to see compliant behavior as positive, admirable, and wise on the part of "good patients" and noncompliant behavior as negative, deplorable, and unintelligible on the part of "problem patients." Noncompliance, from this view, is considered a rejection of advice, a negation of professional expertise, or an obstruction to the helping process.

It seems probable that health professionals having this view would be less likely to search out barriers to noncompliance that might include their own actions or nonactions.

A fourth guideline in analyzing a situation involving apparent noncompliance is to be cautious in attributing causation of noncompliance or in making predictions about levels of compliance based on any one characteristic of a client. Compliance is poorly related to sociodemographic characteristics or stable personality traits (Kasl 1978).

Insufficient knowledge may concern the *purpose* of the recommendation made by the prescriber; sometimes previous experience has been negative because of incorrect *use* of treatment remedies. For example, one client having an acute exacerbation of eczema (duration 35 years) was told to take prednisone in decreasing amounts (5 times, 4 times, 3 times, 2 times, and then 1 time on five succeeding days). His initial resistance became understandable when it was learned that he had developed "terrible stomach pain and a personality change" during prior use of this medication. Exploration revealed that he had taken all the required number of pills at one time each day. Suggestions to space the pills and to use antacids were accepted; he later reported no side effects. This same person, for the first time, complied with directions to wear gloves at night following application of ointment to his hands, after he learned that gloves increased absorption of the medicine: "Never before has anyone told me . . . that makes sense."

Assessment should also lead to a determination of the proper focus of compliance-increasing strategies. It was said earlier that the notion of compliance as self-care may be too restrictive for situations in which compliance with medical regimens cannot be achieved without the assistance of others. The combination of marked disability and chronic illness makes the conceptualization of compliance as a self-care ability inappropriate if the major concern is congruence of the client's treatment with provider recommendations.

Strauss and others (1984) describe two roles of family members in relation to compliance: those of controlling (commanding, manipulating, shaming, reminding) and of assisting. This conceptualization of family roles retains the primary focus on the client as the agent of compliance and may be adequate in situations in which the client's disabilities are not marked. When abilities are markedly diminished, the family member may be the most important agent of compliance and should become the focus of compliance-increasing strategies.

Additional case data about Mrs. Z. and her father illustrate the multiple factors that influence compliance with a treatment regimen for a frail, elderly person. Before describing the problem this family has in managing the treatment regimen, two other aspects of family's involvement need to be mentioned. One is the obvious fact that families have many goals, concerns, and conditions besides managing the illness of one member. The second is that managing the medically prescribed treatment regimen is only part of the work involved in caring for a client. Supervision, assistance, and persuasion to eat and move about, hygiene, diversional activities, and so on, are some of the obvious tasks (see Chapter 2).

Mrs. Z.'s case demonstrates the complexity and the reality of barriers to compliance when client and family members are sharing the work of implementing the regimen. Compliance is affected by the multiple and competing demands and commitments of family members, as well as family member–client interactions. The case also demonstrates the need to focus compliance strategies on all those involved in management of regimens.

Nursing Diagnosis

One of the nursing diagnoses accepted by the North American Nursing Diagnosis Association is *noncompliance*. This diagnosis is used when assessment reveals that the client desires to comply but is prevented from doing so by the presence of certain factors. The diagnosis is not applicable when assessment reveals that the client has made "an informed autonomous

◇ CASE STUDY ◇

Managing a Therapeutic Regimen

Mr. A. moved to his daughter's home more than a year ago, after a month's stay in the hospital for treatment of a life-threatening urinary infection with sepsis. At the time of discharge, he weighed 98 pounds, but now he weighs 115 pounds. Given his 5 foot 11 inch frame, he still appears emaciated. He spends most of his time in bed because of weakness. Although alert and communicative, he often asks his daughter, Mrs. Z., to fully interpret conversations between the home health nurse and himself. On rare occasions, he has unpredictable episodes of confusion.

The physician's prescriptions have consisted of daily Lasix, antibiotics that have varied from once to four times a day, and Tylenol with codeine that is to be taken as necessary. Ordered diet is low-salt, regular. There is daily catheter care, including catheter irrigations, plus monthly change of the indwelling catheter by the nurse.

Mrs. Z., 46, describes her father as stubborn: he had insisted on living alone after the death of her mother. Because he had managed chronic urinary incontinence by self-catheterization for three years, he was distressed by the need for an indwelling catheter. She acknowledges that he is not happy about being "forced" to move from his old neighborhood because he misses his independence and the opportunity to visit with friends at the senior citizens' club. Mrs. Z. describes her husband as being good to her and her father. She works at her husband's shop, where they are very busy, and she does most of her own housework. She goes to great lengths to prevent her husband from knowing the extent of work involved in the care of her father.

Mrs. Z. takes responsibility for administering medications ("I can't trust him"), preparing the diet, and handling some of the catheter management, as well as other aspects of care. On occasion her father does not receive one or more doses because she forgets or finds him asleep when they are due. When he is confused,

she has to argue to persuade him to take the pills. She is unable to manage a four-times-a-day routine with her work schedule at the shop, so she gives him medicine three times a day. She was uncomfortable having a health aide in the house when she was not there and finds that her father often neglects to take the noon pill she leaves for him unless she calls from the shop to remind him.

Managing the low-salt diet is not difficult for Mrs. Z. because she already used salt minimally in food preparation. Mr. A. has gained nearly twenty pounds since coming to his daughter's home. At first he was served meals in bed but now is expected to eat at the table, which he enjoys. There are a snack and water at the bedside for the hours when she is away.

Managing the catheter has been very difficult for both father and daughter. Mr. A. considers the catheter painful, a major handicap, and continually frustrating. He has cut it and removed it twice. A trial self-catheterization was negotiated with the physician, but this lasted only three months until infection recurred. Daily catheter care, which involves cleaning and inspecting the penis and catheter, is stressful for Mrs. Z. Initially she felt she could not look at her father "there" but seemed more comfortable about the irrigations, although she occasionally forgets them. She reluctantly asked her husband to do the daily catheter care until her father gained the ability to manage it himself. She prefers to avoid involving her husband because she does not want him to know the amount of time actually involved in caregiving.

For Mrs. Z., the shifting of roles between assisting and control agent occurs at her father's transitions between confusion and alertness and between states of varying dependency. The organization of time and effort for management of the regimen falls on Mrs. Z. She values her ability to provide care for her father in addition to her commitment to her marriage, home management, and success in the family business.

---

decision not to comply" (Carpenito 1984). Noncompliance is an appropriate diagnosis when it has been clinically validated by the identifiable defining characteristic, "verbalization of noncompliance or nonparticipation" (Carpenito 1984). *Potential noncompliance* is also a possible diagnosis if one or more

situational factors known to be associated with noncompliance are present (see Table 7–1).

Thus, noncompliance is most appropriate as a diagnosis when the client is not following a treatment regimen because of a lack of resources (personal, material, or social) or because of competing de-

TABLE 7-1. Noncompliance

DEFINITION

Noncompliance: The state in which the individual demonstrates personal behavior that deviates from health-related advice given by health care professionals.[1]

ETIOLOGICAL AND CONTRIBUTING FACTORS

Many factors in an individual's life can contribute to noncompliance. Some common ones are listed below.

Situational
    Side-effects of therapy
    Impaired ability to perform tasks (poor memory, motor and sensory deficits)
    Previous unsuccessful experience with advised regimen
    Concurrent illness of family member
    Impersonal aspects of the referral process
    Nontherapeutic environment
    Inclement weather that prevents person from keeping appointment
    Complex, prolonged, or unsupervised therapy
    Expensive therapy
    Nonsupportive family
    Nontherapeutic relationship between client and nurse
    Knowledge deficit
    Lack of autonomy in health-seeking behavior
    Health beliefs that run counter to professional advice
    Poor self-esteem
    Disturbance in body image

DEFINING CHARACTERISTICS

Verbalization of noncompliance or nonparticipation

Associated Defining Characteristics
    Missed appointments
    Partially used or unused medications
    Persistence of symptoms[2]
    Progression of disease process[2]
    Occurrence of undesired outcomes[2] (postoperative morbidity, pregnancy, obesity, addiction, regression during rehabilitation)

---

[1]The use of the nursing diagnosis *Noncompliance* describes the individual who desires to comply, but the presence of certain factors prevents him from doing so. The nurse must attempt to reduce or eliminate these factors for the interventions to be successful. However, the nurse is cautioned against using the diagnosis of noncompliance to describe an individual who has made an informed autonomous decision not to comply.
[2]When these characteristics are considered to be the result of noncompliance, one is assuming that the therapy prescribed has been proved to be effective and is appropriate.

Carpenito, L.J. (1984) Handbook of Nursing Diagnosis, *Philadelphia: J.B. Lippincott Co., pp. 44–45.*

mands (other needs, goals, or concerns) of the client or family. Such demands, commitments, and concerns may compete with those posed by the regimen, as the case study of Mr. M. illustrates. When the client or family caregiver is encouraged to describe daily activities, living conditions, and present concerns, it is more likely that these and other situational factors related to compliance will be identified. For example, the increasing numbers of aged persons make it likely that a particular individual may be more concerned about a loved one's chronic illness than about his or her own health. These etiological factors direct

◇ CASE STUDY ◇
Mr. M.: Competing Demands and Concerns

Mr. M., a 70-year-old business executive, was newly diagnosed with non–insulin-dependent diabetes mellitus (NIDDM). He was educated, alert, and able to solve problems, and he attended classes on diabetes education so he "could learn why and how to follow his regimen." He decided to do home blood glucose monitoring instead of urine testing, but he showed no interest in being compliant about diet and indicated little enthusiasm for changing food intake habits except to omit concentrated sugars.

Only when asked specific questions about his daily schedule, living conditions, and present concerns did he reveal that his attention, energy, and time were completely devoted to his business and to his respirator-dependent wife. His business took most of his daytime hours and he provided direct care to his wife seven nights and four evenings each week. Since her sudden respiratory failure 6 months earlier, he had learned to manage medicines and respirator and oxygen equipment and to perform other specific therapeutic tasks.

He described the dinner hour as "precious time when we can talk about something besides sickness."

Mr. M. identified a number of factors that influenced his noncompliance with diet. First, breakfast was sometimes missed if he slept late. Second, it was difficult to be more consistent in eating lunch at the same time each day because his schedule revolved about his customers' needs, which led to missing this meal frequently. Third, dinner with his wife was the only time either could focus on family matters without interruption, and he did not want to be thinking about what he should be eating at that time. Fourth, he considered his wife's illness and care as more serious and having more immediacy than his own; consequences from his diabetes were seen somewhere in the future, making it easy not to focus on his own care needs. Finally, it was determined that he received little reinforcement from the presence of symptoms or from his physician contact, which was scheduled every three months.

---

the nurse's attention toward strategies that increase the client's use of resources and problem solving to resolve conflicts among competing demands.

If the nursing diagnosis model is used for analysis of client responses to health care recommendations, noncompliance does not refer to those conditions in which directions are not understood well enough to be implemented: recommendations should be clear and specific, so that they make sense to the client. Errors in prescribing and transcribing as well as dispensing medications can also occur (Hulka et al. 1976). These two kinds of errors require different management from an informed and willful choice not to comply.

Encouraging Client Participation

It is generally believed that compliance is increased when clients actively participate in learning and deciding how to implement prescribed regimens. However, insistence by the health care provider on a preconceived or stereotyped notion of the most

desirable level of participation may be inappropriate. A mismatch between an authoritarian provider and an assertive, active learner may result in poor communication and may influence compliance adversely. On the other hand, a passive and nonactive learner can be overwhelmed by the provider who expects active involvement in the learning and communication processes. Some studies using the locus-of-control construct support different approaches to "externals" and "internals" (see the section "Feelings about Personal Control") and suggest that increasing active participation for "externals" may not be appropriate.

One recent study found that participation by clients was not correlated with the intent to adhere among elderly women. The investigators suggest that their sample of elderly women may be one in which assertiveness and active style of learning have not been culturally induced. They also state that such results cast doubt on the hypothesis that participation in decisions leads to increased compliance in all individuals (Chang et al. 1985). Careful assessment will help determine the most appropriate level of participation, and evaluation will serve to determine the effect of a given level of participation.

Tailoring. The minimal outcome of client participation with the nurse in developing a compliance strategy should be that of *tailoring* the treatment to the client's daily behaviors, since this process may help to cue compliance (Haynes 1979). Integrating treatment activities so that they coincide with routine activities, called *rituals,* is an important way of individualizing and enhancing the treatment plan. The daily schedule of eating, arising and retiring, hygiene, favorite television program, and so on, identifies rituals that may be used to incorporate health behaviors into daily life.

Simplifying the Regimen. As a result of discussion between client and nurse, it may become apparent that the client is unable to manage the complexity of the prescribed regimen. Negotiation with the prescribing source may result in better compliance if this barrier is cleared and the regimen simplified. As a general rule, the number of times medications are taken and the number of pills should be held to a minimum.

Providing Reminders. The use of memory aids should not be overlooked. With the high level of illiteracy in the United States today, the ability to read, tell time, and understand numbers must be assessed before such aids are suggested. Calendars, clocks, and individually prepared posters with medication and food reminders can be very helpful. Separating a day's supply of medications can also help the person who has difficulty remembering if a particular dose was taken. The health care provider can reinforce the importance of compliance at episodic visits. Such reinforcement may involve pill counting or attention to client diaries or to other reports of behavior and self-monitoring: all methods that remind the client of the value of compliance and that elicit participation.

Enhancing Coping. The nurse should be very sensitive to clues from individual clients suggesting emotional responses that interfere with learning optimal health behaviors. Situational anxiety, marked depression, and denial are associated with low levels of compliance. These three emotional responses should be interpreted as signals that the client's coping skills are inadequate and that a modification in approach may be more effective. Mrs. T.'s case study illustrates the influence of inadequate coping on compliance.

Contracting. Contracting can be viewed as an educational strategy that engages clients' commitment to learn, to make changes, and to be accountable for their own behavior (see Chapters 11 and 12). Contracting involves the nurse and client in a collaboratively developed written contract with specified goals and methods and explicitly identified incentives. Based on principles of behavioral modification, contracting uses reinforcements to establish and to maintain new or changed behaviors. Contracting has been successfully used as a strategy to increase compliance in various settings and with different types of behavior (Steckel & Swain 1981).

Social Support

It is commonly believed that social support—by significant others or support networks—helps clients cope with chronic illness and reinforces compliant behavior. The increase in self-help groups reflects this belief, as does the current practice of referring people to such groups. In spite of this trend, it is unclear from the literature whether these groups increase compliance behavior.

Although existing and potential social support should be identified, enlisting such assistance is a decision that must include the client; the client's views on the involvement of others should be taken into account. Kasl (1978) cautions that social support be considered part of a broader process of social influence that may guide people in different directions, with effects on disease outcomes, participation levels, interference with or facilitation of medical treatment, and delay in relinquishing the sick role. The client may have very strong opinions about including others, even in a supportive role, in manage-

◇ CASE STUDY ◇

Client Participation

Mrs. T., a 51-year-old practical nurse, was referred to a diabetic education program because she had been unable to manage her weight, then over 200 pounds, and because she needed insulin therapy. She cried as she expressed feelings of failure and shame. She agreed to share information about her living conditions so a plan could be developed to attain two goals: weight reduction and better control of blood glucose levels. An interview revealed the following:

1. She experienced feelings of discomfort ("feeling panic") when visiting the physician.
2. She had had feelings of anxiety and stress since her husband's heart attack 2 years earlier. She had performed cardiopulmonary resuscitation at home at that time.
3. She needed to "keep busy" so she did not have time to worry about her husband. She did this by working twelve-hour night shifts on weekends and maintaining a busy social schedule and housework during the week. Even though she did not have to work for the income it provided, she noted that the activity kept her from worrying: "I'm so afraid to be alone with my husband in case he has another cardiac arrest."
4. She had an excellent knowledge level of calorie and nutrient content of foods and could perform blood glucose monitoring and insulin injections.
5. She actively sought information and help: participa-

tion in many weight reduction programs over the years with successful loss of weight each time.
6. She recognized that maintenance of weight loss was a problem and that she had not learned effective strategies to achieve weight control.

Several situational factors were identified. First, daily insulin therapy was a hazard, given Mrs. T.'s day-and-night schedule. Her schedule also violated the need for consistency in daily activities that were essential in helping her achieve better control. The nurse's planning with the client and physician resulted in these strategies:

1. continued involvement in the diabetic education program to integrate needed changes into her life
2. supportive counseling to help her gain coping skills via referral to a mental health center
3. a month's leave of absence from work as a trial period of consistent daily activities
4. discussion by client and physician of the helping relationship desired by both.

The client followed through on these plans. Six weeks later, the physician reported that Mrs. T. had better control of blood glucose, had shown some weight loss, and was asking for a permanent change in work schedule. It was clear that these outcomes were achieved because Mrs. T. was able to implement changes in her life.

---

ment of the condition. Significant others may be identified by the client as barriers to compliance rather than as facilitators.

Social isolation has been associated with low compliance and a supportive family with high compliance in some studies (Haynes 1979). The study on adherence to medical regimens in elderly women supports the importance of assessing strengths and weaknesses of the individual client's supportive networks (Chang et al. 1985). These authors state that their findings did not support the stereotype that widowed and single people have fewer supportive networks than married persons.

Summary and Conclusions

Compliance is an important area of consideration for researchers and practitioners in chronic illness. Several issues and problems relevant to the development and ethical use of effective compliance strategies have been discussed: barriers to the study of compliance, variables affecting compliance, the state of current knowledge about compliance, impact of differences in expectations of clients and providers, motivation, and ethical issues. Also problematic is the fact that research findings are generally inconclusive about factors that influence compliance or the consequences and utility of any one strategy designed to increase compliance. Several models and theoretical frameworks were presented to provide guidance.

The chapter has proposed that assessment include the client and family's living conditions, demands, commitments, and concerns in order to gain the client's perspective of living with chronic illness and implementing health care recommendations. In this way the provider can more effectively engage the client in problem solving. Assessment and interactions may be directed to the individual client; when assistance is needed or disabilities are marked, family members must be the focus.

The importance of various strategies that increase client participation was noted: tailoring, simplifying the regimen, providing reminders, enhancing coping skills, education, contracting, and social support. An important concern for client and provider is determining the optimal level of compliance appropriate to the situation.

Given the increasing numbers of chronically ill individuals, the importance of adherence to necessary regimens becomes obvious. Responsibility for management falls to the client or family on a day-to-day basis. The provider is responsible for ensuring that the client or family has the needed knowledge, motivation, and skills. Another provider responsibility is helping the client to find ways to make compliance more feasible. Through research, assessment, and strategies that are presented in a nonjudgmental way, the effective performance of compliant behavior can be accomplished.

STUDY QUESTIONS

1. Why is trying to increase compliant behaviors important for clients who are chronically ill?
2. What factors are involved in compliance? Discuss them.
3. Do you agree that *compliance* and *noncompliance* are terms as acceptable as *adherence* and *nonadherence*? Why?
4. How prevalent is noncompliance? What are the problems of trying to determine the extent of noncompliance?
5. What are the methodological barriers to the study of compliance? What is the relationship of single variables to compliance? What conceptual barriers exist?
6. If you were given a choice, which conceptual model would you prefer to support for a study on noncompliance? Explain your preference, citing examples to defend it.
7. How do clients and providers differ in their expectations about participation? Discuss different models that are useful for client participation.
8. What is the difference between internal and external locus of control? How does this difference affect compliance?
9. What are the differences in client and provider perspectives of the facets involved in managing medical regimens?
10. What ethical issues arise when a provider tries to increase a client's compliance? Discuss an ethical approach.
11. How does motivation influence compliance? How does the health belief model affect a client's motivation?
12. What are the strengths and weaknesses of education as a means of increasing compliance?
13. Given a client situation, what factors would you assess to gain a thorough picture of potential compliance or noncompliance? Discuss assessment from this perspective.
14. What are the factors that allow you to use the nursing diagnosis of noncompliance?
15. How can you encourage client participation to increase compliance? Discuss tailoring, simplifying the regimen, and reminders.
16. How could you enhance coping to increase compliance?
17. What are the advantages and disadvantages of contracting? of support groups?

References

Anderson, J., and Kirk, L. M., (1982) Methods of improving patient compliance in chronic disease states, *Archives of Internal Medicine, 142*:1673–1675

Anderson, R. M., (1985) Is the problem of noncompliance all in our head?, *Diabetes Educator, 11*:31–34

Baric, L., (1969) Recognition of the 'at-risk' role: A means to influence health behavior, *International Journal of Health Education, 12*:24–34

Barofsky, I., (1978) Compliance, adherence, and the therapeutic alliance: Steps in the development of self-care, *Social Science and Medicine, 12*:369–376

Barry, V., (1982) *Moral Aspects of Health Care*, Belmont, Calif.: Wadsworth, p. 468

Becker, M., (1976) Socio-behavioral determinants of compliance, in Sackett, D. L., and Haynes, R. (eds.), *Compliance with Therapeutic Regimens*, Baltimore: Johns Hopkins University Press

Becker, M., and Janz, N. K., (1985) The health belief model applied to understanding diabetes regimen compliance, *Diabetes Educator, 11*:41–47

Becker, M. H., and Maiman, L. A., (1975) Sociobehavioral determinants of compliance with health and medical care recommendations, *Medical Care, 13*:10–24

Becker, M. H., and Maiman, L. A., (1978) Models of health-related behavior, in Mechanic, D. (ed.), *Medical Sociology* (2d ed.), New York: Free Press, pp. 539–566

Blackwell, B., (1976) Treatment adherence: A contemporary overview, *Psychosomatics, 20*:27–35

Blackwell, B., (1979) The drug regimen and treatment compliance, in Haynes, R. B., Taylor, D. W., and Sackett, D. L. (eds.), *Compliance in Health Care*, Baltimore: Johns Hopkins University Press, pp. 144–156

Bloom, B. S., (1971) *Taxonomy of Educational Objectives: Cognitive Domain*, New York: David McKay

Carpenito, L. J., (1984) *Handbook of Nursing Diagnosis*, Philadelphia: Lippincott

Chang, L., Uman, G., Linn, L., Ware, J., and Kane, R., (1985) Adherence to health care regimens among elderly women, *Nursing Research, 34*:27–31

Connelly, C. E., (1984) Economic and ethical issues in patient compliance, *Nursing Economics, 2*:342–347

Corbin, J. M., and Strauss, A. L., (1984) Collaboration: Couples working to manage chronic illness, *Image, 16*(4):109–115

Dimond, M., and Jones, S. L., (1983) *Chronic Illness across the Life Span*, Norwalk, Conn.: Appleton-Century-Crofts

Dracup, K. A., and Meleis, A. I., (1982) Compliance: An interactionist approach, *Nursing Research, 31*:32–35

Fawcett, J., (1984) *Analysis and Evaluation of Conceptual Models of Nursing*, Philadelphia: F. A. Davis Co.

Fink, D. L., (1976) Tailoring the consensual regimen, in Sackett, D. L., and Haynes, R. R. (eds.), *Compliance with Therapeutic Regimens*, Baltimore: Johns Hopkins University Press, pp. 110–118

Fink, D., Malloy, M. J., Cohen, M., Greycould, M. A., and Martin, F., (1979) Effective patient care in the pediatric ambulatory setting: A study of acute care clinic, *Pediatrics, 43*:927–935

Gillam, R. F., and Barsky, A. J., (1974) Diagnosis and management of patient noncompliance, *Journal of American Medical Association, 228*:1563–1567

Gordis, L., (1979) Conceptual and methodologic problems in measuring patient compliance, in Haynes, R. B., Taylor, D. W., and Sackett, D. L. (eds.), *Compliance in Health Care*, Baltimore: Johns Hopkins University Press, pp. 23–48

Green, L. W., (1979) Educational strategies to improve compliance with therapeutic and preventive regimens: The recent evidence, in Haynes, R. B., Taylor, D. W., and Sackett, D. L. (eds.), *Compliance in Health Care*, Baltimore: Johns Hopkins University Press, pp. 157–173

Hallel, J., (1975) The relationship of health beliefs, health locus of control, and self concept to the practice of breast self-examination in adult women, *Nursing Research, 31*:137–142

Haynes, R. B., (1979) Determinants of compliance: The disease and the mechanics of treatment, in Haynes, R. B., Taylor, D. W., and Sackett, D. L. (eds.), *Compliance in Health Care*, Baltimore: Johns Hopkins University Press, pp. 49–62

Hellenbrandt, D., (1983) An analysis of compliance behavior: A response to powerlessness, in Miller, J. F. (ed.), *Coping with Chronic Illness*, Philadelphia: F. A. Davis, pp. 215–243

Hingson, R., Scotch, N., Sorenson, J., and Swazey, J., (1981) *In Sickness and in Health*, St. Louis: C. V. Mosby

Hogue, C. C., (1979) Nursing and compliance, in Haynes, R. B., Taylor, D. W., and Sackett, D. L. (eds.), *Compliance in Health Care*, Baltimore: Johns Hopkins University Press, pp. 247–259

Hulka, B. S., Cassel, J. C., Kupper, L. L., and Burdette, J. A., (1976) Communication, compliance, and concordance between physicians and patients with prescribed medications, *American Journal of Public Health, 66*:847–853

Jonsen, A. R., (1979) Ethical issues in compliance, in Haynes, R. B., Taylor, D. W., and Sackett, D. L. (eds.), *Compliance in Health Care*, Baltimore: Johns Hopkins University Press, pp. 113–120

Kasl, S. V., (1974) The health belief model and behavior related to chronic illness, *Health Education Monograph*, 2:433–454

Kasl, S. V., (1978) Social and psychological factors affecting the course of disease, in Mechanic, D. (ed.), *Medical Sociology* (2d ed.), New York: Free Press

Kasl, S. V., and Cobb, S., (1966) Health behavior, illness behavior, and sick role behavior, *Archives of Environmental Health*, 12:246–266

Knowles, M. S., (1970) *The Modern Practice of Adult Education*, New York: Association Press

Levine, S., and Kozlaff, M., (1978) The sick role: Assessment and overview, *Annual Review of Sociology*, 4:317

Marston, M. V., (1970) Compliance with medical regimens: A review of the literature, *Nursing Research*, 19:312–323

Mechanic, D., and Voikart, E., (1961) Stress, illness behavior, and the sick role, *American Sociological Review*, 26:51–58

Moree, N. A., (1984) Nurses speak out on patients and drug regimens, *American Journal of Nursing*, 85:51–54

Parsons, T., (1951) *The Social System*, New York: Free Press

Rotter, J. B., (1966) Generalized expectancies for internal versus external control of reinforcement, *Psychological Monographs*, 80:1–28

Sackett, D. L., (1976) Introduction, in Sackett, D. L., and Haynes, R. B. (eds.), *Compliance with Therapeutic Regimens*, Baltimore: Johns Hopkins University Press, pp. 1–6

Sackett, D. L., (1979) Methods for compliance research, in Haynes, R. B., Taylor, D. W., and Sackett, D. L. (eds.), *Compliance in Health Care*, Baltimore: Johns Hopkins University Press, pp. 323–333

Sackett, D. L., and Snow, J. C. (1979) The magnitude of compliance and noncompliance, in Haynes, R. B., Taylor, D. W., and Sackett, D. L. (eds.), *Compliance in Health Care*, Baltimore: Johns Hopkins University Press, pp. 11–22

Schroeder, P. S., and Miller, J. F., (1983) Qualitative study of locus of control in patients with peripheral vascular disease, in Miller, J. F. (ed.), *Coping with Chronic Illness*, Philadelphia: F. A. Davis

Schwartz, D., Wang, M., Zettz, L., and Goss, M. E., (1962) Medication errors made by elderly, chronically ill patients, *American Journal of Public Health*, 52:2018–2029

Steckel, S. B., and Swain, M. A., (1981) Contracting with patients to improve compliance, *Hospitals: Journal of American Hospital Association*, 51:81–84

Stone, G. C., (1979) Patient compliance and the role of the expert, *Journal of Social Issues*, 35:34–59

Strauss, A. L., Corbin, J., Fagerhaugh, S., Glaser, B., Maines, D., Suczek, B., and Wiener, C., (1984) *Chronic Illness and the Quality of Life* (2d ed.), St. Louis: C. V. Mosby

Szasz, T. S., and Hollander, M. H., (1956) A contribution in the philosophy of medicine, *Archives of Internal Medicine*, 97:585–592

Vincent, P., (1971) Factors influencing patient noncompliance: A theoretical approach, *Nursing Research*, 20:509–670

Wallston, B., Wallston, K., Kaplan, G., and Maides, S., (1976) Development and validation of the health care locus of control scale, *Journal of Consulting and Clinical Psychology*, 44:580–585

Wallston, K., Wallston, B., and DeVellis, R., (1978) Development of the multidimensional health locus of control (MHLC) scales, *Health Education Monograph*, 6:160–170

CHAPTER EIGHT
The Family Caregiver

Introduction

Throughout this book, we have discussed the long-term or permanent nature of chronic illness and its impact on the client. Now we will explore the impact on family members who provide care and support to chronically ill individuals at home. Maintaining chronically ill persons at home is often difficult work and has been shown to have negative physical, emotional, and financial consequences on the primary, or major, caregiver. Even though such home care has proved to be highly cost-effective because caregivers serve as unpaid members of the health team, they receive few services or support that would enhance their ability to continue providing service without associated destructive effects on themselves.

The professional periodically performs specific tasks, but the time spent is usually measured in terms of hours. Often clients can provide much of their own care, but, unlike the infant child who needs less and less care with maturation, chronic illness tends to become progressive, with increasing dependency on the caregiver. Therefore, much of the responsibility for management of both the illness and the household falls to the caregiver (Golodetz et al. 1969). Role responsibilities include those of cook, maid, janitor, launderer, nursing assistant, psychiatrist, and transportation provider. Health-related roles include those of mobility supervisor; overseer/administrator of medications; technician supervising use of special equipment (assistive breathing equipment, catheters, braces, wound care, and so forth); provider of

personal hygiene, such as toileting/incontinence care; manager of transfers, exercises, feeding, and watching; and major communicator and coordinator (Golodetz et al. 1969).

A number of variables influence the decision to assume this caregiving role. These include functional limitations of the client, the caregiver's response to these limitations, family history of interactions and response to crisis, motivation and ability to accept the role, values and attitudes toward this responsibility, and availability of additional support systems (Crossman & Kaljian 1984). The aversion most families have to nursing homes and the sense of reciprocity owed to the now ill individual were two major reasons given for providing home care (Goldstein, Regnery, & Wellin 1981). In another study, identified motivators for giving care were familial obligation (58%), affection (51%), and reciprocity (17%) (Horowitz & Shindelman 1981).

Most studies that focus on families explore ways they cope with the illness or client. Research that examines impact deals primarily with the client as the unit of analysis (*Family Caregiving* 1983) and does not recognize family needs (Hayter 1982). Few studies have been done on how family caretakers are impacted or adapt to the stresses they face (Goldstein, Regnery, & Wellin 1981; Venters 1981). There is a small but growing body of literature on caretakers of impaired elderly persons and some that analyzes the role of caretakers of brain-injured adults. But the literature lacks research on effects on families with chronically ill children or young adults (Hymovich

1984; Strauss et al. 1984). Generalization to this population can only be speculative, even though we can empirically see such application of data.

Because of this limitation, we shall present throughout this chapter a case study involving a family in which the care recipient (client), Tim, is a young man, now age 36, who developed bilateral avascular necrosis of the femoral head three years ago. Increasing intense pain led to profound limitation of motion and gait disturbances. He was forced to stop working and returned to his parents' home, where his mother became his primary caregiver. Tim was not interviewed, but his mother provided input on the way this situation affected her. The designation *Sis* refers to a compilation of comments provided by two of his sisters. At the time these data were collected, Tim and his family were preparing for his seventh surgery: bilateral total hip replacements. Their hope was that this operation would provide adequate relief of symptoms to allow him to move into independent living.

There are a variety of terms used in studies to identify the individual who provides primary care at home: *caretaker, caregiver, informal support system, informal provider,* or *responsor* (one who *respon*ds to client needs and is *respon*sible for client care). All these terms carry the same basic meaning. The following is comprehensive and will serve as our definition: a lay person, usually a close relative of the client, who assumes primary responsibility for the impaired individual's care (Goldstein, Regnery & Wellin 1981).

The Nature of Home Care

Advantages

The lay caregiver role is older than that of professional caregiver, since most families want to take care of their own; there is a social acceptance within the family. In fact, it has been found that most long-term home health services and care are provided by family members (National Center for Health Statistics 1974). Even if institutionalization were considered a more viable alternative for needed care, most long-term

facilities have inadequate numbers of trained professionals to care for this entire client population, nor do most long-term care facilities provide a familylike or meaningful life (Golodetz et al. 1969).

To appreciate the value of family-provided home care, one needs to look at the characteristics of those who become institutionalized. Shanas (1979) studied two groups of elderly individuals who had similar levels of impairment: those who remained at home and those who were institutionalized. Of the elderly who are bedfast in this country, twice as many continue to live at home (10%) as are institutionalized (5.5%). An additional 7% get out of the house only with difficulty but continue to live in the community because of support provided by family. In fact, most housebound elderly persons consider that the social support provided by kin in time of illness enables them to remain at home. Shanas found it interesting that not the number but the regularity and concern of visitors was important to these elderly individuals.

Other researchers have found that services and care provided at home help delay or prevent institutionalization for growing numbers of those who are chronically ill (Brody, Poulshock, & Masciocchi 1978; Crossman, London, & Barry 1981). In fact, given equivalent levels of disability, the critical difference between elderly clients remaining at home and those entering nursing homes was the availability of a spouse or children to provide care (Brody et al. 1978).

Cost of Providing Care

The limited number of studies that examined the value of care from a monetary perspective shows that informal caregivers provide the majority of costly services compared to service agencies (Gurland et al. 1978; Whitfield 1982). One study of cost found that there was less expenditure of public money needed for impaired elderly adults maintained at home, except in cases of extreme impairment. Nevertheless, little funding is allocated for ambulatory or community care despite the increasing amounts provided for construction of proprietary skilled nursing facilities and for payment to acute hospitals for short-term care of chronic illnesses (Brody, Poulshock, &

Masciocchi 1978). Medicare tends to exclude from eligibility persons who require chronic care, rather than short-term, acute care (Nardone 1980) (see Chapter 17).

Characteristics of Family Caregivers

Studies have shown that 60–80% of all care is provided by families to elderly impaired members; most of these providers are spouses or daughters (Gurland et al. 1978; *Hearing on Families* 1980), 21% of these caregivers are 75 years of age or older (Gurland et al. 1978). Older caregivers can provide more caregiving time but have less health, strength, and energy and fewer financial resources than those in younger age categories. Younger caregivers, mostly offspring, have time constraints imposed by family, occupations, and social roles and responsibilities (Goldstein et al. 1981).

Spouses, regardless of sex, usually take on the primary care-giving responsibilities (Crossman & Kaljian 1984; Soldo & Myllyluoma 1983). In most cases, the wife is likely to become the caregiver because women are usually younger than their spouses and, consequently, are less likely to become disabled. In addition, social expectations prepare women more than men for caregiving (Fengler & Goodrich 1979). Although most caregivers had no functional limitations, 7% of elderly caregivers had such limitations and were found to be more vulnerable to health problems (*Family Caregiving* 1983).

The other major group of caregivers are daughters who care for their no-longer-married parents or parents who are too frail to live alone: mostly women who have outlived their husbands and have become dependent on children or others for care. Other caregivers, in decreasing order, are daughters-in-law, sons, other female relatives, other male relatives, and finally nonrelatives (Soldo & Myllyluoma 1983).

Roles of Caregivers

Care giving falls primarily into two categories: care provider and care manager, both roles requiring an initial identification of needed services. Which role is sought is determined by the family's socioeco-

nomic status. Income was found to be the greatest influence since it determines the quantity of services that can be bought (Archbold 1983). Care providers perform services themselves, whereas care managers, who tend to have careers that compete with care giving, manage or arrange for services to be provided by others.

Providers, who expend most of their time and energy on performing physical and personal care, tend to adhere rigidly to solutions and workable routines and have little time to meet the client's psychosocial needs. On the other hand, managers spend extensive time and energy learning which resources are available and arranging for appropriate services. Managers use their own time with care receivers to meet psychosocial needs such as transportation for shopping, bringing visitors, and so on (Archbold 1983).

Problems

Health care providers tend to feel that managing chronic illnesses is essentially a home-based responsibility (Colman, Summers, & Leonard 1982). Families generally also do. Although most care is provided to the elderly by spouses and daughters, mothers usually serve as caregivers in situations in which children are care receivers. This care giving leads to emotional, physical, and financial strain, inconvenience, anxiety, and depression, plus the joint demands of care giving and employment when necessary (*Family Caregiving* 1983).

Services and assistance provided by family increase with the level of impairment of the care recipient (*Family Caregiving* 1983). As an example, the caregiver for a person having Alzheimer's disease can become overwhelmed by the constant care and attention required, necessarily relinquishing relationships or activities with others (Hayter 1982). Often, families do not possess sufficient resources to attend to the complex health and social service needs of their aged relatives (*Hearing on Families* 1980). As we shall see, the caregiver can become the invisible patient.

To maintain the client at home, the primary caregiver must develop management and communication skills and become a master of planning for daily activities and emergencies. Time impositions occur (Watt & Calder 1981), whether both parties share living accommodations or care is provided to someone in a second household. In either case, much independence is lost and many restrictions develop. Those families who have coped well with stresses and problems in the past are better prepared; those that have been dysfunctional become more stressed (Crossman & Kaljian 1984).

Golodetz et al. (1969) provide a poignant picture of a family caregiver:

> She is not trained for her job, a priori. She may have little choice about doing the job. She belongs to no union or guild, works no fixed maximum of hours. She lacks formal compensation, job advancement, and even the possibility of being fired. She has no job mobility. In her work situation, she bears a heavy emotional load, but has no colleagues or supervisor or education to help her handle this. Her own life and its needs compete constantly with her work requirements. She may be limited in her performance by her own ailments. . . .

Problems and Issues of Home Care

Financial Impact

The lack of monetary assistance for the family unit can in itself create financial problems. Public policy ignores caregivers, and support services are limited and spotty (Colman, Summers, & Leonard 1982). When this situation is coupled with decreased income and increased medical expenses, the caregiver often is left in a financial bind (see Chapter 17):

> Sis: Tim had to leave his job as a fisherman. He also lost his insurance and had to go on Medicaid for a long time. The medical care he got then was really bad. There hasn't been consistency in what he needs and should do. He's already had six surgeries, but still is not better. Now his care is better since he's in the experimental program for a new type of hip replacement. Guess you have to be an experiment to get good care if you can't get health care coverage.

> Mom: Getting medical care for Tim was a nightmare. Finally he was examined at County Hospital, where the diagnosis was made. That gave us a whole new

problem to deal with. Dad isn't working full-time, and that helps in giving Tim care. I have to keep my job; it's a necessity.

Public Policy. Even though federal health care policy is meant to help the ill who are in financial need, this policy often causes many financial hardships for family caregivers, especially spouses. The monetary value of family care to the community far exceeds the value of that provided by public agencies (*Family Caregiving* 1983). Most costs for at-home care are not paid by government funds but are out-of-pocket expenses. In 1975 there were about 10 million functionally disabled individuals needing long-term care services. Although one-third of these received such services through public programs, 60% of all care was provided by caregivers at home and without compensation of any kind (Nardone 1980). In fact, 1 million, or 10% of this disabled population, received no care at all (Nardone 1980).

Federal Programs. Most Medicare funds focus on institutional care, with only 2% of the budget spent on home health care services. Prior hospitalization and a physician's orders are necessary in order that services be provided at home. Services that are available focus on client needs, are time-limited, and are provided almost exclusively to individuals living alone. The kind of care that is often needed is not covered if there is a wife at home (Colman, Summers, & Leonard 1982); therefore, the wife receives little with respect to assistance.

Medicaid, which covers more services, including home care, is a program for the indigent, meaning that only people with low income and few salable assets qualify. For families with an incapacitated member to receive assistance, they need to pauperize themselves. Medicaid assistance focuses on meeting client needs at minimal costs. This disregard for the present and future financial needs of care-giving spouses results in impoverishment for the surviving spouse after the impaired individual dies (Colman, Summers, & Leonard 1982). The fear of inadequate finances when alone forces caregivers to continue providing care even when it is not the more favorable option.

Policies that deal with spousal responsibility for medical cost payments tend to be unfavorable to the caring spouse. As an example, let us look at the policy of deeming. *Deeming* assumes that retirement income is available for medical and caretaker expenses of the recipient named on the check. Should the recipient, usually the husband, need to be placed in a nursing home, Medicaid could require that all monies except an amount comparable to the Social Security Insurance (SSI) payment for a single person be "deemed" available to cover hospital costs. Because the remaining amount is generally inadequate to maintain an individual at home, the spouse often feels a need to keep the client at home longer than is healthy for either of them (Colman, Summers, & Leonard 1982).

Social services under Title XIX, meant to maintain independence of the disabled and to prevent institutionalization when possible, does not provide in-home supportive services when there is an able-bodied spouse (Colman, Summers, & Leonard 1982). Given the limited income of most elderly couples, this lack of provided services leads to physical and emotional strain. Even private insurance covers expenses while the client is in the hospital, but not necessary costs at home. Again, this results in home costs becoming out-of-pocket expenses for that family unit (Colman, Summers, & Leonard 1982).

The new reimbursement system of diagnosis-related groups (DRGs), which applies primarily to aged and indigent recipients of Medicare and Medicaid, is not geared to help the family caregiver. Under this system, prolonged treatment, which is often necessary for this population, could be sufficiently unprofitable that hospitals might elect either not to treat these people or to reduce services (Ostrander 1984). Although cost containment is achieved, earlier discharge or higher private third-party payment costs would further impact the limited resources of most Medicare and Medicaid recipients.

Competing Demands

Families often find themselves with many demands that compete with care giving. In fact, middle-aged daughters often find that they are the "women in the middle" with multiple responsibilities to their own family, parent(s), and job (Crossman & Kaljian 1984).

> Sis: We found that the family became divided into camps, and this put extra strain on Mom, especially when we disagreed with her approach. We started to pull further and further away as things got worse till all that was left was Mom providing most of the care.

> Mom: Needless to say, we all thought that Tim's moving into the house would be temporary. There were still four children at home. I overly took care of him at first, but now I let him do more for himself.

Surprisingly, the presence of another impaired individual in the household tends to reduce the primary caregiver's direct responsibilities or to offset additional competing demands (Soldo & Myllyluoma 1983), thus increasing the likelihood that the household would provide care (*Family Caregiving* 1983). In multiperson households where there is an impaired individual, primary caregivers often have a second caregiver available to provide some assistance or relief (Soldo & Myllyluoma 1983).

> Mom: Sometimes I'd notice resentment on the part of my other children and husband when Tim's demands on me are great. They don't realize it, but that increases the stress I feel.

> Sis: Ours is a household where there are other siblings. This means that some of the responsibility can be spread amongst a number of relatives. We sometimes feel resentment and anger for the grief and aggravation Mom has. Some feelings become contagious, like depression.

Employment. Over one-third of all caregivers are employed (Soldo & Myllyluoma 1983), and most of these people are under age 65. Most male caregivers work. A much smaller number of caregivers above age 65 work. In the over-65 age group, the reasons given for not working are either retirement (males) or housekeeping responsibilities (females) (Soldo & Myllyluoma 1983). Studies cite that when women enter the labor force the impact on family care giving is negative, especially in households having no other adult females (*Family Caregiving* 1983).

Inconvenience. As impairment increases, attitudes are found to become more negative in response to growing inconvenience for the caregiver. The decision to institutionalize the ill elderly is usually made because providing continued care becomes overly inconvenient. In fact, inconvenience was the only clear predictor to show a direct relationship to the family's decision to consider institutional placement (*Family Caregiving* 1983). The more impaired or dependent the ill member, the greater the inconvenience.

> Sis: When the patient is an adult child, and there is no necessity for institutionalization, the inability to escape the inconvenience causes hard feelings, stress, guilt on the part of both the caregiver and patient.

Role Changes

With lengthening of life span, there is a growing number of younger old people caring for older old people. This group may be dealing with their own aging or health in addition to caring for a disabled spouse or parent (Crossman & Kaljian 1984). In addition, serious illness brings about changes in family roles that can be difficult to adapt to and accept (Farkas 1980). The caregiver's preexisting relationships alter, and new or unaccustomed duties and responsibilities arise (Golodetz et al. 1969). This awesome responsibility may lead to the need to give up previous activities and contacts (Golodetz et al. 1969).

Role ambiguity can result. Some women find it difficult to take on the role of head of household or to accept responsibility for financial or household management after a lifetime of being dependent (Crossman et al. 1981). Men face handling household chores unfamiliar to them. Family relationships, regardless of which member is the caregiver, change. Conflict and confusion can arise for both: for the caregiver because of fear or lack of experience, for the care recipient because of frustration or anger at role loss (Crossman et al. 1981). Responses can vary greatly, from becoming closer to becoming more distant, isolated, or antagonistic (Farkas 1980). When needed additional support or help is not forthcoming, resentment and dissatisfaction may follow (Farkas 1980).

Spouses. Role problems of care-giving spouses and children are different. One study compared life satisfaction of disabled men and their wives to the national average for people age 65 or older. It found that care receiver and care giver both scored lower than the average (Fengler & Goodrich 1979). Husbands' scores were explained by lower financial status and health. Wives' lower scores were attributed in part to their husband's illness. There was an interesting relationship between husbands' and wives' scores: the highest-scoring wives had the highest-scoring husbands, and lower-scoring wives the lower-scoring husbands (Fengler & Goodrich 1979).

Offspring. Children have a great deal of difficulty dealing with role reversal. Providing personal care for a parent can be emotionally difficult (Crossman & Kaljian 1984). In addition, children must accept their parents' mortality as they watch them deteriorate (Crossman & Kaljian 1984). Long-standing interpersonal problems compound the difficulty and increase the tension of providing care (Crossman & Kaljian 1984).

Generally, one child takes primary responsibility for an aging parent, an arrangement that frequently leads to problems with other siblings. The major caregiver may resent the limited help brothers and sisters provide (Crossman & Kaljian 1984). Siblings who do not face day-to-day care-giving problems and frustrations may be critical of the care provided or feel that the caretaker exaggerates the difficulties (Crossman & Kaljian 1984).

Emotional Strain

All caregivers acknowledged that they felt a great deal of strain from the responsibilities of care giving, with emotional strain being the most severe (66%), followed by physical strain (47%), and finally financial strain (31%). Again, there are some differences in factors identified as stressful by spouses and children. Emotional strain manifests in many ways, including feelings of isolation, anxiety, guilt, resentment, and frustration (Crossman et al. 1981).

> Mom: My faith has been my mainstay. Without it this would have been a shattering experience. Once

though I really lost my cool. He was impossible to deal with. He had caused all the family members to back off almost completely.

Sis: We pulled ourselves away as things got worse and worse. I think this only increased Mom's sense of isolation and frustration. The whole family felt resentment when Tim caused Mom grief and aggravation.

Isolation. Among care-giving wives, there is a prevailing sense of social and emotional isolation, a sense of being prisoners in their own homes (Crossman et al. 1981). These caregivers report that they find no one to talk to who will understand. They suffer from the loss of a previous close and loving relationship with their spouse; yet, because their husbands are still alive, they are not allowed to grieve (Lezak 1978). In situations in which husbands were able to provide companionship and to continue to serve as confidants, these women were able to maintain a high morale (Crossman et al. 1981).

Anxiety. Many factors lead to anxiety among caregivers. Threatened loss of security, end of dependency on partner, being alone, and concern over money and one's own health have all been identified as anxiety-provoking factors (Farkas 1980). All caregivers identify concern over the health condition of the care recipient as causing most anxiety (Cantor 1980). For spouses and children the hierarchy of anxiety-provoking factors differs. Spouses identified anxiety about finances as second, followed by the morale of the ill spouse, and finally, ability to obtain help. Children, and other caregivers, ranked obtaining sufficient help second, with finances being the lowest cause of anxiety (Cantor 1980).

Guilt. Guilt feelings grow from anger and frustration provoked by the situation. Illness often is unexpected and requires the abrupt cancellation of long-anticipated retirement plans (Crossman et al. 1981). Since it is considered inappropriate to be angry about circumstances that are not within one's control, guilt can result. The ongoing difficulties and

problems of maintaining an incapacitated individual can lead to life's becoming extremely difficult for both spouses. The strain can become so severe that the caregiver may wish for the death of the recipient or resent the person's living presence (Crossman et al 1981). Again, since this is not socially acceptable behavior, guilt results.

Sis: Resentment is very, very much the response when an adult child patient is indigent and must return back home for care—just at the time when the parents are beginning to feel free from parental obligations.

Physical Strain

In a number of ways, illness in one family member can result in physical impact on other members. When it does, it can create a problem not only for the caregiver but for the dependent client (Mace & Babins 1981). Some kinds of physical strain are related to accompanying emotional stress, such as the fatigue that accompanies the combination of depression and inadequate sleep (Mace & Babins 1981). This can be followed by various illnesses that are associated with exhaustion, depression, nervousness, fatigue, and a draining of limited physical and emotional resources (Farkas 1980).

A majority of care-giving wives have been found to have at least one chronic illness (Crossman et al. 1981). Interviews with women who care for brain-damaged husbands (having Alzheimer's disease, Parkinson's disease, or a cerebrovascular accident [CVA]) indicate that they face back-breaking lifting, urine-soaked sheets, long enema stints, and interrupted sleep (Colman, Summers, & Leonard 1982). Considering that many of these caregivers are themselves elderly and often frail, it is not surprising that they break down physically under the strain of a twenty-four-hour, seven-day work week. Only when incontinence and lack of sleep become overwhelming do these women surrender.

In families in which interactions became unidirectional, both giver and receiver of care feel a sense of irksomeness. Those families that *perceived* the care giving as disruptive had numerous health crises (Archbold 1980).

Interventions

Continuing in familiar surroundings has the obvious advantages of maintaining a meaningful quality of life. Society as a whole also benefits since home care is a means of containing across-the-board medical costs. Yet, as we have seen, stresses superimposed on the family, as well as the work and energy requirements necessary to manage long-term illness at home, can have a negative impact on the caregiver. Without relief from the continuous responsibility, from the physical and emotional strain, and from the ongoing financial burden, the family caregiver may be overwhelmed:

> Sis: Remaining at home contributes to an overall sense of optimism for Tim and Mom, especially since there is an end in sight. We feel that if he's at home, he's not too bad off. If he were in really bad shape he'd be in the hospital, right? That's a funny, interesting rationalization that I think lots of people make.

Since most families provide care willingly, it is unfortunate that to date helping the caregiver manage in this role has received little attention. This condition is changing slowly, as various types of respite programs evolve. Many agencies and facilities for older persons have developed a greater sensitivity to the caregiver and find that programs that provide respite and support for the family unit help to minimize the negative impact on the caregiver and to delay institutionalization. Caregivers for elderly clients are beginning to realize that they can help themselves and are forming self-support groups in which common problems are identified, problem solving occurs, and eventually an advocacy stance develops. In addition, the health professional, through assessment and creative problem solving, serves to ease the burden faced by this group of silent care providers. These recent, albeit limited, developments are beginning to have an impact that will lead eventually to increasing legislative change and financial support.

Respite

Respite, which is "any service, whether it be day care, home care, or brief periods of institutionalization, that provides intervals of rest and relief for the caregiver" (Crossman et al. 1981), has been identified as essential for individuals having the responsibility of providing continuous home care. Most respite programs discussed in the literature focus on elderly family units, but the concept is valuable for any family involved in continuous care for long-term illness.

> Sis: I think respite is the primary role that additional family members need to play for the benefit of both the patient and the caregiver.

> Mom: Even a day or two away when I know someone else is taking over makes a world of difference for Dad and me. We need some time to ourselves.

Short-Term Institutional Placement. Planned short-term hospital admissions provide in-facility professional care for the client in conjunction with intermittent relief for the caregiver. Such programs are valued by caregivers and health care professionals as a means of keeping incapacitated clients in their homes long after independent living would otherwise be impossible (Robertson, Griffiths, & Cosin 1977). These programs prevent the threshold of family tolerance from being exceeded as a result of unrelieved strain, physical and mental deterioration of the client, and hardened attitudes of relatives.

Long-Term or Rehabilitation Facilities. Families of veterans can have brief periods of respite at nursing home care units set up for such services (Ellis & Wilson 1983). When families request admission to one particular program, they are evaluated and screened by the admission team. Medical evaluation of the client's current health status is required since the program is designed to manage only stable health conditions during the respite period. Persons whose conditions worsen during the program are transferred out of the unit. In spite of this feature, a much greater than expected number of clients were found to need maximum nursing care. Consequently, total-care patients are now limited to a maximum of three at any one time. Other findings are that caregivers often experience a great deal of guilt about seeking respite; strong nursing leadership is necessary because many of these patients are very demanding; and persons having Alzheimer's disease have the least successful referrals because they are fearful and forgetful and tend to wander. However, the program, which reinvigorates the caregiver, is considered valuable since it delays more costly admissions, helps keep families together, and minimizes costs.

Another in-hospital respite program, begun in 1978 with the help of a small grant, uses beds in a rehabilitation intermediate care unit (Huey 1983). This program is available to families with incomes no greater than $40,000 per year. Geared to be flexible, respite is provided for a maximum of six weeks per year in two-week blocks for clients who do not have acute illness or need skilled nursing care. Referrals, which must be made at least two weeks ahead, require financial disclosure and a current medical report. Families are required to provide sufficient medication for the entire planned period of stay, to furnish plans in case acute illness occurs, and to take the client home on the specified date. While in the unit, clients can be involved in the regular program of the facility, participate in regular therapy sessions, and continue with senior center programs. Identified problems include delays in paper work, some discrepancy between family's and physician's reports of the client's status, demands of some clients for "room and maid" services, and occasional difficulty with staff spending either too much or too little time with the respite clients. Overall, the program does provide a needed service of relief for caregivers.

Combined Supplemental Services. Short-term placement can be combined with other services to assist the caregiver. One program, begun in 1964 and evaluated in 1975, is part of a Continuing Care Program in Oxford, England (Robertson, Griffiths, & Cosin 1977). The program assists family caregivers by furnishing in-home family support, community services, plus regular short stays in long-term hospitals. Most of the clients, who are over 75 years of age, are so severely incapacitated that hospitalization would be necessary if their families did not receive additional flexible, individually appropriate supporting services. Hospital beds are categorized as *floating* (three-day, two-night every two weeks to the same ward), *intermittent readmission* (longer periods of time but less frequent intervals), *holiday* (two-week admissions to allow for vacations), and *acute or unplanned* (episodic care for new illnesses, emergency surgery, or change in status). Support services include assistance with physical care and activities of daily living (ADL) and any necessary home services such as cleaning, food shopping, and so forth. Evaluation, by families and professionals alike, rated the program from useful to essential in providing sufficient caregiver relief to keep this very dependent population at home.

The Respite Project, initially a pilot study funded by a private foundation, demonstrates the benefits of a coordinated system of support services for older care-giving wives (Crossman et al. 1981). These women, whose husbands are participants in a day care program, receive both in-home respite care and overnight respite at no cost. Ten to fifteen wives receive four hours of weekly respite from a full-time registered nurse. Respite provided by a nurse rather than a health aide allows for coordinated comprehensive care, ongoing health assessment and teaching, and continuous interpretation of changes in the husband's behavior and functional ability. This regularity of service supplies an unexpected bonus of emotional support that intermittently available home services provided by other agencies cannot supply.

The overnight respite care available in conjunction with this project is housed in a building that was formerly a seminary, modified and licensed as a six-bed adult group residential facility. Functioning as a retreat, the facility maintains a greater sense of normalcy than an institution would. Run from Thursday morning (when the husbands leave for their day care) through Monday morning, it requires advance reservations. Wives can select from twenty-four hours to four days of uninterrupted time away from their care-giving duties. The retreat is staffed by round-the-clock nurses who know the husband through the day care program or the weekly at-home respite service. Surveys indicate that none of these wives had had a vacation for at least three years, and that both husband and wife benefited from a break from the intensity and stresses of their twenty-four-hour-a-day relationship.

The Administration on Aging Models Projects has funded alternative family support projects such as the Natural Supports Program in New York, New York (Colman, Summers, & Leonard 1982). This program, which has no eligibility requirements, helps by supplementing, not substituting for, family caregiving. Focus is on the needs of the entire family. Included are respite services, home care, self-help groups, counseling, assistance in negotiating the bureaucracy, help with access to entitlement programs, skills training, and peer support for caregivers. These services allow the family to survive while continuing to care for loved ones at home.

Day Care Centers. Adult day care centers are a growing phenomenon that furnishes a viable alternative to nursing homes for the dependent client. Day care provides social experiences for invalids, and many provide various kinds of client-centered continuity of care. Centers can include features such as case management to overcome fragmentation, meals, health services, and counseling. Some of these programs provide transportation services that can accommodate wheelchairs; others require that the family provide transportation for the client, precluding some elderly caregivers who cannot transport clients to the center from using the services. Although some centers provide respite and supportive services for the family unit, most do not (Colman, Summers, & Leonard 1982), although some relief from responsibility is possible during the day.

Sis: Day care centers would be very beneficial for families of severely handicapped or long-term incapacitated children, also. I wonder if these programs explain to families that they are not there to be an intrusion, but to help. I know that my family would not allow outside help, nor would Tim allow anyone to come in and help him. It's a dilemma.

One study (Rathbone-McCuan 1976), which focused on families utilizing a day care program, found that families often felt that the aged person was creating some degree of emotional strain on the family unit. These families wanted to avoid institutionalization and needed assistance in order to continue to function. Most (69%) felt that day care served as a *family* service by reducing tension, supplementing the burden of care, and preventing further emotional dependence by the client on the family unit. The other families felt that the aged person benefited more than the family did. This author concluded that day care programs benefit families by assuming part of the physical burden of day care, providing psychological support by assuring the family that its incapacitated member is cared for socially and medically, and allowing the family to keep an aged person at home.

Various means of maximizing day care to meet the needs of different clients have been suggested. Maggie Kuhn, founder of the Gray Panthers, suggested combining day care of children and old people in the same facility (*Hearing on Families* 1980). In this way, elders can provide loving care and act as surrogate grandparents. Kuhn also suggests that it would be economically more feasible for Medicare to authorize someone to stay with an older ill person at home if the cost did not exceed 95% of institutional care. Having such a support person to perform daily tasks necessary to maintain the client at home would allow the caregiver some respite, especially in the case of elderly women who might not otherwise be able to maintain their spouses at home.

In-Home Respite. Home care has expanded phenomenally in recent years, although it receives only 2% of Medicare funds (Griffith 1984). Providers can be proprietary or nonprofit extensions of hospital services or local health departments. The growth in home care has been influenced by earlier discharges plus the increase in technically more complex therapies. Federal and state regulations mandate reimbursement of the services of certified home care agencies. Although home care is funded to meet the needs of clients, a few programs provide some respite services to families.

Services provided by visiting nurses or home health aides are helpful to caregivers (Goldstein et al. 1981), especially when only intermittent support is needed by caregivers who have other resources (such as family and friends) to help them carry the burden of care. The visiting nurse supplements physical and emotional services that help to maintain the client, the caregiver, or the home. Services include homemaking as well as monitoring both the client's and caregiver's health status, taking vital signs, changing catheters, and so on. The caregiver also receives practical and emotional support and reassurance.

One program that specifically provides in-home respite started in 1980 through state funding (Hildebrandt 1983). Referrals are made by families, community nursing agencies, or the county social services department, often in response to family emergencies. Interestingly, self-referrals by families usually occur only after they are "burned out." Designed to be affordable, the program is based on sliding scale fees. When a family requests respite, a nurse practitioner goes to the home and designs, with the family and the dependent individual, a plan of care including activities of daily living, interests, likes, dislikes, and so forth. Trained respite workers are assisted by an on-call nurse practitioner. This program provides service for up to seventy-two hours at a time with respite foster home care encouraged if more time is needed.

At-home services are not always available. When monies to pay for such assistance come from the government, a Catch-22 situation results when allocated fees do not correspond to current costs of services. Caregivers who wish to pay the difference to gain in-home assistance find that any money they provide is deducted from the amount the government pays to that agency (Colman, Summers, & Leonard 1982). This arrangement effectively blocks getting needed help. Even when individuals can afford to pay the entire amount out of pocket, another problem may arise. Often finding a qualified nurse or other worker who is willing to care for such clients is difficult because the work is so hard that few are willing to take it on (Colman, Summers, & Leonard 1982).

Self-Help

Successful care giving requires satisfactory handling of interpersonal interactions of caregiver and care receiver, as well as finding ways of caring for oneself. Caregivers are finding ways of meeting their own needs through self-help groups or by learning, often with professional help, to care for themselves in other ways. Self-help groups, mentioned throughout this book, evolved because the health care system was not meeting client and family needs. Early self-help groups served individuals having chronic illnesses: cancer patients, chronic respiratory patients, and others. But now groups that provide support for caregivers are emerging. These groups help with problem solving and provide information, referrals, and direct support (counseling, locating financial assistance, crisis help, home visits, and so on). Groups also educate professionals and the public and facilitate research (Eisdorfer & Cohen 1981).

Self-Help Groups. Groups supply mutual emotional and practical assistance, counteract the isolation that arises from loss of friends and family, and allow for day-by-day support through sharing of similar experiences (Colman, Summers, & Leonard 1982). Several types of groups provide support for caregivers (Mace & Babins 1981). *Sharing groups* use a skilled person who facilitates discussions or provides therapy for participants. *Peer support groups*, generally voluntary in nature, provide mutual help, not therapy. Advocacy and activism can also be the basis for groups or may constitute part of the function of a group that serves other purposes as well. Advocacy occurs through educating others (discussions, writing to legislators), combining resources with groups having similar goals, or sharing written information.

Many groups serve care-giving wives. The support and caring gained in these groups provide relief of tension through laughter, new and understanding friendships, and supportive telephone networks. Problem-solving techniques are applied to many issues, such as developing ways to meet one's own health needs or finding ways to retain money needed for one's own survival during and after a spouse's illness. In some groups, members eventually become strong enough mentally and emotionally that they become advocates working to effect legislative change. Two such support groups in the San Francisco Bay area that have been effective in meeting the needs of their members are discussed here.

Wives Support Group. A Wives Support Group was started in 1977 in Marin County, California, with funding under Title V, Older Americans Act, Senior Community Employment Program (Crossman et al. 1981). Participants were women whose husbands attended a day care program, plus some others referred by other agencies. During the early formative days, before participating in the monthly meetings, a wife was visited by one of the coleaders, who assessed her situation, explained the purpose and content of the meetings, and helped her determine which needs should be addressed first. New members are now contacted by a current participant, a practice that increases the self-esteem of the group member and provides a personal connection for the new member. Free expression of feelings, in a nonjudgmental atmosphere in which no advice is given, is encouraged. Meetings average about fifteen to twenty participants. Monthly educational meetings cover topics of interest to the members, such as financial preparation for institutionalized care and physiological and psychological aftereffects of strokes. The Respite Project, mentioned previously, is an outgrowth of needs identified by this support group. Members are also active in working toward gaining legislative and financial support for caregivers.

The Family Survival Project. The Family Survival Project in San Francisco is financed by state funds through the Mental Health Association. Membership costs are nominal. This program, geared to meet the needs of brain-damaged adults and their caregivers, provides mutual support and information sharing. Their book, *The Family Survival Handbook*, provides a valuable guide to legal, financial, and social problems these families encounter (Petty et al. 1981). Working mostly with families of people having Alzheimer's disease, the project also serves those having other mental impairments, such as Parkinson's disease, cerebral vascular accidents, and head injuries. Members receive monthly newsletters informing them of meetings and activities throughout the greater San Francisco Bay area that would be of interest or benefit to them. Support and direction are also available via telephone.

Handling the Impact of Care Giving. In addition to groups, caregivers have other resources to help them. Books written specifically to help caregivers include direction, information, and guidance. These books, such as *The 36-Hour Day* (Mace & Babins 1981) and *I Love You But You Drive Me Crazy* (Watt & Calder 1981), can also help the professional in planning interventions.

The reality of a situation may include the awareness that home care giving is not possible or might not be beneficial (Watt & Calder 1981). Before assuming this role, individuals need a thorough awareness of the factors involved. It is unrealistic to assume that the condition will be temporary. The health professional may need to assist in such planning, since taking care of a chronically ill individual may continue for years. It is a good idea to consult free printed material, community workers or agencies, health or social service departments, and other resources to determine what is involved and what kind of help is available.

Managing Interpersonal Interactions. Caregivers must have realistic expectations of the care-giving role (Watt & Calder 1981). Expectations are events that we guess, expect, or assume will happen. Caretakers often have many expectations that are not realistic. One can expect the client's illness to be temporary, can assume there will be improvement of functioning level, or guess that care giving will continue for only a limited period of time. One can assume that personal reserves of energy and resources are endless and expect never to become angry, feel guilty, or become exhausted. Such expectations often are different from actual circumstances. There are many unknown factors, and changes that have an adverse impact on care giving do occur.

> Sis: People need to be made aware of setbacks that can happen. They should almost assume that they will happen. It would help if the health professional would somehow mediate when there is a problem communicating. There is a need for clearly established communication about wants and needs from the onset and periodically throughout the course of the illness.

Prevention can balance unrealistic expectations. When possible, extensive planning should precede assuming responsibility for care giving. Circumstances such as limited health or inadequate resources should be considered. A reasoned decision can be reached if the trajectory of the illness is known (see Chapter 2) and available resources are researched. The health professional can help by teaching, counseling, and assisting in gaining information on community agencies, health and social service departments, finances, and other factors (Watt & Calder 1981). Such efforts ensure more realistic expectations of the care-giving role.

Attitudes of both the care receiver and the caregiver influence interpersonal interactions. It is important to realize that working with care receivers requires differentiating between wants and needs. Ignoring the distinction can lead to disappointment, complaints, and distrust. Frequent irritating requests can be a means of gaining attention that could be given in other ways, thereby leading to fewer demands. The care receiver's preferences must be respected if they are reasonable and do not consume every waking hour. At times the care receiver prefers to be alone, and that wish should be respected. Care receivers who cannot acknowledge that they have a chronic illness present problems, since they do not

try to live the most normal life possible within illness limitations. Such individuals often need help.

Learning to Take Care of Yourself. Taking time away from the twenty-four-hour responsibility of care giving is essential if one is to retain health and to revitalize oneself (Mace & Babins 1981). This requires help from others, such as friends, family, or neighbors, and may require willingness to compromise some details of care or housekeeping. An individual who is willing to oversee an ill person for a full day may not be willing to clean and cook as well. The not-quite-so-immaculate house may be a price worth paying for the rest or opportunity to participate in an enjoyable activity. When people offer to help, let them help. Someone to buy groceries, fix a faucet, or babysit, and so forth, can break the never-ending responsibility. When asked, specify the help you want and need. The neighbor who offers to help should be allowed to help, but not to the extent that the offer will not be repeated.

The caregiver also needs to devote time and energy to enhance his or her own self-esteem, to avoid a sense of entrapment, and to shift the burden of care briefly. Such attention to self helps maintain one's sense of well-being and revitalizes energy that can later be used in providing for the care receiver. But many caregivers feel guilty about such activities. This is unfortunate, since feeling guilty about meeting one's own needs accomplishes little. An occasional indulgence or gift can lift one's spirits immensely. Friendships and social contacts should be continued, and isolation avoided. Avoiding isolation may require time and energy spent at church, in discussion groups, or with those who share common interests. A revitalized self becomes a more effective caregiver (Mace & Babins 1981). Determine your preferences and which activities are meaningful to you and then work toward creating time for them (Watt & Calder 1981). These respite choices may include being alone in the house, going on an outing, or working on a project.

Time and money management is also essential (Watt & Calder 1981). One needs to have a realistic idea of the costs of living, charges for services (hospital, home aide, equipment), and so on. The care-giving spouse needs to know what services are affordable. Children who are providing care need to know not only their parents' financial resources but the extent of financial help the family is willing and able to contribute. Record keeping is necessary for all costs of care: health care costs, gas, food, time, and others. Such records keep one abreast of expenses and indicate whether one is managing satisfactorily.

Should one's coping skills be overwhelmed, outside help may become necessary. The caregiver should recognize warning signs that problems are getting out of hand. These signals can include increased alcohol consumption, changes in eating patterns, excessive use of medication, loss of sleep, emotional liability, thoughts of suicide (Mace & Babins 1981). The hardest step is acknowledging that one needs help; next most difficult is extending the effort to seek help.

Assessment. Horowitz (1982) noted that the involvement of professionals in providing services for chronically ill family members does not push the family out of the care-giving role. She found that the strongest predictor of care-giving commitment among adult children is parent need, followed by their feelings for the parent, gender, marital status, and finally the extent of planning that is undertaken. She points out that professionals can help caregivers master ways of managing older relatives at home, but this assistance requires adequate assessment of family needs and capabilities, including both structural resources (economic and social) and dynamic factors (past experiences, attitudes, affective influences). This assessment is highly important because it has been found that once care giving is accepted, the family feels an ongoing responsibility (Cantor 1980).

The manner in which families cope with long-term care giving also should be assessed. Fengler and Goodrich (1979) looked at how coping is influenced by income, role overload, and companionship. They found that families who considered their incomes adequate to meet needs suffered less role overload. If low income necessitated that more work be added

to their current responsibilities, caregivers often became extremely exhausted and in some instances suffered from emotional collapse. Low income also contributed to more isolation since there was less time to spend with friends, neighbors, and others. Isolation was also increased for women whose husbands were no longer capable of being confidants or companions. These women were forced to spend more time on care-giving responsibilities, limiting time available for meaningful activities and friends. Professionals can assist in this process, but only after making a thorough assessment. Teaching and counseling are effective ways by which caregivers can learn how to gain skill in handling problems that they face.

Counseling

Counseling gives families support and information that they need (Lezak 1978). Counseling services can be combined with other programs such as day care programs or self-help groups. Some of the information that caregivers need to work on during counseling includes the following:

1. Role of emotions: Anger, frustration, and sorrow are natural emotions. When they result in wishing the client would die, then guilt can ensue, further complicating matters.
2. Caretaker's health: Continuing to provide care requires maintaining one's own health, despite the common notion that one must be self-sacrificing. Self-care includes rest, occasional self-indulgence, and respite from responsibilities.
3. Caretaker decisions: The ultimate decision maker when conflicts arise with client or other family members is the primary caregiver.
4. Role changes: Switching roles can be emotionally distressing for all concerned and can promote intrafamily conflicts. Mutual sharing of concerns helps all to understand the naturalness of such dissension.
5. Lack of improvement: Since little that the family does results in improvement, there is no reason to feel guilty.

6. Dependent children: Divided loyalties arise when the welfare of dependent children is threatened, especially when the client's behavior is abusive. Behavioral management techniques may help, but if they do not, then the children must be protected from abuse.

Summary and Conclusions

Not only is the client impacted by chronic illness, but the family caregiver is affected as well. The care provided to the client continues for long periods of time and is given willingly. In spite of the work involved, the cost-effectiveness of providing care at home, and the ability of maintaining people out of institutions, such efforts receive limited financial and service support.

Giving home care is a strenuous role: the toll extracted can be extensive. There may be inadequate finances resulting from loss of income, medical costs, and lack of public funding. Other responsibilities, such as family or job, can compete with care giving, thus impacting on the caregiver. Care giving may be inconvenient and impact on roles negatively. Emotional strain includes isolation, anxiety, and guilt. Physically the caregiver can be adversely impacted, creating a problem for caregiver and care receiver alike.

Since most caregivers prefer to continue in this role, the most important way of helping is to support and sustain the caregiver. This can be done through respite programs and support groups and by teaching the caregiver to help himself or herself. Thorough assessment by the health care provider can provide direction for obtaining help.

One issue that has not been discussed in this chapter is the health provider's responsibility to serve as a client advocate. This requires gaining information and staying abreast of legislation that could serve the needs of this unsung group of people. Increased support (financial, physical, and emotional) will allow care to continue at home, enhancing the quality of the client's life.

STUDY QUESTIONS

1. What are the advantages for the client of being cared for at home? for the caregiver? for the community and society?
2. Who are the primary providers of home care? What are the major roles they take on? How are their other roles affected?
3. How is the caregiver affected by taking on this role? In what ways are caregivers impacted?
4. How does public policy adversely affect caregivers?
5. What kinds of respite programs have been developed for caregivers so that they can continue in this

role? What are the advantages of each of these programs? Can you identify any disadvantages?
6. What contributed to the growth of self-help groups for caregivers? What kinds of groups are there and how do they function?
7. In what ways can caregivers help themselves handle the impact of caregiving?
8. Identify a family situation in which there is a caregiver–care recipient relationship. Discuss how you would go about helping this family unit.

References

Archbold, P., (1980) Impact of parent caring on middle-aged offspring, *Journal of Gerontological Nursing,* 6(2):79–84

Archbold, P., (1983) Impact of parent-caring on women, *Family Relations, 32*:39–45

Bregman, A., (1980) Living with progressive childhood illness: Parental management of neuromuscular disease, *Social Work in Health Care, 5*(4):357–387

Brody, E., (1966) The aging family, Paper presented at the 19th annual meeting of the Gerontological Society, New York, 1966

Brody, S. J., Poulshock, S. W., and Masciocchi, C. F., (1978) The family caring unit: A major consideration in the longterm support system, *The Gerontologist, 18*(6):556–561

Cantor, M., (1980) The entry of the formal organization on the informal support systems of older Americans, Administration on Aging Grant No. 90-A-1329, New York: Fordham University

Cantor, M., (1983) Strain among caregivers: A study of experience in the United States, *The Gerontologist, 23*(6):597–604

Caregivers—A 1984 "Sleeper," (1984) *OWL Observer, 3*(1):1,7

Colman, V., Summers, T., and Leonard, F., (1982) Till death do us part: Caregiving wives of severely disabled husbands, *Gray Paper #7,* Washington, D.C.: Older Women's League

Craft, M., (1979) Help for the family's neglected "other" child, *Maternal-Child Nursing, 4:*297–300

Crossman, L., and Kaljian, D., (1984) The family: Cornerstone of care, *Generations VIII,* 4:44–46

Crossman, L., London, C., and Barry, C., (1981) Older women caring for disabled spouses: A model for supportive services, *The Gerontologist, 21*(5):464–470

Eisdorfer, C., and Cohen, D., (1981) Management of the patient and family coping with dementing illness, *The Journal of Family Practice, 12*(5):831–837

Ellis, V., and Wilson, D., (1983) Respite care in the nursing home unit of a veterans hospital, *American Journal of Nursing, 83:*1433–1434

Family Caregiving and the Elderly: Policy Recommendations & Research Findings (1983) N.Y. State Office for the Aging, March

Farkas, S. W., (1980) Impact of chronic illness on the patient's spouse, *Health and Social Work,* pp. 39–46

Fengler, A., and Goodrich, N., (1979) Wives of elderly disabled men: The hidden patients, *The Gerontologist, 19*(2):175–183

Goldstein, V., Regnery, G., and Wellin, E., (1981) Caretaker role fatigue, *Nursing Outlook,* January, pp. 24–30

Golodetz, A., Evans, R., Heinritz, G., and Gobson, C., (1969) The care of chronic illness: The "responsor" role, *Medical Care, VII*(6):385–394

Griffith, E., (1984) Home care today, an interview, *American Journal of Nursing, 84*(3):340–349

Gurland, B., et al., (1978) Personal time dependency in the elderly of New York City: Findings from the U.S.–U.K. cross national geriatric community study, *Dependency in the Elderly of NYC,* Community Council of Greater New York

Gwyther, L., and Matteson, M., (1983) Care for the caregivers, *Journal of Gerontological Nursing, 9*(2):92–95, 110, 116

Hayter, J., (1982) Finding a balance: Helping the families, *Journal of Gerontological Nursing, 8*(2):81–86

Hearing on Families: Aging and Changing, (1980) before Select Committee on Aging: House of Representatives, 96th Congress, Washington, D.C.: United States Government Printing Office, Publication No. 96–242

Hildebrandt, E., (1983) Respite care in the home, *American Journal of Nursing, 83:*1428–1431

Home health—The need for a national policy to better provide for the elderly, (1977) Washington, D.C.: General Accounting Office

Horowitz, A., (1982) Predictors of caregiving involvement among adult children of the frail elderly, Paper presented at the 35th annual meeting of the Gerontological Society of America, Boston, Mass., November

Horowitz, A., and Shindelman, L. W., (1981) Reciprocity and affection: Past influences on current caregiving, Presented at the 34th annual meeting of the Gerontological Society of America, Toronto, Canada, November

Huey, R., (1983) Respite care in a state-owned hospital, *American Journal of Nursing, 83:*1431–1432

Hymovich, D. P., (1984) Development of the Chronicity Impact and Coping Instrument: Parent Questionnaire (CICI:PQ), *Nursing Research, 33*(4):218–222

Lezak, M., (1978) Living with the characterologically altered brain injured patient, *Journal of Clinical Psychiatry, 39:*592–598

Mace, N. L., and Babins, P. V., (1981) *The 36-Hour Day,* Baltimore: Johns Hopkins University Press

McKeever, P., (1983) Fathering the chronically ill child, *Maternal-Child Nursing, 6:*124–128

Nardone, M., (1980) Characteristics predicting community care for mentally impaired older persons, *The Gerontologist, 20*(6):661–667

National Center for Health Statistics (1974) *1968–1974 Nursing Home Survey,* Washington, D.C.: United States Department of Health and Human Services

Nevin, R., Easton, J., McCubbin, H., and Birkebak, R., (1979) Parental coping in raising children who have Spina Bifida Cystica, *Zeitschrift Kinderchirurgie, 28*(4):417–425

Oppenheimer, J., and Rucher, R., (1980) The effects of parental relationships on the management of cystic fibrosis and guidelines for social work intervention, *Social Work in Health Care, 5*(4):409–419

Ostrander, V., (1984) Editorial: Let's reform health care system says AARP leader, *The American Nurse, 16*(5):4, 15, May

Petty, D., Bosshardt, J., Gibson, D., and Snyder, M., (1981) *Family Survival Handbook*, San Francisco: Family Survival Project of the Mental Health Association of San Francisco

Rathbone-McCuan, E., (1976) Geriatric day care: A family perspective, *The Gerontologist, 16*(6):517–521

Robertson, D., Griffiths, A., and Cosin, L., (1977) A community-based continuing care program for the elderly disabled, *Journal of Gerontology, 32*(5):334–339

Robinson, B., and Thurnher, M., (1979) Taking care of aged parents: A family cycle transition, *The Gerontologist, 19*(6):586–593

Ross, J., (1979) Coping with childhood cancer: Group intervention as an aid to parents in crisis, *Social Work in Health Care, 4*(4):381–393

Safford, F., (1980) A program for families of the mentally impaired elderly, *The Gerontologist, 20*(6):656–660

Sager, A., (1982) Improving the provision of long-term care, *Aging*, United States Department of Health and Human Services, March–April

Shanas, E., (1979) The family as a social support system in old age, *The Gerontologist, 19*(2):169–174

Shanas, E., and Maddox, G., (1976) Aging, health, & the organization of health resources, in Binstock, R. and Shanas, E. (eds.), *Handbook of Aging and the Social Sciences*, New York: Van Nostrand Reinhold

Soldo, B., and Myllyluoma, J., (1983) Caregivers who live with dependent elderly, *The Gerontologist, 23*(6):605–611

Stephen, B., (1984) When an elderly parent is lucky, *San Francisco Chronicle*, February 27, 1984, p. 15

Strauss, A., Corbin, J., Fagerhaugh, S., Glaser, B., Maines, D., Suczek, B., and Wiener, C., (1984) *Chronic Illness and the Quality of Life* (2d ed.), St. Louis: C.V. Mosby

Stroker, R., (1983) Impact of disability on families of stroke clients, *Journal of Neurosurgical Nursing, 15*(6):360–365

Teresi, J., Bennett, R., and Wilder, D., (1978) *Person Time Dependency and Family Attitudes*, New York: Columbia University

Venters, M., (1981) Familial coping with chronic and severe childhood illness: the case of cystic fibrosis, *Social Science and Medicine, 15A*:289–297

Watt, J., and Calder, A., (1981) *I Love You But You Drive Me Crazy*, Vancouver, B.C.: Forbes Publications

Whitfield, S., (1982) Maryland state office for the aging family support demonstration program, *Financial Incentives for Informal Caregiving*, New York City: Community Council of Greater New York

Zarit, S., Reever, K., and Bach-Peterson, J., (1980) Relatives of the impaired elderly: Correlates of feelings of burden, *The Gerontologist, 20*(6):649–660

Bibliography

Chowanec, G., and Binik, Y., (1982) End state renal disease (ESRD) and the marital dyad: A literature review, *Social Science and Medicine, 16*:1551–1558

Hanson, S., Sauer, W., and Seelback, W., (1983) Racial and cohort variations in filial responsibility norms, *The Gerontologist, 23*(6):626–631

Kimbill, C. P., Klieman, C. R., Rosenbaum, E. H., Van DenNoort, S., Wisher, W. J., Murphy, J. P., and Ganz, R. N., (1981) Chronic illness? Help the family cope, *Patient Care*: June 30, 1981, pp. 23–24, 29, 32, 34–36, 38–39, 42–43, 46, 48–49, 52–53

Stoller, E., and Earl, L., (1983) Help with activities of everyday life: Sources of support for the noninstitutionalized elderly, *The Gerontologist, 23*(1):64–69

CHAPTER NINE

Body Image

◇ CASE STUDY ◇

Change in Body Image

F.B., now 70 years of age, was just a teenager when she suffered a severe sunburn on her shoulders after a day at the beach. Initially painful, the burn soon healed and F.B. continued to enjoy her summer activities. By the time school started in the fall, however, some lesions appeared on her shoulder where the original sunburn had been. F.B. paid little attention to these lesions; she was excited about returning to school and, anyway, her clothing covered them. The lesions did not go away but began to spread onto her neck. She became sensitive about her appearance and changed the way she dressed in an attempt to hide the lesions from her classmates.

Because F.B. had a Christian Science background, she made no attempt to seek medical intervention, and the lesions remained. Over the years there were periods of remission and exacerbation, but as F.B. grew older

the lesions became worse and spread to other parts of her body, mainly to areas that were more likely to be moist. Because the lesions were causing her physical discomfort, F.B. finally sought medical attention for her condition and was diagnosed as having Darier's disease.

Although F.B. was extremely careful about body hygiene, the lesions often left an unpleasant odor and intermittently areas became infected. Knowing that the lesions became worse with exposure to sun, heat, makeup, and synthetic materials, F.B. stayed at home more and more. She was embarrassed by the odor created by the lesions and medications and also by the change in her appearance. Many difficulties have confronted this client, one of which has been a lifelong change in her body image.

Introduction

Body image serves as a standard or frame of reference that individuals use when relating to themselves and their physical and social environment. Body image influences others' reactions and also affects emotions, perceptions, attitudes, and personality. It determines the limits we place on ourselves and those others impose. Body image is a dynamic process that influences the way the individual functions.

Historical Background

Understanding body image is important for those in the health profession. Although the concept has been discussed in the literature since the 1880s, not until Schilder first presented his work in 1935 did a new understanding of this concept arise. In his book *The Image and Appearance of the Human Body*, Schilder (1950) explores the dimensions of body image: "The image of the human body means the picture of our own body which we form in our mind, that is to say the way in which the body appears to ourselves." Schilder believes that the perception of one's body is based on a tridimensional image influenced by physiologic, psychologic, and social experiences.

Definitions

Definitions of body image, though varied, share similarities. Common to many of the definitions is the belief that body image develops in response not only to multiple sensory input (visual, tactile, proprioceptive, and kinesthetic) but also to the actions and attitudes of others. Beeken (1978) states, "Body image ... is the interaction between physical and emotional stimuli. It is formed by the interaction between the perceptual pool and the experiential pool." In addition, it is based on both conscious and unconscious information. According to Norris (1978), "Much of the auditing of subjective experiences that makes and modifies the body image is unconscious and no one can describe his or her own total body image."

Although the concept of body image encompasses one's view of the physical structure of his or her body, it includes more than a perception of one's physical appearance. Perceptions of function, sensation, and mobility, as well as feelings and thought, also become incorporated into the body image one holds (McCloskey 1976).

The terms *self-concept* and *body image* are frequently used interchangeably, suggesting that these two concepts are inextricably interwoven (Jenkins 1980). The similarity between these two concepts is that they are related to one's experiences with others and one's view of self in terms of self-esteem, self-image, personality, and identity.

Another similarity among the definitions of body image lies in the notion of reality and ideality. The idea presented here is that the ideal image of oneself and the real image must coincide or be compatible. If a discrepancy exists between what is idealized and what is real, a conflict in body image that may affect personality and health may develop. If, for instance,

F.B.'s idealized view of herself includes tanned, intact skin rather than the real picture of one whose skin lesions become worse with sun exposure, a conflict can arise.

Development of Body Image

Body image is not static but changes and develops through the stages of the life cycle. The development of body image begins in infancy. Newborn infants have no concrete concept of body image, responding to life on the sensory or feeling level. The initial foundation for the formation of body image begins when, during the later part of infancy, infants begin to separate themselves from their mothers. In other words, the initial struggle with the concept of body image begins as the infant starts to identify self as separate from the significant other (O'Brien 1980). Crucial to the development of body image throughout infancy is stimulation.

Awareness of body image expands during childhood, becoming dependent on the reactions of many, rather than a few. School children compare themselves with their peers in the classroom, playground, and other youth-oriented activities. In addition, the reactions of other adults—teachers, youth group leaders, or other parents—become important. This period of childhood finds the child's body image ever evolving as the child begins to develop and refine physical, motor, learning, language, and social skills. Also at this time the child becomes more aware of sexual differences, moving from a period of play with children of either sex to a time when play involves only children of the same sex. At around the age of 12 children begin to accept themselves as unique persons (Murray & Zentner 1979).

Adolescence is a time of exquisite body image sensitivity. Numerous and rapid body changes occur at this time, causing the adolescent to become preoccupied with self and body characteristics. Although such physical changes are important, the meaning that the adolescent gives to them and the way the adolescent uses his or her body may be more important. In addition, peer group recognition, acceptance, and comparison have great significance. Consequently, body image is in a constant state of revision as adolescents attempt to achieve perfect balance with their perceived view of the acceptable. Once the identity tasks are completed in adolescence, body image becomes more stable.

With adulthood, this increased stability is incorporated into the adult's sense of self. The adult is more likely to maintain this body image, regardless of whether it is positive or negative, because it affects the individual's participation in daily life. This is not to say that adults cannot change their body images; rather, changing becomes more difficult because "the person perceives others' comments and behavior in relation to his already established image in order to avoid conflict and anxiety within himself" (Murray & Zentner 1979). Roberts (1978) believes that "an adult's self-image becomes a dynamic interrelationship between three vital components: self-concept, identity and personality." Consequently, an adult who has formed a well-integrated body image is more likely to react positively to life events.

Revising one's concept of body image accompanies the aging process. Confronted by changes that gradually develop as one ages, the adult once again has to redefine body image as these visible, and not so visible, changes occur. Wrinkling of skin, graying and thinning of hair, and changes in body contour are among the visible alterations that remind people of their aging. Frequently, aged clients find incorporating these changes into a viable body image difficult, especially when society places more value on the attributes of youth.

Impaired sensory input due to a decrease in visual and auditory acuity can interfere with the elderly adult's interactions with the environment. The aged client may prefer to limit participation in social and family activities (because of an inability to hear or understand conversations), rather than to wear a hearing aid, another visible sign of deterioration. Other changes that normally accompany aging involve reproductive functions. Although sexual activity can continue, sexual response in all phases of the cycle is slowed. This change in sexual response may lead elderly persons to believe that they are no longer capable of enjoying sexual activity. All these changes

can effect a change in body image (Murray & Zentner 1979).

Although body image changes throughout the life cycle, periods of stability occur. Body image functions to provide the individual throughout life with a sense of personal identity: "It acts as a standard or frame of reference which influences people's ability to perform and the ways in which they perceive themselves, measure their continuity through life, and identify their mastery of the world" (Norris 1978).

Influences on Body Image Concept

Changes that occur during growth and development are among the factors that influence the concept of body image. Others include one's body boundary, factors that influence this boundary, cultural influences, and multiple internal and external phenomena. Reactions of others also influence this concept.

Body Boundaries

One's *body boundary* is the amount of space the individual perceives the body as occupying (Fawcett & Fry 1980). Body boundary affects the individual's interrelationship with the physical environment and differs among individuals. For some, body boundaries are well defined and separate from the surrounding environment. Others, however, cannot clearly delineate the limits of their body boundaries. An obvious example of the latter is a client who has had a stroke resulting in paralysis. Here, although the body remains intact, the individual cannot recognize that the paralyzed limb belongs to him or her.

Sexual differences also influence body boundaries. Women are said to have a more definite body boundary sense than men. Such a characteristic may stem from the fact that women receive more of their identity from their body and its function because of the importance placed on such physical attributes as breasts, legs, facial features, and hair. Men, on the other hand, are more likely to achieve an identity from their accomplishments than from their bodily attributes. Because of this emphasis on body the woman may more quickly arrive at a realistic concept of her body and its boundaries than her male counterpart (Murray 1972a).

Body boundaries can affect interpersonal relationships. It is thought that those individuals with a well-integrated sense of body boundary interact differently from those who have poorly defined boundaries. Certainly individuals who are aware of their body's boundaries are better able to judge whether a given space can be entered; the way the person enters the space can determine the quality of one's interactions with those within that space (Castledine 1981).

Although body boundaries influence one's concept of body image, an interplay occurs between the two. Consequently, whatever affects one will probably affect the other. A chronic illness is one of many factors that can affect both.

Cultural Influences

One's cultural background must also be considered when discussing the concept of body image because it influences which physical and personality traits are deemed acceptable. Obviously, differences among cultures exist, but even within the same culture acceptable attributes may vary. Often these differences are related to societal expectations. Frequently the predominant cultural social group sets the standard by which others are judged. Consequently, within the United States, although tremendous cultural diversity exists, the youthful, slender, attractive, athletic body is prized, and intelligence, friendliness, and success are admired personality traits (Murray 1972a).

Internal and External Influences

One's sense of body image is also affected by internal and external influences (Esberger 1978). *Internal influences* are those sensations that develop in response to systemic physiologic occurrences within the body, including sensations arising from metabolic, neurologic, endocrine, or hormonal changes. These internal influences have a profound effect on the developing body image of the infant, and they continue to exert their influence throughout the life cycle, although external influences also become important later.

Although external influences are many, a few are worth noting. One such external influence is that of the environment, which can encompass many factors and may include weather, availability of light, surrounding decor, clothing, or people currently present. Whether one is male or female may also have an external influence on one's concept of body image. Obviously, differences between male and female body image are partly related to anatomic structure and body function. In his study of sex differences, Fisher (1964) found evidence that "women may have a more clearly articulated and stable body concept than men."

Another external influence relates to topological experiences, including sensations such as touch, taste, pain, thermal changes, and one's reactions to them. Other such experiences concern the surface characteristics of one's body (Norris 1978). Relating these findings to F.B., it is possible that many external influences may be affecting her concept of body image. Certainly she must be selective in the environment into which she places herself. Her topological experiences are, additionally, distorted by the long-term effects of the skin lesions and their result of changing the body's surface.

Interaction with Others

Reactions of and experiences with others can also affect one's concept of body image. In most instances the groups that exert most control over one's body image include one's parents and other family members, significant friends, and peer groups (O'Brien 1980). These people's attitudes frequently determine one's perception of self. In incorporating the opinions of others, the individual will "measure himself against the ideal as well as the disapproved characteristics" (Dempsey 1972). Thus, the more positive the opinions held by others, the more likely is the individual to develop a positive body image concept.

Others who may be less significant, such as teachers, neighbors, health care providers, and society as a whole, can also influence an individual's body image. Unfortunately, these experiences are frequently based on more superficial personal qualities (bodily appearance or appropriate behavior), and yet they may have a great effect on the individual. Other people's opinions are important, and we respond to their perceptions whether they are positive or negative. The individual reacts "to the way he thinks others see him . . . at the same time projecting to others his own body image. Thus, the way in which others perceive an individual will be influenced by both the image he/she really projects and the image perceived by their own body images" (Esberger 1978). Interpersonal experiences can influence the role to which one is assigned, as well as determining many other aspects of oneself, including body image: "It is probably because body image is such a central concept of the human experience that it is (therefore) such an excellent indicator of a person's general health" (Castledine 1981).

Chronicity and Body Image

One can say that modern technology has contributed to a significantly expanded life expectancy. Many who earlier might have had an untimely death or shortened life are now living longer. However, with increased longevity comes the risk of chronic illness and disability. A chronic illness may necessitate prolonged medical care, lifelong medication, or a change in life-style (for example, in one's job, activities, or physical environment). Regardless of the causative factor leading to the chronic illness or whether it is manifested outwardly (for example, skin rash) or internally (diabetes, for example), the person must incorporate a new image of self. Since adapting to a changed body image may not be easy without appropriate intervention, and since available literature is limited and primarily approaches the problem as it relates to acute illnesses, the intent of the remaining portions of this chapter is to address the issue of body image and its relation to chronicity.

Body Image Problems Resulting from Chronicity

Many problems or conflicts arise when an individual's body image is threatened by a chronic illness. Although it is not unusual for disturbances to develop, a conflict is more likely to occur when the individual has difficulty accepting and adapting to the changes.

External Changes

One of the problems that may arise from a chronic illness is physical disfigurement. Certainly the more visible or extensive the disfigurement, the greater the perceived threat to one's body image. Then the individual must cope not only with personal feelings about the disfigurement but with the responses of others, as well (see Chapter 4).

Facial disfigurement is one example of an external alteration that can be extremely threatening to one's body image and to others in the environment. Obviously the face is the most expressive and highly visible part of the body. Murray (1972a) notes, "There is less connection with the body image when an attribute is looked upon as a tool than when it is looked upon as a personal characteristic." In actuality, however, the face is both a tool and a personal characteristic: as a tool, it serves as one of the basic verbal and nonverbal means of communication; as a personal characteristic, it identifies the individual. Thus, when F.B. discovered that the skin lesions were beginning to appear on her face, she took extreme care to camouflage them because of the value her adolescent peers placed on facial features.

Other external alterations that may affect the individual depend upon the extent of involvement and the meaning the individual and society attach to these alterations (Norris 1978). Skin changes can alter one's image of self. The lesions caused by psoriasis are just one example; another is the skin wrinkling and the appearance of brown, or liver, spots accompanying aging.

Visible bodily changes may also necessitate that the individual revise body image. Again the meaning or impact of the change determines the necessity for such revision. Certainly any illness that causes a woman to lose a breast interferes with the way she views herself. If a particular feature or body part is viewed as being especially attractive (for example, attractive hands), and this attractiveness is changed by chronic illness (such as arthritis), body image is threatened.

Joint swelling and changes associated with many rheumatic diseases may also create problems for the individual. Poor dental hygiene or the presence of a malocclusion may be extremely damaging to an individual's perception of self. A young man once noted that having his teeth straightened was the most significant event of his life because it allowed him to smile and laugh without covering his mouth. What a tremendous effect this had not only on his body image but on his entire view of himself and his worth as a person!

Functional Limitations

Body image can also be altered by the presence of a functional limitation. Limitation of function occurs when there is a loss of a body part or a change in the functional capability of the entire body or a part of it (Norris 1978). Any number of chronic illnesses can cause such a disability. Residual effects of other illnesses, such as a fracture or joint disturbance, are contributing factors. Loss of function can lead to decreased mobility, which in turn can foster feelings of dependence and loss of control over the environment and oneself, disrupting one's image of oneself. Rubin (1968) points out that "loss of a complex, coordinated and controlled functional activity which has been achieved and integrated into the personal system is to lose or be threatened with the loss of self."

Loss of function can also affect an individual's ability to perform. Since much of one's identity is tied to the ability to participate in various activities, the loss of the ability to do so may be viewed as a threat to one's body image (Rubin 1968). For example, a woman may question her femininity or sexual attractiveness if her ability to participate in sexual activity is limited by joint immobility caused by hip involvement from rheumatoid arthritis (see Chapter 10). The ability to move and participate in a meaningful way is essential to one's sense of well-being; consequently, any limitation of one's functional ability may alter one's concept of body image.

Body image is threatened when the individual attaches great importance to the body part changed or lost because of chronic illness or disability. Different body parts have different meanings: whereas one individual might view a part as having little significance, another might attach great value to it (Norris 1978).

Although we associate more extensive involvement with a greater degree of disturbance in body image, for some individuals even a minor loss can prove to be devastating. The important factor is the symbolic meaning of the change to the individual (Esberger 1978). Even when a chronic illness produces no visible physical disfigurement, the individual can feel extremely threatened if the body part or function is held in high esteem. It is well known that a hysterectomy may prove disastrous for some women, whereas others imbue the procedure with little importance. The difference obviously lies in the fact that some women see the uterus as essential to their femininity, and its removal, therefore, as a distortion in their body image.

The consequence of experiencing a myocardial infarction (MI) also illustrates the importance an organ can have in determining whether one's image of oneself is threatened. Although changes produced by an MI are not physically visible, the symbolic meaning of the heart is so great and varied and its purpose so strongly attached to life that few survive an MI without some aspect of their body image being threatened.

Another variable to consider is the meaning the treatment or rehabilitation plan has for the individual (see Chapter 18). If the individual sees the positive benefits of active participation in the treatment program, the likelihood that chronic illness or disability will cause a changed body image is reduced.

Temporal Influences

The period during which an alteration in the body occurs may also influence one's body image (Roberts 1978). In the presence of a slow, progressive disease or a gradual change in body image, the individual has time to incorporate the new body image and its resultant changes (O'Brien 1980). When the changes of a chronic illness develop over time, the individual is given warning of what may likely occur and opportunity to acknowledge and integrate the change over a longer period of time.

Unfortunately individuals who are victims of sudden, traumatic illness have no warning of the events to come, and therefore relatively little time or opportunity to cope with the change (Beeken 1978). The sudden alteration may have a greater impact on the individual, thereby making resolution of the changes in body image more difficult. A person who loses functional ability through the long-term effects of rheumatoid arthritis may incorporate these changes into a revised body image more easily than one who suddenly becomes a hemiplegic as a result of a stroke. It must be recognized, however, that for some individuals even knowing what is likely to occur may not help them to adapt to the changes, because of the many other variables involved.

Influences of Other Aspects of Self

Self-esteem, identity, behavior, personality, and self-concept are closely intertwined with one's concept of body image. Consequently any or all of these factors may become distorted if the individual fails to accept and adapt to the bodily changes accompanying chronic illness. Failure to adapt may depend on the individual's preillness image. Beeken (1978) believes that "an individual with a fairly affirmative body image will probably react more positively to the condition rather than one who perceived this body image negatively pre-injury."

Cultural/Social Influences

Several years of teaching experience have demonstrated to this author that the capacity for a successful revision of body image following a chronic illness depends on one's cultural or social background. Each cultural and social group establishes its own norms governing the acceptable, especially in terms of physical appearance and personality attributes. If, then, a chronic illness causes an individual to differ from the group, the person may be ignored or avoided (see Chapter 4). The attitudes of others are quickly sensed; when one cannot meet group expectations because of a chronic illness or disability, the individual's body image is likely to be threatened. The cultural or social group can also covertly or overtly discourage the individual from using public places. F.B. let her hair grow long and wears it in a bun to avoid subjecting herself to the inspection and scorn of hair stylists. She also sews many of her own clothes because in the past she found that salespersons became uneasy when they discovered that she was going to try clothes on "that" body.

The Health Team Members

The success an individual has in adapting to a new body image also depends on the members of the health team. Differences in perspectives of a chronic illness or disability by the client and members of the health team are not unusual (Leonard 1972). If for some reason the health team, or even one individual within it, views the change with revulsion, the client's concept of body image will probably incorporate that revulsion. Likewise, if the client views the bodily changes as significant in some way and the health team views them as just another example of the benefits of modern medicine in saving or prolonging life, conflict arises. The client may not comply with the treatment regimen or may otherwise attempt to make others acknowledge that the changes are important. The more the health team can help the client adapt to changes, the more likely it is that there will be an acceptable outcome in the integration of a constructive body image change.

For example, individuals who have needed colostomies can benefit from talking about the surgery's effects on the body before and after surgery. Providing willing assistance with stoma care until the person is ready to undertake self-care, as well as positive feedback as self-care is initiated, is a way health professionals can assist these clients in developing positive body images related to their colostomies and themselves.

Impact of Poor Adjustment

Inability to adjust to a changed body image may be manifested by the client's experiencing a variety of physical or psychological symptoms. Physical symptoms can include vague subjective complaints of illness that may or may not be associated with the chronic illness. Intractable pain is another common complaint. Chronic fatigue may indicate that the client is unable to accept the reality of the changed body image and expends a disproportionate amount of energy denying its existence (Libbus 1982). Other physical symptoms related to psychological problems can also occur.

Psychological problems may be as varied and frequent as physical complaints; therefore, one must consider these problems in relation to the individual's concept of body image. Anger or resentment may focus on the family or health care provider. The person may also appear depressed, especially if unable to complete the grieving process for the idealized body image because of the constant reminder of the changed bodily state. Anxiety may appear in patients in whom "a discrepancy between the perceived disturbed physical state and the previously established model yields emotional tension" (Henker 1979). Denial, as mentioned previously, is another common psychological response, as are feelings of guilt. Although these are the most common psychological problems that occur, others may develop in the person having a chronic illness.

Interventions

The goal of intervention is to help the client adapt successfully to body image changes that are taking place as a result of having a chronic illness. Many factors determine the effectiveness with which the chronically ill individual adapts to changes in body image. Regardless of whether the change results from surgery, an accident, or a disease process, the client of necessity must incorporate a new self-concept. However, adapting to a new body image is not necessarily a static process.

As the variables that originally influence the adaptation process change, the client's perception of self changes as it is again threatened. The chronically ill person is continually reintegrating a new image of self, especially during periods of illness exacerbation or remission or at times when the chronic illness that caused the original change in body image is again confronted. At such times clients may need to rework their body image.

Stages in Restructuring Body Image

The client must work through four stages to integrate physical or functional changes into a restructured body image; as originally proposed by Lee (1970), they include impact, retreat, acknowledgment, and reconstruction. Individuals proceed through these stages in different ways and may return to the first stage as they revise their body image. Familiarity with the behavior that typically occurs during each of these stages will help the professional to evaluate the client's progress, predict the likelihood of recovery, and determine appropriate interventions.

During the *impact* stage, attention again focuses on the body part or disease entity causing the chronic illness. While the client is unaware of a threat to body image, he or she directs energy primarily toward coping with the disease. Consequently, a client having rheumatoid arthritis who experiences an exacerbation of the disease will turn attention to alleviating the symptoms rather than concentrating on the disfigurements that result from the disease.

During the *retreat* stage, the client becomes aware of the body changes that have occurred. However, the reality of the situation, coupled with a lack of emotional energy, becomes so overwhelming that the client retreats psychologically. The retreat phase provides the client with a "rest period during which forces are reorganized and strengthened and a point of readiness is reached for the work ahead" (Lee 1970). Denial regarding the presence of bodily changes is the behavior manifested by the client and may range from feelings of indifference to those of euphoria.

Acknowledgment is the period when the reality of the chronic illness and the losses that have occurred are faced. Mourning for the idealized body image may occur as the client acknowledges the losses. To redefine the self-image, the individual may need solitude. This is also a time, however, when the client needs to discuss events surrounding the illness, the disability, and body image changes that are occurring. The reactions of others, including the professional's verbal and nonverbal responses, during this period are crucial to the client's progress.

Once the client has successfully acknowledged the threat to body image, *reconstruction* can begin. During this final stage, the client begins to assimilate a new image of self and to incorporate it into daily activities of living. Adaptation to the changes imposed by chronic illness may require time, because the amount of energy the client can devote to a successful reintegration may be limited. For some, it may never occur. Murray (1972b) recognizes this point and comments that "adaptation is not always positive or growth-promoting. There are those individuals who will permanently avoid the reality of having undergone change in the body." But for most, the reconstruction phase is positive, bringing about an adjustment to adaptive devices or technical procedures, a reorientation in the social aspects of life, and, finally, a reintegration of the client's body image (Lee 1970).

Factors Influencing Adaptation

Knowledge of these stages is not sufficient to help clients adapt successfully to the problems that arise from an alteration in body image. The professional must also consider the various factors that influence adaptation if intervention is to be successful.

Age.   Among those factors influencing adaptation is the client's age. Body image changes in an adolescent will be viewed differently from those occurring in a young or elderly adult. Adolescence is a time when attention normally focuses on the body and how it compares with those of the peer group. At this developmental stage, body image change may be devastating and extremely threatening.

One can say that bodily change can be as devastating to an adult as it is to an adolescent, even though the variables influencing the response may be different. Body image in the adult is well developed and provides a basis for identity. Therefore, an adult may find change no easier to accept than an adolescent does, because it interferes with the individual's well-established self-image.

Adaptation to changes in body image for the older individual may also be complicated by the necessity to cope with the changes that accompany aging (Norris 1978). An illness that creates changes during this period in one's life may be overwhelming. If the changes in any way affect the elderly individual's independence, acceptance may prove impossible. Elderly individuals may also be dealing with the fears that develop because they are no longer useful in a society that (1) values physically attractive, independent people and (2) has not successfully identified a place or role for the healthy aged, let alone those who have a chronic illness.

Sex.   A client's sex is another variable that determines appropriate intervention, especially when the body image change is closely associated with perceived "masculine" or "feminine" characteristics. A woman, therefore, who has a mastectomy may have difficulty adapting to body image changes because "such loss, by its very nature, interferes with her female body image" (Jenkins 1980). Likewise, surgery, drug therapy, or disease that interferes with a man's ability to perform sexually may disrupt his view of himself as a man, thereby slowing his adjustment to a revised body image (see Chapter 10).

Coping Mechanisms.   Previous and current coping mechanisms are aspects of a client's personality that affect the manner in which adaptation occurs. In most instances, the client's coping with the present situation depends on the success with which the individual has handled other life stresses (O'Brien 1980). Thus to initiate useful intervention, the health professional must assess previous and current coping mechanisms. Even when the client does not appear to have adequate coping strategies, O'Brien (1980) believes that an important first step is to regard the client as coping.

Prior Experience.　Since past experiences exert a tremendous influence upon the client's ability to adapt to current changes, knowledge of some aspects of the client's past may help the intervention process. Areas that may provide useful information include the client's past experiences with illness and hospitalization and previous alterations in body image. Becoming aware of the amount of disparity between the preillness and current images of self may also facilitate intervention. Successful intervention is predicated on the health professional's understanding of what the chronic illness, body image changes, and management plan mean to the client, since these factors dramatically influence the client's compliance with a medication regimen or rehabilitation program (Roberts 1978).

Assessment

A thorough assessment is a prerequisite to appropriate and successful intervention. This assessment is made to determine the client's perceptions of the chronic illness and its effects on body image. It entails observing the client to assess the nature of the threat and interviewing the client to assess the meaning of the threat (McCloskey 1976). In addition, interviewing the family or significant others is necessary because their responses are important to the client's adaptation to the illness and to body image changes.

Assessing the stage of recovery the client has reached is of primary importance for planning intervention. If, for instance, the client is still in a state of denial, making realistic teaching or rehabilitation plans may be impeded. On the other hand, the threat of the illness and its effects on the client's body image may make the client very receptive to help. At this point, teaching and counseling may be instrumental in helping the client to begin to adapt to these

changes, thereby promoting a more rapid return to a higher level of functioning. Once clients reach a stage of receptiveness to the health professional's assistance, a therapeutic relationship can begin to be established. This relationship, in turn, may have the effect of helping the client accept the changes that have occurred, thereby facilitating progression through the recovery process.

It is the purpose of assessment, which occurs throughout the client's recovery, to compile a complete client profile. More specifically, the health professional seeks information that will facilitate intervention. Areas worth consideration include the following:

1. Assessing the client's definition of the current situation
2. Determining the client's knowledge of the chronic illness
3. Ascertaining the significance the client assigns to the altered body part and the client's attitude toward it
4. Discovering the client's assessment of others' responses to the changes

The greater the number of internal and external strengths and the more positive the indications of adaptation, the more likely it is that the client will be able to begin to revise and to adapt to a changed body image. For effective intervention, assessment should include finding both positive and negative indicators of the client's adaptation to a changed body image, as well as ascertaining the client's internal and external strengths. Although internal strengths depend on such factors as the client's previous self-esteem, body image, and concept of self, assessment should also take into account factors that clients perceive as particular strengths. External strengths encompass many phenomena, most importantly the support of family and significant others. Care providers must also assess the psychosocial background (religion, cultural orientation, social groups, occupation, and so on) and the effect of body image changes on interactions with relevant groups.

A complete client assessment must include the family or significant others because of the importance of their reactions and support to the client's adaptation. Assessment is accomplished by interviewing the family and observing its verbal and nonverbal interactions with the client (Leonard 1972). Family dynamics illustrate "who are supportive and concerned, [and] who are unable to cope themselves with the relative's illness" (O'Brien 1980). Valuable to successful intervention is discovering the following:

1. Meanings the family attaches to the chronic illness and body image changes
2. Perceived physical, psychological, or social losses experienced by them and by the client
3. Financial stresses that are present

It is important to realize that the family, like the client, may be experiencing many reactions to chronic illness and bodily changes. Incorporating assistance, via support for the family, into the intervention plan allows them, in turn, to be supportive of the client.

Specific Interventions

The success of intervention depends on establishing a therapeutic, supportive professional relationship. If this relationship is to be therapeutic, health care providers must identify their feelings about working with clients whose chronic illnesses encompass bodily changes. A study by Billie (1977) indicated that clients who reported a more positive body image were more likely to comply with posthospitalization recommendations, a necessity for any chronically ill individual. Therefore, if the health professional is unable or unwilling to help clients work through their feelings about a changed body image, little therapeutic success can be expected. Acceptance of the client by the health professional, like that by the family, is important in facilitating the client's acceptance of self.

The health professional also must understand the varied dimensions that result from changes in body image, since such changes involve more than altered appearance. The person having a chronic illness that results in bodily changes needs a health care provider who is willing to act as an advocate (see Chapter 13) and to provide consistent ongoing support and care. This role requires commitment, but it also increases the probability of successful intervention.

Communication. Numerous interventions assist the client and family to adapt to body image changes. Providing the client with the opportunity to talk about the body image changes as they relate to the chronic illness is beneficial. The climate for such discussions should be nonthreatening and conducive to sharing. Acceptance by the health professional, demonstrated by a willingness to listen, is extremely important (Marten 1978). In addition, clients must feel encouraged to express both positive and negative emotions. They need to talk about their emotions and experiences; through such discussions they are able to integrate a new picture of self. Consistent support by the health professional can ensure a positive outcome. Family members should also have an opportunity to analyze and express their feelings, either with or without the client present. Providing opportunities for such expressions is beneficial to the growth of both the client and the family.

Touch. Touching that is not perfunctory is an important intervention through which the health professional can demonstrate acceptance (Ernst & Shaw 1980). The need for touching and being touched often supersedes the need for talking about the condition. Touch, therefore, provides an effective nonverbal sign of care and concern. Used therapeutically, it can alleviate the stress and anger associated with redefining body image and can help the client feel more positive about bodily changes.

Positive Emotions. Providing an atmosphere that is conducive to positive emotions is another valuable intervention. Norman Cousins (1983), in his work *The Healing Heart*, suggests that positive emotions supplement the healing process. Whether expressed as "laughter, hope, faith, love, will to live, cheerfulness, humor, creativity, playfulness, confidence, [or] great expectations," positive emotions have great therapeutic value.

Self-Help Groups. Experience has shown that providing an opportunity to link up with community and self-help groups can be instrumental in recovery. These organizations give the client an opportunity to be with others who have the same problem and to share not only their fears and frustrations but also their successes. This group involvement helps some persons to regain the confidence to socialize and to be with others. Self-help groups especially designed for the adolescent are extremely beneficial to the process of developing an acceptable image of self.

Self-Care. Assisting clients to regain control and feelings of self-worth is fostered by helping them to assume responsibility for self-care as soon as it is feasible. The sooner the client looks at, touches, or manipulates the involved part, the sooner the adjustment process can begin. Involving the client in the planning of care and in the setting of short- and long-term goals is also important. When clients can understand, determine, and participate in self-care, they gain a sense of control over the chronic illness and resultant bodily changes.

Teaching. Educating the client about the chronic illness is also beneficial because knowledge dispels myths that impede adjustment (see Chapter 12). The knowledgeable client and family can select viable alternatives that are most appropriate for the specific aspects of their disease and adaptation, including body image changes.

Summary and Conclusions

Body image is an important concept for the health professional to understand. Many definitions have been proposed, all integrating the concept that body image serves as a frame of reference that individuals use in relating themselves to the physical and social environments. Body image is not static: it changes as the individual passes through the various stages of the life cycle. One's sense of body image is also influenced by body boundaries, culture, internal and external environment, and experiences with others.

In the presence of a chronic illness one's sense of body image can be threatened, particularly when physical disfigurement occurs. However, one's sense of body image also changes in the presence of a functional limitation or when the changed or lost bodily part has great importance to the individual. Other factors that influence adaptation include the reactions of the client's cultural or social group, family, and caregivers. Inability to adjust to changed body image can result in various physical and psychological problems.

Successful intervention depends on the health professional's understanding of the recovery process. Other variables that can influence intervention include the client's age and sex, perception of the future, coping mechanisms, and past experiences with illness. A thorough assessment of the client is, therefore, necessary for successful intervention. Once the professional has assessed how well the client is adapting to a changed body image, it is possible to develop a plan of care. Establishing a therapeutic relationship with the client and family and helping the client to participate in the care are two beneficial interventions.

Success in adapting to body image changes varies. Awareness of factors that influence such change and knowledge of actions that are effective can help maximize adaptation.

STUDY QUESTIONS

1. Briefly describe the development of body image during the various phases of the life cycle.
2. Discuss the ways that cultural background influences one's concept of body image.
3. Body image can be threatened by a functional limitation. Explain.
4. What signs or symptoms might indicate an inability to adjust to a changed body image?
5. Identify and describe the four stages of the recovery process.
6. Describe the importance of family in the client's adaptation to a changed body image.
7. List factors that determine the client's success in adapting to a changed body image.
8. Describe four different actions the helping professional can use when intervening on behalf of the client.

References

Beeken, J., (1978) Body image changes in plegia, *Journal of Neurosurgical Nursing, 10*:20–23

Billie, D. A., (1977) The role of body image in patient compliance and education, *Heart and Lung, 6*: 143–148

Castledine, G., (1981) In the mind's eye . . . , *Nursing Mirror, 153*:16

Cousins, N., (1983) *The Healing Heart*, New York: W. W. Norton

Dempsey, M. O., (1972) The development of body image in the adolescent, *The Nursing Clinics of North America, 7*:609–615

Ernst, P., and Shaw, J., (1980) Touching is not taboo, *Geriatric Nursing, 10*:193–195

Esberger, K., (1978) Body image, *Journal of Gerontological Nursing, 4*:35–38

Fawcett, J., and Fry, S., (1980) Exploratory study of body image dimensionality, *Nursing Research, 29*(5):324–327

Fisher, S., (1964) Sex differences in body perception, *Psychological Monograph: General and Applied, 78*(14):1–22

Henker, F. O., (1979) Body image conflict following trauma and surgery, *Psychosomatics, 20*:812–820

Jenkins, H. M., (1980) Self-concept and mastectomy, *Journal of Obstetrics, Gynecologic and Neonatal Nursing*, 38–42

Lee, J. M., (1970) Emotional reactions to trauma, *Nursing Clinics of North America, 4*: 577–587

Leonard, B., (1972) Body image changes in chronic illness, *Nursing Clinics of North America, 7*:687–695

Libbus, K., (1982) Psoriasis and body image, *The Nurse Practitioner, 7*:15–18

Marten, L., (1978) Self-care nursing model for patients experiencing radical changes in body image, *Journal of Obstetrics, Gynecologic and Neonatal Nursing, 7*:9–13

McCloskey, J. C., (1976) How to make the most of body image theory in nursing practice, *Nursing 76, 6*:68–72

Motta, G., (1981) Stress and the elderly: Coping with a change in body image, *Journal of Enterostomal Therapy, 8*:21–22

Murray, R. L. E., (1972a) Body image development in adulthood, *The Nursing Clinics of North America, 7*:617–630

Murray, R. L. E., (1972b) Principles of nursing intervention for the adult patient with body image changes, *The Nursing Clinics of North America, 7*:697–707

Murray, R. B., and Zentner, J. P., (1979) *Nursing Assessment: Health Promotion Through the Life Span*, Englewood Cliffs, N. J.:Prentice-Hall

Norris, C. M., (1978) Body image: Its relevance to professional nursing, in Carlson, C., and Blackwell, B. (eds.), *Behavioral Concepts and Nursing Intervention*, New York: J. B. Lippincott

O'Brien, J., (1980) Mirror, mirror, why? *Nursing Mirror, 150*:36–37

Roberts, S. L., (1978) *Behavioral Concepts and Nursing Throughout the Life Span*, Englewood Cliffs, N.J.: Prentice-Hall

Rubin, R., (1968) Body image and self-esteem, *Nursing Outlook, 16*(6):20–23

Schilder, P., (1950) *The Image and Appearance of the Human Body*, New York: John Wiley & Sons

Bibliography

Blaesing, S., and Brockhaus, J., (1972) The development of body image in the child, *The Nursing Clinics of North America, 7*(4):597–607

Dropkin, M. J., (1979) Compliant behavior and changed body image, *American Journal of Nursing, 79*:1249

Hagglund, F., and Piha, H., (1980) The inner space of the body image, *Psychoanalytic Quarterly, 49*:256–283

Hauser, S., Jacobson, A., Noam, G., and Powers, S., (1983) Ego development and self-image complexity in early adolescence, *Archives of General Psychiatry, 40*:325–332

Henderson, L., and Gartland, G. J., (1978) Testing disorders of body scheme in stroke rehabilitation, *Physiotherapy Canada, 30*:192–194

McDowell, D., (1983) The special needs of the older colostomy patient, *Journal of Gerontological Nursing, 9*:294–296

Ullman, M., (1964) Disorders of body image after stroke, *American Journal of Nursing, 64*:89–91

Wilson, D., (1981) Changing the body's image, *Nursing Mirror, 152*:38–40

Wineman, N. M., (1980) Obesity: Locus of control, body image, weight loss, and age-at-onset, *Nursing Research, 29*:231–237

CHAPTER TEN
Sexuality

◇

Introduction

Sexuality is one of the most natural and fundamental aspects of our lives, an early and basic element of our identity as human beings. It is integral to self-concept and, as such, is intrinsically involved with self-esteem and body image. It encompasses the whole person and is the sum of personality traits, ignitions behaviors, physical functioning, and communications.

The need for intimacy and love, for touch and body contact, begins in utero and follows us throughout life (Morris 1972). Calderone (1974) suggests that sexual needs are a natural and inherent aspect of human existence and that the expression of sexuality is part of the whole person, an aspect of dignity as a human being. Sexuality transcends genitality and encompasses many kinds of expressions. It has biological, psychological, and sociocultural components.

Chronic illness does not destroy one's sexuality. It may change one's perceptions of oneself as a sexual being or the ways in which one functions sexually, but it does not alter the universal lifelong need to be close to others, to be touched, and to communicate one's feelings. Adaption to illness is a developmental crisis with many ramifications, not the least of which are sexual concerns and functioning (Bullard et al. 1980; Mitchell 1982; Harris, Good, & Pollack 1982; Papadopoulus et al. 1983).

For many, sexuality and sexual expression mean being alive (Lamb & Woods 1981). Being sexual plays an important part in the adjustment to chronic illness (Berkman, Weissman, & Frielich 1978; Sadoughi,

Lesher, & Fine 1971; Cole 1975). Sexual expressions may change with personal needs and interpersonal experiences as a result of the limitations that affect sexual behaviors. Nursing has an obligation to help clients in their adjustment to these limitations if they want such assistance. The purpose of this chapter is to provide information that will assist nurses in this important aspect of nursing care.

Definitions of Terms

Human sexuality is a complex biological, psychosocial phenomenon. Clarifying some relevant terminology will provide a better understanding of the process. The word *sex*, in the biological sense, refers to the structural and functional qualities of being male or female. For purposes of this chapter, abnormal biological sex will not be addressed. *Sex* includes the following:

1. Genetic sex, as revealed by the chromosome count of 46XX or 46XY
2. Gonadal sex: the presence of ovaries or testes
3. Hormonal sex: the androgen-to-estrogen balance
4. Morphology of the internal reproductive organs and the external genitalia (Money 1972)

Sexuality is the quality of being sexual, capable of having sexual feelings and capacity (Katchadourian 1979). The term also refers to other aspects of an individual and includes behavior or expected behavior. Broadly defined, this includes any activity of an individual, including subjective experiences and those that can be observed. The behavior can have an erotic component in the form of arousal, with or without physiological concomitants (Katchadourian 1979). It includes the interpersonal, emotional, and nongenital facets of eroticism.

Gender, or sexual identity, relates to the biological sex of a person: male or female. It also includes the personality component of one's identification of one's own gender (Katchadourian 1979). It answers the question, What sex am I? According to Money and Ehrhardt (1972), *gender identity* is the private experience of gender role, whereas *gender role* is the public expression of gender identity.

Role, according to sociologists, is the set of societal expectations related to the way an individual in a given position should behave in fulfillment of that position. *Gender,* or *sex role,* can be defined as "everything a person says or does to indicate to oneself or others that one is male, female or ambivalent. It includes mannerisms, deportment, and demeanor and may or may not include sexual arousal and responses" (Money & Ehrhardt 1972).

Linked with sex role and identity is *sex object choice.* It refers to the choice for one's sexual activity. Although this choice is fluid during early childhood development, by adolescence most people have reached a choice decision, usually heterosexual. There are many styles of final resolution of object choice, with a state of settlement ultimately made in adulthood (Katchadourian 1979).

Developmental Aspects

Human sexuality is present from conception, when sex is genetically determined, through old age (see Table 10–1) as part of a continuum. Life-cycle tasks are interdependent, yet failure to complete the psychosexual tasks at one age impedes healthy adaption and retards growth (Erikson 1963). When ill, a person may well regress to an earlier stage. Knowing the psychosexual tasks inherent to the developmental process assists sick or disabled persons to maintain their identity as sexual beings (Schain 1980).

The infant receives pleasure and sexual gratification through oral satisfaction. Through infancy and the preschool years, the child's growing awareness and mastery of the physical self include awareness of anatomical differences between male and female. Genital behavior and exploration are extended to other children, often of the opposite sex (Kolodny et al. 1979). According to Kolodny and associates (1979), inherent in many cases of adult sexual problems is a history of negative parental reactions to the discovery of childhood sexual activity. Along with awareness of the physical self, most children move from a dependency on mother through seeing the opposite-sex parent as a role object to establishing gender identity with the same-sex parent (Erikson 1963). The child's growing awareness of sex roles within the family structure (Maccoby & Jacklin 1974) is influenced by parental attitudes, values, responses, and behaviors. These factors influence the child's perspective of the sexual self.

The school years are a time when children focus beyond themselves and their own bodies and gain satisfaction and pleasure from mastering skills and knowledge that will be used in later years. Teachers, neighbors, and others are added as role models. Parental attitudes regarding sex are reflected by their beliefs, the physical control they demonstrate, and their approach to their child's sexual behavior, all of which can influence their children's views even into adulthood (McNab 1976).

During adolescence, physical maturation progresses rapidly, with girls developing earlier than boys (Marshall 1975; Kolodny et al. 1979; Woods 1979). Strong sexual urges are present and attempts at self-identity are made through projection on a love object. Impulse control must be mastered, as well as adjustment to physiological changes and secondary sex characteristics. It is now that the choice of love object is usually defined, either a heterosexual or a homosexual object (Simon & Gagnon 1967). If well concluded, this phase results in a strong sense of self.

A desire for intimacy and a close emotional relationship with another person, including sexual intimacy (Woods 1979), are characteristic of early adulthood (Erikson 1963). Acceptance of one's body image greatly affects one's ability to relate to a sexual partner. This is a time of involvement in parenthood

TABLE 10-1. Sexual Development through the Life Cycle

Age span	Sexual development
Conception to birth	Sex is genetically determined at conception. Gonad hormonal secretion between the seventh and twelfth weeks results in biological sex determination. Brain sex typing is influenced by the hypothalamus around the time of birth (Money & Ehrhardt 1972).
Infancy	An infant's source of pleasure is primarily oral; the sexual drive is through sucking. Male infant erections are believed to be genital excitement (Woods 1979). Parental behavior and cues influence gender role expectations. Girl infants are more likely to be rewarded for being "good" and are more aware of visual and verbal stimuli. Boy infants are more exploratory and physically active and do not touch the care provider as much as girls do (Money & Ehrhardt 1972).
Early childhood	There is a growing sense of body awareness and self-control; the child can differentiate male and female anatomy, including genitals. The parent of opposite sex becomes the role object, and there is early awareness of sex roles; sex role modeling begins (Maccoby & Jacklin 1974). Genital exploration extends to other children (Kolodny et al. 1979); the child realizes that he or she can be like same-sex parent (Erikson 1963)
School age	Teachers and neighbors also become role models. Pleasure and satisfaction expand beyond one's own body into development of skills and education. Girls show higher verbal ability and attention to details, in contrast to boys' ability to analyze and score higher in arithmetic reasoning. Girls' grades tend to be higher, but boys do inch up; by high school they test higher (Maccoby & Jacklin 1974). Parental attitudes, beliefs, and approach to the child's sexual behavior influence the child's views and can be the basis of later sexual problems (Kolodny et al. 1979).
Adolescence	Rapid and profound biological changes lead to physical maturity, with girls maturing earlier than boys (Marshall 1975). Impulse control between sexual urges and proscribed behaviors must be mastered. Adjustment is made to physiological changes (menses for girls, ejaculation for boys). Choice of love object is usually defined (Simon & Gagnon 1967). Role confusion usually occurs for youngsters who have not achieved proper sexual identity earlier in life (Erikson 1963).
Early adulthood	The desire for intimacy, including sexual intimacy, which requires adjustment and adaptation to one another (Woods 1979), is often developed in marriage. The tasks of parenthood and vocational effectiveness become important. Successful adaption allows the individual to be committed to concrete relationships, affiliations, and partnerships rather than distancing self from others (Erikson 1963).
Middle adulthood	In addition to learning to separate from offspring and showing a widening concern for others, many adjustments occur during this developmental phase (Erikson 1963). These changes influence sexuality and include concerns over body image changes, menopause, changes in sexual response, and plans for retirement. One's own values, self-concept, and assets and limitations are also reviewed (Dresen 1975).
Old age	Although sexual involvement may be limited by declining physical capacity, lack of a sexual partner, and chronic illness, the desire for sexual activity usually continues for many older individuals (Pfeiffer & Davis 1972; Rolf & Kleemack 1979; Christenson & Gagnon 1965). This can range from desire for intercourse to satisfaction with a close, caring relationship.

and vocational effectiveness. The middle adult years are characterized by caring and concern for others. Physiological changes that influence sexuality occur and necessitate adjustments: visible body changes, menopause, and changes in sexual responses. Old age is a time of declining physical capacity. When it is coupled with lack of a sexual partner or chronic illness, sexual involvement becomes limited. Yet people continue to desire sexual activity (Pfeiffer & Davis 1972; Rolf & Kleemack 1979; Christenson & Gagnon 1965), manifested as desire for continued intercourse or physical contact with others.

Sexual Health

At the World Health Organization (WHO) meeting on sexuality and health programs, *sexual health* was defined as "the integration of the somatic, emotional, intellectual, and social aspects of sexual being, in ways that are positive, enriching and that enhance personality, communication and love" (WHO 1975). Included in this concept are three basic elements:

1. A capacity to enjoy sexual and reproductive behavior in accordance with a personal and social ethic
2. Freedom from fear, guilt, shame, and false information that inhibit sexual response and impair a sexual relationship
3. Freedom from organic diseases and disabilities that interfere with sexual and reproductive functions (WHO 1975).

Maddock (1975) adds these criteria to judge sexual health:

1. Congruency between one's gender identity and a sense of comfort with the range of sex role behaviors
2. Ability to carry on an effective interpersonal relationship with both sexes, including the potential for love and commitment
3. Capacity to respond to erotic stimulation so as to make sexual activity stimulating and a positive experience

4. A high correlation between sexual behavior and congruency with one's value system.

Although chronic illness and disability affect sexuality and sexual functioning, these problems are by no means limited to sick persons. Masters and Johnson (1970) reviewed their work with 790 persons, both single and married, who were physically healthy adults with a variety of sexual dysfunction problems, most "psychogenic" in origin. Like Masters and Johnson, Levine (1976) found that sexual dysfunction among married couples had an emotional component often reflecting marital discord. Communication skills were found to be important, a factor noted by Masters and Johnson (1970). In their treatment program for sexual dysfunctions, they suggest that in the middle class, sex is an expression of intimacy.

Although many sexual problems are termed *psychogenic*, dysfunction can actually be an early symptom of illness. Sparks, White, and Connelly (1980) found hormonal difficulties in 107 patients who were labeled psychogenic. The controversy between psychogenic and organic is still unclear among renal patients (Procci et al. 1981). It is suggested that an early symptom of multiple sclerosis is sexual dysfunction due to disruption in spinal cord tract messages (Valleroy & Kraft 1984). Among diabetics, there is a high correlation of neuropathy that may or may not precede the dysfunction (Kolodny et al. 1974; Ellenberg 1979; Kolodny 1971).

Physical impairment often affects sexual expression through lack of energy, fear, and the general debility of chronic illness (Stockdale-Woolley 1983; Papadopoulos et al. 1980; Harris, Good, & Pollard 1982). Impairments may be due to pain and/or difficulty with mechanical function (Yoshimo & Uchida 1981; Maruta & Osborne 1978). They might be affected by metabolic dysfunction (Procci et al. 1981), vascular problems (Bray, Frank, & Wolfe 1981), neurological (Berkman et al. 1978; Frank & Boller 1981; Valleroy & Kraft 1984), neurovascular (Kolodny et al. 1974; Ellenberg 1979), or self-esteem and body image disturbances, as often noted in cancer patients (Jusenius 1981; Lamb & Woods 1981). The list is long (see Table 10–2). The dysfunctions are mainly erectile difficulties in men, arousal or lubrication problems in

Disorder	Mechanism for dysfunction	Effect on sexual function
A. Neurologic		
I. Spinal cord surgery, trauma	1. Interference with afferent and efferent traits in spinal cord	M: Erection and/or ejaculation
Disc surgery		F: Orgasm and/or lubrication
Sympathectomy	2. Interference with spinal nerves	B: Sexual dysfunction often an early sign
Multiple sclerosis		
II. Cerebral cortex	Affects limbic center	B: Libidinal changes; increase or decrease or changes in sexual behavior
Lesion in temporal or frontal lobe		
Trauma		
Epilepsy		
B. Vascular	Interferes with blood flow to penis	M: Erectile difficulties
Atherosclerosis of lower part of body		
Trauma		
Sickle cell		
C. Endocrine		
Addison's disease	Impaired feedback mechanisms between adrenals and pituitary; affecting androgens, general debility and fatigue	B: Decreased libido
Cushing's syndrome		M: Erection
Hypothyroidism		F: Lubrication
Diabetes mellitus	Neuropathy, angiopathy	M: Impotence
		F: Possible lubrication
D. Liver disease	Build-up of estrogens due to inability of liver to conjugate estrogen; general debility	M: Decreased libido; impaired erection
		F: Often impaired libido
E. Systemic diseases		
Renal	Metabolic, general debility	B: Decreased libido
Pulmonary	General debility, fatigue	M: Erection
Cardiac	General debility; may have vascular involvement; depression and medications are involved	F: Lubrication
Arthritis	Pain, body mechanical problems, impaired body image	
Cancer (see also Surgical conditions and Local genital disease	Pain, general debility, body image, localized disfigurement or damage to sexual organs	
F. Local genital disease (female)		
I. Vulva and vagina		
Infection	Irritation to genital organs; pain on coitus	Decreased libido
Senile vaginitis		Dyspareunia
Allergies to spermicide sprays		Possible vaginismus
Leukoplakia		

TABLE 10-2. Continued

Disorder	Mechanism for dysfunction	Effect on sexual function
II. Pelvic		
Pelvic inflammatory disease	Damage to genital organs, general disability, fatigue, pain in abdomen, pelvic areas	Dyspareunia: can lead to decreased libido
Endometriosis		
Tumor, cysts		
Prolapsed uterus		
III. Other		
Tight clitoris	Prevent rotation of clitoris, pain on stimulation	Orgasm impaired
G. Local genital disease (male)		
I. Conditions producing pain on coitus		
Preorgasm	Damage to external genital organs	Decreased libido
Penile trauma	Pain	May have impotence problem
Balanitis		
Phimosis		
II. Conditions causing irritation during sexual response		
Urethral pathology	Damage to reflex mechanisms	Erectile problem
Prostatitis		Premature or retarded ejaculation
III. Conditions affecting testicular function		
Orchitis	Decreased androgen level	Decreased libido
Tumor		Possible impotence
Trauma		
Contraction		
H. Surgical conditions		
I. Damage to genitals and nerve supply (males)		
Radical prostatectomy	Destruction of nerves involved with sexual function (pudendal, sacral)	Impotence
Anterior-posterior resection		
Abdominal aortic procedure		Possible ejaculation and impotence
Lumbar sympathectomy, other prostate surgery		Ejaculation Retrograde ejaculation
II. Damage ro sexual organs (female)		
Vulvectomy	Mechanical problems	Decreased libido (psychogenic)
Obstetrical trauma	Fibrotic scans, body image problems	Impaired lubrication Dyspareunia

Adapted from Kaplan, H. S., (1974) The New Sex Therapy, *New York: New York Times Book Company.*
Only a partial listing; B= both; M= male; F= female.

women, and declining libido. However, problems with ejaculation, orgasm, and reproductive ability are not uncommon, especially in neurological disorders.

Our society has become more permissive about sexual expression in general and less critical of sexual behavior among physically disabled and ill persons (Schmidt 1982). Yet attitudes have an emotional and value component and are difficult to change. If we truly are to accept the concepts of sexual health as previously stated, our challenge is to accept the sexuality of our clients and their partners as real and to assist them in expressing their desires for sexual contact and closeness, although that expression may be different from previous methods.

The Physiology of the Sexual Response

Female sexual response has two phases: arousal, or lubrication, and orgasm (see Figure 10–1). During the arousal stage, the walls of the vagina moisten, followed by clitoral and labial swelling; the outer one-third of the vagina contracts, while the inner two-thirds expand; breasts swell, and nipples become erect (Kaplan 1974). In the ill or disabled woman, there may be alterations in the changes in the genital area. Orgasm consists of a series of reflex, involuntary contractions of the muscles surrounding the vaginal inlet, perineal floor, and pelvic muscles. Deep pressure proprioceptors within the perineal and vaginal musculature, as well as sensory receptors, probably transmit orgastic sensations to the brain for pleasure and awareness (Kaplan 1974).

Although it has been stated that orgasm has only one component mediated by the sympathetic nervous system, Graber and Kline-Graber (1979) suggest that it has both a sensory (afferent) component and a motor (efferent) component. They think that in an orgastic woman the pubococcygeal muscles do not effectively contract, but they are unclear as to the mechanism.

In men, the sexual response is also biphasic, with erection and ejaculatory components (see Figure 10–2). Erection involves both sensory and psychic inputs and occurs as a result of vasocongestion within the corpora cavernosa and the corpora spongiosum of the penis. At the same time, the skin of the scrotum tenses, and the testes elevate. As in women, nipples become erect. The parasympathetic nerves are involved in reflexogenic erection, erection produced by direct stimulation of the genitals, whereas the sympathetic erection center mediates erection caused by mental stimuli (Boller & Frank 1982). Weiss (1972) suggests that both centers act synergistically to produce erection. Erection requires intact neurologic and vascular reflexes. However, psychogenic erection can be found in individuals with disruptions of the spinal cord, even at the sacral nerves (Comarr 1970).

The first part of ejaculation is called *emission*. Prior to ejaculation, semen must be expelled into the prostate urethra, a process dependent on the hypogastric sympathetic nerves. Once this occurs, it is difficult for a man to control ejaculation. This condition has been termed *ejaculatory inevitability* by Masters and Johnson (1970). Ejaculation is under parasympathetic control, is mediated by nervi erigentes (pelvic nerves), and involves contraction of the bulbocavernosus and ischiocavernosus muscles (Boller & Frank 1982). With disruption to the spinal cord, this phase of sexual response is usually lacking, although spinal cord patients often report a "para-orgasm," a feeling very much like genital orgasm that occurs with sexual excitement (Glass 1976).

Masters and Johnson have graphically depicted the human sexual response (see Figure 10–3). During the *excitement stage*, vasocongestion of the pelvic organs occur. This includes psychic and reflexogenic stimulation, which produces lubrication or an erection. During this period, heart rate, blood pressure, and breathing increase. Both sexes develop a flush of the face, neck, and trunk. The *plateau stage* is marked by increased sexual tension with heightening vasocongestion. *Orgasm* occurs by a neural reflex arc once threshold has been reached or exceeded. Following orgasm is a *resolution phase*.

With resolution, the male enters a refractory pe-

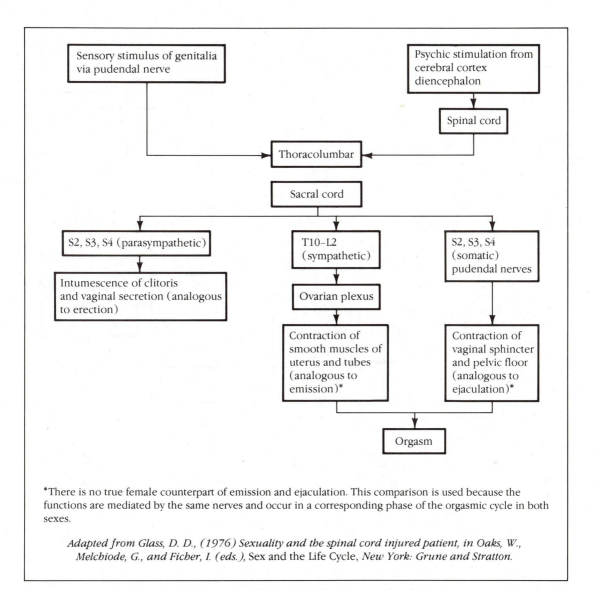

*There is no true female counterpart of emission and ejaculation. This comparison is used because the functions are mediated by the same nerves and occur in a corresponding phase of the orgasmic cycle in both sexes.

Adapted from Glass, D. D., (1976) Sexuality and the spinal cord injured patient, in Oaks, W., Melchiode, G., and Ficher, I. (eds.), Sex and the Life Cycle, New York: Grune and Stratton.

FIGURE 10-1. Mechanism for female arousal and orgasm

riod during which further ejaculation is impossible, although erection may be maintained. There is great variability in the duration of this period among individuals. With aging, the time lengthens, as does the latency period during which the male is unable to have an erection. Females have the potential of being multiorgasmic, without dropping below the plateau stage of arousal. During resolution, the anatomic and physiological changes of the excitement and plateau phases are reversed (Kolodny et al. 1979).

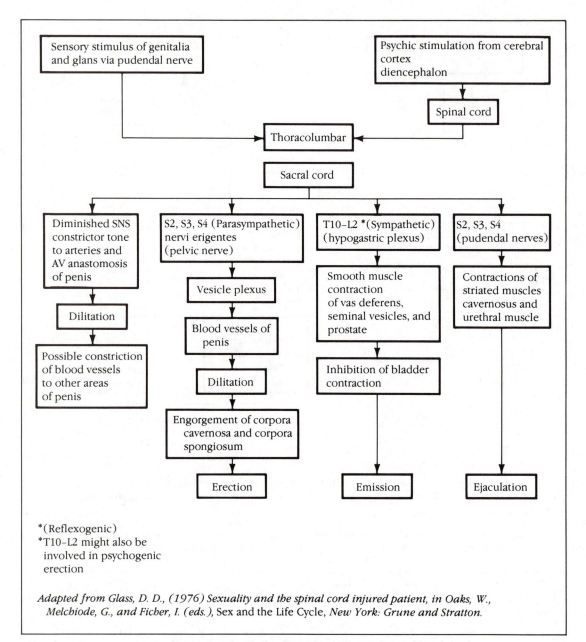

FIGURE 10-2. Mechanism of erection and ejaculation

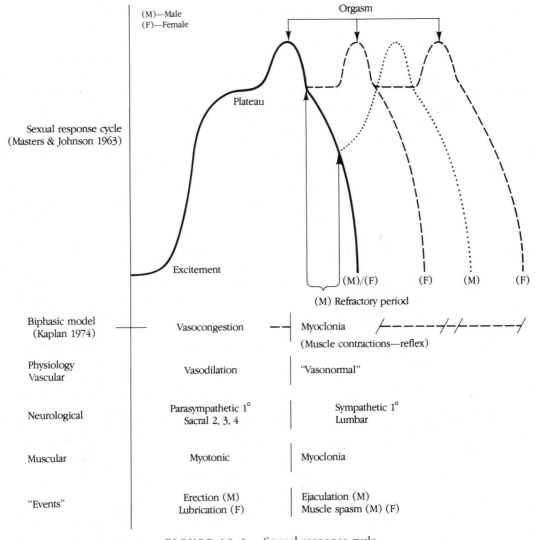

FIGURE 10-3. Sexual response cycle

Effects of Chronic Illness on Sexual Health

Irreversible illness and disability have significant impact on many facets of life. With illness, one must deal with the direct (physiologic) and indirect (psychosocial) effects of impairment. The perceptions of illness of clients and those involved with them influence behavior, functioning, and coping. One's values, culture, and sex role patterns are also involved with adaptation. The interrelationship among these factors has a definite effect on sexuality. This section presents a broad overview of general principles related to sexual functioning and chronic illness.

Psychosocial Effects

Underlying many illnesses is depression, an emotional state in which low energy and fatigue are present. This same lack of energy is associated with extreme stress and loss. Illness, a state of loss of one's prior good health, is indeed stressful and, in fact, constitutes a deep personal insult. Sexual energy (libido) is diminished, although the mechanism through which this occurs is not clear (Kaplan 1974). It has been suggested that the endocrine system undergoes physiological changes that accompany stress, and that depression affects brain catecholamine functioning (Kaplan 1974). Another hypothesis is related to neuroendocrine response; during depression, plasma control levels increase. Through a feedback system, the hypothalamus-pituitary system decreases the release of gonadotropic hormone, resulting in decreased testosterone production, which depresses libido (Stockdale-Woolley 1983; Kaplan 1974).

Illness can sap physical as well as emotional energy. In a study of 112 women having rheumatoid arthritis, Yoshimo and Uchida (1981) found that 50% of the participants had decreased libido, much of it related to decreased physical energy. This same lack of energy is found among clients with chronic pulmonary disease who experience hypoxia and respiratory insufficiency (Stockdale-Woolley 1983; Kass 1972). Lack of energy and decreased libido have been reported in studies of people with multiple sclerosis (Valleroy & Kraft 1984; Lilius, Valtonen, & Wickstrom 1976).

Untreated renal failure produces changes in sexual functioning for both sexes. In one study, 90% of anemic men and 80% of anemic women reported decreased sexual desire and lowered physical energy levels (Levy 1973). Abram and associates (1975) and Short and Wilson (1969) found that frequency of intercourse declined among individuals with chronic renal failure. These authors concluded that multiple psychogenic factors such as role reversal, dependency, economic burden of chronic illness, postdialysis lethargy, and age, as well as physiologic effects, caused the decreased energy.

In the limited research on sexuality of stroke victims, there is confusion about the finding of libidinal changes following stroke. Bray, Frank, and Wolfe (1981) and Ford and Orfiren (1976) report no change in desire after stroke, especially among individuals less than 60 years old. Goddess, Wagner, and Silverman (1979) found that libido was more diminished after strokes affecting the dominant hemisphere; Kalliomaki, Markannen, and Mustonen (1961) reported that of the 105 persons in their study, 37.8% suffered decreased libido if the lesion was in the left hemisphere and a 16.9% decline with right-sided lesions.

Fear has a definite impact on sexual functioning. Among 66 married clients with chronic nonmalignant pain, 68% of the women and 88% of the men reported a decrease in the frequency of intercourse, in part related to fear of pain acceleration (Maruta & Osborne 1978). Fear of pain is also reported by Swinburn (1976) and Yoshimo and Uchida (1981) in their work with arthritic persons. Among those who have cardiac disease, fear of pain, another heart attack, or sudden death deters sexual relationships (Mehta & Krop 1979; Block, Maider, & Horsely 1975; Papadopoulus et al. 1983). Concerns were noted by client and partner. Sadoughi, Lesher, and Fine (1971) report a high correlation between fear of pain and decreased sexual activity in their study of a chronically ill population with disabilities that included arthritis, amputation, stroke, and emphysema.

Persons with limited mobility, either anatomical (as with amputation), physiological (as with neurological problems in spinal cord injury or stroke), or associated with multiple joint involvement (as with arthritis), seem to be less sexually active. Swinburn (1976) notes that joint deformity affects sexual practices among his client population, whereas Conine and Evans (1982) report that pain is a greater impedance to sexual intimacy than deformity. Wheelchairs often get in the way of sexual overtures (Glass 1976). Persons whose limbs are paralyzed or deformed may abstain from sex because they are unable to position themselves as they formerly did (Cole 1975). Spasticity usually does not interfere with sexual activity, according to Romano and Lassiter (1972), although they also point out that when adductor spasm is severe, intromission may be impossible for the female client (see Chapter 5).

People are expected to be in control of bodily

functions, especially bladder and bowel functions. When these functions are beyond one's control, and especially when the marital or sex partner has to care for the client, sexual activity has been known to decline or to cease (Glass & Padrone 1978). Changes in attitude regarding sex can also occur among spouses of ostomate patients (Kolodny et al. 1979; Burnham, Leonard-Jones, & Brooke 1977).

Conditions that affect sensory function can affect sexual behavior. For example, it is postulated by Wiig (1973) that aphasics having relatively good receptive comprehension exhibited the least problem with sexual adjustment, irrespective of expressive language ability. Wiig conjectures that a client's inability to interpret body language affected sexual responses.

Few studies address sexuality in persons having congenital hearing or sight deficits (Kolodny et al. 1979). Hearing impairment affects one's psychosocial development. Deficits in the realm of communication and social skills may predispose deaf persons to sexual adjustment problems (Fitz-Gerald & Fitz-Gerald 1977).

Visual clues are important for sexual expression. When vision is impaired, through either congenital or acquired blindness, there may be effects on sexuality, although in this area, too, there is a paucity of research (Kolodny et al. 1979). Specially tailored sex education as well as parental and teacher attitudes may well affect outcomes related to blind persons' attitudes toward their sexuality. When blindness is acquired, attention to feelings of helplessness, depression, impaired self-esteem, and underlying disability must be addressed (Fitzgerald 1973).

Tied into these effects is the impact of chronic illness on body image and self-esteem (see Chapter 9). Body image is the way in which one sees one's body: one's own mental image of the self (Woods 1979). Body image is a fluid concept and is affected by one's perceptual apparatus of sensory experiences, along with attitudes and overtones expressed by others. Shontz (1974) identifies functions of body image that define the concept:

1. It is a *sensory register* for integrating basic materials of cognitive and perceptual operations.

2. It is an *instrument for action*, mediating all activities.
3. It is *the source of all drives* and needs, including food, water, air, sleep, sex, and shelter.
4. It functions as a *stimulus to the self* on conscious and subconscious levels.
5. It is a *stimulus to others* and is an individual's first point of control with others.
6. It functions to *create the impression of a private world* where personal decisions are made.
7. It is an *expressive instrument* reflecting one's individuality.

When there is an insult to the perception of one's body, body image disturbance occurs. The distortion of self results, as a major assault to self-esteem and body integrity. The way in which individuals see their own bodies also affects their self-concepts. A negative self-concept and diminished self-liking usually cause a person to feel unattractive or unlovable. These negative effects have been demonstrated with clients who have amputations (Reinstein, Ashley, & Miller 1978) and among cancer patients (Lamb & Woods 1981; Woods 1975), ostomates (Druss, O'Connor, & Stern 1969), and the spinal cord–injured (Fitting 1978). Feeling ugly influences the sexual self-concept and in turn sexual behavior (Woods 1979).

Whether body disruption is obvious to others (as with mastectomy or amputation), is invisible (as with a prostatectomy or hysterectomy), or results in loss of function (as with a spinal cord injury), the important factor to be assessed is the effect of the loss of that part of function on one's physical integrity, sense of wholeness, and definition as a sexual being (Derogatis 1980).

Although many disease states and disabilities affect both the psychogenic and psychologic aspects, cancer, because of its broad effects on nearly every body system, probably best shows the direct and indirect effects (see Table 10–3).

Physiologic Effects

It is impossible to discuss all the direct sexual dysfunctions that can result from chronic illness or disability. Many of these are specific to the pathology of

TABLE 10-3. Effect of Cancer on Sexuality

Site	Dysfunction Organic	Psychologic*	Reproductive effect on fertility	Impact on partner
Cervix	Hysterectomy shortens vagina, usually no dysfunction, treatment of in situ with cone, resulting in no dysfunction	Sometimes	Unable to have children with hysterectomy or x-ray therapy, which will thicken vagina	May think he will contract cancer, be affected by x-ray therapy, think he caused cancer
Endometrial	Radical hysterectomy, usually no dysfunction	Sometimes	As above	As above
Ovary	In premenopausal women with bilateral oophorectomy, resulting in menopausal symptoms	Sometimes	If bilateral oophorectomy	As above
Vulva	Simple can cause introital stenosis. Radical includes clitorectomy and often has decreased range of motion and lupus erythematosus	Usually, especially altered body image	Patient usually postmenopausal	Usually
Breast	Absence of nipple arousal	Usually includes altered body image	None, unless oophorectomy and hormonal treatment were once used	Usually
Prostate	Radical resulting in impotence, retropubic and suprapubic resulting in retrograde ejaculation, hormonal manipulation and orchiectomy can alter libido	Usually altered self-image, estrogen hormone resulting in gynecomastica	Yes	Usually afraid she might develop cancer
Testicular	Retroperitoneal lymph node dissection usually resulting in retrograde ejaculation and can cause erectile dysfunction	Yes, if bilateral orchiectomy resulting in decreased libido and sexual responsiveness	Often	Usually

TABLE 10-3. Continued

Site	Dysfunction Organic	Dysfunction Psychologic*	Reproductive effect on fertility	Impact on partner
Bladder	Local-seldom; cystectomy in female includes anterior vagina, uterus, and urethra. Male includes prostate, bladder, urethra	Yes, altered body image with urinary incontinence	Usually yes if x-ray therapy, often patient is older male	Yes
Colon-Rectal	If anterioposterior resection, sacral nerve involvement, results in erectile dysfunction	Yes, especially with ostomy	None, unless x-ray therapy done, sometimes with chemotherapy	Yes
Leukemia	Chemotherapy and its effects may affect erection	Sometimes, especially with fatigue	Chemotherapy affects ovulation and spermatogenesis; rebound after treatment stopped	Usually, especially if patient has decreased energy and function; may take it as rejection
Hodgkins	Libido and ability affected	Usually	As above, x-ray therapy affects testicle and ovarian function; contraception should be used because effects of chemotherapy on ovarian function and sperm maturation not understood	

Adapted from Lamb, M. A., and Woods, N. F., (1981) Sexuality and the cancer patient, Cancer Nursing, 4:138–139.

*It is often difficult to determine the difference between psychologic and physical dysfunction since they are interrelated.

the disease; others result from the individual's psychosocial response (see Table 10–2). Several disease states with known sexual impact will be discussed in depth.

Diabetes Mellitus. Estimates of impotency among male diabetics range from 29% to 60% (Kolodny et al. 1974; McCullock et al. 1980). Libido remains intact, but erectile dysfunction may gradu-

ally increase over a 6- to 24-month period (Kolodny et al. 1974; Krosnick & Poldolsky 1981). There is no loss of the ability to ejaculate or to be aware of orgasmic sensations, nor is there a change in measures of circulatory testosterone between diabetic and nondiabetic men (Kolodny et al. 1974).

There is general agreement that the primary pathogenesis is neuropathy, involving microscopic damage to nervous fibers (Ellenberg 1971). Faerman and

◇ CASE STUDY ◇

The Diabetic Client

T.R. is a 63-year-old male who has had type II diabetes for years. Until 5 years ago, he was using an oral hypoglycemic agent, but he is now taking 25 units NPH and 10 units regular insulin every day. His fasting blood sugar averages 180. He has had peripheral neuropathy for 5 years but has no other long-term complications.

At onset of his neuropathy, T.R. began to have orgasmic dysfunction with inability to maintain erection. Over a 2-year period, the problem advanced to complete inability to have an erection. His desire remained intact. This was a blow to his self-concept because he had always thought of himself as a "ladies' man" and otherwise took care of himself by maintaining his weight and physique.

On several occasions, he discussed his sexual difficulty with his nurse practitioner, who compiled a sexual history, tested hormone levels, and discussed penile implant with him. He was referred to the urology clinic and the sexual dysfunction clinic for assessment of penile implant, which he ultimately had. The healing process went more slowly than he had anticipated, which was discouraging to him and to his female companion. After 3 months the healing was complete and the prosthesis device was deemed successful. T.R. wonders why he waited "so long" to pursue coitus actively again.

---

associates (1973) found histologic changes in autonomic nerve fibers in the corpora cavernosa of impotent diabetic men at autopsy. Ellenberg (1971) and Kolodny and collaborators (1974) discovered a high correlation between diabetic neuropathy and erectile dysfunction. Because of the microvascular angiopathy that diabetics experience, Tyler and associates (1983) suggest that a combination of nerve and vascular damage affects potency in diabetic men. Ellenberg (1979) proposes that other vascular pathology, such as atherosclerosis or peripheral vascular disease, which limits blood supply to the penis, might affect the male diabetic's potency. Regardless of cause, if impotency appears early in the course of the disease, even with good blood glucose control, prognosis for reversal is poor, especially when neuropathy is present (Kolodny et al. 1979).

Where impotence is irreversible and definitely organic in origin, one of two types of penile prosthesis has proved beneficial (Scott, Bradley, & Timm 1973; Small 1978). A "new" old drug, Yohimbine, is currently being tested. Yohimbine is an alpha-adrenergic blocker that stimulates norepinephrine release and thus decreases vasoconstriction of penile blood flow. To date, the results are nonconclusive (Morales et al. 1982).

Until 1971, no one studied the effects of diabetes on women. In a matched sample study of 125 diabetic and 100 nondiabetic women, 35.2% of the diabetic women reported being anorgasmic a year prior to the study. Interestingly, they all had previously experienced orgasm, whereas 6% of the nondiabetic women had always been anorgasmic. Kolodny (1971) concluded that the cause was organic rather than psychogenic. In a study of 82 insulin-dependent women and 47 controls, Tyler and coresearchers (1983) found that the diabetic women were slower to achieve vaginal lubrication. Ellenberg (1977) found no difference in orgasm and libido between diabetic and nondiabetic women. In summary, evidence for sexual dysfunction among diabetic women is contradictory and nonconclusive. Brooks (1977) suggests that there is a high likelihood of dysfunction where automatic neuropathy is present.

Diabetic women do seem more susceptible to vaginal infections, probably through a combination of increased leukocytes and elevated tissue concentrations of glucose that provide an excellent medium for bacteria. Monilia, the most common vaginal infection for diabetic women, produces decreased lubrication, pruritis, and tissue tenderness that may make intercourse painful and exudes a malodorous discharge. The reported infections may have an effect on sexual activity (Bagdade, Root, & Bulger 1974). Kolodny and associates (1979) suggest that women experiencing orgasmic problems who were previously orgasmic might benefit from the increased stimulation of a vibrator.

Chronic Renal Disease. The degree of diminished libido, erectile dysfunction, arousal (in women), and intensity of orgasm seem to be related to the degree of disease (Abram et al. 1975; Steele, Finklestein, & Finklestein 1976). Procci and coresearchers (1981) reported that 50% of clients having uremia complained of impotence and decreased coital frequency. They found no difference between clients receiving dialysis and those not receiving such therapy. Levy (1973) and Abram and associates (1975) found a worsening of sexual function among both sexes who were being dialyzed. Levy (1973) reported that women who had renal transplant returned to their premorbid sexual functioning, whereas a significant percentage of the men did not.

A correlation between the absence of nocturnal penile tumescence (NPT) and uremia was observed by Parker and associates (1977) and Procci and collaborators (1981). The former suggest that the absence of NPT might be related to the metabolic effects of the disease, whereas the latter suggest that age is a factor.

In a study by Berkman, Katz, and Weissman (1982) in which 50% of the men had severe sexual dysfunction and 22% had moderate dysfunction (erection and ejaculation dysfunction for both groups), there was a high correlation between declining sexual function and uremic neuropathy. Uremic men have decreased testosterone levels regardless of dialysis or control of the renal failure (Lim & Fang 1975). After successful transplant, testosterone levels return to normal, accounting for the increased libido, but other sexual dysfunctions do not improve (Lim & Fang 1975).

In women, chronic renal failure results in menses changes and infertility. Decreased lubrication and atrophic vaginitis may be due to an estrogen deficiency. With successful transplant, fertility improves, and normal pregnancy may be possible (Feldman & Singer 1974).

Spinal Cord Injury or Lesion. The level of the cord injury and presence of complete or incomplete lesion determine the type of dysfunction the person

experiences. In a review of the literature based on 1,296 male spinal cord injury impaired individuals, 35% were found able to engage in intercourse, 77% could have erection, and in 10% ejaculation was preserved (Tarabulcy 1972).

Generally speaking, clients having a lesion in the cauda equina (L2 and below) experience loss of erection but can possibly ejaculate (Boller & Frank 1982). Among a sample of 20 males with lumbar injuries, 8 were able to have psychogenic erection, but none was able to have reflexogenic erection (Comarr 1975). Seven had successful coitus and five achieved orgasm. For injuries above the lumbar area and complete, psychogenic erections occur infrequently, although reflexogenic and spontaneous erections are common. However, erection has a short duration, and orgasm is rarely achieved (Boller & Frank 1982). Fertility is generally impaired, although the mechanism is not clear. Usually there is impaired spermatogenesis, possibly due to recurrent infections or temperature-regulation impairment in the scrotum (Comarr & Bors 1955).

As with other areas of sexual functioning and disability, females with cord injuries have been studied less than males. In general, irrespective of the level of injury, intercourse is more possible for women than men. According to Kolodny and collaborators (1979), this finding reflects the fact that women do not require intense vasoconstrictive changes to engage in coitus. Although typical orgasm is absent in women with complete cord lesions, heightened arousal can be obtained by tactile stimulation of body parts innervated by spinal cord segments above the lesion (Griffith & Trieschmann 1975). Within 6 to 12 months, menses returns to normal, and these women have no more difficulty with conception or delivery than ablebodied women (Comarr 1966; Goller & Paeslack 1972). Pregnancy might be complicated by automatic dysreflexia, urinary tract infections, and premature labor (Goller & Paeslack 1972).

Adverse Effects of Medication on Sexual Function

Table 10-4 summarizes the effects of a number of drugs (by categories) on sexual dysfunction. Much

TABLE 10-4. Some Drugs That Affect Sexual Function

Drug or drug category	Libidinal change	Impotence (male) or lubrication (female)	Gynecomastica or galactorrhea	Climax changes	Menses change	Hormonal change
I. Diuretics						
a. Thiazide		Impotence				
b. Spironolactone	High doses	Impotence	Gynecomastica		High doses	Antiandrogenic properties
c. Furosemide		Impotence				
II. Antihypertensives						
a. Propanolol (beta-adrenergic)	Occasional decrease	Impotence				
b. Methyldopa	Decrease	Both	Gynecomastica	F: anorgasmic M: decrease or slow ejaculation		
c. Vasodilators	Decrease with high doses					
d. Clonidine		Impotence				
e. Reserpine	Decrease		Gynecomastica	Decrease or no ejaculation		
III. Psychotropic						
a. Phenothiazines	Yes	Both	Both	Decrease or no ejaculation		
b. Thioridazine		Impotence	Galactorrhea	Decrease or no ejaculation	Yes	Increases testosterone levels
c. Trifluoperazine			Gynecomastica	Decrease or no ejaculation	Yes	
d. Haldol		Both	Both	Decrease or no ejaculation		
e. Lithium	Yes	Impotence				Decreases testosterone levels

f. Tricyclic antidepressants	Yes		Occasional impotence	Gynecomastica	
g. Benzodiazepines oxazepam	Yes	Yes		Galactorrhea	
IV. Barbitals	Yes	Yes	Both		
V. Aminoglycosides				Gynecomastica	Increases estrogen and decreases testosterone levels
VI. Alcohol			Both		Decreases testosterone levels
VII. Cimetadine				Gynecomastica	Decreases sperm count
VIII. Anticholinergics			Some decreased lubrication, impotence		
IX. Flagyl	Yes				
X. Antiandrogens					
a. Clofibrate	Yes		Impotence	Gynecomastica	
b. Estrogens (in men)			Impotence	Gynecomastica	
XI. Steroids	Yes				
XII. Others					
a. Heroin, cocaine	Increase libido (small dose)		Impotence		
b. Marijuana			Impotence with large amounts	Gynecomastica	Decreases testosterone levels

Adapted from Kolodny, R.C., Masters, W. H., Johnson, V. E., and Biggs, M. A., (1979) The Textbook of Human Sexuality for Nurses, Boston: Little, Brown; Kaplan, H.S., (1974) The New Sex Therapy, New York: New York Times Book Company; Soyka, L. F., and Mattison, D. R., (1981) Prescription drugs that affect male sexual function, Drug Therapy, 11:46–58; Wise, T. M., (1984) How drugs can help or hinder sexual function, Drug Therapy, 14:51-63.

more is known about the effects of medications on men than on women, primarily because erection and ejaculation are visible and therefore more measurable than female dysfunctions, which tend to be subjectively reported (Kolodny et al. 1979).

Soyka and Mattison (1981) reviewed the 100 most commonly prescribed drugs in 1979. Four consistent findings were changes in libido, gynecomastica, impotence, and retarded or absent ejaculation. Three drugs (Amitriptyline, Cyclobenzaprine, and Imipramine) caused testicular swelling.

Although one tends to think of drugs as having a negative effect on sexual activity, they can also enhance function. For example, birth control pills allow women to enjoy sexual relations without fear of pregnancy. If used properly, the "pill" is considered 99% safe (Woods 1979). "Once a month" and morning-after postcoital drugs for men and women are being studied (Bennett 1974; Dierassi 1970). Chemical contraception has contributed to better understanding of sexuality in our society as well as greater enjoyment of sexual activity for both men and women.

Many drugs used for treatment of hypertension affect sexual function. Often compliance with the medication is a problem because high blood pressure is a "silent" disease. If sexual side effects occur, compliance becomes more problematic (Blackwell 1973). Kolodny and coresearchers (1979) suggest the following guidelines when starting the client on antihypertensive therapy:

1. Obtain a good sexual history as a baseline of function.
2. Do not assume that sexual symptoms are automatically drug-related. Be alert to psychological factors, other illnesses, or use of alcohol that might underlie the dysfunction.
3. Be certain to inquire about sexual problems at each visit. Such inquiries will determine dosages that can be tolerated and will be helpful in assessing sexual difficulties before the patient continues treatment.
4. Be willing to work with the patient to adjust drugs or dosages. Often blood pressure control therapy

uses a combination of drugs that have different actions and therefore are less likely to be synergistic.

Whether or not to inform a client about drug-related side effects on sexual function remains a question. Some believe that suggestions cause the problem; others prefer to be forthright. The point is that the patient must know that the effects are reversible. Careful inquiries and the genuine concern of the care provider can often offset the problem of noncompliance (see Chapter 7).

Another category of drugs that cause sexual side effects are the phenothiazines, along with other antipsychotic drugs. Again, compliance is a problem because of sexual side effects (Story 1974). Chlorpromazine, the prototype phenothiazine, can block ovulation and cause menstrual irregularities, galactorrhea, gynecomastica, or decreased testicular size (Meltzer & Fang 1976).

Long- and short-term use of alcohol affects sexual function. Acutely, it is a central nervous system depressant, interfering with pathways of reflex transmission for sexual arousal (Farkas & Rosen 1976). Blood alcohol levels well below intoxication levels suppress erection (Farkas & Rosen 1976). Gorden and associates (1976) suggest that alcohol lowers circulatory testosterone levels in healthy young men.

Men who are chronic alcohol users display reduced libido, even with allowances for age. Approximately 40% are impotent and 5% to 10% have ejaculatory difficulties (Lemere & Smith 1973). One study of alcoholic women revealed that 30% to 40% had difficulty with arousal, and 15% experienced reduction in the intensity or frequency of orgasm (Kolodny et al. 1979). Sexual problems in men are caused in part by a decreased testosterone rate, as well as protein binding of testosterone. Spermatogenesis is also impaired (Van Thiel 1976). Alcoholic women are more susceptible to cirrhosis than men, and the endocrine system probably is affected in a parallel manner (Morgan & Sherlock 1977).

In addition to hormonal disturbances, nutritional problems found in alcoholics result in anemia (Straus

1973) and peripheral neuropathy (Morgan & Sherlock 1977). If the alcoholic has chronic liver disease, other physiological problems plug into the causes of sexual dysfunction.

Effects of Illness on the Sexual Partner

Prior to illness or disability, it is likely that the individual was active in various social roles, contributed to the household, and was able to express sexuality in socially acceptable ways. Illness, with its many ramifications, changes former ways of functioning, often affecting interpersonal relationships, especially with those closest to the client. Sexual relationships seem to be generally impaired.

There was a decline in sexual activity among 78% of the chronically ill men studied by Sadoughi, Lesher, and Fine (1971). Yet 42% believed that their spouse wanted more sex. There was a greater decline in interest among men in this study than among women, a finding that may indicate why women clients tended to think their spouse was satisfied with the marital relationship.

Yoshimo and Uchida (1981) reported that more than 50% of the women in their study refused the sexual advances of their spouses. They noted a high correlation between disability and dissatisfaction with sex life for both the patient and her spouse (60%). Patients were anxious about their own desire as well as that of their spouse.

Harris, Good, and Pollard (1982) examined the sexual beliefs of 96 women who had gynecologic cancer and the attitudes of their partners. Sexual activity and discussions about sex declined after surgery. Partners often felt guilty and thought that they caused the disease. These beliefs, along with fear of causing more pain and concern for the health of their spouse, were cited as major reasons for decreased sexual activity.

Among cardiac clients and their spouses, 51% expressed fear of resuming sexual activity, despite the fact that 72.6% of these couples resumed sex at a mean of 10.8 weeks after myocardial infarction (Papadopoulos et al. 1980, 1983). Concerns include fear

(previously discussed), attractiveness, safety, and the quality of sexual expression now, compared to the premorbid expression.

In a study of 32 clients receiving home hemodialysis, 77% reported sexual dissatisfaction and genital function that resulted in less demonstrated affection and decreased sexual intercourse (Berkman, Katz, & Weissman 1982). Abram and coresearchers (1975) reported that 45% of their subjects had decreased libido, potency, or both. Clients cathected and withdrew from their spouse to preserve their own diminished physical energy. Wives generally denied psychological effects on sexual function and tended to be defensive and protective toward their husbands.

The effects of chronic lung disease on life in general and on sexuality were examined in 128 clients (Hanson 1982). Of these, 67% considered the most detrimental aspect of their illness to be the effect on the sexual aspect of their marriage. Only 40% thought that the emotional impact on their marriage was worsened, and many thought the disease had brought them emotionally closer to their spouse.

In instances in which illness necessitates surgery that results in physical deformity, the role of the partner is vital to the adjustment process. For example, in a study of 60 women undergoing mastectomy, the majority (70%) undressed in front of their partners before surgery. During the 3-month period following surgery, that proportion declined to 35%. The follow-up study made 8 years after surgery revealed that 53% still undressed in front of their partners. Before surgery, 76% were nude during sexual activity, whereas only 45% were 8 years after surgery. However, 50% reported more tenderness from their partner with sex after the mastectomy than before. This study (Frank et al. 1978) concluded that the women who adjusted better were those whose partners accepted their new body image. Similar findings were reported by Jusenius (1981) and Burnham, Lennard-Jones, and Brooke (1977) (see Chapter 9).

Other problems for the couple include their own roles: passivity, dependence (especially if they formerly were independent), economic burdens, shame, anger, fear of abandonment and rejection, loss of friends, and fear of death. Glass (1976) proposes the question, Can a 24-hour-a-day, 7-day-a-week caregiver also be a lover? In summary, when one member of a sexual relationship is affected by illness, the partner also incurs the effects.

The Social Impact on Sexuality

Our society looks upon youth and beauty with favor, expecting vigor and sexual expression among this population. Many people equate illness with old age, despite the fact that illness—indeed, chronic illness—affects all age groups. Although our society has begun to look more favorably and even realistically at the sexual needs of the elderly, there still persists the erroneous belief that being old, ill, or disabled ends the need for sexual expression.

This attitude is particularly prevalent toward persons who are institutionalized. Paradowski (1977) studied 155 residents who were chronically ill and institutionalized. He reports that 35% were involved in an active relationship, and 25% said that they would like to be part of a heterosexual dyad. Many of the unattached individuals reported that they masturbated. In a study of 63 residents of a nursing home, the majority believed that sexual activity was appropriate for other elderly people in nursing homes but not for themselves. Men and women had different beliefs about why the opposite sex would want sex (Wasow & Loeb 1979). Their beliefs, no doubt, were affected by their cultural upbringing. Authors of both studies suggest that institutions should offer more privacy and opportunities for those who desire a sexual relationship.

Our society includes many subcultures, which contribute certain values, attitudes, and learned behaviors to their members. Religion often enters into cultural life-style, further affecting beliefs. Kinsey, Pomeroy, and Martin (1948) suggested that religious affiliation was not so strongly correlated with sexual practices as was religiosity, even among persons of the same faith.

There is a new phenomenon in our society related to the openness of homosexuality. Gay men and lesbians comprise 10% of the population (Raphael & Robinson 1980). With aging, they describe decreased libido, much as the heterosexual population does. Likewise, sexual expression continues to be an important part of their aging, with improved communication skills being stressed to enhance the emotional intimacy part of their relationships (Kimmel 1978; Robinson 1979). A problem confronting sick or elderly homosexuals who are institutionalized is insensitivity to the existence of their partners. Although space for conjugal visits is seldom provided for heterosexual couples (Paradowski 1977), private space for homosexuals is never considered (Brossart 1979). Brossart also suggests that homosexual partners are often denied access to intensive care units and that often nursing homes admit only one member of a homosexual couple.

A new health problem facing our society is acquired immune deficiency syndrome (AIDS). AIDS is found primarily among young gay men, especially those having multiple partners. Others at risk to develop this fatal disease are intravenous drug abusers, prostitutes, and individuals who need multiple blood transfusions, such as hemophiliacs. A small but growing number of heterosexuals have also contracted this disorder, and several have died; most of these cases have followed blood transfusions.

Providing Sexual Health Care

Nurses and other health providers are social beings who have a set of values and beliefs about sexual practices. How do we, or should we, treat chronically ill persons whose ways of expressing sexuality differ from our own? Regardless of our own perspective, to be effective in working with clients and their sexual concerns, it is important not to create for the couple or client a conflict with their values.

Various studies indicate that sex plays an important part in adjustment to chronic illness (Berkman,

Weissman, & Frielich 1978; Sadoughi, Lesher, & Fine 1971; Conine, Disher, & Gilmore 1979). It is suggested that better sexual adjustment is related to better social, physical, and psychological functioning necessary for successful rehabilitation (Berkman et al. 1978). Among spinal cord–injured persons, the degree of sexual adjustment was found to be highly correlated with success in vocational training and employment (Conine, Disher, & Gilmore 1979). Sick or disabled individuals who view themselves as desirable and enjoy sexual behaviors that do not entirely depend on genital function have learned to value personal assets rather than to focus on disabilities (Cole 1975).

Research further indicates that clients have sexual concerns that they want to discuss, and that they expect the health care provider to initiate the discussion (Bullard et al. 1980; Harris 1982; Papadopoulos et al. 1980). Finally, studies indicate that they want their sexual partner included in the counseling (Bullard et al. 1980; Hock 1977; Hartman, MacIntosh, & Englehardt 1983). Workshops in human sexuality do reflect changes in attitudes regarding sexual behavior, knowledge, and comfort in talking with clients about their sexual concerns (Frazer et al. 1982; Mims, Brown, & Lubow 1974).

Given this information, it seems only fitting that nursing be involved in this aspect of a client's adjustment to illness. For the nursing profession, like other health professions, dealing with sexual health is a relatively new domain. There is an increasing concern among nursing educators that students receive accurate information to help them in this important role.

On the basis of her study of 124 nurse educators at ten nursing schools, Fontaine (1976) made the following recommendations;

1. Hold faculty workshops on human sexuality to examine attitudes and beliefs about sex.
2. Support textbooks that examine the relationship between illness and sexual functioning.
3. Include in course content alterations in health that affect life patterns, including sexual functions.

The nurse's ability to deal with a client's sexuality depends on acceptance of her or his own sexuality, as well as acceptance of the client's (Zalar 1975). Being comfortable with one's own sexuality allows for more sensitivity to client concerns. When the nurse conveys, verbally and nonverbally, such comfort, the client feels some leeway for the expression of feelings about the impact of illness on sexuality. The nurse who is aware of such sexual concerns also is aware of times when the client does not want to discuss sex (Payne 1976).

The Golden and Golden study (1980) found that clients want direction and support in reestablishing sexual functioning or relationships. They make the following suggestions to health care providers:

1. Be comfortable in discussing sexual issues.
2. Know where to refer the patient and his or her partner if your knowledge is inadequate or your values based on cultural and religious beliefs differ.
3. Initiate discussion of sexual concerns at various stages of illness and treatment:
   a. When the diagnosis is being made.
   b. When treatment planning occurs.
   c. Early on, and later along the road to recovery.

The PLISSIT model is a good format to help the patient and family with sexuality. It was devised by Jack Annon, a sex therapist in Honolulu (Annon 1976). This hierarchical model moves in accordance with the nurse's skills and the setting in which treatment is to occur. The model starts with simply giving *permission* (P) for certain behaviors such as masturbation, fantasies, or feelings. The second step is giving *limited information* (LI) related to the problem, such as telling a cardiac patient that sudden death during intercourse almost never occurs. Step three involves *specific suggestions* (SS). Here the nurse gives specific recommendations regarding a problem that has been clarified by good history taking, so that the suggestion is relevant and appropriate to the client's illness and concerns. Last comes *intensive therapy* (IT), such as sensate focus exercises (Masters & Johnson 1970). If such therapy is beyond the nurse's capabilities, referral of the couple to a professional with

◇ CASE STUDY ◇
Using the PLISSIT Model

Mr. G. is a 55-year-old man who has a history of angina and hypertension. Two weeks ago he had a myocardial infarction. He and his wife of 30 years have enjoyed a close relationship. Sex has been enjoyable for both of them. However, Mr. G. has been the more dominant partner, and their coital activities have been rather traditional. They both have concerns that this illness will terminate their sex life. They are afraid of sudden death or pain if they try to resume sexual activity. In addition, Mr. G. is taking a thiazide diuretic and a beta-adrenergic blocker to control his hypertension.

The nurse first initiated a discussion about sexual concerns and obtained the G.s' permission to proceed. The hospital's program for sexual activities was discussed, and the first stage was reviewed with them. Here, Mr. G. learned that masturbation is *permissible*. *Limited information* about cardiac activity was then given. For example, the nurse was able to tell them about the outcomes of the Hellerstein and Friedman (1970)

study on heart rate and sexual activity, as well as informing them that with conjugal sex, Ueno (1963) found only 0.6% coital deaths among the 5,559 deaths he investigated.

Specific suggestions were made, including reviewing the remainder of the cardiac sexual activities program, suggesting that they wait 2 to 3 hours after eating before engaging in coitus, taking a nitroglycerine tablet just prior to intercourse to prevent chest pain, and that Mrs. G. should take the superior or side-lying position so that her husband would not incur cardiac stress by the isometric effects of the male-superior position. In taking their history, the nurse learned that although Mrs. G. has enjoyed sex, she has had a difficult time with orgasm and she wonders if this situation can be changed. In this case, the nurse suggested the names of two sex therapists whom she felt might provide *more intensive therapy* to assist this couple in this more complicated realm of their sexual functioning.

---

more advanced training may be appropriate. The way the PLISSIT model works is illustrated by Mr. G.'s case study.

Components of a sexual history should include the nature of the problem or concerns about the marital or interpersonal relationship, previous ways of sexual expression (for example, they may not enjoy oral-genital sex), other physical health problems, medications, and use of alcohol. It is important to understand the persons' attitudes about their own bodies (Hammond & Stuart 1980). The quality of the relationship should also be assessed. The affective tone of the relationship determines couples' perception of their sexual relationship (Frank, Anderson & Robinstein 1978). If premorbidity problems existed, the stress of illness probably heightens the problems in the sexual arena or produces a deterioration or break in the relationship (Glass 1976).

In further assessing the sexual functioning of any chronically ill person, three parameters must be considered. First is the psychological realm, involving depression, regression, self-esteem, and body image.

Next are the specific aspects of physiologic functioning that can alter sexual functioning and response. Factors to consider include the disease state, which may alter sexual organs, medication, technical trappings of treatment such as a body cast, or changes in anatomy, as with radical pelvic surgery. The third area is that of organic enjoyment, in which physical functioning is intact, but the milieu is less than satisfactory. Fatigue, fear of odors or pain, decubitus, or deformities may create a less than satisfactory environment for pleasure (Wise 1977).

Good communication is foremost when working with sexual problems: between client and nurse and client and partner (Kolodny et al. 1979; Mooney, Cole, & Chilgren 1975; Lamb & Woods 1981). Communication provides a means of discussing and defining each person's perspective of intimacy and its relation to sexual needs. Leviton (1978) defines *intimacy* as a close relationship with another, a desire to be with and enjoy that individual, perhaps a desire to hold and be held, a desire to share and confide or both. In a sexual relationship, intimacy may range from being nonexistent to reaching an extreme high. Not only does intimacy vary, but so do sex acts; illness interferes with only some of them. Although illness may impose a change in actual sexual behaviors, the intimacy between the couple might be heightened if they are working harder to have a good relationship. Good communications can help the client experience empathic gratification, a feeling of adequacy by pleasuring his or her partner (Cole 1975).

In working with clients and their sexual concerns, it is important not to create in the couple or client a conflict with personal values. Remember that many people do not want to discuss sexuality (Curry 1970), but, on the basis of the findings discussed, the nurse should open the door for discussion by using a statement such as, "Many people who have experienced _____ have concerns about their sexual functioning. Do you have any problems or concerns that you would like to discuss?"

In addition to fostering communication and opening the door to discussion about sexual concerns, Lamb and Woods (1981) make these suggestions:

1. Provide anticipatory guidance. By offering information, aid the client and partner to cope more realistically with problems. This can help dispel myths.
2. Validate normalcy of sexual functioning. This helps the client to focus on alternative expressions and what might be prudent or possible, given the limitations that the illness or disability imposes.
3. Educate beyond the anticipatory. This might include interventions to lessen pain, prevent pain, decrease spasms, affect timing, increase function, or improve appearance or control.
4. Counsel about alternative techniques for sexual expression such as approaches, techniques, positioning, masturbation, imagery, touching, massage, and cuddling. Here the nurse must be knowledgeable about the couples' values, attitudes, and beliefs.
5. Refer to those with a high level of comfort or more expertise as needed. This includes serving as a client advocate.

Many clients benefit from good counseling and accurate information (Melynk, Montgomery, & Over 1979; McLane, Krop, & Mehta, 1980). However, we must accept the fact that we will not always be successful for a myriad of reasons, such as continued denial or lost self-esteem of the client, desire to retain established beliefs or behaviors by the couple, or a partner who is negative or sabotages efforts at sexual readjustment (Glass 1976).

Isolation from sexuality and its paths toward intimacy can be disabling. By teaching our clients and their partners new ways to express closeness and intimacy, by helping them discover new options and erogenous zones, by working with them to accept their bodies and themselves as valuable, lovable human beings, we can help to enrich and enhance their lives (Cole 1975).

Summary and Conclusions

Sexuality and intimacy are basic aspects of our lives. From genetic determination through old age, people find sexual gratification in many ways. Chronic illnesses can alter the opportunity and means for sexual expression. Such changes can result from interference with various physiological responses of men and women, from iatrogenic effects of treatment, or from the psychosocial effects that accompany many illnesses.

The health professional can assist the client and partner in dealing with sexual difficulties, if the client wishes such help. To be effective, professionals must be aware of their own sexuality. In addition, an adequate sexual history should be obtained as the basis of any intervention. Suggested here is the PLISSIT model, which is a useful format for helping the client and family to deal with identified sexual problems. Inherent in this approach, as in most other interventions, is the need for effective communication skills. The health professional can, through sensitive involvement, contribute to the clients' retaining of their sexual selves to help enhance their lives.

STUDY QUESTIONS

1. What does the word *sex* connote? What are the differences between gender identity, gender role, and sex object choice?
2. How would you explain why the steps in psychosexual development as described by Erikson are not mutually exclusive?
3. In what ways do the following affect sexual functioning: lack of energy? body image distortion? altered mobility?
4. How do the following chronic conditions affect libido or sexual functioning, including causes: diabetes mellitus? CVA? hypertension? male and female spinal cord injuries? myocardial infarction?
5. What are the various factors that affect sexual expression among alcoholics?
6. What is (are) the effect(s) of chronic illness on the sexual partner of the client? What are some of the concerns of sexual partners?
7. How does the way in which the sexual partner accepts or rejects the client's new body image affect the client's adjustment to the illness? the partner's? Explain your answer.
8. How does our society respond to the sexual needs of the chronically ill? the aged? homosexuals? Explain your answer.
9. Should the nurse or the client and partner initiate discussion about sexuality? Explain your answer.
10. Why is it important to incorporate the client's values and beliefs in sexual counseling?
11. What does the acronym *PLISSIT* stand for? How can the nurse use this format to counsel the client?
12. What constitutes a satisfactory sexual adjustment to chronic disease or disability? In what ways can a satisfactory sexual adjustment contribute to positive rehabilitation?

References

Abram, H. S., Lester, L. R., Sheridan, W. F., and Epstein, G. M., (1975) Sexual functioning in patients with chronic renal failure, *Journal of Nervous and Mental Disease, 160*:220–226

Annon, J., (1976) The PLISSIT model: A proposed conceptual scheme for the behavioral treatment of sexual problems, *Journal of Sex Educators and Therapists, 2*:1–15

Bagdade, J. D., Root, R. K., and Bulger, R. J., (1974) Impaired leukocyte function in patients with poorly controlled diabetes, *Diabetes, 23*:9–15

Bennett, J. P., (1974) Chemical contraception in the male, in *Chemical Contraceptives,* New York: Columbia University Press

Berkman, A. H., Katz, L. A., and Weissman, R., (1982) Sexuality and life-style of home dialysis patients, *Archives of Physical Medicine and Rehabilitation, 63*:272–275

Berkman, A. H., Weissman, R., and Frielich, M. H., (1978) Sexual adjustment of spinal cord injured veterans living in the community, *Archives of Physical Medicine and Rehabilitation, 59*:22–23

Blackwell, B., (1973) Patient compliance, *New England Journal of Medicine, 289*:249–252

Block, A., Molder, J., and Horsely, J., (1975) Sexual problems after myocardial infarction, *American Heart Journal, 90*:536–537

Boller, F., and Frank, E., (1982) *Sexual Dysfunction in Neurological Disorders,* New York: Raven Press

Bray, G. P., Frank, R. S., and Wolfe, T. L., (1981) Sexual functioning in stroke survivors, *Archives of Physical Medicine and Rehabilitation, 62*:286–288

Brooks, M. H., (1977) Effects of diabetes on female sexual response, *Medical Aspects of Human Sexuality, 11*(2):63–64

Brossart, J., (1979) The gay patient: What should you be doing? *RN, 42*(4):50–52

Bullard, D. G., Causey, G. G., Newman, A. B., Orloff, R., Schnaube, K., and Wallace, D. H., (1980) Sexual health care and cancer: A needs assessment, *Frontiers of Radiology Therapy and Oncology, 14*:55–58

Burnham, W. R., Lennard-Jones, J. E., and Brooke, B., (1977) Sexual problems among married ileostomists, *Gut, 18*:673–677

Calderone, N. S., (1974) *Sexuality and Human Values,* New York: Association Press

Christenson, C. V., and Gagnon, J. H., (1965) Sexual behavior in a group of older women, *Journal of Gerontology, 20*:351–356

Cole, T. E., (1975) Sexuality and physical disabilities, *Archives of Sexual Behavior, 4*:389–403

Comarr, A. E., (1966) Interesting observations on females with spinal cord injury, *Medical Services Journal, 22*:651–661

Comarr, A. E., (1970) Sexual function among patients with spinal cord injury, *Urology International, 25*:134–168

Comarr, A. E., (1975) Sexual function in spinal cord injury patients: Diagnosis and therapy, *Urology, 1*:1–18

Comarr, A. E., and Bors, E., (1955) Spermatocystography in patients with spinal cord injuries, *Journal of Urology, 73*:172–178

Conine, T. A., and Evans, J. H., (1982) Sexual reactivation of chronically ill and disabled adults, *Journal of Allied Health, 11*:261–270

Conine, R., Disher, C., and Gilmore, S., (1979) Physical therapists' knowledge of sexuality of adults with spinal cord injury, *Physical Therapist, 59*:395–398

Curry, H. L. F., (1970) Osteoarthritis of the hip joint and sexual activity, *Annals of the Rheumatic Diseases, 29*:288

Derogatis, L. R., (1980) Breast and gynecologic cancers, *Frontiers of Radiation Therapy and Oncology, 14*:1–11

Dierassi, C., (1970) Birth control after 1984, *Science, 169*:941–957

Dresen, S. E., (1975) The sexually active middle adult, *American Journal of Nursing, 75*:1001–1011

Druss, R. G., O'Connor, J. F., and Stern, L. O., (1969) Psychologic response to colectomy, *Archives of General Psychiatry, 20*:419–427

Ellenberg, M., (1971) Impotence in diabetes: The neurological factor, *Annals of Internal Medicine, 75*:213–219

Ellenberg, M., (1977) Sexual aspects of the female diabetic, *Mt. Sinai Journal of Medicine, 44*:495–500

Ellenberg, M., (1979) Sex and diabetes: A comparison between men and women, *Diabetes, 2*:4–8

Erikson, E. H., (1963) *Childhood and Society*, New York: Norton

Faerman, K., Glaser, L., Fox, D., Jadzinsky, M. N., and Rapaport, M., (1973) Impotence and diabetes, Eighth Congress of the International Diabetes Federation, Brussels, Belgium, July 15–20, 1973

Farkas, G. N., and Rosen, R. C., (1976) Effects of alcohol and elicited male sexual response, *Journal of Studies on Alcohol, 37*:265–272

Feldman, H. A., and Singer, I., (1974) Endocrinology and metabolism in uremia and dialysis: A clinical review, *Medicine, 54*:345–376

Fitting, M. D., (1978) Self-concept and sexuality of spinal cord injured women, *Archives of Sexual Behavior, 7*:143–156

Fitz-Gerald, D., and Fitz-Gerald, M., (1977) Deaf people and sexual, too! *SIECUS Report, 6*(2):13–15

Fitzgerald, R. G., (1973) Sexual behavior in the blind, *Medical Aspects of Human Sexuality, 7*:60–61

Fontaine, K. L., (1976) Human sexuality: Faculty knowledge and attitudes, *Nursing Outlook, 24*:174–176

Ford, A. B., and Orfiren, A. P., (1976) Sexual behavior and the chronically ill patient, *Medical Aspects of Human Behavior, 8*:10–30

Frank, D., Dornbush, R., Webster, S., and Kolodny, R. C., (1978) Mastectomy and sexual behavior, *Sexuality and Disability, 1*:16–25

Frank, E., Anderson, C., and Rubinstein, D., (1978) Frequency of sexual dysfunction in normal couples, *New England Journal of Medicine, 299*:111–115

Frazer, J., Albert, M., Smith, J., and Dearner, J., (1982) Impact of a human sexuality workshop in the sexual attitudes of nursing students, *Journal of Nursing Education, 21*(3):6–13

Glass, D. D., (1976) Sexuality and the spinal cord injured patient, in Oaks, W., Melchiode, G., and Ficher, I. (eds.), *Sex and the Life Cycle*, New York: Grune and Stratton

Glass, D. D., and Padrone, F. J., (1978) Sexual adjustment in the handicapped, *Journal of Rehabilitation, 44*:43–47

Goddess, E. D., Wagner, N. N., and Silverman, D. R., (1979) Poststroke sexual activity of CVA patients, *Medical Aspects of Human Sexuality, 13*:16–30

Goldberg, S., and Lewis, M., (1972) Play behaviors in the year old infant: Early sex differences, in Bardwhich, J. M. (ed.), *Readings on the Psychology of Women*, New York: Harper and Row

Golden, J. S., and Golden, M., (1980) Cancer and sex, *Frontiers of Radiation Therapy and Oncology, 14*:59–65

Goller, H., and Paeslack, V., (1972) Pregnancy damage and birth complications in children of paraplegic women, *Paraplegia, 10*:213–217

Gordon, G. G., Altman, S., Southren, A., Rubin, E., and Lieber, C., (1976) Effect of ethanol administration on sex hormone metabolism in normal men, *New England Journal of Medicine, 295*:793–797

Graber, B., and Kline-Graber, C., (1979) Female orgasm: Role of puboccogeus muscles, *Journal of Clinical Psychiatry, 40*:348–351

Griffith, E. R. and Trieschmann, R. B., (1975) Sexual functioning in women with spinal cord injury, *Archives of Physical Medicine and Rehabilitation, 56*:18–21

Hammond, D. C., and Stuart, F. M., (1980) Workshop on sexual dysfunction, University of Utah, Salt Lake City, Utah, June 11–15

Hanson, E. I., (1982) Effects of chronic lung disease on life in general and on sexuality: Perceptions of adult patients, *Heart and Lung, 11*:435–441

Harris, R., Good, R. S., and Pollard, L., (1982) Sexual behavior of gynecologic cancer patients, *Archives of Sexual Behavior*, *11*:503–510

Hartman, C., MacIntosh, B., and Englehardt, B., (1983) The neglected and forgotten sexual partner of the physically handicapped, *Social Work*, *28*:370–374

Hellerstein, H. K., and Friedman, E. H., (1970) Sexual activity and the post coronary patient, *Archives of Internal Medicine*, *125*:987–999

Hock, Z., (1977) Sex therapy and marital counseling for the disabled, *Archives of Physical Medicine and Rehabilitation*, *85*:413–417

Jusenius, K., (1981) Sexuality and gynecologic cancer, *Cancer Nursing*, *4*:479–484

Kallomaki, J. L., Markannen, T. K., and Mustonen, V. A., (1961) Sexual behavior after cerebral vascular accident, *Fertility and Sterility*, *12*:156–158

Kaplan, H. S., (1974) *The New Sex Therapy*, New York: New York Times Book Company

Kass, I., (1972) Coitus induced bronchospasm, *Medical Aspects of Human Sexuality*, *7*:48

Katchadourian, H., (1979) *Human Sexuality*, Berkeley: University of California Press

Kimmel, D., (1978) Adult development and aging: A gay perspective, *Journal of Social Issues*, *34*:113–130

Kinsey, A. C., Pomeroy, W. S., and Martin, C. E., (1948) *Sexual Behavior in the Human Male*, Philadelphia: W. B. Saunders

Kleeman, J. A., (1971) The establishment of core gender identity in normal girls, *Archives of Sexual Behavior*, *1*:103–116

Knorr, D., and Bildingmaier, F., (1975) Gynecomastia in male adolescents, *Clinics in Endocrinology and Metabolism*, *4*:157–171

Kolodny, R. C., (1971) Sexual dysfunction in diabetic females, *Diabetes*, 557–559

Kolodny, R. C., Kahn, C. B., Goldstein, H. H., and Barnett, D. M., (1974) Sexual dysfunction in diabetic men, *Diabetes*, *23*:306–309

Kolodny, R. C., Masters, W. H., Johnson, V. E., and Biggs, M. A., (1979) *The Textbook of Human Sexuality for Nurses*, Boston: Little, Brown

Krosnick, F., and Poldolsky, S., (1981) Diabetes and sexual dysfunction: Restoring normal ability, *Geriatrics*, *36*:92–100

Lamb, M. A., and Woods, N. F., (1981) Sexuality and the cancer patient, *Cancer Nursing*, *4*:137–144

Lemere, F., and Smith, J. W., (1973) Alcohol-induced sexual impotence, *American Journal of Psychiatry*, *130*:212–213

Levine, S. B., (1976) Marital sexual dysfunction, *Annals of Internal Medicine*, *84*:448–453

Leviton, D., (1978) The intimacy–sexual needs of the terminally ill and the widowed, *Death Education*, *2*:261–280

Levy, N. B., (1973) Sexual adjustment to maintenance hemodialysis and renal transplantation, *American Society of Artificial Internal Organs*, *19*:138–143

Lilius, H. G., Valtonen, E., and Wickstrom, J., (1976) Sexual problems in patients suffering from multiple sclerosis, *Scandinavian Journal of Social Medicine*, *4*:41–44

Lim, V. S., and Fang, V. S., (1975) Gonadal dysfunction in uremic men: A study of hypothalamo-pituitary-testicular axis before and after renal transplantation, *American Journal of Medicine*, *58*:655–662

Maccoby, E. E., and Jacklin, L. M., (1974) *The Psychology of Sex Differences*, Stanford: Stanford University Press

Maddock, J. W., (1975) Sexual health and health care, *Postgraduate Medicine*, *58*:52–58.

Marshall, W. A., (1975) Growth and sexual maturation in normal puberty, *Clinics in Endocrinology and Metabolism*, *4*:3–25

Maruta, T., and Osborne, D., (1978) Sexual activity in chronic pain, *Psychosomatics*, *19*:531–537

Masters, W., and Johnson, V. E., (1970) *Human Sexual Inadequacy*, Boston: Little, Brown

McCullock, D. K., Campbell, I. W., Wu, F. C., Prescott, R. J., and Clarke, B. F., (1980) The prevalence of diabetic impotence, *Diabetalogia*, *18*:279–283

McLane, M., Krop, H. L., and Mehta, J., (1980) Psychosexual adjustment and counseling after myocardial infarction, *Annals of Internal Medicine*, *92*:514–519

McNab, W. L., (1976) Sexual attitude development in children and the parents' role, *Journal of School Health*, *46*:537–542

Mehta, J., and Krop, H., (1979) The effect of myocardial infarction on sexual functioning, *Sexuality and Disability*, *2*:115–121

Meltzer, H. Y., and Fang, V. S., (1976) The effect of neuroleptics on serum prolactin in schizophrenic patients, *Archives of General Psychiatry*, *33*:279–286

Melynk, R., Montgomery, R., and Over, R., (1979) Attitude changes following a sexual counseling program for spinal cord injured persons, *Archives of Physical Medicine and Rehabilitation*, *60*:601–605

Mims, F. H., Brown, L., and Lubow, R., (1974) Human sexuality course evaluation, *Nursing Research*, *25*:187–191

Mitchell, M. E., (1982) Sexual counseling in cardiac rehabilitation, *Journal of Rehabilitation*, *48*(4):15–18

Money, J., (1972) Sex reassignment therapy in gender identity disorders, *International Psychiatry Clinics*, 8:197–210

Money, J., and Ehrhardt, A., (1972) *Man and Woman: Boy and Girl*, Baltimore: Johns Hopkins Press

Mooney, T. O., Cole, T. M., and Chilgren, R., (1975) *Sexual Options for Paraplegics and Quadraplegics*, Boston: Little, Brown

Morales, A., Surridge, D., Marshall, P., and Fenemore, J., (1982) Nonhormonal pharmacological treatment of organic impotence, *Journal of Urology*, 128:45–47

Morgan, M. Y., and Sherlock, S., (1977) Sex related difference among 100 patients with alcohol liver disease, *British Medical Journal*, 1:939–941

Morris, D., (1972) *Intimate Behavior*, New York: Random House

Papadopoulos, G., Beaumont, C., Shelley, S., and Larrimore, P., (1983) Myocardial infarction and sexual activity of the female patient, *Archives of Internal Medicine*, 14:1528–1530

Papadopoulos, G., Larimore, P., Cardin, S., and Shelley, S., (1980) Sexual concerns and needs of the post coronary patient's wife, *Archives of Internal Medicine*, 140:38–41

Paradowski, W., (1977) Socialization patterns and sexual problems of the institutionalized chronically ill and physically disabled, *Archives of Physical Medicine and Rehabilitation*, 58:53–59

Parker, R. A., Bennett, W. M., Harris, R. L., Barry, J., and Porter, G. A., (1977) Nocturnal penile tumescence: Objective method for evaluation of impotence in chronic renal failure, *Clinical Dialysis Transplant Forum*, 7:34–38

Payne, T., (1976) Sexuality of nurses: Correlations of knowledge, attitudes and behavior, *Nursing Research*, 25:286–292

Pfeiffer, E., and Davis, G. C., (1972) Determinants of sexual behavior in middle and old age, *Journal of the American Geriatric Society*, 20:151–158

Procci, W. A., Goldstein, D. A., Adelstein, J., and Massry, S. G., (1981) Sexual dysfunction in the male with uremia: A reappraisal, *Kidney International*, 19:317–323

Raphael, S., and Robinson, M., (1980) The older lesbian: Love relationships and friendship patterns, *Alternative Lifestyles*, 3:207–229

Reinstein, L., Ashley, J., and Miller, K., (1978) Sexual adjustment after lower extremity amputation, *Archives of Physical Medicine and Rehabilitation*, 59:501–503

Robinson, M., (1979) The older lesbian, Master's thesis, California State University, Dominguez Hills, Carson, California

Rolf, L. L., and Kleemack, D. L., (1979) Sexual activity among older persons, *Research on Aging*, 1:389–399

Romano, M. D., and Lassiter, R. E., (1972) Sexual counseling with the spinal cord injured, *Archives of Physical Medicine and Rehabilitation*, 53:568–575

Sadoughi, W., Lesher, M., and Fine, H. L., (1971) Sexual adjustment in chronically ill and disabled population: A pilot study, *Archives of Physical Medicine and Rehabilitation*, 52:311–317

Schain, W., (1980) Sexual functioning, self-esteem and cancer care, *Frontiers of Radiation Therapy and Oncology*, 14:12–19

Schmidt, G., (1982) Sex and society in the eighties, *Archives of Sexual Behavior*, 11:91–97

Scott, F. B., Bradley, W. E., and Timm, G. W., (1973) Management of erectile impotence: Use of implantible penile prosthesis, *Urology*, 2:80–82

Shontz, F. C., (1974) Body image and its disorders, *International Journal of Medicine*, 5:461–472

Short, N. J., and Wilson, N. P., (1969) Roles of denial in chronic hemodialysis, *Archives of General Psychiatry*, 20:433–437

Simon, W., and Gagnon, J. H., (1967) Homosexuality: The formulation of a sociological perspective, *Journal of Health and Human Behavior*, 8:177–185

Small, M. P., (1978) The Small-carrion penile prosthesis, *Urology Clinics of North America*, 5:549–562

Soyka, L. F., and Mattison, D. R., (1981) Prescription drugs that affect male sexual function, *Drug Therapy*, 11:46–58

Sparks, R. F., White, R. A., and Connelly, P. B., (1980) Impotence is not always psychogenic, *Journal of the American Medical Association*, 243:750–755

Steele, T. E., Finklestein, S. H., and Finklestein, F. O., (1976) Hemodialysis patients and spouses: Marital discord, sexual problems and depression, *Journal of Nervous and Mental Disease*, 162:225–237

Stockdale-Woolley, R., (1983) Sexual dysfunction and COPD: Problems and management, *Nurse Practitioner*, 8:16–18

Story, N. L., (1974) Sexual dysfunction resulting from drug side effects, *Journal of Sexual Research*, 10:132–149

Straus, D. J., (1973) Hematologic aspects of alcoholism, *Seminars in Hematology*, 10:183–194

Strauss, A., (1976) *Chronic Illness and the Quality of Life*, St. Louis: C. V. Mosby

Swinburn, W. R., (1976) Sexual counseling for the arthritic, *Clinics on Rheumatic Diseases*, 62:122–123

Tarabulcy, E., (1972) Sexual function in the normal and in paraplegia, *Paraplegia*, *10*:201–208

Tyler, G., Steel, J. M., Ewing, D. J., Bancropft, J., Warner, P., and Clarke, B. F., (1983) Sexual responsiveness in diabetic women, *Diabetologica*, *24*:166–176

Ueno, O., (1963) The so-called coition death, *Japan Journal of Legal Medicine*, *17*:333–340

Valleroy, M. L., and Kraft, H., (1984) Sexual dysfunction in multiple sclerosis, *Archives of Physical Medicine and Rehabilitation*, *65*:125–128

Van Thiel, D., (1976) Testicular atrophy and other endocrine changes in alcoholic men, *Medical Aspects of Human Sexuality*, *10*:153–154

Wasow, M., and Loeb, M., (1979) Sexuality in nursing homes, *Journal of the American Geriatrics Society*, *27*:73–79

Weiss, H. D., (1972) The physiology of human penile erection, *Annals of Internal Medicine*, *76*:792, 799

Wiig, E. H., (1973) Counseling the adult aphasic for sexual readjustment, *Rehabilitation Counseling Bulletin*, *17*:110–119

Wise, T. M., (1977) Sexuality in chronic illness, *Primary Care*, *4*:199–207

Wise, T. M., (1984) How drugs can help or hinder sexual function, *Drug Therapy*, *14*:51–63

Woods, N. F., (1975) Influences on sexual adaptation to mastectomy, *Journal of Obstetric and Gynecological Nursing*, *4*:33–37

Woods, N. F., (1979) *Human Sexuality in Health and Illness*, St. Louis: C. V. Mosby

World Health Organization, (1975) Education and treatment in human sexuality: The training of health professionals, *WHO Technical Report Series*, No. 572, Geneva: WHO

Yoshimo, S., and Uchida, S., (1981) Sexual problems of women with rheumatoid arthritis, *Archives of Physical Medicine and Rehabilitation*, *62*:122–123

Zalar, M., (1975) Human sexuality: A component of total patient care, *Nursing Digest*, November–December, pp. 40–43

PART THREE

Impact of the Health Professional

CHAPTER ELEVEN

Change Agent

Introduction

Coping with change is a facet of life for everybody in today's society, but it can be especially troublesome for chronically ill people, who frequently must make permanent major changes in their life-styles. Indeed, many of the effects of chronic illness described in Parts I and II are in fact changes. The chronically ill must accept such changes as altered levels of independence and vigor as innate characteristics of their disorders. Conversely, they often must choose whether or not to change some aspect of their lives in order to follow medical advice. The purpose of this chapter is to explore change, whether imposed or chosen, as a framework for understanding and helping the chronically ill client.

Historical Perspective

The process of change has been studied in relation to individuals as well as to groups and institutions. For example, studies on change relating to individuals and families deal primarily with various psychotherapeutic approaches as change tactics (Benne 1976; Watzlawick, Weakland, & Fisch 1974; Fisch, Weakland, & Segal 1982). The literature focusing on larger groups often addresses change in work environments and changes at the community level (Brooten, Hayman, & Naylor 1978; Lancaster & Lancaster 1982; Mauksch & Miller 1981). Nursing literature that

describes change as a clinical tool is limited. The focus of the following discussion is applying change theory to chronically ill individuals and their family and support networks. Several strategies and their application are presented. One strategy and its relation to the nursing process is proposed as a clinical tool for the practitioner. The issue of change in the work place and community, which is often needed to further the interests of the chronically ill client population, is addressed in the works cited.

Lippitt (1973) has defined *change* as "any planned or unplanned alteration in the status quo in an organism, situation, or process." This definition has features in common with definitions of education, so the two must be differentiated. Educational interventions are "those that rely heavily on transmission of information and instructions as a means of changing behavior" (Dunbar, Marshall, & Hovell 1979). Education, consequently, is one form of change; the change process may certainly include educational interventions, but it is not limited to them. Change should be viewed as a metaframework, an "umbrella" under which problems and a variety of approaches can be organized. The use of change theory to analyze and intervene in a client problem provides the professional with a rich understanding of this concept and a broad array of management choices.

Change, as advocated in this chapter, is consistent with the philosophy of holism. People's choices and behaviors are related to their beliefs and feelings. Also, individual clients, even isolated ones, are enmeshed in larger social systems. Change theory allows the professional to account for all these factors in decision making. The change process culminates in an *integration* of changes into the client's daily existence; change theory combines knowledge and skills training with the support needed to sustain new perceptions, attitudes, and behavior.

The Change Process

Change can be unconscious or conscious. Unconscious change, called *drift*, can be so imperceptible that it is recognized only after it occurs (Reinkemeyer 1970). Conscious change may be an individual process, or it may be accompanied by other processes.

Drift

Drift is a series of small changes in a situation that go unnoticed. The cumulative effect of such changes may be great, and it is sometimes perceived as a sudden event. Change of this sort can be problematic for the chronically ill client. For example, slowly deteriorating family relationships may be recognized only after a crisis. Another common example of change by drift is the gradual laxity of personal health care habits. All practitioners have seen clients who, for a variety of reasons, slowly lose their enthusiasm for health routines.

Conscious Process

As a conscious process, change varies among individuals and groups in respect to the planning and deliberation that are involved. Conscious change is apparent to people who are changing.

Lewin's View. Kurt Lewin (1958) described a model of conscious change having three stages: unfreezing, moving, and refreezing. Schein, who had a background in Gestalt therapy, elaborated on Lewin's model, describing the psychological mechanisms for each of the three phases (1969). During *unfreezing*, people's beliefs and perceptions are shaken about

particular situations, about themselves in those situations, or about others involved in the situations. Individuals may react in several ways: experiencing feelings of inadequacy that motivate change or wishing to effect a change without experiencing a sense of inadequacy. Once *open* to new ways of viewing one's state, the individual is ready for the next stage of the model: moving. During the *moving* phase, the person actually tries out different perceptions, actions, and standards. These new views and values are part of a process of redefining the situation. For example, understanding for the first time that a half-empty glass is also half full results from this redefinition process. Exploration during the moving phase may or may not be conscious; but conscious or not, cognitive redefinition is essential. Schein notes that the moving phase is allied with Gestalt learning theory. The third phase, *refreezing*, occurs when the new responses are integrated into the person's personality and significant relationships.

Behaviorist View. Behaviorists are also students of change, and they offer a different perspective of conscious change. Behaviorists differ from Schein in that they do not consider cognitive redefinition important to achieving behavior change. Rather, reinforcement theory is used to evolve methods for changing behavior.

One behaviorist, Steckel (1982), outlines both respondent and operant conditioning. *Respondent conditioning* is based on passive association of two events by an individual; it does not include a reward system. Aversive therapy, such as that employed in some smoking cessation programs, is an example of this type of conditioning. Smokers who receive electrical shocks as they light cigarettes begin to associate the unpleasant experience with lighting the cigarette. Presumably, this association decreases the desire to smoke. *Operant conditioning* differs in that it incorporates rewards. A fundamental principle of operant conditioning is that behavior that is followed by a favorable consequence is likely to be repeated on future occasions when the same conditions prevail. In operant conditioning the individual can reproduce the favorable consequences by operating on the environment. Contingency contracting, a change strategy based on operant conditioning, is discussed later in this chapter.

The reader must appreciate both the expanded Lewin view and the behaviorist view of the change process. To provide effective support during change, one must understand and apply methods from both perspectives.

Problems and Issues Relating to Change

Problems and issues pertinent to change affect professionals and clients in an interrelated manner. Although the issue of ethics is largely a professional one, the way one manages the ethics of change affects clients. The other issues addressed are intrinsic to the client population, but they clearly affect the professional's management decisions.

Professional Ethics and Change

Because of the ethical implications of the process of change, the topic is addressed briefly here. The result of the change process is some modification of a person's life; indeed, that modification is the *goal* of planned change. The professional must guard against using knowledge of the change process either to manipulate the client or to deprive the client of the right to make independent decisions.

Power and Decision Making. Power is a factor that enters the change process. One might ask whether anyone has the right to intervene in client choices, even when a client lacks information to make valid decisions. The professional, by virtue of education and experience, has knowledge that can broaden the client's decision-making base. To allow a client to make decisions ignorant of the consequences or risks is viewed by many as irresponsible professional behavior (Rappsilber 1982). But does eliminating the client's ignorance fulfill the professional's responsibility, or should compliance with a medical plan be the goal?

The legitimate goal of change is a mixture of eliminating ignorance and encouraging compliance. Although client and family satisfaction with the choices made is most important, the professional should work to remove all possible barriers to following sound medical advice. All tactics available to support medically advised changes or acceptance of imposed changes should be offered to the client.

In the final analysis, the choice to change belongs to the client, and the professional must honor this choice. Accepting such decisions is difficult for many professionals, who genuinely want to assist the client but are unwilling to accept choices that result in noncompliance. Health professionals regard their service as valuable, but clients do not always share that value. This incongruence can occur whether or not client and professional share socioeconomic strata and ethnicity.

How Much Information? Providing information is another issue that can gnaw at the conscience of the professional. How much information is appropriate? If given too little, the client acts in ignorance. If given too much, a person may be overwhelmed and unable to make any choices. Must the client be aware of all the information underlying the professional's decisions?

Jonsen (1979) points out that information must be shared in ways appropriate to the individual situation. Some clients want detailed information; others are unable to accept all the aspects of their status. For example, the mother of a child with newly diagnosed cystic fibrosis may be so preoccupied with learning how to care for her child in the here and now that she cannot digest information about future events. The professional must determine, sometimes by trial and error, the extent of information necessary to maintain the client's motivation, right to know, and sense of competency. Otherwise, the client may be unable to act because of anxiety related to overwhelming or insufficient information.

Client Dependency. At times clients must depend on others' choices. Decisions made by others, such as family members, on behalf of the frail elderly, debilitated adults, or children are often based on values or beliefs different from those of the professional. This difference may cause an ethical conflict between the decision maker and the caregiver.

In cases in which decisions are clearly not in the individual client's best interests or are made without regard to the individual's dignity, power-coercive change is in order. (Power-coercive strategies will be discussed shortly.) Legal sanctions may become necessary when efforts to implement health-promoting or health-maintaining choices are refused and the client's status is jeopardized.

Resistance to Change

People resist change because they strive to maintain consistency and predictability in their lives. The professional as change agent must be sensitive to sources of client resistance. Clients' resistance to changes is based on real or imagined consequences (Klein 1969). Advice to exercise may be ignored because setting aside time is difficult. Advice to change dietary habits may go unheeded because the individual likes the forbidden food, finds eating pleasurable, and wants to continue to eat. When the cost outweighs benefits, the client will not adopt the suggested change. The professional must either work to increase the attractiveness of the benefits or attenuate the cost in some way.

People also resist changes that threaten their integrity, that is, the "sense of self-esteem, competence and autonomy enjoyed by those . . . who feel that their power and resources are adequate to meet the usual challenges of living" (Klein 1969). Individuals need to protect those feelings that promote a sense of security. As one diabetic man says, "I feared that if I followed *all* the rules and regulations, I'd end up a goody-goody, sapped of my spirit and independence" (Pray 1983).

The professional works to help the client maintain integrity by acknowledging the client's power and independence whenever possible, by making a real investment in the relationship, and by helping the client set and achieve realistic goals. When another person makes such an investment in an individual's

well-being and the outcome is successful, the client's worth and competence receive validation.

People may resist change because they feel alienated from the professional (Klein 1969), especially when there is distance between the professional's theoretical knowledge and the client's experiential knowledge. Conflicts may arise because professional and client actually view problems differently or because they cannot make themselves understood by one another. Cultural and societal differences exemplify this kind of alienation.

Clients may resist changes that must be imposed because of altered or deteriorating health status. Such resistance may be manifested by defenses such as denial, overcompensation, and rationalization. Often resistance to imposed change is accompanied by resistance to new health care habits in which the client is able to exercise choice. Most health professionals have encountered clients such as those with obstructive lung disease who rationalize continued smoking "because stopping wouldn't help anyway."

Demoralizing Effect of Change

The need for consistency, autonomy, and competence has been mentioned. Change associated with chronic illness often threatens satisfaction of these needs and can lead to loss of hope and courage. Deterioration of vigor, mobility, or comfort is common among people having chronic illnesses. Such losses may reduce their pursuit of work, hobbies, and social activities. Thus, the change in one's physical status can have implications for that person's relationships to loved ones and community: The sense of belonging is threatened, as is the sense of integrity.

The day-to-day management of many chronic illnesses such as cystic fibrosis, diabetes, rheumatoid arthritis, spinal cord injuries, renal failure, and chronic obstructive lung disease is complex and time-consuming. Committing time and energy to a complicated survival or management regimen further limits one's ability to pursue leisure, work, and social activities. In addition, many aspects of the care required for these diseases are intrinsically unpleasant. Mist treatments and postural drainage required by the person with cystic fibrosis not only take time but involve handling sputum. Most people find this process unpleasant, at least initially.

Erosion of Support Systems

Day-to-day management demands of chronic illness affect not only ill individuals but those around them as well. Well-established family traditions may be shaken by an individual's loss of health or inability to manage the disease. The family who has always enjoyed late Sunday morning brunch must take into account a new factor when a diabetic member requires morning insulin and an early meal. The couple who enjoyed hiking and golf together may have to adapt to less strenuous exercise if one of them develops rheumatoid arthritis or peripheral vascular disease.

Norms such as role definitions are also shaken. The stricken wife who has always taken care of the housework now finds increasing need for help with her chores as her incapacity from multiple sclerosis increases. The husband who has been the sole support of the family and who is disabled by renal failure will have to relinquish that role to his wife. Both the impaired sick role (see Chapter 3) and disease trajectory (see Chapter 2) are affected.

Customs that govern shared pleasure and work are part of the glue that holds families and loved ones together. When these customs are threatened, so, too, is the nurturing that the chronically ill client receives from his support network. The extreme example of this phenomenon is caretaker burnout. When the chronically ill person's needs are great and assistance in care is not, the caretaker can suffer physically and emotionally (see Chapter 8). Goldstein, Regnery, and Wellin (1981) have noted that the caretaker role affects virtually all aspects of the caretaker's life. The stress of this responsibility can become so great that the caretaker may abandon the client.

Society's Resistance to Integration of the Chronically Ill

The term *resistance* in this context reflects passive more than active resistance. Society is more indifferent to the needs of the chronically ill than openly hostile to them. Nevertheless, the stigma associated with chronic illness and disability can be viewed as a function of society's fear. Being in the presence of the chronically ill or disabled person can make a well person feel especially vulnerable and uncomfortable. The denial that operates around one's own susceptibility to illness can be threatened. Human history reflects a tendency to exclude or shun the less able person (see Chapter 4).

Social institutions that once cared for the chronically ill in the home have also been disrupted. In the past, the extended family, the wife who worked in the home, the close-knit neighborhood and church group all supported the care of the chronically ill. Indeed, close neighbors, family, and church members provided not only respite for caretakers but stimulation and caring for the sick person. These supports are less available in today's society, and they have not been adequately replaced.

The lack of facilities, ranging from architectural barriers to insufficient respite care centers and other support services, indicates societal indifference and a consequent lack of funding. Society seems to have other priorities than the needs of the chronically ill or the disabled. This area demands intervention by the health professional. Aligning oneself with volunteer organizations already interested in such causes places the professional in contact with an established support group. Organizing a consciousness-raising campaign and negotiating or lobbying for changes on the community level could have an impact on this source of resistance.

Interventions Based on Change Theory

The results of change, some theories of the mechanisms of change, and resistance to change have been addressed. This section discusses strategies to effect change.

Facilitating Change

A person who deliberately promotes a change process is a *change agent* (Mauksch & Miller 1981). The skilled change agent consciously uses a variety of strategies and tactics to promote the process. Strategies are overall master plans for managing change; tactics are activities designed to carry out portions of the plan (Mauksch & Miller 1981). Chin and Benne (1976) have devised three general categories of strategies differentiated by underlying assumptions.

Normative-Reeducative Strategies. Schein's elaboration of the Lewin model, introduced earlier, refers to normative-reeducative strategies. According to this model, people have and exercise rational choice, but sociocultural norms, with their underlying values and perceptions, also are important. While the client's knowledge level and skill learning are attended to, so too are the psychosocial implications of the proposed change. This strategy is indicated when the client's feelings, attitudes, values, or significant relationships oppose the change.

Normative-reeducative change has several defining qualities. First, clients are involved in defining problems and developing solutions. The way they see themselves and the task enters into the relationship with the change agent. Second, the relationship between the client and change agent is collaborative, with approximately equally distributed power. Third, nonconscious factors are brought to light and explored. Clients' feelings, beliefs, and assumptions that direct their behavior enter the problem-solving process. Finally, both change agents and clients use methods from the behavioral sciences in this process.

Empirical-Rational Strategies. In empirical-rational strategies, the change agent operates on the assumption that people are rational and make choices that promote their best interests if they have such choices. This strategy is effective when the client's values and beliefs do not conflict with the proposal. This author views the three-stage Lewin model as appropriate to empirical-rational change. Unfreezing is not likely to be difficult since, by definition, the client's values and norms are in harmony with the change. The client has to acquire information or skills and integrate them into selected life choices (moving and refreezing).

The empirical-rational strategy is characterized by a power imbalance between change agent and client because knowledge is power, and the change agent is the expert. The inadequacy of this strategy has been demonstrated many times by investigators who show that having more knowledge does not necessarily lead to changed behavior (Edwards 1980; Haynes 1979; Korhonen et al. 1983; Mazzuca 1982).

Power-Coercive Strategies. As the name implies, force of some sort is intrinsic to power-coercive strategies. Political and economic sanctions are frequently chosen. For example, legislating access to public buildings for people confined to wheelchairs is power-coercive change. Moral sanctions can also be invoked. Exploiting guilt or shame is a coercive strategy often used by health professionals: "Why aren't you exercising?" Although meting out punishment in response to some undesirable behavior reduces the frequency of that behavior, the effects are short-lived. The client may avoid the change agent who employs this strategy (Steckel 1982).

Contingency Contracting. Contingency contracting is presented as a fourth strategy because it does not fit readily into any of the three categories described by Chin and Benne. At first glance, one might assume that this strategy is a power-coercive one, but closer examination reveals significant differences.

In *contingency contracting*, behavior is examined for situations that prompt it, for consequences that reinforce it, and for ways in which complex behaviors can be introduced a step at a time. Behavior that supports the client's goals is prompted and reinforced; behavior contrary to client goals is not reinforced, and situations that stimulate such behavior are eliminated or altered whenever possible. As the name implies, the reward is contingent on the performance of a desired behavior. A contract outlining the terms of the agreement is developed (Steckel 1982).

Unlike those of power-coercive strategies, the goals in contingency contracting are the client's. Another difference is control of the consequences of behavior: In power-coercive strategies, change agents or representatives apply sanctions; in contingency contracting, professionals may participate in the rewards, but rewards may also be designed to exclude the professional. Finally, the client participates in identifying means as well as goals and rewards. This degree of client participation divides the power between client and professional much more evenly than do power-coercive strategies.

Contingency contracting shares many characteristics with normative-reeducative change. The major distinction is that contingency contracting's nonconscious elements *per se* assume less importance since the focus is on behavior and environment.

The Change Agent's Role

In matters of choice, the change agent assists clients in making informed decisions, works to alter unacceptable or unpleasant aspects of the choice, and supports the client's efforts to achieve personal goals. Imposed changes that are problematic generally represent some sort of loss. The change agent in these situations supports the grieving process and explores the meaning of the loss in practical terms. Modifying those losses that are amenable to adaptation helps to restore the client's sense of control and consistency.

The change agent always uses empathy and facilitative communication. In addition, the agent examines the situation, selects the appropriate strategy, and, in collaboration with the client, selects tactics consistent with the strategy. Most tactics involve techniques from problem solving, teaching, and operant conditioning. The change agent has been described as a "facilitator/logician" who identifies the support needed to propel a change and then provides this support (Bailey 1983).

Applying Change Theory to a Client Situation

The method described here combines steps of the problem-solving process used in nursing (assessment, planning, intervention, and evaluation) with Lewin's phases of change (unfreezing, moving, and refreezing). It primarily uses tactics consistent with normative-reeducative change. A case study involving a 57-year-old woman with a 1-year history of non-insulin-dependent diabetes mellitus illustrates the use of the change process in an ambulatory setting.

Unfreezing. During the unfreezing phase of the change process (see Table 11-1), the client becomes open to new perceptions, attitudes, and behaviors. Careful assessment is in order at this point for several reasons. In the discussion that follows, the term *client* refers to the individual and to the individual's support system unless otherwise noted.

1. Minimize the need for change in the client's life. Disease management must be tailored to honor habits, norms, and the character of satisfying relationships so long as such individualization is within the limits of safety.
2. Determine which problems in the client's life are amenable to change. Experiencing success helps maintain motivation. Focusing on *realistic* change projects is critical.
3. The health professional must operate on knowledge rather than assumptions of the client's priorities and concerns. Assumptions can leave client needs untouched. Lauer, Murphy, and Powers (1982) found that nurses and cancer patients in one study differed considerably when asked to rate the importance of informational items and the problems they introduced for patients.
4. Selection of appropriate change strategies depends on a full understanding of the client's situation, including attitudes and choices. For informational needs, empirical-rational change should suffice. When there is conflict between disease management and client attitudes, beliefs, relationships, or group norms, then the normative-reeducative strategy is in order. If only behavior is not congruent with disease management, then operant conditioning is an option available to the change agent and client.
5. Referral may be necessary to satisfy client needs. Identifying when a different health care professional better meets client needs may relieve or prevent client frustration.

Assessment. The goal of the unfreezing phase is to determine what changes would lead to optimum disease management and to identify the forces that promote and inhibit these changes. This identification of

TABLE 11-1. Unfreezing

Assessment	Planning	Intervention	Evaluation
Goal: Identify forces that promote and inhibit change process.	Goal: Develop a plan to support change and modify resistance	Goal: Assist client to achieve/strengthen motivators to change	Goal: Determine effect of intervention and extent of unfreezing
Assessment factors	Interpretation of assessment factors	Methods as appropriate	Client's verbal and nonverbal communication
Understanding of disease	Attractiveness of various changes	Selection of most attractive change	Comfort in discussing feelings, pro and con
Understanding of medical plan	Motivators	Supportive listening and investment	Willingness to help solve problems
Usual daily routines	Client's level of confidence	Discussion of inaction	Discusses goals
Changes proposed for routines	Client's support systems	Discussion of unrealistic fears	Discusses means
Feelings and attitudes about these changes	Client's perception of change compared to reality	Discussion of safe variations in self-management	Explores barriers
Others' feelings and attitudes toward the changes	Resistance compared to goals	Discussion of goals and resistance	Client and professional comfort with expectations
Goals held		Selection of realistic goals with client	
Motivators present		Discussion of client-professional relationship	
Evidence of resistance			

change-promoting and inhibiting forces was introduced by Lewin, who referred to the process as a *force field analysis* (Lewin 1958). In work with the chronically ill, the professional identifies these forces by interviewing client and loved ones. Separate interviews yield information that would not otherwise be divulged; joint interviews provide the opportunity to observe family interaction. This perspective is critical to a realistic force field analysis.

The professional must evaluate the client's understanding of the illness and of the medical plan and a description of the client's usual day. Has the illness been explained adequately? What has the client read about it? Have other friends or family had the illness, and how did they manage? Can the client list all points of self-care? Do client and family understand the rationale for the medical plan? What are the day's usual activities? How are weekday routines different from those on weekends? What are the differences in individual perceptions on these points?

Client and family members' beliefs and attitudes must also be explored. Beliefs give rise to attitudes, and attitudes held by people close to us can sway us (Mauksch & Miller 1981). Beliefs are the basis of the *health belief model*, which attempts to explain personal health decisions. According to this model, decisions are functions of the client's perception of the following:

1. Level of susceptibility to the illness or condition
2. Severity of the consequences of the illness, either physical or social

3. Potential benefit to be derived from a given health action
4. Balancing of physical, psychological, financial, or other barriers related to the health action against the benefits (Rosenstock 1974)

At this point in the assessment, changes in lifestyle necessary for ideal management become clear and should be validated with the client to reach consensus about what is necessary for ideal management. If realistic changes are to be accomplished, the professional must identify client goals and motivators for and resistance to change. From among all these factors, the professional can determine the optimal place and time to initiate the change process.

Planning and Intervention. Having identified driving and restraining forces in the assessment, the professional next attempts to strengthen the driving forces and minimize the restraining ones. The professional's goal is to engage the client's willingness to try different ways of viewing and solving problems. The true test of the change agent's skill during unfreezing is the ability to ferret out those openings in the client's resistance and to provide the support needed to move the client away from the *status quo.* Several factors should be considered:

1. If multiple changes are indicated, relative resistance to them must be noted. If possible, focus first on the project that is most appealing or least noxious to the client. This emphasis increases the probability of success, which in itself is motivating.
2. The cause of low motivation must be ascertained. Some clients have little motivation because they do not appreciate their long-term peril; others use suppression to deal with high anxiety about their health. Still others recognize the health threat but feel helpless about altering the trajectory. Once the cause of low motivation is determined, the professional can explain the probable consequences of inaction or bolster the client's feeling of hope and confidence. Sometimes both steps are appropriate.
3. Combating the struggle with chronic illness requires that the professional boost client morale

by emphasizing client supports, both inside and outside the health care system, including knowledge of community resources.
4. Unrealistic fears or misconceptions must be allayed to promote the client's confidence. Is the client's perception of the illness and treatment realistic? Are there false notions about the future or present? Are there ways to vary home management that are safe and more agreeable to client and family?
5. The professional must compare client's goals to client's resistance. What is the likelihood that attainable goals can be achieved in the face of resistance? The client may need to alter one or the other to avoid further discouraging experiences. Breaking down long-term goals into short-term steps gives guidance to the change process and increases the probability of success.

The most difficult factors to unfreeze are the client's attitudes and beliefs, which change only as a result of experience. The onus is on the professional to arrange necessary experiences; for example, placing a positive value on urine testing might result from first trying and then finding such a test useful. When an experience indicates that the client will derive no benefit from a course of action, the professional must be ready to make another suggestion that could be a more effective way of achieving the desired goal.

With all these factors in mind, goals and means to achieve them must be explored. The client-professional relationship requires that both reach an understanding about the contribution each will make. The client's responsibilities and authority are clarified in this way. The professional can confirm that the client's frustrations and fears have been acknowledged and at the same time acknowledge the client's strengths.

Evaluation. The professional must determine whether the client is willing to engage in a change process. This is done by considering whether the client's verbal and nonverbal communication indicates openness (for example, whether the individual discusses negative and positive feelings with apparent ease). The change agent cannot single-handedly

◇ CASE STUDY ◇

L.S.: Unfreezing

Assessment of L.S. In the year before L.S. began this project, she had experienced several changes, including her diagnosis of diabetes and the development of painful peripheral neuropathy in her hands and feet. Six months later, her mother, with whom she lived, died suddenly. Her only other relative was her daughter, who lived 125 miles away. There was weekly telephone contact, but she saw her daughter only about four times a year. At this time she still had painful feet, was hyperglycemic, and was receiving daily insulin injections with the possibility of needing insulin twice a day. At the time of her diagnosis, L.S. had seen a diabetic educator, had learned to give herself insulin, and recognized the relationship between obesity and her diabetes. She subsequently lost 20 pounds and now had a stable weight of 145 pounds (height: 5 feet).

Restraining forces: In spite of lost weight, L.S. still required insulin. She was grieving the loss of her mother, who had been a companion and source of encouragement. She was tired of testing her urine "because the tests are always positive for sugar anyway." She was faced with the possibility of a second daily insulin injection, even though she had lost weight in the hope of no longer needing insulin. Her coworkers, who encouraged her to eat sweets at staff meetings, did not know she had diabetes, and she felt that a presupper injection would jeopardize her relationship with them. L.S. mildly resisted exercise because of her painful feet. She was discouraged and inconvenienced by her current condition.

Driving forces: L.S. was aware that change was necessary since her daily regimen was not managing her diabetes. She was open to examining her dietary habits. Her understanding of her diabetes was accurate, and she was aware of her physician's instructions regarding a nutritious diet with no concentrated sweets, continued weight loss, exercise, twice-daily urine testing, and daily insulin injections. Her goals were to be pain-free, insulin-free, and in better control of her diabetes. These goals and a sense of helplessness and loneliness during the previous year motivated her to seek help.

Planning and intervention. Weighing the driving and restraining forces and the fact that L.S. sought help indicated at least minimal openness to change. She had a need to feel that she could have some control over her situation.

To preserve credibility, the professional avoided giving false hope. L.S.'s first two goals were not immediately attainable. Her peripheral neuropathy had not resolved and was refractory to medication. She had not responded to weight loss with the usual reduction in insulin requirement. There could be no guarantee that the goals of eliminating the pain of neuropathy and of discontinuing insulin could be reached. However, better diabetic control was probably attainable. Her many restraining forces worked against this goal attainment.

All these factors, her frustration at seeing her condition worsen in spite of efforts, and the blow of her mother's death were discussed with L.S. Acknowledging that the power to make choices was clearly L.S.'s allowed the professional to state concern about some of these choices. Specifically, the professional was concerned about the potential danger of L.S.'s not revealing her diabetes to coworkers, her withdrawal and increasing isolation following her mother's death, and the inadequacy of her support system. Nurturing could be provided during the change process, but the need to cultivate support outside this relationship was also explored.

The discussion led to an agreement to meet eight to ten times over a period of three months to try ways to meet L.S.'s goals. More specifically, L.S. agreed to keep a food diary over the following week, and the professional agreed to arrange to show her a teaching film on diabetes she had requested. Jointly, they planned to analyze the food diary by the basic four food groups.

Evaluation. After three meetings, the professional had succeeded in establishing a working relationship with L.S., who voiced a willingness to engage in some change. Some attainable goals were established. L.S. was comfortable asserting her limits with the professional and with carrying the responsibility for her decisions. She also showed willingness to hear other points of view.

create change in someone else. The client must be willing to identify goals and discuss means and barriers to reaching them. A willingness to discuss specifics of effecting one change is a beginning. Persistent problems in any of the areas discussed are manifestations of resistance and are treated accordingly.

If the terms of the relationship are not acceptable to all parties, they should be renegotiated until a satisfactory arrangement is reached. Sometimes the

TABLE 11-2. Moving

Assessment	Planning	Intervention	Evaluation
Assessment in the moving phase overlaps evaluation in the unfreezing phase.	Goal: Effect a specific plan with the client	Goal: Continue to maintain motivation	Goal: Identify progress toward goal achievement
	Always collaborative, never imposed	Acknowledgment of client's efforts	Review of evaluation tool(s)
	Specific goals behaviorally stated	Empathetic listening to feelings	Acknowledgment of changes proceeding
	Logistics included (how? where? by whom? how often? with what?)	Continued exploration of safe variations in self-management	Exploration of difficult areas
		Continued content and skills teaching	Exploration of feelings toward success and difficulties
	Rewards identified if desired		
			Exploration of new change projects
	Evaluation tools (diary, verbal report, etc.) identified		Others' responses to change
	Plan for specific teaching clarified		New needs for teaching skills and content
	Communication channels identified		Effectiveness of communication channels
	Family communication		
	Professional		
	Physician		
	Community resources explored		

most effective way to deal with a family group is to work primarily with the person most stressed and most committed to seeking change (Fisch, Weakland, & Segal 1982), since change in one person in the family system is certain to have an impact on the others. For example, if a client who has obstructive lung disease continues to smoke, working with a nagging family in reducing the pressures they place on the client may be beneficial. When such pressure lessens, the client may no longer feel the need to assert autonomy in self-destructive ways.

The case study of L.S. illustrates the collaborative nature of the normative-reeducative strategy. In this strategy, power to make arbitrary demands of the

client does not reside in the change agent role. Change occurs because its value is demonstrated to professional and client.

Moving. During the moving phase of the change process (see Table 11-2), the client tries different ways of viewing and handling situations. When the professional determines that unfreezing has occurred, the process of moving begins. The professional's role in this phase is to orchestrate new approaches to the client's problems. The client participates by expressing ideas and opinions. Progress may be rapid when the client is motivated and experiences no conflict. If only knowledge and skills are lacking, a teaching program representing empirical-rational change can be planned and implemented with the client and family.

When normative-reeducative strategies are indicated, the professional's challenge is to help the client launch changes identified in unfreezing while gaining the experiences necessary to continue to unfreeze attitudes, beliefs, and role definitions. Trials to test the validity of various solutions to problems the individual is experiencing or to family interaction and coping difficulties should be encouraged. Clients may use the professional or others as models when trying out new attitudes and values. Since clients generally need to discuss changing perceptions, attitudes, and values as they emerge, professionals can encourage such discussion by using communication techniques to elicit changes implied in clients' conversations. The normative-reeducative process helps clients clarify their stance and validates the importance of clarification.

The professional should encourage launching some change that is likely to succeed in order to enhance the client's belief in the ability to change. The importance of helping the client experience success cannot be overemphasized, especially when previous experiences have been demoralizing. If motivation and courage to seek new solutions to problems are to be maintained, repeated failure must be avoided.

When the strategy selected is contingency contracting, the professional's role is to help identify the behavior that is the client's goal and to classify it into steps. As described earlier, each step is then reinforced until the overall goal is reached (Steckel 1982).

A number of tactics are effective with any strategy. One such tactic is cuing, a behaviorist concept, and its variations. A *cue* is a signal that stimulates behavior (Steckel 1982); for example, some people associate finishing a meal with lighting a cigarette. Sending reminders cues desirable behavior: reminders may be sent to encourage clients to keep appointments or to ensure that they take medication at the appropriate time (Dunbar, Marshall, & Hovell 1979). *Tailoring*, fitting a prescribed regimen to the client's unique

circumstances, also incorporates cuing. Finding a convenient time for administration of medication may well connect it to some daily event that then becomes a cue (Dunbar, Marshall, & Hovell 1979). Whether cuing occurs or not, fitting a regimen to the client's circumstance reduces disruption of the client's daily life.

Feedback is another tactic that is effective in promoting choices conducive to health. Haynes, Taylor, and Sackett (1979) noted that when drug serum levels were reported to clients, their compliance with medication regimens increased. Dunbar, Marshall, and Hovell (1979) cite studies that indicate that self-monitoring increases compliance to treatment programs. Sonksen, Judd, and Lowy (1980) found that home blood glucose monitoring improved the home management techniques of diabetics. On the other hand, Nathan's work (1983) indicated that monitoring and home management deteriorated when close supervision by a health team was discontinued.

Teaching, a time-honored tactic, is the focus of Chapter 12. Other tactics usually appropriate regardless of strategy are *supportive listening* and *celebration* when the client reports a success.

Planning and Intervention. Planning in the moving phase requires that the client and professional be committed to a specific trial solution. Again, details are planned explicitly, tactics are selected, evaluative tools are chosen, and communication channels are identified. The use of community resources for financial support, supplies, respite care, and the like are appropriate considerations at this point.

Once the plan is in effect, the professional's goals are to provide emotional support during the trial, to help fine-tune the solution being tested, and to provide information and skills training necessary to implement the plan. During this phase, clients' efforts must be acknowledged by others, including professionals, family, and friends. Clients must also be able to express their negative and positive feelings about the new solution; expression of these responses guides the fine-tuning that occurs during intervention. Minor changes in the plan smooth out problems that could not have been anticipated. Finally, new

◇ CASE STUDY ◇
L.S.: Moving

Planning and intervention. For the sake of clarity, only changes in L.S.'s dietary habits are described here, although many changes eventually took place. The decision about dietary changes had been initiated during the unfreezing phase. L.S. recorded her food intake, and it revealed inconsistent eating times as well as insufficient foods from the following groups: milk, vegetables, and bread. With this information, L.S. elected to increase her vegetable intake; in the following week, her food diary revealed an increase in vegetable intake. L.S. next elected to improve the regularity of meal times and to invite a neighbor for tea and a homemade sugar-free treat.

After achieving these goals in her dietary management, L.S. decided to purchase a sugar-free snack to take to a staff party at work. These events had always been a strain because of the pressure from coworkers to eat sweets. This party was much more pleasant, and L.S. felt less alienated from her coworkers. She reported, "I felt kind of in with them."

During the eighth week, because of urine test results, L.S. began to reshuffle her meal and snack patterns to prevent glycosuria. She had begun sporadic urine testing earlier and was now testing three times daily. Clearly, her dietary management was much improved. Her weight remained stable.

Evaluation. Over the eight-week period L.S. made many changes recorded in her diary, which she chose to expand. It now included not only food intake but urine test results, leisure activities, chores, and social contacts. The professional always listened attentively to the information presented and helped L.S. interpret it in light of her goals. She felt no pressure from the professional to incorporate all this information.

L.S.'s sense of control increased greatly over this time. Initially she was very discouraged but had now progressed to testing various meal patterns in light of urine test results. Her grief work continued, and she was able to inventory her mother's belongings and to dispose of them.

Other areas of improvement included a modest exercise program of using an exercycle occasionally and adding an evening insulin injection after she had learned to take the materials to work in a way that maintained her privacy. Another area in which L.S. made progress was in cultivating a support system. During the moving phase, she began not only to accept invitations but to extend them.

An area that remained problematic was L.S.'s comfort level. She began to use distraction to cope with her pain but continued to fear the regular use of nonnarcotic analgesics. She would not discuss this point with her physician.

---

skills and knowledge are frequently necessary to implement a new solution.

Evaluation. After the trial has been started and fine-tuned, its effectiveness must be evaluated. The point of evaluation is to decide whether to proceed with the solution being tested, to modify it, or to begin again. This represents a major decision point in the change process. Usually, the client has several changes concurrently in motion, and the extent of challenge must be evaluated. If some changes are particularly difficult, others can be temporarily abandoned, and the converse is also true. The maxim here, as always, is to help the client to see progress and to enjoy successes.

The professional must explore not only the client's response to change projects but the responses of family and even coworkers. The adequacy of communication channels among the client, health team, and loved ones must be ascertained. Needs for further teaching must also be identified. When none of these parameters indicates the need for further work, the client has moved to the refreezing phase of change.

Several change tactics were used during the planning and intervention phase of L.S.'s dietary project. The diary served as a self-monitoring tool that also provided feedback from the professional. Feedback about dietary adequacy led L.S. to learn about nutrition and the relationship of food intake to insulin

TABLE 11-3. Refreezing

Assessment	Planning	Intervention	Evaluation
Assessment in the refreezing phase overlaps evaluation in the moving phase.	Goal: Identify mechanisms to stabilize change Future checkpoints for client self-evaluation Minimizing anticipated threats to change Ongoing support from loved ones, for loved ones	Goal: Provide closure for the relationship Review of work done Review of changes made Review of plan for stabilization Review of accessibility of health care team	Goal: Assess comfort with continuing independent function Stated level of confidence in independent decision making Stated level of confidence in maintaining new health practices Demonstrated ability to make decisions consistent with goals Demonstrated level of support

injections. The project proceeded in small, achievable steps. The professional spent a considerable amount of time listening to and celebrating with L.S.

The overall strategy for this change was normative-reeducative. The change involved L.S.'s relationships with others, the values she held about specifics of dietary management, and her beliefs about her own ability to change. Planning was collaborative, and L.S.'s limits were honored.

Refreezing. The refreezing phase begins when the changes are acceptable to the client and others who are affected by them. The professional's role in this phase is to help anticipate and plan for future threats to new behaviors, to conduct a final evaluation of the changes' impact on the client's life, and to provide for closure on this project, if not on the relationship (see Table 11-3).

Planning and Intervention. The professional's goal during the refreezing stage is to identify with the client those mechanisms that will stabilize the accomplished changes. Since change has not occurred by drift, establishing checkpoints for the future will help the client monitor for reappearance of old problems and behaviors. This process may not include the professional or may be associated with follow-up visits, depending on the nature of the relationship.

Another stabilizing factor is planning ways to deal with predictable threats to the change. Threats that emerged during the moving phase are likely to recur, and threats that were not present during moving may be anticipated. Exercise routines and diets, for example, are affected by holiday schedules. Parts of a regimen that require the time and energy of another person may be difficult to arrange at busy times. Help provided by others runs the gamut from dependency for total care to assistance with procedures such as postural drainage and percussion. The task here is to *plan* ways to handle these situations without abandoning the new behavior.

For the client who depends on others to perform health routines, the need for support is obvious. Even the client whose management is independent needs continued support and consideration from those who are close. The professional may want to use anticipatory guidance to help the family plan methods

◇ CASE STUDY ◇
L.S.: Refreezing

Planning and intervention. Since L.S. attributed her previous ability to cope to her mother's encouragement, the major thrust at stabilizing L.S.'s changes focused on her need for supportive others. To allow L.S. more independence while she was still seeing the professional, the last three meetings spanned a period of six weeks. She had also been supported in her efforts to reestablish acquaintances and friendships throughout the project.

Positive changes that L.S. reported at the last meeting were that she was still eating three meals daily with special attention to vegetable intake, that her weight was stable at 145 pounds, and that she had maintained her urine testing two to three times per day. She had achieved glycemic control sufficient that the physician no longer advised the second insulin injection. L.S. had discussed her diabetes with her supervisor at work. Areas in which change had not been accomplished were

discouragement about her pain, avoidance of exercise because she did not feel well, and increased social withdrawal since the moving phase. Some behaviors appeared to have refrozen; others did not.

Evaluation. Evaluation was speculative since the relationship between L.S. and the professional was designed to be short-term. L.S. maintained many new health habits consistent with new goals, as noted. However, she showed some reversion to old ways in that final meeting. The most worrisome implication is that it may have reflected an increase in L.S.'s use of avoidance coping. During the moving phase L.S. had become an aggressive, constructive problem solver. She had developed a measure of confidence in her ability to devise and try new solutions to old problems. In the final meeting some of the old problems seemed to have been reasserting themselves.

---

for coping with imaginary conflict scenarios. Support for family members must not be overlooked. Continued use of community resources, the health care team, and nurturing from other family and friends should be explored and encouraged.

The plan in the refreezing phase is future-oriented, so intervention may be devoted to closure for the project or the relationship, including a review of the work invested in the changes made by both professional and client. Reviewing the plan for stabilization may also be appropriate, as may reiterating the accessibility of support to the client and family.

Evaluation. If the professional has a short-term relationship with the client, evaluating the refreezing phase will be speculative. One may infer probability of refreezing from the client's confidence in decision making and ability to maintain new behavior and demonstrated capacity to make decisions consistent with stated goals. Finally, the support and encouragement available to the client are critical to predicting the extent of refreezing.

If the client and professional have an ongoing relationship (for instance, if the professional works in a clinic), evaluation of refreezing is easier and more

precise. One can ascertain the extent to which new behaviors, attitudes, or role relationships have actually become norms in the client's life. Another factor that can be examined under these circumstances is the long-term impact of the changes: Have the client's vigor and comfort improved, or deterioration at least slowed? If not, one could legitimately question the value of the complicated treatment regimen.

The Change Process in Episodic Settings

Although much of the health care delivered to people having chronic illness occurs in ambulatory care settings, professionals working in acute care hospitals also have large numbers of clients with chronic illnesses. Change as a framework for decision making can also be helpful in that environment.

The principles used for decision making are the same. For example, in the unfreezing phase, the approach involves minimizing restraining forces and maximizing driving forces. A significant difference, though, is the length of the client-professional relationship, since the client usually remains in this setting for a short period of time. The change process cannot usually be observed from beginning to refreezing. Forcing the process is not likely to result in sustained, integrated changes. Indeed, most changes cannot possibly be integrated until they are tested and modified in the client's daily life. These factors make referrals to community agencies for follow-up doubly important.

This framework, applied to the acute setting, lays out the stepwise nature of change. Once professionals accept that the process of change cannot be pushed, they more readily adopt reasonable, achievable goals with clients. If the client has progressed only to the unfreezing phase by discharge, acceptance and appropriate referral are the best choice. Reaching unfreezing may represent giant strides for client and professional and may not reflect unsatisfactory management.

Summary and Conclusions

The change process has been described as a tool for clinical decision making for health professionals. Change may be imperceptible or a conscious, sometimes anxiety-laden process. The phases advance from unfreezing to moving to refreezing. In all phases, the change agent's goal is to strengthen driving forces and to weaken restraining forces, especially during unfreezing and moving.

Several strategies are useful for implementing these approaches. Normative-reeducative strategies are indicated when values, attitudes, or significant relationships are in conflict with the proposed changes. The empirical-rational strategies work when the client's needs are primarily informational. Power-coercive strategies are used when a dependent client needs a strong advocate. Behaviorist techniques, based on operant conditioning, are effective when the client's stated knowledge, attitudes, and values are in concert with change, but the client's behavior is not.

Since families and supportive others are important to the management of a person's chronic illness, normative-reeducative change is most often the strategy of choice. It takes into account the changes in role relationships and family norms often seen with chronic illness.

The change process is applicable to any sector of the health care delivery system by a variety of professionals and can be used to temper the professional's expectations of the client and of self. More helpful, realistic interventions by the professional result.

Whatever the nature of the change, helping the client respond to it can and should be planned. Planned change is deliberate, is collaborative, has direction, and involves integrating the old with the new. Planned change takes into account implications of the change at all levels of the client system. Based on scientific principles (Menke 1977; Brooten, Hayman, & Naylor 1978), the process has as its goal the improved functioning of that client system.

STUDY QUESTIONS

1. What are the historical highlights relating to change as a strategy for health care providers?
2. How does drift differ from conscious change?
3. How does Lewin's model differ from the approach of behaviorists? What are the components of each?
4. Discuss professional ethics in relation to change.
5. What factors influence resistance to change?
6. How does change demoralize people? erode support systems?
7. What are the differences between normative-reeducative strategies, empirical-rational strategies, power-coercive strategies, and contingency contracting?
8. How could each of the strategies in question 7 be used to create change? What conditions and factors would influence your choice?
9. What roles and behaviors are appropriate for a change agent?
10. If you were managing a client's situation in which change was important, how would you determine the change needed, the strategy to be used, the way your plan would be carried out, and the means of evaluation you would use?

References

Bailey, B. J., (1983) Using change theory to help the diabetic, *The Diabetes Educator, 9*(3):37–39, 56

Benne, K., (1976) The current state of planned changing in persons, groups, communities and societies, in Bennis, W., Benne, K., Chin, R., and Corey, K. (eds.), *The Planning of Change* (3d ed.), New York: Holt, Rinehart & Winston

Brooten, D. A., Hayman, L., and Naylor, M., (1978) *Leadership for Change: A Guide for the Frustrated Nurse*, New York: Lippincott

Chin, R., and Benne, K., (1976) General strategies for effecting changes in human systems, in Bennis, W., Benne, K., Chin, R., and Corey, K. (eds.), *The Planning of Change* (3d ed.), New York: Holt, Rinehart & Winston

Dunbar, J. M., Marshall, G. D., and Hovell, M., (1979) Behavioral strategies for improving compliance, in Haynes, R. B., Taylor, D. W., and Sackett, D. (eds.), *Compliance in Health Care*, Baltimore: Johns Hopkins University Press

Edwards, V., (1980) Changing breast self-examination behavior, *Nursing Research, 29*:301–306

Fisch, R., Weakland, J. H., and Segal, L., (1982) *The Tactics of Change: Doing Therapy Briefly*, San Francisco: Jossey-Bass

Goldstein, V., Regnery, G., and Wellin, E., (1981) Caretaker role fatigue, *Nursing Outlook, 29*:24–30

Haynes, R. B., (1979) Strategies to improve compliance with referrals, appointments and prescribed medical regimens, in Haynes, R., Taylor, D. W., and Sackett, D. (eds.), *Compliance in Health Care*, Baltimore: Johns Hopkins University Press

Jonsen, A. R., (1979) Ethical issues in compliance, in Haynes, R. B., Taylor, D. W., and Sackett, D. (eds.), *Compliance in Health Care*, Baltimore: Johns Hopkins University Press

Klein, D., (1969) Some notes on the dynamics of resistance to change: The defender role, in Bennis, W., Benne, K., and Chin, R. (eds.), *The Planning of Change* (2d ed.), New York: Holt, Rinehart & Winston

Korhonen, T., Huttunen, J., Aro, A., Hentinen, M., Ihalainen, O., Majander, H., Siitonen, O., Uusitupa, M., and Pyorala, K., (1983) A controlled trial on the effects of patient education in the treatment of insulin-dependent diabetes, *Diabetes Care, 6*:256–261

Lancaster, J., and Lancaster, W., (1982) *Concepts for Advanced Nursing Practice: The Nurse as Change Agent*, St. Louis: C. V. Mosby

Lauer, P., Murphy, S., and Powers, M., (1982) Learning needs of cancer patients: A comparison of nurse and patient perceptions, *Nursing Research, 31*:11–16

Lewin, K., (1958) Group decision and social changes, in Maccoby, E., Newcomb, T., and Hartley, E. (eds.), *Readings in Social Psychology*, New York: Holt, Rinehart & Winston

Lippitt, G. L., (1973) *Visualizing Change: Model Building and the Change Process*, La Jolla, Calif.: University Associates

Mauksch, I., and Miller, M., (1981) *Implementing Change in Nursing*, St. Louis: C.V. Mosby

Mazzuca, S., (1982) Does patient education in chronic disease have therapeutic value? *Journal of Chronic Disease, 35*:521–529

Menke, E., (1977) Persistence, change and crisis, in Hall, J., and Weaver, B. (eds.), *Distributive Nursing Practice: A Systems Approach to Community Health*, Philadelphia: Lippincott

Nathan, D. M., (1983) The importance of intensive supervision in determining the efficacy of insulin pump therapy, *Diabetes Care, 6*:295–297

Pray, L. M., (1983) My struggle with acceptance, *Diabetes Forecast*, May–June, pp. 14, 16

Rappsilber, C., (1982) Persuasion as a mechanism for change, in Lancaster, J., and Lancaster, W. (eds.), *Concepts for Advanced Nursing Practice: The Nurse as Change Agent*, St. Louis: C.V. Mosby

Reinkemeyer, A., (1970) Nursing's need: Commitment to an ideology of change, *Nursing Forum, 9*(4):340–350

Rosenstock, I. M., (1974) Historical origins of the health belief model, *Health Education Monographs, 2*:328–335

Schein, D., (1969) The mechanisms of change, in Bennis, W., Benne, K., and Chin, R. (eds.), *The Planning of Change* (2d ed.), New York: Holt, Rinehart & Winston

Sonksen, P. H., Judd, S., and Lowy, C., (1980) Home monitoring of blood glucose: New approach to management of insulin-dependent diabetes patients in Great Britain, *Diabetes Care, 3*:100–107

Steckel, S. B., (1982) *Patient Contracting*, Norwalk, Conn.: Appleton-Century-Crofts

Watzlawick, P., Weakland, J., and Fisch, R., (1974) *Change: Principles of Problem Formation and Problem Resolution*, New York: W.W. Norton

CHAPTER TWELVE
Teaching

Introduction

Health professionals have found that teaching is an important method of increasing knowledge and achieving behavioral changes that help clients cope with chronic diseases. However, teaching does not always guarantee attainment of the long-term adaptation necessary for effective management. Even when teaching initially seems successful, problems may arise indicating that the desired integration of behavior, knowledge, and skills was not accomplished. This chapter addresses many of these problems and explores possible solutions.

Review of the Teaching-Learning Process

Teaching intended to create change in a client's adaptation to chronic illness is a planned activity individualized to the learner's abilities, needs, resources, and support systems. To achieve a positive outcome, this teaching process becomes an interaction between the health educator and one or more clients. It encompasses several steps: (1) assessment, (2) planning, (3) implementation, and (4) evaluation.

Information collection in a teaching-learning *assessment* helps the teacher plan and implement teaching activities. Assessment data should include information about the learner's readiness and ability to learn, the learner's previous knowledge of the subject, what the learner wants to know about the subject, any incorrect information or misconceptions held by the learner, and educational needs of both learner and family.

Planning involves developing goals; determining when, where, and how the teaching process will occur; and developing a method of evaluation. It should be noted that successful outcomes are more likely when the learner is involved in the planning phase of the teaching process. *Implementation* is the actual process of teaching and utilizes a variety of teaching methods and tools. *Evaluation* enables the teacher to ascertain whether learning has occurred; it is basically a feedback loop determined by the method of evaluation developed during planning.

Review of Teaching-Learning Principles

Individual client education plans are based on identified teaching and learning principles (Pohl 1978) (see Table 12-1). These principles are not reviewed here; presumably the reader has some familiarity with them. In-depth information about the teaching-learning process, the principles of learning, and the principles of teaching is available in the teaching texts listed in the references and bibliography at the end of this chapter.

Learning Styles: Pedagogical versus Androgogical Learning

Learning is classified as either *pedagogical* or *androgogical* on the basis of various assumptions

TABLE 12-1. Teaching and Learning Principles

1. Perception is necessary for learning.
2. Conditioning is a process of learning.
3. Learning often occurs by trial and error.
4. Learning may occur through imitation.
5. Concept development is part of the learning process.
6. Motivation is necessary for learning.
7. Physical and mental readiness are necessary for learning.
8. Active participation is necessary for effective learning.
9. New learning must be based on previous knowledge and experience.
10. Learning is affected by the individual's emotional climate.
11. Repetition and reinforcement strengthen learning.
12. Success reinforces learning.
13. Good teacher-learner rapport is important in teaching.
14. Teaching requires effective communication.
15. Learning needs of clients must be determined.
16. Objectives serve as guides in planning and evaluating teaching.
17. Planning time is required for effective teaching and learning.
18. Control of the environment is an aspect of teaching.
19. Teaching skill can be acquired through practice and observation.
20. Evaluating effectiveness is a part of teaching.

Summarized from Pohl, M. L., (1973) The Teaching Function of the Nursing Practitioner *(2d ed.), Dubuque, Ill.: Brown*

about the characteristics of the learner. Originally, pedagogy was defined as the art and science of teaching children, and androgogy as the art and science of helping adults learn. However, pedagogy and androgogy can be seen as the two ends of a spectrum, with actual teaching-learning interactions falling somewhere in between (Knowles 1980).

Knowles (1980) lists several assumptions that underlie pedagogical learning. The first is that the learner is in a dependent role; the teacher takes full responsibility for determining the content, the point at which topics are introduced, the manner in which they are presented, and the student's success in learning the material. The second assumption is that learners' experiences have limited value, whereas the experiences of the teacher or other experts are highly valuable to the student. The third assumption is that people are ready to learn when society says they ought to learn. And the final assumption is that learners see education as a process of acquiring content that will be useful at a later time in life. According to the assumptions of pedagogical learning, the teacher, without input from the learner, develops the teaching plan in terms of material to be taught and the time, place, and technique of teaching. The teacher devotes little attention to the learner's past experiences, thoughts, and feelings about the material that needs to be taught.

Androgogical learning is based on a different set of assumptions (Knowles 1980): (1) as persons mature, they move from dependency to increasing self-direction, but different people do so at different rates; (2) as people mature, they accumulate an increasing reservoir of experience that provides a rich resource for learning; (3) people become ready to learn when learning is necessary for coping with a real-life problem or task; and (4) learners consider education a process of developing increased competence to achieve their full potential and want to apply any knowledge they gain to their present living situation. In using these assumptions, the teacher takes into consideration the learner's past experiences, the learner's need for self-direction, and the learner's desire to learn about a particular topic.

Nurses and other health educators use assumptions from both models in client education, although pedagogy predominates. However, careful assessment should be made to determine which set of assumptions is most appropriate to meet the needs of the individual client.

Problems and Issues of Teaching Clients

Since management of a chronic illness is a lifelong undertaking, and since the management plan is often quite complex, successful learning is important to maximize outcomes. When teaching has not achieved desired change, evaluation requires determining the cause. Problems addressed in teaching texts used by health professionals are generally taken into consideration and teaching interventions modified to compensate for them. But other problems occur that are not addressed in standard texts; causes appear more elusive, and clients may be considered noncompliant, but rarely is the ineffectiveness of the teaching considered. Increased awareness of teaching's role as a contributing factor in poor learning performance could enhance the health professionals' ability to evaluate long-term outcomes and to seek long-term solutions.

The tendency to use the pedagogical learning model more than the androgogical model may be based on time and other constraints such as limited awareness of the learner's autonomy and values. The learner is often assumed to be dependent and likely to benefit from teaching. Although assessment occurs, the client's prior experiences (as factors that could potentiate learning) and self-identified learning needs receive less emphasis. The teacher assumes responsibility for determining content and implementing the teaching plan, assuming that the learner will use presented material later. Often this approach leads to successful outcomes.

But the pedagogic method is not always effective. Long-term problems seem to emphasize the importance of androgogic learning—that is, encouraging client self-direction and responsibility. Androgogic teaching plans more readily take into account what the client is ready and willing to learn in order to cope with client-identified long-term needs or problems. In addition, more complete integration of prior experiences allows tailoring of teaching plans to variations in rates of learning and differences in life-style and need.

Regardless of which teaching model is determined more effective for long-term success, the health professional must be more sensitive to potential problems. Sensitization leads to the achievement of more positive outcomes for the client whose "lack of learning" surfaces after discharge from the acute setting.

Common Problems of the Learner

If teaching is to lead to successful change, obstacles within or related to the learner must be identified and eliminated. Common learner problems include lack of readiness, physical and emotional obstacles, language barriers, and lack of motivation. The acute or chronic nature of the disease is not a factor. However, because of the characteristics of chronic illnesses, learner problems may be more frequently present in individuals having such conditions.

Lack of Readiness. *Readiness* is the learner's ability in terms of physical and mental development; readiness in both respects is necessary for effective learning (Pohl 1973). Physical readiness depends primarily on the state of the individual's neuromuscular system and is relevant chiefly to learning physical skills. Performing procedures that require fine motor coordination is impossible for the person who lacks such coordination. Mental readiness depends on the state of the individual's intellectual development; the learner must have sufficient capacity for the learning task, as well as adequate ability to perceive ideas, verbalize thoughts, and conceptualize information needed for learning. If learning is to occur when physical or mental readiness is lacking in the learner, the teaching process must be adapted to the individual's developmental stage or intellectual abilities.

Physical Obstacles. Discomfort, energy limitations, and decreased physical mobility are among the physical obstacles that can hinder learning for any ill person (Narrow 1979; Bille 1981). Pain and nausea are just two of many symptoms that produce *discomfort*. Such symptoms draw the client's attention toward ways of gaining comfort and therefore away from learning about self-management techniques. For example, clients having advanced neoplastic disorders experience pain that is quite severe; until that pain is relieved, learning is blocked.

Clients who have severe energy limitations may focus on meeting basic physiological needs. For example, individuals having chronic obstructive pulmonary disorders often use their limited energy levels to perform basic activities of daily living, with little reserve left for attention to learning activities. However, one must be careful not to assume that no learning has occurred because no obvious involvement has been noted. Individuals may be learning what needs to be learned, but on their own terms.

Physical limitations involving decreased mobility may hamper learning. This is especially true of motor skills that require involvement of the affected extremity. A client having severe rheumatoid arthritis may have difficulty mastering a physical skill requiring use of the hands.

Eliminating physical obstacles to learning is desirable but not always possible. The nurse-educator should assess these obstacles so that the teaching plan will provide necessary adaptation. Premedication may relieve nausea or pain, timing for high energy levels can provide available reserves for learning, and modification of equipment can compensate for lost physical mobility. In short, timing of teaching and plan flexibility allow individuals to circumvent physical obstacles.

Emotional Obstacles. Numerous emotional obstacles affect readiness or ability to learn. These include denial of the condition, anger, depression and withdrawal, and anxiety. In addition, lowered self-esteem may impede learning.

Denial is a normal coping mechanism that individuals use when they face overwhelming situations. For instance, denial occurs when a serious or irreversible illness is diagnosed. Clients often think, "This might happen to others, but not to me," or "It can't be as bad as my doctor says it is." Teaching self-care management is ineffective during denial because affected individuals cannot yet accept the presence or seriousness of the illness and place little value on learning to understand and manage the condition.

Anger is often present when the client begins to accept that something is wrong and that the identified chronic illness is really present. Hostility against health care providers and family is a common reaction during this phase of coping with illness. Teaching efforts are often met with angry responses or signs of hostility. The teacher should realize that anger is a normal reaction and should not argue with, or belittle, the feelings of the learner (Bille 1981). More effective would be working with the client to resolve the anger and then beginning the teaching process.

Depression is also a coping mechanism that clients having chronic illnesses use. Depression is a reaction to the loss of valued health and well-being. Withdrawal sometimes results from this depression. While experiencing depression, clients tend to give little attention to ongoing activities, demonstrate a decreased ability to concentrate, and spend time sleeping or sitting quietly by themselves (Miller 1983). Although these responses are not necessarily negative, the client displays little interest in learning about the illness or about self-management during depression or withdrawal.

Anxiety associated with illness can obstruct learning. Fear based on an identifiable factor, such as pain or surgery, can lead to anxiety that is more free-floating. Should anxiety be unrelieved, it can become severe. Severe anxiety, in turn, limits an individual's perception of events that are occurring; attention focuses on relieving the anxiety rather than on learning (Redman 1980). For example, a newly diagnosed diabetic may be unable to master the skills of diabetic self-care, such as urine testing and diet control, because of anxiety over self-administering insulin injections.

When lowered self-esteem is displayed by persons having chronic illness, it may become an obstacle to the teaching-learning process. Lowered self-esteem leads to doubts about abilities or to feelings of inferiority, ineffectiveness, or insignificance. Consequently, lowered self-esteem can impede the client's ability to set goals or the client's sense of competence (Miller 1983). Individuals who have low self-esteem may not believe that they are capable of performing the self-care tasks required for management of chronic illnesses. In turn, their confidence about mastering such tasks decreases.

Dealing with emotional obstacles to learning requires identifying them during the assessment process. Initially, teaching must focus on coping with and managing the activities of today rather than on following a future self-management plan. Learning to deal with present-day activities can sometimes help clients decrease fear and depression and increase confidence in their ability to manage the illness.

Language Barriers. Language barriers have several sources (Bille 1981; Narrow 1979). First is a difference in primary language between the learner and teacher. When teacher and learner use different languages, someone should be located who can speak the client's language so that the teaching plan can be implemented. Second, the learner may have limited mastery of the language used by the health educator. Health care providers sometimes forget that clients do not know the meaning of many medical words used daily in health care agencies. Lack of familiarity can be overcome by using terms more familiar to the learner. Third, the extent and type of the client's educational background influence the person's comprehension of the teaching plan. Assessment of language limitations caused by lower educational attainment leads to identifying an appropriate language level for the learner.

The reader is cautioned to remember that lack of response to teaching does not necessarily indicate limited learning capability. Rather, limited response can reflect fear of appearing "dumb" by acknowledging that terms being used are unfamiliar. Feedback can assure the teacher that the client understands the terminology being used.

Motivation. Motivation is essential if learning is to occur. Motivation increases when the individual develops a desire to understand the illness, to begin self-care, to find ways to avoid complications, to please others, or to enjoy a higher level of wellness (Narrow 1979). Behavior that indicates an individual's motivational level may be difficult to identify without a thorough assessment.

Redman (1980) lists general principles of motivation that are applicable to teaching-learning situations:

1. Incentives motivate learning.
2. Internal motivation lasts longer and is more self-directive than external motivation.
3. Learning is most effective when the learner feels a need to know.
4. Motivation is enhanced by the organization of the material.
5. Success is more predictably motivating than failure.
6. A mild level of anxiety is useful in motivating individuals, but severe anxiety is incapacitating.

Although these principles help in motivating the client, adequate incentive to learn may be lacking if the individual has no internal inducement based on self-need.

Developmental Level and Life Cycle Influences on Learning

Age-related differences can influence ability to learn. These differences are most apparent when teaching a young child or an elderly person, and they point out the need for some consideration of the influence of an individual's developmental level on the teaching-learning process.

Factors That Influence Learning in the Young. The teaching-learning process involving a young child has problems that are not present in working with an adult. These problems are due to the physical and intellectual development level of the child. To promote effective learning, one must assess the child's developmental level in terms of communication ability, level of understanding, attention span, memory, and physical ability to perform necessary tasks. After a thorough assessment of the child's abilities, one can make an informed decision about whether the teaching should primarily involve the child alone, the family (or person responsible for the child's well-being), or both the child and the family.

Ability to communicate, capacity to understand concepts, and attention span vary among children, even children in similar age groups. As a child's ability to communicate increases, the effectiveness of the teaching-learning interaction with that child increases correspondingly. Children must have sufficient vocabulary to ask questions, verbalize understanding, and clarify and verify the information being taught. The child's ability to understand concepts is closely related to communication ability. Normally, at about age 5, the child begins to talk comprehensively, asks the meaning of words, is capable of memorizing, and is able to follow three-step directions in the proper sequence (Schuster & Ashburn 1980). These skills progress rapidly as the child grows older.

The ability to attend is considered an important factor in the learning process (Schuster & Ashburn 1980). Since attention span increases with age, the older the child, the longer the attention span. To promote maximum learning, teaching should be planned in segments that accommodate the child's actual attention span. For example, teaching a toddler or preschooler is best done in five- to ten-minute segments, whereas teaching a school-age child may involve thirty- to forty-minute segments.

Since learning cannot occur without the retention and recall of past experiences, memory plays a major role in learning. Memory is also necessary for conceptualization (Schuster & Ashburn 1980). Obviously, the younger the child, the more limited the memory; therefore, teaching must be geared at an appropriate level for the child, given that child's ability to remember the material.

Physical growth is another consideration in teaching the young child. The very young child, who has not developed fine motor coordination, cannot master the same kinds of tasks that the older, more coordinated child can. When teaching a physical skill to a child, the nurse educator must determine if the child's motor skills have progressed to an appropriate level for mastery. Insufficient motor development impedes learning and produces frustration and a sense of failure for both the learner and the teacher (Schuster & Ashburn 1980).

Factors That Influence Learning in the Elderly.
Older people are motivated to learn and to engage in activities that they consider meaningful but do not perform well when learning tasks they view as irrelevant or unnecessary (Hogstel 1981). Older people learn better when they can pace learning so as to monitor both the rate and amount of incoming stimuli. They tend to be cautious and hesitant in new learning situations and commit omission errors rather than performance errors, reflecting a need to be certain of the outcome of their activities before acting. Factors that affect ability to learn in the elderly are related to physiological and memory changes that occur with aging.

Physiological Changes Affecting Learning. Although sensory changes occur throughout the entire life span, decreases become apparent in the middle years and are progressive throughout the remainder of an individual's life. For example, the sense of touch is decreased in the elderly person (Hogstel 1981) so that evaluating externally applied heat becomes difficult. Should heat be applied to joints affected by rheumatoid arthritis, a burn may result.

Change in visual abilities begins in middle age and continues into the older years, although most older people retain good to adequate visual acuity (Kornzweig 1979). Color discrimination, especially of the blue-violet hues, decreases because of yellowing of the lens (Storandt 1979), although discrimination of red-yellow hues continues. Depth perception is also altered as a result of decreased elasticity of the lens (Storandt 1979). Nursing educators must confirm that older adults can read any written teaching material presented and also must consider colors that they use for teaching purposes.

Age-related hearing loss, called *presbycusis,* is more apparent in high tones (Storandt 1979; Hogstel 1981). Presbycusis also influences speech intelligibility, impeding comprehension. When communicating with older individuals who have hearing losses, the teacher should sit or stand directly facing the learner, talk slowly, enunciate clearly, and eliminate background noises such as radios or television. Voice volume should not be raised, since this change tends also to raise the tone, and higher tones are the most difficult for older people to hear.

Endurance and muscle strength also gradually decrease with aging (Hogstel 1981), although most older people can continue to perform daily activities. Changes in endurance and strength affect physical skills that are involved in learning activities and exercises related to the client's particular chronic condition. Also present in some older persons is a decreased sense of balance, particularly when rising quickly or acting rapidly (Hogstel 1981). Balance should be considered in relation to activity level of the individual, and individuals should be instructed to get up or to begin activities slowly.

Cardiovascular changes that accompany aging include decreased cardiac output and stroke volume; these changes do not adversely affect the individual's ability in daily functioning. Some older people develop atheroscleroses (Hogstel 1981) with associated decreased blood flow to the brain that alters cognitive functioning or decreases alertness; the individual's ability to absorb and process information can, therefore, be affected. Assessing the individual's level of cognition and alertness should precede teaching; after each teaching-learning session, retention of the material, especially by individuals known to have cognitive impairment, should be evaluated.

Memory Changes.   Although older persons seem to undergo minimal impairment of their ability to recall events of the distant past, a weakening in short-term memory or in the recall of recently learned information tends to occur. The greatest memory change associated with aging seems to be related to the type of recall used to form new associations (Hogstel 1981). Since some decrease in short-term memory apparently occurs, the dissemination of information needs to be planned at a slower pace and be reinforced more frequently.

Lack of Compliance

The issue of noncompliance to a prescribed therapeutic plan has been identified by health care providers as a significant problem in working with chronically ill individuals. Even when health care educators provide specific and thorough teaching to improve health and manage illness, clients often do not follow the plan presented. The complexity of factors that influence compliance has been extensively studied, but many of these studies have conflicting results. Although problems related to compliance exist, these issues will not be addressed in this chapter; the reader will find a more extensive discussion of noncompliance in Chapter 7.

Locus of Control.   One theory that seems to influence compliance is *locus of control,* a construct based on the assumption that an individual's beliefs about factors that influence health may be related to that individual's health behaviors (Smith & Carson 1981). People having an internal locus of control ("internals") are individuals who believe that their health is largely determined by their own behaviors and actions. "Externals" believe that their health is determined by factors outside their control, such as fate, chance, or other people; consequently, they tend to feel powerless or helpless in managing their illness. It is important that the client's beliefs about control of his or her health status be ascertained before teaching begins. If the client is an "internal," teaching may need to encourage client follow-through on necessary externally imposed regimens. If the client is an "external," teaching interventions and strategies should be geared toward assisting the individual to become more "internal" in relation to health care beliefs, or assuring the client that the health professional will be accountable for some aspects of regimen such as scheduling appointments, validating performance, and so forth.

Sociological Influences on Compliance.   The degree of compliance the client demonstrates may be influenced by sociological factors. Interestingly, the literature indicates that client noncompliance is widespread among all socioeconomic groups and occurs in the well-educated client as well as in the illiterate and indigent client (Sarnecky & Sarnecky 1984). However, socioeconomic factors may make compliance more difficult for some clients.

In a study of clients in a chronic renal disease program and their families, Korsch and Negrete

(1980) identified characteristics that were predictive of clients who were at high risk for poor adaptation to the identified treatment program, and specifically predictive of clients who were at high risk for non-compliance with posttransplant immunosuppressive therapy. These characteristics were low family income, absence of a father in the home, a sense of being less happy than other families, poor understanding of the medical condition, and less trust in the medical profession.

Financial Resources. Chronic illness can drain the client and family financially (see Chapter 17). Since most families have financial limitations, economic resources necessary to maintain the treatment regimen may be inadequate in relation to other needs and expenses; clients may begin to seek ways to decrease health care costs. Consequences of this effort to balance needs and finances can result in decreasing or omitting medication dosages, not purchasing needed supplies, reduced compliance with treatment regimens, or discontinuation of the treatment plan (Miller 1983).

Time. Time, like money, is finite for most people. Many treatment plans for chronic illness, such as managing an ulcerative colitis or a cystic fibrosis regimen, are very time consuming. In view of other tasks and activities, the client may decide to modify, adjust, or totally omit the plan of care designed to control symptoms or exacerbations if the time requirements of the regimen are extensive (Strauss et al. 1984).

Life-Style versus Needed Change. A conflict between a client's life-style and identified needed change may cause the individual to abandon the treatment plan. Clients may determine that, even though they understand the risks and results of not managing their symptoms or illness, they would rather accept those risks than institute a change in life-style.

Health care providers should assess factors and adapt the teaching plan to accommodate sociological circumstances that place clients at risk for noncompliance. Interventions that compensate for sociological factors include providing additional support (physical or emotional) and scheduling and encouraging more frequent follow-up visits for reinforcement of teaching.

Dependence/Independence Conflicts and Role Loss

Chronically ill individuals often experience dependence-independence conflicts and role losses that influence their self-esteem and can be obstacles to effective teaching and to mastery of self-care management. In addition, client and family may perceive the progress of the illness differently from the health provider so that willingness to learn is affected.

Dependence-independence conflicts arise because the nature of many illnesses requires that the individual become dependent; for example, clients are dependent on medications (such as insulin), machines (such as for dialysis), equipment (for example, portable oxygen), or other people (caregivers who manage activities of daily living). The need to be dependent that results from illness may be in conflict with the life-style preference or personality of the individual. Conflicts can also arise because health care providers encourage independence on the part of the client even when the client may feel a need to maintain more dependence.

Role loss can impact self-esteem and create a feeling of helplessness. Roles can be lost within the family (a mother who can no longer take care of her child), with a career (an individual who can no longer fulfill job responsibilities), or socially (an individual who can no longer attend enjoyed social activities, such as parties or ballgames, because of the illness). Issues that arise from role losses are best resolved prior to implementing a teaching plan.

Family Influences on Learning

Since the family is the chronically ill individual's major support system, family members may have a significant impact on the individual's ability to manage illness. Family attitudes and reactions to the illness and the treatment plan influence the client's ability to learn about it. Family influence may be positive or negative.

Denial by Family Members. Just as clients use denial when they are informed of serious illness, families also cope in this way (Bille 1981). Like the client, the family needs time to overcome its initial reaction and to accept the illness. If a lack of acceptance continues for a long time, it creates an obstacle to learning about necessary aspects of the treatment plan. Prolonged denial by the family may also encourage continuance of the client's denial.

Sometimes the client accepts the illness but the family continues to deny it. This situation creates difficulty for the client in implementing the treatment plan. Without family support, the individual may feel the need to conceal necessary equipment and medications, or may never purchase them. Follow-up doctor or clinic appointments may not be kept, especially if transportation by family is necessary. Individuals may refrain from discussing the illness with family members, thereby being deprived of the emotional support of those persons most important to them.

Overprotection. If families overprotect the chronically ill individual, learning may be impeded. For example, when chronically ill children are overprotected so that there are major activity restrictions, they begin to feel different from other children. This feeling can lead to frustration, anger, loneliness, or even denial. In an attempt to be like their peers, children may avoid learning or using information or skills necessary to manage their disease.

Decision Making. Involvement in the decision-making process promotes learning of a given treatment plan. However, at times the family or health care providers make all the decisions about management of the illness without input from the client, most frequently with children and the elderly. Without input, the client lacks a sense of control and is less likely to be motivated to learn about the plan or to perform appropriate self-management behaviors.

Problems of the Professional as a Teacher

Even when the learner is motivated and ready to learn, ineffective teaching may impede the integration of knowledge and skills necessary for managing the illness. The professional can contribute to inadequate learning in several ways, including managing the teaching-learning process incorrectly and being unable to override inherent limitations or differences in the relationship with the learner.

Inadequate Assessment. Inadequate assessment often has a number of causes: poor interview or communication skills, inadequate observational skills, time limitations, or failure to consider the learner's home or social environment. The health care provider may also be unaware of when an assessment has not been thorough. Nurse-educators often assume that they know what the learner needs to know; therefore, they do not assess the learner's knowledge or identify misconceptions on the part of the learner.

Individualization of the management plan should be based on each client's personal situation. Clients do not always inform health care providers of problems or limitations that exist in the home or involve their social situation. Therefore, both of these areas should be assessed before development and implementation of the teaching plan. Unless the home environment and social situation are adequate for carrying out the management plan, the client is not likely to follow that plan.

Other Factors That Impede Teaching. Developing and carrying out a teaching plan can be impeded by cost limitations, time constraints, lack of support from the agency administration or physician, and environmental limitations of the teaching setting.

Cost Limitations. As agencies become more cost-conscious, budgets are cut and "nonessential" services are omitted (Redman 1980). Education, unfortunately, sometimes falls into the category of "nonessential." Although the cost of client education is often minimal, some financial support is necessary for the purchase of teaching materials and for salaries. Inadequate or outdated teaching materials obstruct the teaching process. Without adequate financial support, educators, whether involved full or part time, cannot afford to continue teaching.

Time Limitations. Time limitations in the clinical setting pose a major problem for teaching. Usually, diagnostic procedures, activities of daily living, treatments, visits by the physician or various therapists, and other tasks have priority over teaching. It is often assumed that teaching occurs when the client is not busy with this myriad of other activities. As a result, teaching is sometimes neglected or occurs immediately before the client's discharge from the facility, making assimilation of information difficult (Bille 1981).

Lack of Support. Efforts extended toward providing quality teaching often do not receive support from the agency administration or the physician. Unless the administration believes that teaching is as important as other tasks, it probably will be done only in an unplanned, sporadic manner. Some physicians do not want their patients to be fully informed of their condition; others prefer to do all required teaching themselves. Although the physician may do an excellent job of teaching needed information, time limits make effective evaluation difficult. Without the involvement of other health care providers, the client may not receive needed reinforcement or answers to questions that arise when the physician is not present (Bille 1981).

Environmental Limitations. Control of the environment, such as providing privacy, is the responsibility of the teacher in the teaching-learning situation. In a hospital, teaching often occurs in the client's room, which may be shared, with only curtains separating the areas. Since all conversations may be heard by others, learners become reluctant to ask questions and clarify information, or are embarrassed that someone else is hearing all about their problems. Privacy problems may also occur if teaching is performed in the waiting room of a clinic or physician's office while other individuals are within hearing distance. Other environmental factors that the teacher should consider are the temperature of the setting, adequacy of lighting, presence of unnecessary noise, and interruptions. Problems with any of

these factors could lead to less than ideal teaching-learning interactions (Narrow 1979).

Inadequate Evaluation. Another common problem that impedes the teaching-learning process is inadequate evaluation of teaching effectiveness (Narrow 1979). Nurse-educators sometimes believe that transmission of information constitutes teaching and that learning has therefore occurred. A method of evaluation must be developed during the planning step of the teaching-learning process and must follow each teaching session as well as the entire teaching program. Evaluation must include an objective means of determining teaching effectiveness. Asking the client "Do you understand what I have told you?" does not produce an adequate evaluation of learning.

Sociocultural Differences between Teacher and Learner. Sociocultural differences between teacher and learner can impede the teaching-learning process. In this area, the teacher has two responsibilities: (1) being aware of the sociocultural beliefs of the client and incorporating them into the teaching plan, and (2) ensuring that personal sociocultural beliefs or biases do not interfere with teaching (Bille 1981).

Interventions to Improve Teaching

It is assumed that nurse-educators are already familiar with basic teaching methods and tools (see Table 12-2). For those who are not, many excellent teaching texts for health professionals are available that provide detailed discussion and guidance. Yet detailed and accurate teaching during early phases of illness does not always lead to demonstrable application of self-management skills. Lack of change on the part of the learner can be frustrating and disheartening to health professionals who genuinely believe they have provided effective teaching. It becomes easy to blame the client for this lack of change.

The literature provides some assistance to health educators and clients in overcoming persistent learning problems. Included are suggestions for better as-

TABLE 12-2. Frequently Used Teaching Methods and Tools

Methods of client education	Rationale
Demonstration and practice	For teaching skills.
Group discussion	To share information about coping and adapting; for discussing effective management strategies.
Role playing	To present a particular attitude or point of view to the learner through performance of behavior. Role play can be effective in collecting information difficult to obtain otherwise. Often used with children, it can be used in teaching adults.
One-to-one discussion	To facilitate individualization.
Lecture	To give information to a group of persons. Is mainly a one-way communication from the teacher to the learner. Used as a method of providing a great deal of information in a short period of time, but its effectiveness is sometimes questioned because of the lack of active participation by the learner.

Commonly used teaching tools*	Examples
Written material	Books, pamphlets, charts, self-instructional manuals, teacher-developed instruction sheets, or any written information given to the client for the purpose of teaching.
Audiovisual materials	Audiotapes, videotapes, films, slides, closed-circuit television.

*Usually used in conjunction with verbal instruction.
From Narrow, B. W., (1979) Patient Teaching in Nursing Practices, New York: Wiley; and Redman, B. K., (1980) The Process of Patient Teaching in Nursing (4th ed.), St. Louis: C. V. Mosby.

sessment and evaluation, plus some specific teaching strategies that have proven effective in achieving change in people with long-term illnesses.

Improving Assessment and Evaluation

Several strategies suggested in the literature can improve assessment and evaluation, which are essential for effective client education. These strategies address total education programs as well as individual assessment methods and skills. Accurate assessment identifies important problems and issues that will influence the teaching-learning process. Evaluation provides the feedback mechanism necessary for determining weaknesses in the entire process. Evaluation should encompass the effectiveness of each teaching-learning interaction and the effectiveness of the total client education program.

In a study of educational assessment skills of hospital staff, Windsor (1981) stresses the importance of interviewing and observation and suggests that these assessment skills be periodically updated even if they are used regularly. Interviewing is a means of collecting useful assessment information, and observation identifies educational and health behavior deficits. Windsor's study suggests that individuals who

TABLE 12-3. Assessment Criteria for Evaluating Educational Programs

Assessment Criteria Related to Program Planning
    Budget
    Planning advisory group
    Community resources
    Written definition of potential target population
    Written program goals
    Written outline of major content area
    Written learning objectives
    Presence of a coordinator
    Job description for a coordinator responsible for client education

Assessment Criteria Related to Program Implementation
    Educational assessment of client learning needs
    Listing of educational methods used
    Provision for adapting educational methods and materials to learner's needs

Assessment Criteria Related to Evaluation of Client Learning
    Evaluation of client's progress in the program
    Documentation of progress with medical record
    Additional client education arranged for client discharge preceding program completion

Assessment Criteria Related to Program Effectiveness
    Evaluation of extent to which program goals are attained
    Planning advisory group receives evaluation
    Documentation of number of clients who have attained learning objectives

routinely make assessments can improve their accuracy through formal in-service training programs focusing on observation and interview skills. Also suggested was the importance of periodic self-evaluation of these skills.

Knudson, Spiegel, and Furst (1981) studied an educational program for rheumatoid arthritis clients. They suggest the use of a *needs assessment questionnaire* as a valuable tool for ascertaining the motivational level of a client before beginning an educational program. Through the use of a needs assessment, educators can identify those topics and educational activities in which the client is most interested and develop an educational program appropriate to the client's individual needs.

Murdock, Pack, and Palma (1983) developed and tested a model for assessing client educational programs that can be used to evaluate any program before actual teaching begins. They identified eighteen client education assessment criteria as essential components for evaluating existing programs as well as

developing new programs. These eighteen criteria are divided into four categories: program planning, implementation, evaluation of client learning, and program evaluation (see Table 12-3).

The criteria for program planning represent the degree of planning necessary for program implementation. The criteria for implementation can identify learning needs and appropriate educational methods and materials to meet these needs. Criteria for evaluating client learning and criteria for program evaluation help determine whether the goals and objectives of the program are being accomplished. The authors suggest that these criteria can help educators to establish and maintain quality educational programs.

The study done by Lane and Evans (1979) evaluated educational programs for chronically ill people. They proposed using four indicators to determine the effectiveness of such programs on the client's health status and management of illness: physiological measures, compliance, knowledge, and utilization of health services. These indicators are designed to follow each session as well as the complete teaching plan. *Physiological* measures are changes in signs and symptoms toward a less pathologic state. *Compliance* indicators are present when client actions indicate compliance with a planned therapeutic regimen. *Knowledge* indicators evaluate client awareness of pathological process and treatment expectations. Cost-effectiveness of the educational program is measured by *utilization of health services* (hospital admissions, emergency room use, and office or clinic visits). Lane and Evans suggest that these four areas are common to all educational programs, even though knowledge of the disease and its management is useful only in conjunction with the other indicators, because of the low correlation between knowledge and either control or behavior. They recommend that specific outcome goals related to these four areas be developed for each educational program; these goals could then be used in evaluating the educational program.

Combining the Murdock assessment model to evaluate programs before teaching with the Lane and Evans evaluative outcome goals for educational programs would improve both assessment and evaluation of educational programs.

Behavioral Strategies

Educational programs for the chronically ill tend to focus on teaching about the disease process and then presenting a management plan, without incorporating a component for changing client behaviors. This limitation is unfortunate, especially since behavioral strategies have been found effective in teaching the chronically ill. In fact, several authors have stressed that combining dissemination of information with behavioral strategies helps the individual to gain self-management skills (Bartlett 1982; Given, Given, & Coyle 1984; Watts 1980; Becker & Maiman 1980; Hassar 1979).

Behavioral strategies (sometimes referred to as *behavioral therapy* or *behavior modification*) use a systematic approach to analyzing assessed data to find the causes and consequences of existing behav-

ior in order to propose effective behavioral changes. Some authors use the term *behavioral diagnosis* for the process that identifies unwanted behavior and the reinforcers of that behavior. After the behavioral diagnosis, a technique to alter cause, reinforcer, or both is then determined. For clients who possess self-management knowledge but are unable to change their behavior, this strategy is quite effective.

A Model for Behavioral Intervention. Both Mager and Pipe (1970) and Melamed and Siegel (1980) outline behavioral intervention programs. Combining ideas from both these sources enables one to develop a model for effective change (see Figure 12-1). This model requires that ineffective behaviors identified through assessment be defined in behavioral terms and that factors that promote the occurrence of this behavior be analyzed. Such factors can be classified as causes or consequences. During the process of analysis, possible alternatives or solutions should be explored.

Identifying the Problem. Behavioral diagnosis is a sequential process. First, one needs to determine whether the behavior is due to a knowledge deficit: Does the client know the appropriate self-management behavior? If lack of knowledge underlies continued ineffective performance, then teaching can be modified or strengthened to eliminate the difficulty.

Once adequate knowledge has been demonstrated, one must determine whether the behavior is lost or has deteriorated. This step includes finding out whether the behavior is frequent or infrequent. If it is used frequently but is performed incorrectly despite regular use, periodic feedback may lead to improvement. For example, a diabetic who self-injects insulin every day may be using incorrect technique. If the behavior is used infrequently, a regular schedule of practice becomes important. For example, a family member who monitors a client's blood pressure occasionally may need to practice the technique during clinic visits.

When skill performance of the behavior is assured, the individual's potential for carrying out the

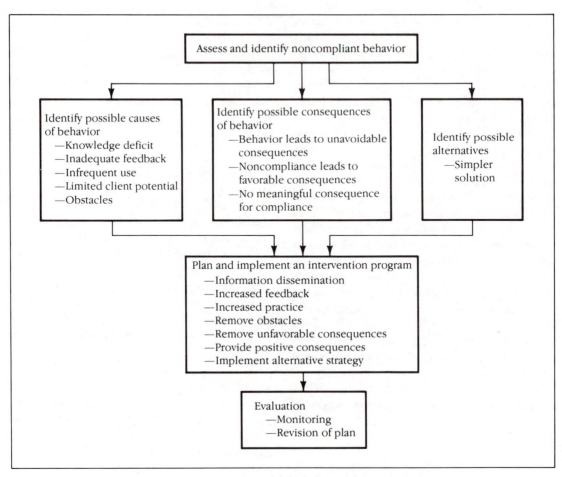

FIGURE 12-1. A model for behavioral intervention

desired performance needs to be assessed as a possible cause of the unwanted behavior. Possible developmental or intellectual deficits or decreased interest that might hamper the individual from performing desired behavior must be determined. The presence of deficits requires modification of the teaching plan so that the client can successfully perform necessary actions. The lack of intellectual interest can be countered by stimulating the client's curiosity in such ways as identifying resources in the literature that the client can pursue and discuss.

The last major cause of unwanted behavior is obstacles to performance of desired behavior. Removing these obstacles allows correction of the difficulty. For example, a diabetic who can and wants to carry out insulin injections and glucometer testing may be prevented from doing so by limited finances. Obstacles, rather than obstinacy, may be the cause.

Up to this point, the model considers only the causes of poor performance. Once causes are ruled out or corrected, then consequences, or lack of consequences, may underlie continued unwanted performance. Analysis of consequences is also sequential, with the more likely being considered and corrected first.

Direct, unfavorable consequences, such as unwanted side effects, can underlie poor compliance and must be removed before satisfactory performance can be achieved. For example, clients who become nauseated every time they use a prescribed medication may be reluctant to use the medication. Solutions in this case include finding a way to control the nausea or selecting another effective medication that does not cause nausea.

The next step, should there be no unfavorable consequences, is to determine whether nonperformance leads to more favorable consequences than would the desired behavior. Arrangements for positive reinforcement for appropriate behavior will correct the basis of such problems. For example, the child who receives more parental attention for refusing medication than for taking it may consider refusal to have a more favorable result. Correcting the behavior requires providing positive reinforcement for taking the medication.

The next step for continued unwanted behavior is to determine whether the consequence is meaningful. If it is not, arrange a favorable result. For example, the client might receive an extra privilege for performing the desired behavior.

A final factor to consider, should neither cause nor consequence appear to influence behavior, is the possibility of alternatives such as a simpler solution to the problem. For example, would another behavior net the same outcome in terms of management of the treatment plan?

Planning and Implementing an Interventional Program. Once the underlying basis of poor performance is identified, a solution can be determined and implemented, with the selected strategy depending on the source of the difficulty. The most practical, economical, and easy solution should be determined. Achieving the greatest results for the least effort is likely to increase self-management.

Several teaching strategies are applicable to the causes that underlie poor performance. For lack of knowledge, information dissemination is appropriate. When skill is inadequate, increased feedback helps, just as increased practice strengthens deteriorating skills.

Should consequences be the basis of poor learning performance, then unfavorable consequences should be removed, positive consequences or reinforcers should be provided, or obstacles to performance should be eliminated.

Finally, if neither cause nor consequence seems to underlie poor learning, then one must attempt to identify and implement an alternate behavior that would net the same outcome.

Evaluation. The final step in using behavioral strategies is to evaluate the entire process. Change in the specific behaviors identified during assessment should be identified, or performance of new behaviors should be clearly demonstrated. Evaluation includes continuous monitoring of client progress and identification and implementation of necessary revisions.

Contract Learning

The use of a contract has also been effective in assisting clients with chronic illnesses to manage their care. Identifying the underlying basis of poor outcomes is not emphasized; rather, reaching agreement about preferred actions is the focus. Often called a *contingency contract,* this tool is a written plan for systematic reinforcement of specified desirable behaviors. The contract may be negotiated between the health care provider and client or may be a *self-contract* in which the client administers his or her own reinforcers, with another person available for support and advice, if needed. A number of elements have been identified as desirable in a contingency contract (Janz, Becker, & Hartman 1984; Steckel 1982); most of them pertain to clarity of statement and intent (see Table 12-4).

Contingency contracting seems to be effective for chronically ill individuals for several reasons. The client becomes involved in the decision-making process regarding the treatment regimen and makes a commitment to behavior change. Everyone has the opportunity to discuss potential problems and solutions. Accountability is fostered through written specification of each person's responsibilities for the

TABLE 12-4. Elements Desirable for Contract Learning

1. Clearly stated goals that are specifically described and agreed upon by all.

2. Responsibilities (behaviors) of each person must be stated in detail, including time and frequency requirements for performance of the behaviors.

3. The required behaviors should be easily observable and measurable to facilitate reinforcement activities.

4. The methods of recording the behavior and the reinforcement should be identified.

5. Positive reinforcers must be clearly specified. This should also include timing and conditions for delivery of the reinforcements.

6. A detailed description of events that will occur if any person fails to fulfill the responsibilities of the contract must be provided.

7. A "bonus clause" may be included to provide additional reinforcers if the client exceeds the outlined responsibilities.

8. Specific dates for contract initiation and termination or renewal should be included.

9. The contract should be signed by all persons involved.

From Janz, N. K., Becker, M. H., and Hartman, P. E., (1984) Contingency contracting to enhance patient compliance: A review, Patient Education and Counseling, 5: 165–178; and Steckel, S. B., (1982) Patient Contracting, Norwalk, Conn.: Appleton-Century-Crofts.

client's health care; the contract elicits a formal commitment from all involved persons. The written document provides an instrument of communication for others involved in the client's care and facilitates evaluation of progress by permitting comparison of activities and outcomes with the precise terms of the contract. Finally, the contingency component provides an additional incentive for achieving goals through reinforcement of the desired behaviors (Janz, Becker, & Hartman 1984; Becker & Maiman 1980). Chapters 7 and 11 also discuss contracting.

Other Strategies

Groups. Numerous authors have addressed the effects of group teaching and group process on the self-management of chronic illness, but success of group programs has been limited except in terms of information dissemination. Groups, however, have been successful in helping the chronically ill for a variety of reasons, such as providing emotional support, presenting alternatives, and sharing.

Two studies (Gross & Brandt 1981; Potts & Brandt 1983) have analyzed the effect of educational support groups: one for clients with rheumatoid arthritis, the other for clients with ankylosing spondylitis. In both cases, the educational support groups were found to increase the client's knowledge about the disease and its treatment. However, the groups had little effect on the client's ability to cope with illness, nor did compliance with prescribed treatment increase.

Rancour and Moser (1980) instituted a self-help group for individuals with arthritis. Although compliance was not evaluated, the group participants displayed more positive self-esteem, had decreased feelings of isolation and helplessness, shared coping strategies with each other, and displayed a higher level of positive thinking. Since feelings of isolation and helplessness are obstacles to both learning and compliance, attitude changes brought about by this group process might result in desired change.

Ross (1984) identified three types of groups that could be used in a health care setting: individually oriented change groups, group-process learning groups, and focused-criterion groups. Individually oriented change groups help reduce client fears, anxieties, and misunderstandings and help overcome resistance. The group facilitator works individually with clients on their specific health problems and helps each member move toward development of a contract for new behavior in carrying out the treatment regimen.

In group-process learning groups, change occurs through the interactions among group members, who help each other overcome resistances, solve problems, and develop alternative health behaviors. The facilitator helps members interact with each other, move toward a contract of change, and adopt more healthy behavior.

Focused-criterion groups are designed to change or eliminate self-destructive behavior. Specific techniques are used in implementing the specific behavioral change. The facilitator encourages behavioral adaptation to some specified norm. Alcoholics Anonymous groups can be characterized as focused-criterion groups.

Self-Instruction. Self-instruction manuals have not been studied extensively as an effective teaching method for chronically ill individuals. However, Behn and Lane (1983) found that such a self-instruction manual was effective for assisting individuals in weight control. The manual included not only information and guidance about diet management but a section on behavior modification that provided behavioral strategies for coping with difficult situations. Information also included factors that might influence behaviors, as well as a plan for identifying, analyzing, and developing solutions to behavioral problems. Individuals were assisted through the manual in self-monitoring and problem solving.

Self-instruction might also be successful with some chronically ill individuals. Before selecting such an approach, the health care provider must make a thorough assessment of the client's motivational level, support systems, abilities in self-control, and educational level. Work with an individual who has desirable characteristics in these areas might indicate to the health professions that a self-instructional manual of this type could be effective.

Discharge Planning. Discharge planning can incorporate teaching to gain effective outcomes. One discharge planning program, identified as a way of decreasing hospitalizations for chronically ill individuals, used a six-step plan (Huey et al. 1981), the *METHOD discharge plan*. Each letter in the word *METHOD* stands for one step that needs to be considered. Note that some of these steps actually involve teaching:

- *M—Medication:* The client will know his or her medication's name, purpose, effect, dosage,

schedule, precautions to take, and side effects that should be reported.
- *E—Environment:* The client is informed that adequate homemaking and transportation services and emotional and economic support will be ensured. Physical hazards in the home will be corrected.
- *T—Treatments:* The client or family member will know the purpose of treatments and will be able to demonstrate the correct technique and to report any problems that develop.
- *H—Health Teaching:* The client will be able to describe the way the disease affects his or her body, to list the keys to health maintenance, and to name signs and symptoms that require medical attention.
- *O—Outpatient Referral:* The client will know when and where to keep appointments and whom to call for medical help. The client and referral agencies will have copies of the discharge instruction plan.
- *D—Diet:* The client will be able to describe the appropriate diet and its purpose, to name restricted foods, and to describe some typical menus.

Although this teaching strategy does not involve mechanisms to assist clients in modifying their behavior, it does present a structured plan for giving the necessary self-management knowledge to client and family. The plan allows the health care educator to provide needed support services (physical, emotional, and economic), as well as furnishing a copy of the management instructions to all referral agencies. This produces a mechanism by which the persons providing the support services and the persons in the referral agencies can monitor client behaviors and assist with the self-management plan.

Summary and Conclusions

Teaching clients with chronic illnesses about their disease and managing their care can be challenging.

The nurse-educator must be familiar with the general concepts of teaching and learning, as well as issues specific to the chronically ill individual. Because of the long-term nature of chronic illnesses and the complexity of their management, clients often have difficulty mastering and carrying out their treatment plans.

A number of problems make teaching less effective with the chronically ill, including problems inherent in the client, the family, the sociocultural environment, and the teacher. Only if these problems are considered can corrective teaching interventions be identified.

Although knowledge about the illness and its regimen increases the likelihood of clients' managing their own care, knowledge alone does not assure such behavior. Any number of teaching methods and tools are useful, depending on the nature of the subject being taught and on an assessment of the client's learning needs and style. Appropriateness of pedagogic and androgogic techniques also must be considered.

Effective assessment and evaluation by the health educator are prerequisites of effective teaching. Combining information dissemination with behavioral strategies has proved to be an effective process of the teaching-learning interaction. Behavioral strategies based on identified specific causes or consequences of behavior can be developed to assist the client in adhering to a plan.

Contract learning has also been effective for the chronically ill. Contracting does not require identifying the basis of poor outcomes; rather it focuses on agreement about future behaviors by means of a written document that includes all factors of behavior, reinforcer, and responsibility for plan components.

Also mentioned is the value of groups to provide support (although they do not enhance learning) and of self-instruction, as adjuncts to improved teaching for the chronically ill client. Discharge planning could incorporate aspects of a teaching plan to assist the client.

Because teaching is closely tied to compliance (see Chapter 7) and change (see Chapter 11), the reader will find the discussion in the chapters devoted to these topics useful.

STUDY QUESTIONS

1. What are the four steps of the teaching-learning process? Briefly define each.
2. In what ways are pedagogic and androgogic learning different? the same?
3. What are the six common obstacles to learning on the part of the learner?
4. What factors influence learning in a child? in the elderly?
5. What client factors might lead to noncompliance with the treatment regimen?
6. What factors on the part of the teacher can create problems in the teaching-learning process?
7. In what ways can assessment and evaluation be improved? Discuss them.
8. How can behavioral strategies help teach the chronically ill person? Explain the process.
9. What are the desirable elements of a contingency contract? How does contingency contracting differ from behavioral strategies?
10. What value for teaching can be found in groups? self-instruction? How can discharge planning be used to enhance compliance?

References

Bartlett, E. E., (1982) Behavioral diagnosis: A practical approach to patient education, *Patient Counselling and Health Education, 4*:29–35

Becker, M. H., and Maiman, L. A., (1980) Strategies for enhancing patient compliance, *Journal of Community Health, 6*:113–132

Behn, S., and Lane, D. S., (1983) A self-teaching weight-control manual: Method for increasing compliance and reducing obesity, *Patient Education and Counseling,* 5:63–67

Bille, D. A. (ed.), (1981) *Practical Approaches to Patient Teaching,* Boston: Little, Brown

Given, C. W., Given, B. A., and Coyle, B. W., (1984) The effects of patient characteristics and beliefs on responses to behavioral interventions for control of chronic diseases, *Patient Education and Counseling, 6:*131–140

Gross, M., and Brandt, K. D., (1981) Educational support groups for patients with ankylosing spondylitis: A preliminary report, *Patient Counselling and Health Education, 3:*6–12

Hassar, D. A., (1979) Your role in patient compliance, *Nursing 79, 9*(11):48–53

Hogstel, M. O., (1981) *Nursing Care of the Older Adult,* New York: Wiley

Huey, R., Loomis, J., Rosson, T., Owen, D., Kiernan, L., Madonna, M., and Quaife, M., (1981) Discharge planning: Good planning means fewer hospitalizations for the chronically ill, *Nursing 81, 11*(5):70–75

Janz, N. K., Becker, M. H., and Hartman, P. E., (1984) Contingency contracting to enhance patient compliance: A review, *Patient Education and Counseling, 5:*165–178

Knowles, M. S., (1980) *The Modern Practice of Adult Education: From Pedagogy to Andragogy,* Chicago: Association

Knudson, K. G., Spiegel, T. M., and Furst, D. E., (1981) Outpatient educational program for rheumatoid arthritis patients, *Patient Counselling and Health Education, 3:*77–82

Kornzweig, A. L., (1979) The eye in old age, in Rossman, I. (ed.), *Clinical Geriatrics* (2d ed.), Philadelphia: Lippincott

Korsch, B. M., and Negrete, V. F., (1980) Counselling patients and their families in a chronic renal disease program, *Patient Counselling and Education, 2:*87–91

Lane, D. S., and Evans, D., (1979) Measures and methods in evaluating patient education programs for chronic illness, *Medical Care, 17:*30–42

Mager, R. F., and Pipe, P., (1970) *Analyzing Performance Problems,* Belmont, Calif.: Fearon

Melamed, B. G., and Siegel, L. J., (1980) *Behavioral Medicine: Practical Applications in Health Care,* New York: Springer

Miller, J. F., (1983) *Coping with Chronic Illness: Overcoming Powerlessness,* Philadelphia: Davis

Murdock, R. B., Pack, B. E., and Palma, L. M., (1983) A model for assessing patient education, *Patient Education and Counseling, 5:*85–88

Narrow, B. W., (1979) *Patient Teaching in Nursing Practice,* New York: Wiley

Pohl, M. L., (1978) *The Teaching Function of the Nursing Practitioner* (3d ed.), Dubuque, Ill.: Brown

Potts, M., and Brandt, K. D., (1983) Analysis of education-support groups for patients with rheumatoid arthritis, *Patient Counselling and Health Education, 4:*161–166

Rancour, P., and Moser, T., (1980) Group synergy or how to multiply health potential in persons coping with chronic disease, *Health Values: Achieving High Level Wellness, 4:*117–118

Redman, B. K., (1980) *The Process of Patient Teaching in Nursing* (4th ed.), St. Louis: C. V. Mosby

Ross, H. S., (1984) Working with groups in patient education, *Patient Education and Counseling, 6:*105–112

Sarnecky, M., and Sarnecky, G. J., (1984) Better patient compliance through effective instructional planning, *Military Medicine, 148:*221–224

Schuster, C. S., and Ashburn, S. S., (1980) *The Process of Human Development: A Holistic Approach,* Boston: Little, Brown

Smith, B. C., and Carson, H. M., (1981) The relationship of health locus of control to patients with end-stage renal disease, *Patient Counselling and Health Education, 3:*63–66

Steckel, S. B., (1982) *Patient Contracting,* Norwalk, Conn.: Appleton-Century-Crofts

Storandt, M., (1979) Psychological aspects of aging, in Rossman, I. (ed.), *Clinical Geriatrics* (2d ed.), Philadelphia: Lippincott

Strauss, A. L., Corbin, J., Fagerhaugh, S., Glaser, B., Maines, D., Suczek, B., and Wiener, C., (1984) *Chronic Illness and the Quality of Life* (2d ed.), St. Louis: C. V. Mosby

Watts, F. N., (1980) Behavioural aspects of the management of diabetes mellitus: Education, self-care and metabolic control, *Behaviour Research and Therapy, 18*(3):171–180

Windsor, R. A., (1981) Improving patient-education assessment skills of hospital staff: A case study in diabetes, *Patient Counselling and Health Education, 3:*26–29

Bibliography

Adom, D., and Wright, A. S., (1982) Dissonance in nurse and patient evaluations of the effectiveness of a patient-teaching program, *Nursing Outlook, 30:*132–136

Avery, C. H., March, J., and Brook, R. H., (1980) An assessment of the adequacy of self-care by adult asthmatics, *Journal of Community Health, 5:*167–180

Blackwell, B., (1981) Biofeedback in a comprehensive behavioral medicine program, *Biofeedback and Self-Regulation, 6:*445–472

Brough, F. K., Schmidt, C. D., Rasmussen, T., and Boyer, M., (1982) Comparison of two teaching methods for self-care training for patients with chronic obstructive pulmonary disease, *Patient Counselling and Health Education, 4:*111–116

Counte, M. A., Bialiauskas, L. A., and Pavlou, M., (1983) Stress and personal attitudes in chronic illness, *Archives of Physical Medicine and Rehabilitation, 64:*272–275

Craighead, W. E., Kazdin, A. E., and Mahoney, M. J., (1981) *Behavior Modification: Principles, Issues, and Applications* (2d ed.), Boston: Houghton Mifflin

Davis, A. J., (1980) Disability, home care and the care-taking role in family life, *Journal of Advanced Nursing, 5:*475–484

De Hays, W. F. J., (1982) Patient education: A component of health education, *Patient Counselling and Health Education, 4:*95–102

DiMatteo, M. R., and DiNicola, D. D., (1982) *Achieving Patient Compliance,* New York: Pergamon

Glanz, K., and Scholl, T. O., (1982) Intervention strategies to improve adherence among hypertensives: Review and recommendations, *Patient Counselling and Health Education, 4:*14–28

Greene, J. Y., Weinberger, M., Jerin, M. J., and Mamlin, J. J., (1982) Compliance with medication regimens among chronically ill inner city patients, *Journal of Community Health, 7:*183–193

Gregor, F. M., (1981) Teaching the patient with ischemic heart disease: A systematic approach to instructional design, *Patient Counselling and Health Education, 3:*57–62

Heine, A. G., (1981) Helping hypertensive clients help themselves: The nurse's role, *Patient Counselling and Health Education, 3:*108–112

Hoover, J., (1980) Compliance from a patient's perspective, *The Diabetes Educator, 6:*9–12

Iyer, P. W., (1980) A teaching plan for pregnant diabetics, *The Diabetes Educator, 6:*19–21

Jackson, C., (1981) Diabetes: How your patient looks at it, *Nursing 81, 11*(5):82–83

Jones, W. L., Rimer, B. K., Levy, M. H., and Kinman, J. L., (1984) Cancer patients' knowledge, beliefs, and behavior regarding pain control regimens: Implications for education programs, *Patient Education and Counseling, 5:*159–164

Kazdin, A. E., (1980) *Behavior Modification in Applied Settings,* Homewood, Ill.: Dorsey

Keane, T. M., Prue, D. M., and Collins, F. L., (1981) Behavioral contracting to improve dietary compliance in chronic renal dialysis patients, *Journal of Behavior Therapy and Experimental Psychiatry, 12:*63–67

Krulik, T., (1980) Successful "normalizing" tactics of parents of chronically-ill children, *Journal of Advanced Nursing, 5:*573–578

Lewis, S. J., (1984) Teaching patient groups, *Nursing Management, 15:*49–56

Linde, B. J., and Janz, N. M., (1979) Effect of a teaching program on knowledge and compliance of cardiac patients, *Nursing Research, 28:*282–286

Marcuz, L., (1980) To learn, to teach, to grow, *The Diabetes Educator, 6:*16–18

Marks, V. L., (1980) Health teaching for recovering alcoholic patients, *American Journal of Nursing, 80:*2058–2061

Miller, J. F., (1982) Categories of self-care needs of ambulatory patients with diabetes, *Journal of Advanced Nursing, 7:*25–31

Pelczynski, L., and Reilly, A., (1981) Helping your diabetic patients help themselves: A plan for inpatient education, *Nursing 81, 11*(5):76–81

Peters, V. J., (1980) Teaching-learning strategies, *The Diabetes Educator, 6:*23–26

Pruyn, J. F. A., (1983) Coping with stress in cancer patients, *Patient Education and Counseling, 5:*57–62

Roberts, C. R., Hosokawa, M. C., Walts, B., and Mueller, R., (1982) Evaluation of a self-teaching program, *Patient Counselling and Health Education, 3:*161–165

Rottkamp, B. C., and Donohue-Porter, P., (1983) The role of patient needs and preferences for instructional approaches in self-management of diabetes, *Patient Counselling and Health Education, 4:*137–145

Scherwitz, L., Priddy, D., and Vallbona, C., (1983) A three-dimensional model for teaching about hypertension, *Health Values: Achieving High Level Wellness, 7:*25–27

Scott, R. S., Beaven, D. W., and Stafford, J. M., (1984) The effectiveness of diabetes education for non-insulin dependent diabetic persons, *The Diabetes Educator, 10:*36–39

Sponk, V. R. A., and Warmenhoven, N. E., (1983) Patient education in general practice: Opinions of general practitioners, *Patient Education and Counseling, 5:*68–75

Squyres, W. D. (ed.), (1980) *Patient Education: An Inquiry into the State of the Art,* New York: Springer

Stewart, C., (1980) Principles of patient education for the patient with an altered neurological status, *Journal of Neurosurgical Nursing, 12:*179–183

Strodtman, L. K., (1984) A decision-making process for planning patient education, *Patient Education and Counseling, 5:*189–200

Williams, C. L., and Arnold, C. B., (1980) Teaching children self-care for chronic disease prevention: Obesity re-duction and smoking prevention, *Patient Counselling and Health Education, 2:*92–97

Wong, J., Wong., S., and Mensah, L., (1983) A conceptual approach to the development of motivational strategies, *Journal of Advanced Nursing, 8:*111–116

Zangari, M., and Duffy, P., (1980) Contracting with patients in day-to-day practice, *American Journal of Nursing, 80:*451–455

◇

CHAPTER THIRTEEN

Advocacy

◇

Introduction

Nurses and other health professionals who care for the chronically ill are in a position of power in relation to the client (Orgel 1983). Knowledge and understanding of advocacy can lead to effective use of this power for the client's well-being and preclude its being used to the client's detriment. There are no prescriptions for being advocates; rather, health professionals have the challenge of designing a framework for advocacy for the chronically ill.

Definition

To advocate is to plead a cause. Advocacy requires taking one side in a dispute or argument, in contradistinction to assuming a position of neutrality. Defined more narrowly, *advocacy* is "action designed to help the powerless acquire and use power to make social systems more responsive to their needs" (Rogers 1980). This definition prescribes a relationship between provider and client that is not so simple as it sounds. Implicit in this definition is the mandate to protect the clients' right to make decisions and to take actions in their own behalf (Gadow 1983). Clients should consider advocates as allies supporting them and helping them meet their needs.

Advocacy is not deciding or doing for the client; rather, it is providing information and support to help that person make the best decisions possible (Kohnke 1980). Promoting self-management and self-determination to the limit of the client's capabilities is the goal of both advocacy and nursing (Gadow 1983; Orem 1985).

Advocacy, then, is first an attitude the nurse brings to the relationship with clients; it influences values and judgments about clients and enlists the nurse in the client's support. Thus, the nurse becomes coach, teacher, and friend. From this central relationship, advocacy shapes the nurse's actions (Brower 1980) regardless of setting: the physician's, administrator's, or nursing director's office; the state Ombudsman's office; the Department of Consumer Affairs, the state legislature; or hearings conducted by the Congress of the United States.

Assumptions

Several assumptions distinguish the advocacy role from other nursing roles (Gadow 1983):

1. The chronically ill client is a morally capable person responsible for his or her own behavior in relation to self and others.
2. Health care systems frequently obstruct the client's exercise of power by failing to recognize the right to autonomy as a morally capable agent.
3. The appropriateness of the nurse as advocate for the client stems from two factors. First is the nurse's provision of care to the client over time and the mutuality that develops as a result of this care. Second, the nurse has a position within the health care system and a consequent ability to influence others.

Power Deficits and Self-Care

Power Deficits. The chronically ill client who needs the nurse to serve as an advocate is unable to meet his or her own needs in at least one activity necessary for good health and well-being. Normally, human beings care for themselves, but illness necessitates that someone else provide assistance to assure performance of the deficient activity. The necessity of relying on someone else places the client in an extremely vulnerable position. A power deficit prevails, with the client in a subordinate position. Consequently, the person assisting with the activity has more power within the relationship than the client.

Interferences with Self-Care. In the practice of this chapter's primary author, four areas in which dysfunction can lead to the client's lessened power position have been noted. These areas include physiological and psychological limitations, lack of skill, lack of knowledge, and lack of motivation. They do not constitute an exhaustive list; rather, they illustrate power deficits.

Physiological or Psychological Limitations. Physiological incapacitation or psychological dysfunction can exceed the client's conscious ability to correct at a point in time, as the following examples indicate.

1. A client whose spinal cord is severed has no available nerve pathways to carry messages to the legs and is unable to move them.
2. A client having manic-depressive illness becomes psychotically depressed and goes to bed and stays there. If unaided, this person will die.

Lack of Skill. The lack of skill in performing a physical function or activity can prevent the individual from performing necessary activities.

1. The amputation of the dominant hand leaves a client unable to write until the other hand is trained. There is no physiological reason why the client is unable to write, but the muscles of the other hand have not been exercised to take over the lost function.
2. The psychotically depressed client who took to bed for a year finds, as recovery from the depression begins, that ambulation is difficult because of leg weakness. Leg strengthening is required to allow ambulation.

Lack of Knowledge. Without knowledge of available treatments, resources, or the importance of the task to be performed, individuals cannot identify or meet their own needs.

1. A client whose hemiparalysis was caused by a cerebral vascular accident is unable to move around the nursing home because the wheelchair requires two hands to move it forward. The client does not know that some wheelchairs can be driven with one hand.
2. At a psychiatric hospital, a middle-aged woman, diagnosed as depressed, is given electroshock therapy. She is uninformed of other treatment options.

Lack of Motivation. Motivation is a requisite for performing necessary tasks or functions.

1. An individual who has amyotrophic lateral sclerosis has been sitting in the same position day and night for two years because of fear of lying down. She is reluctant to ask her personal attendants to elevate her feet because she does not want to burden them. As a result, morbid fluid retention develops in both lower extremities.
2. A chronic schizophrenic client will not attend an activity because voices are telling him not to attend.

Self-Care and Decision Making. The right of the client to care for self and make decisions relating to that care is a highly valued tenet of nursing in Western industrialized societies (Orem 1985; Gadow 1983). Yet, the ability to act as advocate for oneself in relation to this right is a learned skill, possessed by few. Essentially, the nurse's role of advocate for chronically ill clients is based on both the client's right to self-care (to the extent of that individual's ability) and the right to make decisions affecting this care.

Self-Care Requisites. Orem (1985) delineates self-care for all human beings as follows:

1. The ability to gather and use needed elements from the environment: air, food, and fluid.
2. The ability to excrete waste, urine and feces, and to perform these functions in socially acceptable ways.
3. The ability to provide a clean, safe environment; maintain the skin as a protective barrier; and recognize and maintain a safe, comfortable temperature.
4. The ability to recognize and provide a balance between rest and activity to enrich the human spirit and rest the body and mind.
5. The ability to recognize and provide time and experiences that lead to a healthy relationship with self in solitude and with others through socialization.

Vulnerability and dependency occur when there is a deficit in an individual's ability to provide and maintain any of these five necessities, or when an individual is unable to exercise control over others who provide care in any of these areas. Within the advocacy role, the nurse helps the individual to learn and exercise power and responsibility so that resources that provide for self-care needs can be gathered. In this framework, the nurse is accountable to the client. Good advocacy leads to self-advocacy.

Advocacy by Others. Advocacy, long recognized as an essential aspect of client-centered nursing care, stems from self-advocacy and should only supplement what the individual cannot or will not do. Recent nursing literature (Gadow 1983; Kohnke 1980; Murphy & Hunter 1983; Rogers 1980) has specified the roles and functions of an advocate, though few agree as to which of these roles and functions are appropriate for nurses. In addition, none of these authors specifically addresses the role of advocacy in the care of the chronically ill.

The advocacy relationship requires that the nurse

first assist the client to clarify the personal meaning and value that illness holds. This personal value system becomes the basis for all further decisions. This value system can continue to develop or change from time to time as the client experiences various life changes affected by the illness and subsequent life adaptation.

Murphy and Hunter (1983) suggest that the nurse can serve as an advocate by being a catalyst enabling the client to reach a new acceptance of self. The nurse is in a position to be nonjudgmental in supporting and facilitating the client's struggle to integrate beliefs and behaviors. The nurse also serves to combat feelings of dehumanization that the client may experience. This role is especially important in the care of the chronically ill client since "cure" is rarely possible. The client's adjustment to chronicity may be strongly influenced by the way nurses exercise power: either by advocating self-sufficiency and self-determination or by imposing a paternalistic rule over the client's daily life. The tyranny of the latter has been associated, at times, with the institutional personality syndrome prevalent in long-term care facilities (Underwood 1981).

The Advocate Relationship

Advocacy is a partnership between nurse and client. The nurse achieves such a partnership by using self as therapeutic agent; by employing a sense of humor, values, and personality, as well as knowledge and skill to forge a human connection with that client. Clients can then feel valued because of this connection to someone they trust and care about. This type of advocacy casts the acts of doing and helping in a new light.

Many argue that when nurses become involved in the client's life, they trade objectivity for the client's subjective view. Every new nursing student has experienced, at least once, the hazard of identifying with a client, usually one of similar age, sex, and social characteristics. Crossing the line from the objective to the subjective is not one of movement from

TABLE 13-1. Categories of Problems of Daily Living

Category	Strategies	Example
Prevention of medical crises and their management once they occur.	Rescuing or saving a life.	Providing insulin to a client in diabetic coma.
Control of symptoms.	Protecting from harm.	Assisting a client with amyotropic lateral sclerosis (ALS) to elevate feet.
Carrying out prescribed regimens and managing problems attendant upon carrying out the regimens.	Assisting, helping with a regimen.	Assisting a diabetic client to buy and cook appropriate foods.
Prevention of, or living with, social isolation caused by lessening contact with others.	Control, helping the client continue the regimen.	Arranging needed transportation to allow a home-bound client to leave home.
Adjustment to changes in the course of the disease, whether it deteriorates or has a remission.	Helping the client adapt.	Helping children eat foods to which they are not allergic by using only those foods in meal preparation.
Attempts at normalizing both interaction with others and style of life.	Coordination, organizational gathering, and coordinating resources. Working with friends and family.	Arranging for friends to stay with the cystic fibrosis child so parents can attend a support group.
Funding for treatment or survival despite partial or complete loss of employment.	Finding the necessary funds.	Publicity and setting up bank account to pay for transplant surgery.

less to more personal involvement, but of failing to recognize the essential difference between the client's experience of chronic illness as a completely unique, deeply interior journey, and the nurse's external perception and observation of that experience (Gadow 1983).

When nurses identify rather than empathize, they replace perception of the client's experience with a "movie" of their own responses and feelings in that situation. Nurses who are advocates always remain "the other," external observers, albeit sympathetic, to the client.

Advocacy versus Agency

It is important to distinguish between advocacy and agency. The *agent* acts with and for the client by doing

those things that the client cannot do (or does with difficulty); the *advocate* assists the client to gather the necessary agents and resources. Agents include not only caregivers but family, friends, and even strangers.

Strauss and Glaser (1975) identify several major categories of problems in daily living that arise from chronic illness (see Table 13-1). These authors also identify four types of assistance provided by agents that have a mitigating effect on the stated problems. The *rescuing agent* is one who literally saves a life (for example, assisting a stroke client who is choking while eating in a restaurant). The *protective agent* serves in a supervisory role to ensure continued safety (for example, monitoring a young heart client to prevent undue cardiac stress during play). The *assisting agent* supports the client's self-management (such as when an individual allows an elderly diabetic spouse to perform the daily insulin injection). The *controlling agent* prevents the abandonment of a regimen or treatment (for example, deciding that a diabetic child should eat a smaller meal in order to have popcorn at a movie).

The advocate functions differently. Advocacy begins with the advocate not doing for the client but establishing a relationship that facilitates the helping process by enabling the client to reframe his or her world and decide whether assistance from others is necessary. The advocate helps the client clarify values, test decisions, plan strategies for living, and gather resources.

Since chronic illness effects changes in independence for the client, the advocate must understand the meaning of the illness to the client to determine what help is necessary and what values may have to change to preserve the client's self-love and self-esteem. The client's perspective of this forced dependency is often greatly different from those of family, friends, staff, or physicians (see Chapter 2), who are often unable to step outside the unfolding drama with the rigor required for advocacy. In addition, the advocate knows that love and respect for (and a comfortable relationship with) others allow one to accept help and to give and share with others so as to normalize a new life-style.

The Goal of Advocacy

The goal of advocacy is to redistribute power among the client and family, the professional caregiver, and the health care system (Rogers 1980). Inherent in such a goal is the existence of a partnership, not a relationship dependent on power. A power-dependent relationship develops when one party provides all needed services for another, receiving nothing in return. A client who is to be a partner and not a victim must have an opportunity to reciprocate. When there is no reciprocation, the provider has a disproportionate share of power since the continuing supply of the needed service can be made contingent upon compliance (Kayser-Jones 1981).

To understand the relation of the ill person to those who have the power to help, Kayser-Jones (1981) applied the theory of "reciprocal exchange of valued goods" to chronically ill residents in nursing homes and their caregivers. Financial reimbursement is one commodity available for exchange. Services and friendship are also available as payment for care given, as is a sense of satisfaction. Without means or power to reciprocate, the client who is unwilling to be victimized may begin to use coercion to obtain the needed services, manage without them, or obtain them elsewhere.

By understanding the importance of reciprocation, the advocate can intervene and help eliminate noncooperative or nonproductive behavior. The nurse acting in the advocacy role can help the client identify means of supplementing the subordinate role and can guide the client to understand the importance of reciprocity. In addition, an important advocate function is to explain to other staff members and to the client's family the role that reciprocity plays in helping the client maintain self-worth in relationships.

The Advocate Role

The role of the advocate is essentially a dynamic, ever-changing relationship with the chronically ill individual that depends on identified needs, wishes, and desires. Also influencing this role are the situational variabilities, the inherent requirements of the condition and environment, and the skills of the advocate.

The primary role of advocate, as described in this chapter, is that of trusted confidant: someone who is able to remain connected to the client by empathy and understanding while keeping enough emotional distance to make the client a partner in relationships with the other members of the family, the support group, the health care system, and society.

Functions of the Advocacy Role

In this primary role, the nurse-advocate performs a number of important functions:

1. The advocate assists the client to recognize the needs, wishes, desires, and fears that affect the ability to act either positively or negatively.

2. The advocate clarifies for and reflects to the client perceptions of the effects of these needs, wishes, desires, or fears on his or her ability to act and to relate to others effectively.

3. The advocate helps the client to articulate wishes, desires, needs, and fears in the form of problems that he or she is able to solve.

4. The advocate helps the client discover the roots of the problem by investigation and productive dialogue with other involved persons.

5. The advocate and client jointly devise a plan to resolve the problem to the satisfaction of the client.

6. The advocate keeps the client fully informed and involved, to the extent that prudence dictates, in the problem-solving process.

7. The advocate becomes a consultative resource for strategies for solving the problem.

8. The advocate accepts and supports the client's decision when all the data have been gathered and presented and the options are known. This is an essential and often overlooked advocacy function.

9. The advocate helps the client to implement the plan and to negotiate with others to solve the problem satisfactorily.

10. The advocate coaches and supports the client in efforts to enlist the help of others in resolving the problem. Asking for help requires the willingness to risk being refused. To ask without coercing is more readily achievable if the client has the support of an advocate.

Subroles

Recall for a moment the definition of advocacy: action designed to help the powerless acquire and use power to make social systems more responsive to their needs. It has been suggested that the advocate, in order to act on behalf of the client, be a trusted confidant. The client communicates to the advocate specific needs, wants, and desires; the advocate plays a number of secondary roles while assisting the client in working within a given social system.

The primary role precedes action, whereas the secondary roles are fulfilled during the course of action. Following are the various subroles, defined by this chapter's primary author, that the advocate uses.

Spokesperson. The spokesperson uses personal power to add strength. The role requires strength, personal communication skills, and personal presence. Influence can be increased through appropriate dress and behavior. Spokespersons speak for others and therefore must be comfortable in expressing not only personal views but those of persons they represent. It is important to listen carefully to the client and convey not only the content of the message but its spirit or intent. For this, the spokesperson must know the client well. Many issues have been lost by the presence, the demeanor, the behavior of a spokesperson who has a "take me as I am" attitude.

Broker. The broker directs others to appropriate services in the way an insurance broker helps others determine their insurance needs. The client then can select the preferred plan. "Salesmanship" is a characteristic of a good broker. Knowing the individual's needs and preferences enables the broker to present options in their most favorable light. Integrity earmarks the difference between opportunism and honest persuasion to help the person achieve goals or formulate new goals.

Mediator. Sometimes the achievement of one person's goals appears to require that another person relinquish all hope of achieving his or her own goals. Mediation occurs when negotiation between the two parties is facilitated by the advocate. A skillful mediator can ideally lead both persons to a compromise beneficial to both.

An advocate assuming a mediatory posture temporarily relinquishes allegiance to either party. Arriving at a solution is accomplished by listening, clarifying, suggesting, and soliciting responses until a balance is achieved and both parties believe they have gained.

Teacher. The role of teacher or coach carries with it a certain amount of authority and may be most appropriate at times of imminent crisis when the client is experiencing acute stress and suffers from a diminished capacity to solve problems. The teacher, at these times, uses a calm but directive manner to reassure and facilitate the performance of tasks that might otherwise be neglected.

Consultant. The role of consultant is distinguished from that of teacher since it emphasizes the communication of information in a less directive and more egalitarian manner. Functioning as a consultant implies active soliciting of advice by the client and provision of advice in an objective, nonjudgmental manner by the consultant.

Activist. An activist is a person who is results-oriented and is willing to take calculated risks to solve the problem. The concept is frequently misunderstood because of connotations of the Free Speech movement, strikes, and peace marches of the recent past. An activist is highly motivated to solve a problem. Some problems are more difficult to solve than others. The following story relates to activism on behalf of the chronically ill.

A group of personal attendants of disabled clients took their clients to the Capitol to get support from legislators for a bill that would make the building wheelchair-accessible so that the disabled could testify at hearings in their own behalf. Although this may seem like a rather nonessential service far removed from the day-to-day needs of the chronically ill, it is not. Decisions made by legislators affect every aspect of the chronically ill person's life from the number of hours of attendant care the state will reimburse to the client's right to refuse food. Who can be more eloquent in speaking in their behalf than the disabled themselves? Who would speak for them? In this context, access to the decision makers becomes a significant issue.

Negotiator. A negotiator represents another and bargains for needed goods and services. Negotiation is a learned skill that the client may not have. Services

of a negotiator are especially valuable when the person with whom negotiations will be pursued is in a position of real or imagined power, and the client finds bargaining from a position of strength difficult because of fear of loss of services or of retaliation. The advocate may either elect to negotiate about a problem in general without revealing the identity of the client or pose the problem in a nonconfrontational manner to protect the client's well-being. The advocate becomes the negotiator when it is not in the client's interest to do the negotiating or when the client is physically or mentally unable to do so.

Problems and Issues of Advocacy

Any situation in which people are at a disadvantage due to inability to negotiate their position can be helped by an advocate. Advocacy occurs in the context and setting in which the nurse and client find themselves. A wide range of difficulties impedes satisfaction of the client's advocacy needs.

Client Barriers

Barriers occurring within the client's social system can prevent problem solving. Helping the client remove these barriers is the first challenge to an advocate. The same barriers that prevent interaction with other members of the client's social network continue to operate unless some enlightened person can assist the client in gaining greater self-awareness and in changing the patterns of decision making and interaction with members of the support network. These barriers have been identified by the primary author in her practice and in the training of advocates.

Ambivalence. Ambivalence is immobilizing and prevents clear, directed action. Ambivalence arises from the presence of conflicting emotions. A very ill stroke client finds himself caught between his desire to die rather than be disabled and his unwillingness to leave his wife. His wife too is ambivalent about her husband's dependence upon her. Loving him for the many years they shared together and loving the person he used to be, she finds that her own needs are not being met. She believes she should provide care for her spouse at home, but fatigue may push her to choose nursing home care.

Disagreement with Significant Others. Disagreement between the client and members of the client's personal network concerning decisions made by the client may make resolution of a problem difficult or may lead to ambivalence. Individuals' decisions ultimately affect self, family, and friends. If the family and friends do not support decisions and actions, the client's power is considerably lessened and may hinder resolution of the problem. These factors must be considered when the advocate discusses client options.

Disagreement with Significant Professionals. Ideally, health team members avoid coercing the client, since coercion violates the ethical principle of alternate possibilities (Shelp & Ternes 1980). It is difficult for the health care professional to support fully a client's right to make decisions when the professional disagrees with those decisions, and the client often feels that disapproval.

In one case a client continued to behave in a way that was threatening her health. For reasons of her own, she neglected to ask family members who cared for her to elevate her feet or to ambulate her. She believed that her physician refused to give her medication to reduce edema in her feet and ankles and felt that she needed more exercise. The swollen feet limited her willingness to leave home because they were unsightly. This client's inability to communicate her needs to her family caregivers and to explain her situation to the doctor led to worsening of her health problem.

Many articles in nursing ethics address the issues surrounding selecting a course of action and the role conflicts among professionals regarding the client's right to choose (Annas 1981; Davis 1981; Shelp & Ternes 1980). The client changes and grows only by experiencing personal failures and successes. Often

in discussions of autonomy, other ethical principles conflict with clients' right to decide for themselves. When such conflicts occur, the issue should be discussed openly with the client's permission so that all parties can express their concerns. If possible, a consensus or agreement by involved parties about the nature of the central issues can help health professionals to appreciate the complexities of the problem and to support the decisions made by the client.

Functional Impairment. Clients' disabilities and resulting functional impairments may hinder their ability to be their own advocates or to enlist the aid of an advocate. Even moderate loss of ability, skill, and knowledge can separate clients from those who could help. Isolated clients may be unable to access systems providing home-delivered meals, affordable oxygen, hospital-based monitoring systems, and so forth.

Loss of Credibility. Loss of credibility is a bitter blow often dealt the client by health professionals. The client's acceptance of vulnerability and dependency often appears to the health professional as needless complaining and unwarranted dependence. The advocate who recognizes this dilemma can guide and reassure the client, help in the retention of self-esteem, and assist the client in finding a way through treacherous waters.

This author's experience indicates that the conflict of dependence versus independence is actually a matter of finding the point on a continuum of dependence where the client's needs are met without loss of the respect and credibility of friends, family, and health professionals. The client must answer these questions: How much help do these people think I need? How much can I ask for without being labeled a malingerer? A client's credibility to people the client depends on is often determined by the ability to answer these questions accurately.

Loss of Motivation and Depression. Loss of motivation to care actively for oneself may be manifested as a lack of interest in bettering oneself through self-advocacy. Decreased motivation often

◇ CASE STUDY ◇

A Missed Diagnosis

An obese 46-year-old White housewife became fatigued easily, was lethargic, claimed she had blurred vision and severe headaches (pressure over the left hemisphere), and began to spend an increasing amount of time in bed. After six months she consulted her family physician, who had been trying to persuade her to lose weight and felt that she overate because she was unhappy with her marriage. This physician began treating her for middle-age depression, telling her she was "fair, fat, forty,

and unloved." Six months later, when she blacked out and fell, she returned to the same physician. He still believed that she was depressed but changed her medications.

Only because a neighbor was able to convince a prominent pathologist in the community of the client's credibility was she referred to a neurosurgeon. A brain scan revealed a tumor, which was later surgically removed.

---

accompanies depression and is accompanied by a fine web of excuses. The advocate learns over time to recognize the client who appears accommodating yet graciously but firmly declines to participate in any activity suggested. One of the first cues is often the professional's sense of fatigue and frustration and a sudden recognition that he or she is doing all the work.

Often when such inertia is discovered, referral to a support group or to a professional counselor may be the most appropriate intervention. Until someone helps them recognize and work against this depression, clients often remain unaware of their role in what they perceive as a hopeless situation.

It is well to remember that depression has a number of causes other than nonacceptance of an illness. Depression is a side effect of some pharmaceuticals used to treat certain chronic illnesses. Sometimes the disease itself is characterized by symptoms of depression. To summarize, then, lack of motivation, evidenced by poor eating and hygiene habits, withdrawal, inertia, and feelings of hopelessness, can occur. When the advocate's skill has no effect in building trust and confidence and motivating the client to act, then referral for evaluation by a mental health professional is the nurse-advocate's best course.

Advocate Barriers

Some barriers to building a trusting relationship with clients for the purpose of understanding their needs

and wishes lie within the advocate and the advocate's professional network. These barriers prevent the advocate from relating to the client or contributing the advocate's best skills to the relationship. Many possible barriers exist. Those presented here were found by this author to be most frequent and troublesome.

Stereotyping and Prejudging. Prejudice among health professionals is a serious barrier. Not only does prejudice impede advocacy but it frequently causes mistreatment of clients. When health professionals are blinded by their own biases, they are unable to see clearly. Assessment by nurses and diagnosis by physicians are only as accurate as the health professional's ability to see.

Advocacy requires that the caregiver inspire trust and confidence. How can a client trust if the advocate has already determined the nature of the client's problem before consulting the client?

In the case study above, the client's lack of credibility to the physician caused him to ignore or disbelieve the personal testimony of a severe pressure inside the cranium. The neighbor acting as the woman's advocate persuaded another physician that she was reliable and deserved a fair assessment. It is frightening to imagine what could have occurred if the client had not had a neighbor who was able to intervene on her behalf.

Disagreement among Health Professionals. The chronically ill person relies greatly on physicians, nurses, and other caregivers for support and encouragement. Each of these caregivers may have considerable influence on the client's opinions and decisions and may act as the person's advocate. Confusion can arise from conflicts about treatment among these various individuals. Therefore, it may become essential to elicit the cooperation of all health team members to reach a consensus in supporting the client's decision-making process. The nurse-advocate acting as a negotiator can aid other health professionals to reach a consensus and support the client.

Conflict of Interest. Nurses usually are employed by agencies who contract with clients to provide health care services. Under these circumstances, the nurse is in the position of "serving two masters" (Greenlaw 1980). Contractual responsibility is to the employer because of an agreement to provide nursing services for a paid wage. Therefore, the employer has the right to expect the nurse to follow the policies and procedures of the agency and to be a cooperative and productive member of the work force. The employer's goals are the guiding principles for the agency. Ideally, one of those goals is delivering not only cost-effective but quality services to clients.

On the other hand, nurses have an ethical responsibility to provide high-quality nursing care. This responsibility is supported by licensing requirements for safe care. In addition, nurses have a Code of Ethics to practice according to their consciences.

These two sets of obligations can create direct conflict between the nurse's sense of responsibility to practice in a safe manner and contractual factors such as working cooperatively with other employees and maintaining positive relationships with physicians who provide needed referrals for the employing agency or hospital.

A conflict of interest can arise when the professional has opposing obligations to the hospital and to the client. The nurse in this case may face a choice between two mutually exclusive actions. Now, a nurse who chooses to act for the client as an advocate may perceive a conflict with the goals of the agency or hospital. Greenlaw (1980) suggests that the nurse's professional standards require that the client's health and rights override any duty to an employer.

Although this may be the ideal, the decision to uphold the client's rights may pose a threat to the agency; the administration may consider replacing the nurse to serve the hospital's best interest. The risk of losing employment, current and future, is a very real barrier to the nurse's ability to advocate for clients. The nurse must become wise in the ways of organizations and learn to be an advocate for her clients skillfully without jeopardizing such employment. Safeguards presented later in this chapter can reduce the nurse's risk of sanctions.

Overinvolvement. Overinvolvement is another potential barrier to the nurse's ability to be an advocate. When the nurse becomes overly involved in a client's life, the line between nurse and client fades, and the nurse can no longer distinguish the client as separate from self.

Overinvolvement is not simply a matter of degree of caring for the client, for the nurse cannot care too much. It is a difference in perception. Nurses lose their perception of the client as separate from their personal subjective world. The client becomes part of that world and takes on emotional characteristics of one of the characters dear to the nurse: parent, child, sibling, spouse. When this occurs, the nurse loses sight of the client as a separate individual and becomes overly invested in linking her or his positive self-image to successful advocacy, a process familiar to helping professionals. This process, which Karpman (1968) called the *games triangle* (rescuer-victim-persecutor triangle), takes the decision-making process out of the hands of the client. Kohnke (1980) applied this model to ineffective use of the nurse-advocate role, as, for example, when the nurse helps make a decision (rescue) for a reluctant client (victim) and then is reluctant to be held responsible when the client places blame (persecutor) on the nurse for making a poor decision.

This kind of overinvolvement requires that at some point the nurse withdraw from the client to avoid becoming angry or resentful toward the client.

Such intense feeling can become emotionally and physically exhausting. Frequently, the nurse finds that she or he is missing days from work or beginning to avoid the client. At that point, the nurse has long since lost perspective on the situation as it actually is and needs a peer or coworker to restore perspective.

Time and Energy Limitations. Although advocacy is a proper activity for nurses caring for people who are chronically ill, employment as a staff nurse may leave the potential advocate time- and energy-poor, necessitating developing time management skills. Acting as an advocate diverts time from expected nursing duties. Implicit in this perspective is the assumption that advocacy is not the nurse's primary activity. Rather, the employing agency perceives the nurse's primary responsibility as providing ongoing assessment of client status, assisting the person with self-care activities, and performing prescribed procedures and treatments. The advocate who neglects nursing duties for the sake of advocacy becomes vulnerable to sanctions by an administration whose focus may differ from that of the nurse and therefore may disapprove the nurse's making advocacy a priority.

Time available for nursing advocacy remains limited for another important reason. Access to clients is determined to a large extent by the nursing functions that are paid for by third-party payers (insurance companies, Medicare, and Medicaid). The payers determine which duties are reimbursable, often without nursing input; since advocacy is not in the realm of reimbursable duties, it remains an unpaid function. Consequently, the nurse must advocate as an adjunct to her regular duties when time and energy permit.

Social and Cultural Barriers. Social and cultural differences between advocate and client can be barriers to the advocacy process. These differences may make it difficult for nurse-advocates to intervene with those clients whose values are markedly different from their own. The inclusion of humanities and social sciences as prerequisites or requirements for nursing education broadens nurses' background for understanding other social groups and cultures.

When Clients Are Not Their Own Legal Agents

Although an in-depth analysis of guardianship or conservatorship is beyond the scope of this chapter, some discussion of the impact of legal agency on the client-advocate relationship is in order.

At times chronically ill clients cannot care for themselves physically or mentally or perform the necessary steps to ensure their personal safety in a complex society. At these times clients may elect to appoint a legal representative or the court may appoint a legal guardian or conservator. Conservators usually assume responsibility for such persons, ensuring that their needs are met, or conservators may manage the estate or finances. In both cases, whether they are selected or appointed, the probate court oversees the conservators' and guardians' performance. Therefore, if a client is being neglected or wishes another conservator, the probate court investigates and takes appropriate action.

The advocate must determine whether the client has a legal agent and whether the agent was voluntarily selected by the client or appointed by the court. Clients who have guardians are not their own agents and cannot enter into agreements except those specified by the court. An advocate must know the client's status before acting as an advocate or becoming immersed in a legal morass.

A legal agent can be a friend, family member, or public guardian. In any case, unless the conservator is a health professional, he or she will most likely be unfamiliar with the medical disability of the client and the needs that arise from it. Qualifications of public guardians vary widely from state to state: some are trained in personal financial management; others have no training.

There are problems associated with working with a client's legal agent; many can be avoided by identifying the person who is the legal agent and including this person, from the beginning, in any decisions made by and for a client. Assuming that a conservator is concerned with the client's well-being may, at best, win a valuable colleague; at worst, it diffuses a potential adversary as the nurse attempts to advocate for a client. Determining the effectiveness of the client's relationship with the conservator may be a first step in teaching the client self-advocacy.

Irresolvable Problems

Sometimes problems that have no solution arise. At other times, clients perceive difficulties to have solutions that, in fact, are not practical. Two factors can render a problem irresolvable: distortion and necessity for higher resolution.

Distortion.   At times an individual's perception of a situation is distorted; the problem may not exist as the client sees it. The solution most obvious to the client may not be relevant to the "real problem" the nurse or others perceive. On the other hand, the client may believe a problem has no solution, although it may be readily resolved, and therefore refuse to make efforts toward resolution. The task of redefining the client's problems in solvable terms is a prerequisite to solving them.

Need for Higher Resolution.   Most problems can be solved to some degree, but not all solutions are within the grasp of the advocate. It is important that nurse-advocates realistically assess their ability to help the client and recognize problems that should be referred to someone else, especially when problems are at the legislative, regulatory, or policy-making level. In such circumstances, focusing on the immediate facility is ineffective.

For example, in nursing homes in the state of California the facility is paid by Medicaid for residents' room fees. Residents receive a nominal fee each month for personal needs allowance and incidental expenses. The fee paid to the facility does not cover supplemental services such as laundry or some medications. When residents must pay for laundry expenses, they often complain since this expense limits the allocated allowance available for inciden-

tals such as candy, cigarettes, birthday cards, or note paper. The criticisms of nursing homes by advocates, family, clients, and sometimes staff for charging these laundry fees do not take into account that these laundry charges are within an "acceptable" range approved by the state. In addition, allowance fees paid to residents are determined and controlled by legislation. Taking this complaint to the individual facility does not solve the problem. Rather, such complaints only create hard feelings and more frustration.

A more effective approach would be to focus on the passage of legislation that would prohibit the use of a resident's personal needs allowance for pharmaceuticals and laundry fees and would provide room rate fees that include incidental costs. Solving a problem at the appropriate level involves determining the source of the problem and the factors that led to its development.

Interventions

The preceding sections have discussed the roles and functions of the advocate and the problems the advocate encounters. This section presents a model for advocacy by nurses.

Toward a Model for Advocacy by Nurses

The advocacy model presented here is adapted from a description of the advocacy process developed by Terri Brower (1980). The model has been formulated to complement the nursing process (see Table 13-2) and is appropriate for both acute and skilled facilities.

This advocacy model has three phases. In the first phase, the nurse and client build and define their relationship, establishing rapport, building trust, and setting limits. The acceptable amount of dependency the client will be allowed to demonstrate without censure is determined. At times the client takes charge, and the nurse assumes a less directive but supportive posture. At other times, the client is in a learning mode, and the nurse teaches advocacy skills.

TABLE 13-2. Advocacy Model

Goal	Objectives	Activities
Phase I A supportive relationship with client is developed.	Client will begin to trust nurse-advocate for support, advocacy, and decision making.	1. Advocate listens empathetically. 2. Advocate states client's observations, feelings, and desires in an honest, nonthreatening manner.
Client and advocate have and abide by a written agreement.	Client and advocate will agree upon roles and activities in advocating for client's self-interest.	1. Client and advocate both state their expectations. 2. Areas of disagreement are discussed and compromises made.
Problem is identified.	Client and advocate will state problem in concrete, observable terms.	1. Advocate encourages client to state problem from a personal perspective. 2. Advocate directs and assists client to restate problem in terms that can be observed and validated. 3. Advocate encourages client to visualize and articulate the ideal situation.
Phase II Plan is developed to the client's satisfaction.	Client will be able to articulate problem in terms of unmet expectations or needs.	1. Advocate directs client to decide what must change to achieve the desired effect.
	Client will have access to information needed for decision making.	1. Advocate evaluates client's readiness to participate in finding information. 2. Advocate, on the basis of client's knowledge, ability, skill, and motivation, assists client in obtaining needed information. 3. Client participates in obtaining needed information.
	Client will decide whether to take action to make the desired change or to take no action.	1. Advocate assesses client's readiness for making the decision (grasp of information, objectivity, motivation to solve problem). 2. Advocate informs client of all options.
	If taking action, client will decide the most effective action.	1. Advocate reviews all information accumulated, including available resources and possible avenues of recourse.

TABLE 13-2. Continued

Goal	Objectives	Activities
		2. Advocate presents options and possible consequences of various actions.
		3. Advocate honestly relates to client the extent to which the advocate can participate in each option.
	Course of action will be determined and plan made.	1. Advocate praises and supports client's decision even if the advocate would not have chosen it.
		2. Advocate presents available resources, time frames, and any other information needed for a workable plan.
		3. Advocate assesses client's ability and readiness to participate and consequent role of advocate in complementing client.
Plan is implemented with maximum participation by client and support by advocate.	Action taken will directly address the problem defined by client and advocate.	1. Advocate supports client in carrying out plan.
		2. Advocate participates in activity to whatever extent is deemed necessary according to their contract.
Phase III Degree to which problem is solved is determined and new goal is set.	Client will determine whether problem has been corrected satisfactorily.	1. Advocate provides honest feedback about success of plan, praising aspects deserving recognition.
		2. Advocate encourages client to correct aspects that were unsuccessful.

Ideally, they arrive at a partnership for action. Also during the first phase, the client and nurse begin to examine the situation and to separate fact from misconception or distortion. A definable, observable problem will be identified by the client and nurse; the nurse and client contract for the degree of participation acceptable to both.

During the second phase, the work of problem solving begins. Goals are set and a course of action

planned. The client's readiness, ability, and motivation to solve problems that arise are assessed, and the time and energy commitment that the nurse can and will make is specified. The advocate participates in each step of the process, providing support, encouragement, and information to complement the client's need for assistance in decision making and action. The client who determines a course of action is more likely to be committed to the selected course.

The advocate must then accept the client's decision even if the advocate cannot condone the option or does not want to participate in it. This position can be difficult for the advocate.

A word of caution is necessary: Once a plan is determined, it is well to let the client "sleep on the decision" unless there is an urgent need for action. Delay allows the client time to change his or her mind and to realize that the advocate has not been coercive. Delay also provides clients the opportunity to be sure that they made the decision themselves. If they did, they are less likely to blame the advocate should the outcome be less satisfactory than expected.

The advocate and client then collaborate on a method for carrying out the option, keeping in mind the client's resources and ability. Clients who feel unable to cope with the selected method may find reasons not to fulfill their function in the plan. This problem often can be prevented if the advocate sincerely tries to tailor the method to the client's skills and motivation. As an example, a client who finds speaking to strangers impossible should not have to consider the option of testifying before a state legislature. This method certainly does not maximize the client's strengths. In addition to carrying out the actual plan of action, success or failure should be noted. Attention to the process used is important at this juncture since in the third phase it will determine future action.

The skill of negotiating effectively for the client may be necessary when other people are involved in the problem. The goal at this time should be to resolve the problem to the client's benefit. Teaching the art of skillful and effective negotiation is beyond the scope of this chapter.

In phase three, the client and nurse evaluate the performance and assess the results. Measures of success that were set up jointly by the advocate and client during the first phase are used. The evaluation tool should focus on a means of determining whether the problem has been resolved to the client's satisfaction. During the evaluation phase, the attainment of realistic goals should be approximated, and the process and methods used should be evaluated. The client and advocate can take pleasure in successes large or small. The client can then proceed toward realistic plans for further action growing out of the evaluation.

Developing Power in the Work Setting

To act in the best interests of their clients and avoid termination, nurses must acquire skill in the art of surviving in a bureaucracy: developing personal and political power and the ability to influence others.

The New Employee. Exercise of power depends on length of tenure in the position. The nurse who is new in an agency must observe the "Rules for Rookies" found in the nursing lounge in a community hospital:

1. Know your job duties and perform them well. Remember, it doesn't matter how good you are; how well you perform as part of the team is what counts.
2. Don't let anger and fear drive you to impulsive actions that you may regret.
3. Never criticize or challenge your superiors or colleagues at meetings when others are present.
4. Don't try to do everything or to be all things to all people.
5. Learn from mistakes and putdowns. Figure out better tactics for the next try.
6. Don't disparage any success you achieve. Publicize.

The new nurse must undertake advocacy cautiously. Observing these six rules will help the new employee gain credibility. Often it is important to have a mentor or friend who has more experience and in whom one can confide. Many colleagues can be gained through active membership in the professional nurses' associations, in which the joys and frustrations of the work can be shared in a safe, supportive environment. The novice advocate can also benefit from determining the potentially useful structures or persons within the work organization. In every organization some individual usually stands out as being particularly skilled at getting things done. Making a connection with this person to learn his or her methods is a way to develop these skills in the particular work setting.

The Long-time Employee. Many nurses with years of experience have never contemplated the possibility of changing hospital policy to improve quality of life for the client. Should he or she decide to advocate some change, the long-time employee has one advantage over the neophyte: a history of service to the institution. The long-time employee who begins to believe that change and improved conditions are possible can draw on an established network for assistance. It is well to avoid coercion; a simple request often suffices. Enlisting support may take time.

Nurses who avoid both being defensive and projecting a judgmental attitude find many people willing and able to follow them into this new role. The most efficacious technique is to build on small successes.

Summary and Conclusions

A thorough knowledge of advocacy can help the practicing nurse to serve his or her clients better. To do so requires a working knowledge of advocacy, the roles and functions of an advocate, and ways to apply this knowledge in the work setting. The potential advocate must be aware of the relationship that needs to exist between advocate and client and acknowledge that the client has the final voice in decisions.

Problems that can impede the individual in the performance of the advocate role include barriers erected by client and advocate that impede the development of a trusting relationship. Advocacy is also affected when clients cannot act as their own legal agents, when administrative policy conflicts with client considerations, and when irresolvable problems arise.

The advocacy model serves as a means of integrating advocacy with the nursing process. Through this model, the advocate develops a relationship with the client while identifying the problem, acts to help the client reach a solution, and teaches the client to evaluate results. The potential advocate needs also to master guidelines to advocacy that balance meeting the client's needs with meeting the nurse's responsibility to the employing agency. It must again be emphasized that the client decides the actions to be taken with the advocate's support.

Nurses who try to act as advocates are perceived negatively if they do not learn to get and keep power in their pursuit of excellence. They must avoid becoming isolated or finding themselves the object of criticism and close scrutiny. Nurse-advocates' ability to intervene effectively is lost when their hands are tied.

In some sense, all nurses who wish to advocate are swimming upstream, going against the tide, at least at the beginning. If they are able, through power of persuasion, to convince others of their credibility and the rightness of their actions, the tide may turn.

STUDY QUESTIONS

1. How do you define advocacy? the advocate role of the nurse? What assumptions underlie any discussion of this role?
2. What factors influence power deficits? Discuss their relationship to advocacy.
3. Under what circumstances will an advocate intervene to help another person?
4. What is the difference between advocacy and agency?
5. What are the primary role and functions of an advocate? What are the subroles? Discuss them.
6. What client barriers prevent problem solving? Discuss each.
7. How do barriers within the advocate impede functioning in this role? Discuss each of these advocate barriers.
8. What is an irresolvable problem? How can such problems be handled?
9. Given a client situation, how would you implement advocacy through Brower's advocacy model?
10. As an employee in a hospital, how would you function to maximize your opportunities to work as an advocate?

References

Annas, G. J., (1981) Invasion of privacy, *Nursing Law and Ethics, 2*(2):3

Brower, T. H., (1980) Advocacy: What it is, *Journal of Gerontological Nursing, 8*(3):141–143

Davis, A. J., (1981) Compassion, suffering, morality: Ethical dilemmas in caring, *Nursing Law and Ethics, 2*(6)

Gadow, S., (1983) Existential advocacy: Philosophical foundations of nursing in ethical problems, in Murphy, C. P., and Hunter, H. (eds.), *Ethical Problems in the Nurse-Patient Relationship,* Boston: Allyn and Bacon

Greenlaw, J., R.N., J.D., (1980) To whom is the nurse accountable? *Nursing Law and Ethics, 1*(1):3

Karpman, S., (1968) Script drama analysis, *Transactional Analysis Bulletin, 7*(26):39–43

Kayser-Jones, I. S., (1981) *Old, Alone and Neglected: Care of the Aged in Scotland and the United States,* Berkeley, Calif.: University of California Press

Kohnke, M. F., (1980) The nurse as advocate, *American Journal of Nursing, 80*(11):2038–2040

Murphy, C. P., and Hunter, H., (1983) Existential advocacy: Philosophical foundations of nursing, in *Ethical Problems in the Nurse-Patient Relationship,* Boston: Allyn and Bacon

Orem, D. E., (1985) *Nursing: Concepts of Practice,* New York: McGraw-Hill

Orgel, G. S., (1983) They have no right to know: The nurse and the terminally ill patient, in Murphy, C. P., and Hunter, H. (eds.), *Ethical Problems in the Nurse-Patient Relationship,* Boston: Allyn and Bacon

Rogers, J. C., (1980) Advocacy: The key to assessing the older client, *Journal of Gerontological Nursing, 6*(1):33–36

Shelp, E. E., and Ternes, C., (1980) Moral integrity for nurses, *Nursing Law and Ethics, 1*(9):2–8

Strauss, A. L., and Glaser, B. G., (1975) *Chronic Illness and the Quality of Life,* St. Louis: C.V. Mosby

Underwood, P., (1981) "Advocation of self-care deficit theory to the community based elderly." Paper presented at Self-Care Deficit Workshop sponsored by St. Luke's Hospital, San Francisco, April 1981.

CHAPTER FOURTEEN

Research

Introduction

Research is increasingly recognized as an important component of the professional nurses' role. In recent articles in professional journals, authors encouraged nurses to identify problems in their clinical practice that lent themselves to research, to conduct or collaborate in research investigations, and to utilize research findings more fully in their clinical practice (Downs 1984; Haller, Reynolds & Horsley 1979; Kirchhoff 1983; Morse & Conrad 1983).

Practitioners who work with the chronically ill often are dissatisfied with the limited impact of their interventions, yet they may not be aware of research findings that offer possible solutions to their problems. Nurses and other health care providers also may not consider conducting research studies to gain a better understanding of their clients' health problems or to test the effectiveness of treatment approaches. Without the active pursuit of new knowledge, treatment of chronic health problems can become very routine, and practitioners may feel pessimistic about the potential benefits of their treatment efforts.

Research-Based Nursing Practice

The ultimate goal of nursing, like that of other health disciplines, is to promote health and quality of life and to prevent premature death, illness, disability, and suffering. Chronic illness, such as that of Mr. Wil-

son in the case study, presents a persistent challenge to this goal. Other chapters in this text discuss many of the problems imposed by chronic illness and offer suggestions as to how nurses might assist chronically ill clients and their families to maintain optimal functioning and quality of life. Many questions regarding chronicity remain unanswered, however, and nursing research is crucial to building a knowledge base for professional practice. Nursing research can contribute significantly to the understanding of chronic health problems, as well as assisting practitioners to identify the most effective strategies for their clients' successful adaptation to long-term illness.

Documenting Cost-Effectiveness

In addition to building a stronger base of clinical knowledge, nursing research can help improve the cost-effectiveness of long-term health care. This has important implications for the chronically ill, since the present economic climate has seriously limited funding for long-term care. Fagin (1982) reviewed a number of studies that demonstrate how innovative nursing practices can directly benefit clients and result in cost savings as well. Several of these studies show that periodic nursing home visits, as well as other types of educational and counseling programs for the chronically ill, can improve the way clients manage their symptoms and decrease emergency room visits, hospitalization, and absenteeism from work. Ventura and others (1985) conducted a detailed

◇ CASE STUDY ◇
Mr. Wilson

Mr. Wilson's admission to the hospital was no surprise to the nurses on Unit 6-South. For several months, he had periodically been brought to the emergency room in severe respiratory distress. Since his wife's stroke last year, Mr. Wilson, an emphysemic, had been having increasing difficulty managing his medical regimen. He had missed several clinic appointments, and nurses noticed that he was becoming increasingly forgetful and resistant to help.

Mr. Wilson is a 64-year-old retired carpenter and, before his wife's stroke, he had spent a good deal of time in his workshop, making toys for his grandchildren. Recently, having taken over most of the light household chores, he found little time for the toy making he so enjoyed. With daily visits from his daughter and help from the local medical pool for his wife's care, Mr. Wilson managed the daily routine fairly well, although his coordination was becoming quite poor and he frequently could not remember how to proceed with household tasks. Mr. Wilson's greatest worry was that he would be unable to continue caring for his wife at home. He tried to avoid thinking about this problem, since emotional upsets made him very short of breath.

Mr. Wilson's current respiratory crisis appeared to have been precipitated by a letter from his insurance company, advising him that coverage for his wife's home care would end in one month. Soon after receiving the letter, he began coughing and wheezing and was brought to the emergency room by his daughter.

The nurses on 6-South had no difficulty in initiating emergency treatment for Mr. Wilson, but long-term care was a real dilemma. Mr. Wilson's daughter suggested that her parents temporarily move in with her. Although very much opposed to this idea, Mr. Wilson accepted the offer, since there seemed to be no other solution.

---

cost analysis of a nurse-conducted health-promotion program for patients with peripheral vascular disease. These investigators found that the program dramatically cut the costs of health care services, even when costs of implementing the new program were included in the analysis.

Several studies have demonstrated the cost-effectiveness of home care for the chronically ill (Fagin 1982; Hammond 1979; Martinson 1978). In Martinson's studies of nurse-coordinated home care for children dying of cancer, hospital care was found to be approximately 18 times more expensive than home care. Parents' participation in the home care program also emphasized the improved quality of care that could be provided through a home hospice orientation and the parents' emotional rewards from caring for their dying child at home (Martinson 1978).

Other studies have focused on evaluating the cost and quality of health care when nurses are substituted for other health care providers. Overall, these studies indicate that when nurse-midwives, pediatric and adult nurse-practitioners, and clinical nurse-specialists are appropriately substituted for physicians, costs can be lowered without sacrificing the quality of care (Fagin 1982). Findings from such studies can be used in the political arena to influence legislation that impacts on the chronically ill. The nursing profession also benefits from documenting its cost-effectiveness, as third-party reimbursement and the scope of nursing practice are strongly influenced by economic considerations.

Need for Use of Findings

In order for research to have a positive impact on nursing practice, nurses in clinical settings need to become aware not only of research relevant to their areas of practice but also of how to utilize findings effectively to benefit their clients. Although the basic idea of using research findings to improve patient care is accepted in nursing, individual practitioners actually may have considerable difficulty in obtaining needed information and assessing its usability (Barnard 1980; Krueger, Nelson, & Wolanin 1978). Similar problems in research utilization are experienced in most professional disciplines, but their particular significance for nursing comes from the profession's pressing need for a stronger base of scientific knowledge for practice.

Historical Perspectives

Since the early 1900s, research in the health fields has undergone considerable growth and change. In the early part of the century, health research consisted primarily of privately funded medical investigations that searched for cures for infectious diseases. With the discovery of antibiotics, X rays, and other diagnostic techniques during World War II, infectious diseases were brought under control and attention turned toward chronic conditions, including heart disease, strokes, and malignancies, which rapidly became the major health problems (DHEW 1979). Also, interest in mental disorders increased during the post–World War II years because of both the large numbers of veterans with combat-related mental problems and the discovery of tranquilizer drugs, which offered hope for advances in mental health research.

From the 1940s to the mid-1960s, research on chronic diseases flourished in medical centers, as investigators attempted to discover the causes of specific diseases as well as effective treatments and cures. During this time, federal funding for health research increased substantially. The National Institutes of Health (NIH) and the National Institute of Mental Health (NIMH) were established to provide leadership for this research. The mandate of the national institutes was to conduct research and to encourage outside research on significant health problems by funding extramural projects through competitive grants.

The National Cancer Institute was the first NIH institute established that centered on a specific category of disease. It was followed by institutes for

heart and lung diseases, allergy and infectious diseases, and mental disorders (NIMH) in the 1940s, and by institutes for arthritis and metabolic disorders, neurologic problems, eye diseases, and environmental health problems in the 1950s and 1960s (Larson 1984).

Since the mid-1960s, health research has taken a much more multidisciplinary approach, integrating psychologists, sociologists, public health researchers, nurses, and other health care providers into the medical research community. Also, emphasis on prevention in health research has increased. The preventive focus emanated from a greater awareness of the role of environmental, psychosocial, and behavioral risk factors in the cause and progression of chronic disease. The 1979 Surgeon General's report on health promotion and disease prevention (DHEW 1979) stimulated the federal government to sponsor prevention-related research. For example, during the 1980s, these included demonstration projects for control of hypertension and other health promotion programs (NCHS 1983).

Although the greatest portion of federal health research funds continues to be allocated to biomedical research, government agencies support a substantial number of social and behavioral studies. Many studies on chronic illness and aging are eligible for funds from the National Institute on Child Health and Human Development, established in 1969, and the National Institute on Aging, established in 1974 (Martinson 1983). A number of private foundations and associations also have begun to fund research on chronic care.

Development of Nursing Research

Nursing has only begun to demonstrate its potential in health research. During the formative years of the NIH research program, nursing studies focused primarily on personnel and professional activities rather than on client-centered health problems. However, clinical nursing research has shown progressive growth in the past two decades. Table 14-1 shows the major historical highlights of this trend.

TABLE 14-1. Historical Highlights

	Legislation; agency development	Major nursing research activities
1920–1930s		A few case studies and patient-centered care plans appear in nursing literature.
1940s		Surveys on nursing needs and resources: Goldmark Report, Committee for the Grading of Nursing Schools Study, Brown's "Nursing for the Future" publication.
		World War II prompts increased collection of data on nursing personnel resources and stimulates interest in documenting nursing practices. After World War II, articles suggesting the need for systematic evaluation of nursing techniques appear in the literature.
	Division of Nursing Resources; U.S. Public Health Service (1948)	Agency is mandated to investigate nursing supply and distribution, quality and costs of nursing education, job satisfaction and turnover, patient and personnel satisfaction with care. Studies lead to published guidelines for institutions on techniques for studying nursing activities. Several nursing "activity" studies completed.
1950s		ANA conducts study of nursing activities and publishes document on functions, standards, and qualifications for nursing practice.
	Nursing Research Grants and Fellowship Program; U.S. Public Health Service (1955). Administered under NIH	Grants provide funding for study and development of clinical graduate programs in nursing. Fellowships are awarded to a few nurses for doctoral studies in nursing-related disciplines. Sociological studies of nurses' personality traits, professional socialization, career mobility, and educational opportunities are published.
1960s	Institutional Training Grant Program; U.S. Public Health Service (1962). Administered under NIH until 1963, then transferred to Division of Nursing	Grants increase funding for training of nurse-scientists in disciplines related to nursing. Studies are conducted on nursing education, with increased emphasis on health research and patient care issues.
	Faculty Research and Development Grants Program; Division of Nursing (1959-1966)	Grants provide funds for research development in 19 nursing schools and 3 other agencies. Clinical studies are initiated on interpersonal aspects of care, death and dying, and other topics.
1970s	Research Development Grants Program; Division of Nursing (1968-1977)	Funds are provided to 20 schools of nursing for research development. There is increased emphasis on generating knowledge base underlying nursing practice, development of nursing theory.

TABLE 14-1 Continued

Legislation; agency development	Major nursing research activities
	WICHE Delphi Study of clinical nursing research priorities identifies need for greater utilization of research in nursing practice, as well as development of valid and reliable research instruments; it also suggests more studies of the impact of nursing interventions on patient welfare.
	National Academy of Science survey of doctoral programs in nursing (1977–1978) finds variability in quality of nursing research training and recommends further strengthening of faculty research productivity and comprehensive program for strengthening existing doctoral programs in nursing.
Nursing Research Grants Program; Division of Nursing (component of biomedical and behavioral research grants program authorized under U.S. Public Health Service)	Grants are made available for individual nurse-investigators, as well as research-oriented conferences and institutional research projects. Increased numbers of nurses conduct clinical studies and obtain funding from Division of Nursing, NIH institutes, and private sources.
1980s Nursing Research Grants Program; Division of Nursing	Grants for development of nursing research continue. Types of grants are expanded to include individual nurse-investigator projects, program (cluster) grants for collaborative studies, new investigator awards, research on research utilization, doctoral program development, and small business grants.
	ANA (1981) identifies five priorities for nursing research: 1. promoting well-being and competency for personal care 2. preventing health problems throughout the life span 3. decreasing negative impact of health problems on coping abilities, productivity, and life satisfaction 4. ensuring care needs of vulnerable population groups 5. designing and developing more cost-effective health care delivery systems
	Institute of Medicine Report on Nursing and Nursing Education (1983) emphasizes the need for increased funding of nursing research and better integration of nursing research into scientific community; it advocates a federal center for nursing research. Nursing groups lobby for increased federal funding and creation of an NIH institute for nursing research.

TABLE 14-1. Continued

Legislation; agency development	Major nursing research activities
	ANA Cabinet on Nursing Research develops position paper for nursing research development (1984). Strategies are outlined for (1) ensuring an increased supply of nurse-scientists; (2) generating knowledge concerning well-being and health, nursing interventions, effective delivery of services, excellence in nursing education, and impact of nursing on health policy; (3) disseminating results of nursing research; (4) developing environments that support nursing research and inquiry.
	By 1984, more than 4,000 nurses have doctoral degrees. Doctorally prepared nurses are employed in many clinical settings as well as in universities. Nurses become more active in the political arena and are appointed to national health advisory councils.

Source: Compiled from information in articles by Jacox (1980), Gortner (1980, 1983b), and Larson (1984) and from general information available from the American Nurses Association and the Division of Nursing.

In late 1984, the ANA Cabinet on Nursing Research policy statement included several goals, strategies, and priorities for development of nursing research during the 1980s and 1990s. General goals include

1. Increasing the supply of nurse scientists
2. Generating knowledge about the well-being and optimal functioning of human beings, the effective delivery of nursing services, excellence in nursing education, and the impact of the profession on health policy
3. Disseminating the results of nursing research to clinicians, the scientific community, the public, and policy makers, and increasing the utilization of research findings
4. Developing environments that support nursing inquiry and research.

At the present time, the future of nursing research looks promising, although the profession continues to lack adequate funding for research development; nurses currently receive only 0.8% of federal research and development funds (Larson 1984). Although legislators have become more aware of the need for increased funding for nursing research, nurses must be more politically active and persuasive if they are to compete successfully for research support.

Areas of Chronicity Research

Several broad areas of research can contribute to the knowledge base needed in chronic care nursing. Research studies to determine how various environmental, psychosocial, and behavioral factors influence specific chronic illnesses and disease progression are especially important. An example of this type of research would be a longitudinal study of the course of illness among chronic lung disease patients who quit smoking versus those who continue to smoke. Other studies might focus on identifying environmental stressors that exacerbate disease symptoms or how different social support systems help clients cope with environmental stressors or the disease process.

Another important area of research is the impact of chronic illness on clients and their families. Many of the chapters in this text present research about such impact relative to the chapter's topic. Dimond and Jones (1983) point out the need to study the impact and consequences of illness at different developmental life stages, since chronic conditions pose very different problems and require different coping strategies in childhood, adolescence, mid-adulthood, or old age. Longitudinal cohort studies are very useful in this type of research, since the investigator can select a specific disease and can describe how individuals at different life stages experience it.

A third major area of research is the impact of nursing on the course of illness and the patient's adaptation. Clinical trials, in which different intervention strategies are tested, are crucial for nursing practice. This type of research can clarify which interventions are most effective for which clients, illnesses, or stages of illness. Nurses also can conduct studies to compare the costs and benefits of different types of interventions and nursing care delivery systems. Cost-effective services can assure higher quality care for the chronically ill and can help guarantee the appropriate use of nurses in the health care system.

Major Methodologies in Nursing Research

Various methodologies are used to conduct nursing research studies, many of which are appropriate for research on chronic illness. To avoid confusion, it is helpful to conceptualize nursing studies as either *observational* or *interventional* studies. Observational studies of chronic illness are intended to gain information about the illness, client adaptation, or other phenomena relevant to nursing practice. Investigators may seek to better describe the phenomena under investigation (descriptive research) or may study relationships among variables to predict or explain

events (correlational research and hypothesis testing). Observational studies are essential in building theories and determining the rationale underlying nursing practice.

Nursing intervention studies evaluate or "test" the effectiveness of innovative nursing practices or compare the outcome of different interventional strategies. The interventions tested should be based on sound rationale or theories previously developed from observational studies. An example of this process would be a study to determine whether a nurse-conducted support group for adolescent diabetics results in improved management of diet and medication and better control of the disease. The theory underlying the intervention in this example would have been developed from a long series of observational studies in which the positive effects of social support networks on coping and health status had been well documented.

Qualitative and Quantitative Methods

There is much confusion about qualitative and quantitative methods in nursing research. Although these methods are often discussed as though they represented separate and mutually exclusive research perspectives, they actually reflect only different approaches to data collection and analysis. Table 14-2 outlines and compares some of the major features of qualitative and quantitative research methods.

It is important for nurses to avoid strong biases against either research method, since both play an important role in nursing research (Goodwin & Goodwin 1984; Hoeffer & Archbold 1983; Knafl & Howard 1984; Swanson & Chenitz 1982). Quantitative methods are especially useful in research testing hypotheses and evaluating programs in which measurements of outcome criteria must be very exact. Qualitative methods, on the other hand, often provide in-depth information that cannot be gained by quantitative methods and, thus, are very important in generating theories (Goodwin & Goodwin 1984; Swanson & Chenitz 1982).

Many nursing studies of chronic illness and long-term care exemplify the effective use of quantitative

TABLE 14-2. Major Features of Qualitative and Quantitative Research Methods

	Qualitative Methods	Quantitative Methods
Purposes	Gathering information about a relatively unknown phenomenon; conceptualization and theory formulation; supplementing quantitative data to increase sensitivity and understanding of clients' problems; developing research instruments.	Gathering information to describe or explain phenomena when variables can be defined clearly and operationalized; testing theory; validating research instruments; formal hypothesis testing.
Types of studies	Observational studies: anthropologic or ethnographic studies, case studies, surveys using open-ended interviewing techniques or clients' diaries. Intervention studies: less frequent, though qualitative data can be collected and studied to assess the impact of interventions.	Observational studies: formal surveys, using questionnaires with coded response options such as rating scales. Intervention studies with experimental or quasi-experimental designs. Expected outcomes of intervention are measured or are categorized, using precoded formats.
Data collection	Often by participant-observation. Investigators use field notes to collect narrative information or record selected data from audiotapes or videotapes. Information also can be collected from medical records, diaries, and other documents.	Survey data collected by mailed questionnaires or by telephone or face-to-face interviewing. Data in intervention studies collected by observation, participant-observation, medical record review, or other recordings. Specific protocols for intervention and data collection used.
Data generated	Narrative descriptions (from clients' statements or observers' recordings). Information not coded into numerical categories but studied for its substantive meaning. Information subjected to content analysis or grounded theory methods are used to identify meanings; typologies may be developed. Statistical tests do not apply.	Numerical data or information grouped into categories. Various descriptive or inferential statistics may be used, depending on the level of data (nominal, ordinal, interval, ratio) and purpose of the study (descriptive, explanatory, hypothesis testing).
Strengths	Qualitative data may provide much in-depth information concerning clients' subjective experiences or other observable phenomena, and thus are especially useful in theory construction. Case studies are often easier to conduct in practice settings than are full-scale surveys or randomized experiments.	Quantitative data may be easier to interpret, since they are numerically coded. More useful for hypothesis testing, since outcomes are more clearly defined and measured. Procedures for assessing validity and reliability of survey instruments are well developed. Threats to validity in quasi-experimental research studies can be assessed, and control can be established through study design or data analysis.
Weaknesses	Procedures for assessing validity and reliability of data are less developed than those for quantitative data. Methods of data collection often are less precise and not universally accepted. Funding agencies may consider qualitative methods "weaker" than quantitative methods.	Information obtained may provide limited answers to theoretical questions or may not adequately explain phenomena. Well-controlled studies may be difficult to implement in practice settings. Usually need larger sample of subjects for research questions to be answered, especially if results are to be generalized to wider population.

research methods. In a recent study by DeVon and Powers (1984), quantitative methods were used to determine whether the beliefs of hypertensive clients about compliance and their psychosocial adjustment could predict their control of hypertension. Standardized instruments were used to measure beliefs, adjustment, and blood pressure ratings; statistical tests were applied to the data to answer the research questions. Another study (Dimond 1979) used quantitative methods to investigate the relationship between social support variables and clients' adaptation to maintenance hemodialysis. In this study, questionnaires and rating scales were developed to measure the different dimensions of social support, adaptation, and medical status. This method allowed a detailed analysis of how different types of social support relate to clients' adjustment and health status.

Corbin and Strauss's study (1984) of couples' management of chronic illness is an example of the effective use of qualitative methods in nursing research. In this study, narrative information was collected from 60 couples through unstructured interviews over a period of 2 years. The information was then organized into a meaningful conceptual framework to explain how couples manage illness. Theory and guidelines for how nurses might assist such couples to achieve effective collaboration resulted from this study.

Chenitz's study (1981) of elderly persons' responses to nursing home admissions is another good example of qualitative research methods. In this study, nurse participant-observers recorded descriptive accounts of elderly individuals' interactions with staff in the nursing home. Different interactional styles were identified and compared to gain insight on how elderly persons accept or resist nursing home admission. Hypotheses regarding the predictors of successful nursing home adaptation were subsequently developed.

Combining Methodologies

A number of investigators encourage the use of both quantitative and qualitative methodologies in a given research study (Goodwin & Goodwin 1984; Hoeffer

& Archbold 1983; Swanson & Chenitz 1982). Combining the two methods can often provide a more comprehensive and meaningful data analysis. Qualitative information from open-ended interviews, for example, can supplement findings from a quantitative analysis and help the researcher better understand the substantive meaning of statistical associations (Hoeffer & Archbold 1983). Using a combination of qualitative and quantitative methods also helps to cross-validate research findings. This is a great advantage, since no single measurement strategy or method is perfectly reliable or valid (Goodwin & Goodwin 1984).

Problems in Chronicity Research

Despite the potential benefits of research into chronic illness, only a limited amount of this research is actually being conducted by practicing nurses, partly because clinical research is still fairly new to nursing. Most nurses are not prepared to conduct research studies related to their practice, and too few nurses are researchers to provide leadership for these endeavors (Bergstrom et al. 1984). Furthermore, chronic health problems are very complex and more resistant to intervention than are most acute health problems. As a result, fewer nurses may be attracted to chronic care nursing settings and those that are may be less interested in conducting research.

While funding for research on chronic illness is available from a variety of sources, studies that focus on tertiary preventions (such as quality of life) are less likely to receive financial support than those directed toward prevention or cure of specific diseases. Nurses who conduct such research may be constrained by cost considerations and may have to curtail the scope of their investigations.

A number of surveys have examined nurses' utilization of research findings in practice. Overall, these studies indicate that most nurses are unaware of research studies in their clinical areas and that

◇ CASE STUDY ◇
Trying to Validate Pet Therapy

Sally W., a baccalaureate nurse, was recently employed in a new rehabilitation center. She noticed that many of the elderly clients brought to the center were withdrawn, and that they were very difficult to engage in treatment. Aware of reports of successful pet therapy for the elderly, Sally attempted to interest the staff in setting up a study to determine if including a pet in the program would increase elderly persons' receptivity to treatment. While the staff expressed interest in pet therapy, they saw no need for a research study. One of the nurses commented that "research is for doctors, not nurses." Others reminded Sally of the difficulty in obtaining funding, as well as permission, for research. The head nurse told Sally that she could not be given "time off" for research, but suggested that Sally ask for permission to bring a pet to the center.

---

they rarely attempt to actually apply research findings (Hefferin, Horsley, & Ventura 1982; Kirchhoff 1983; Lelean 1982). Many practice settings do not encourage nurses to utilize research. A survey by Lindemann and Schantz (Lindemann 1984) revealed that only 27% of nursing administrators are committed to introducing results of research to their practice settings. Whereas 39% of the surveyed administrators stated that they were committed to research utilization in general, only 23% of the hospitals had research review committees and only 7.4% actually had positions for nurse researchers.

Conducting Research in Practice

Gaining Support from Colleagues. The case discussing pet therapy illustrates some of the problems nurses face when they try to introduce research in service settings. One of the most obvious problems is other health workers' lack of understanding and appreciation for nursing research (Todd & Gortner 1982). Many staff nurses, as well as other health care providers and administrators, view nursing as a "service-rendering" rather than a "knowledge-generating" profession and do not recognize the potential benefits of nursing research. In such instances, the nurse who wishes to conduct research will need a considerable amount of time in order to change the attitudes of the staff. Without such changes, it will be very difficult to gain access to clients for research

studies, and the staff may resist the nurse-investigator's projects.

Nurses may have particular difficulties in gaining support for research in chronic care institutions that have a very strong biomedical research tradition. Behavioral research often is not regarded highly in these institutions, and nursing investigations that focus on the psychosocial and behavioral aspects of chronic illness may be viewed with much skepticism. Staff nurses in large medical research centers also may be reluctant to collaborate on nursing research projects because of previous negative experiences in research; many of these nurses have been required to collect data for physician-sponsored research projects without financial compensation or other acknowledgment of their contributions. These experiences have often led to resentment and fear of exploitation in research projects (Robb 1981).

Even when nurses recognize the value of nursing research, they may be reluctant to participate actively because of their limited knowledge and skills in research. Since few nursing education programs adequately prepare their graduates to participate in nursing research studies, many staff nurses are intimidated by research terminology and procedures (Morse & Conrad 1983) and fear being observed and criticized (Gortner 1982). Practicing nurses also may be unaware of their rights and responsibilities as research participants. Though guidelines for nurses' participation in research have been published by the American Nurses Association (ANA 1975, 1980), specific research policies have not been established in many institutions and agencies.

Limited Resources for Research Development. Another problem that accentuates the difficulties of practicing nurses with research is the limited availability of research resources in clinical practice settings. Nurses who work in university-affiliated institutions may have fairly good access to library resources, nurse researchers, and others who can assist them in grant writing, funding, and the general conduct of research studies. However, most nurses in chronic care settings are not so fortunate. These settings may be not only physically isolated from research centers but also psychologically cut off from the mainstream of research. Without adequate link to those who can provide guidance and support for research activities, nurses may have great difficulty planning and conducting research in a clinical setting, leading to possible discouragement.

Conflicts between Research and Service Needs. Nurses who work in clinical practice settings may have difficulty in handling the conflict between the competing demands of research and service (Todd & Gortner 1982). At the personal level, nurses may experience role conflict because of the different interactional behaviors required of research versus clinical practice. When collecting data for research purposes, for example, the nurse must attempt to maintain objectivity and not bias the client's responses, whereas the nurse who functions as a practitioner intentionally attempts to influence the client's feelings and responses in order to effect positive adaptation. To be successful as both a nurse-investigator and clinician, the nurse must be capable of adapting to multiple roles without compromising the integrity of research findings or the quality of care provided the client.

Competing demands for time by research and service activities may also present a problem in the practice setting. Since patient care must normally be given first priority, the research project may require substantial personal time from the nurse investigator

and other staff members. Even when the staff have strong commitments to nursing research, demands for prolonged periods of extra time may create interpersonal tensions and conflict. Obtaining funding for a nursing research project can greatly ease this problem. This allows staff to be compensated for overtime or allows research assistants to be hired to collect and analyze data.

In clinical settings where staffing patterns are very good or where research projects are funded, administrators may release nurses during clinical time to participate in research activities, which can facilitate the completion of research projects. Clinical release time policies may create interpersonal conflicts among the nursing staff, however. Nurses who are not participating in the research activities may resent others' release from clinical duties. Traditional behavior norms of a service setting, which include that nurses always be accessible to each other in the clinical area, may make using clinical release time very difficult. Nurses may be expected to be "on call" for clinical emergencies while actively involved in their research activities. They also may be expected to return to the nursing unit to complete their "fair share" of clinical work, even when they have been granted clinical release time for research activities (Davis 1981).

Nurses who wish to be successful in meeting their research goals obviously need to be very politically sensitive and capable of promoting support from their peers. Since a research orientation conflicts with the traditional service norms, it will probably be necessary to implement structured in-service programs in order to introduce research values into the service setting.

Other Realities of the Workplace. Other factors in clinical practice settings create obstacles for aspiring nurse-investigators. Financial constraints and administrators' concerns about cost-effectiveness usually restrict the time allotted to research activities as well as the funds available for nursing research projects. In many service settings, staff resources for clinical activities also may be quite limited. Under these

◇ C A S E S T U D Y ◇

Integrating Research into Practice

Joel S., a 35-year-old R.N., had been employed at Green-lawn Mental Health Clinic for several years. He worked very diligently to develop his therapeutic skills and prided himself on being open to new treatment approaches that might help his chronically ill clients. After attending a seminar on nursing research, Joel was eager to begin applying research findings to his clinical practice. However, locating studies relevant to his clients' problems seemed to be rather difficult. In addition, several of Joel's colleagues were pessimistic about the new

venture, stating that they didn't understand statistics and they "couldn't really do research" in the clinic.

Undeterred, Joel organized a luncheon forum for mental health workers interested in research. While many of the staff were too busy to attend these sessions regularly, a small core group began reviewing research studies and discussing possible applications. A nurse researcher from the university was invited to visit the clinic and make suggestions for staff learning activities.

---

conditions, treatment may focus mainly on crisis management instead of prevention, and research on clients' chronic health problems is likely to receive a very low priority.

Utilizing Research to Improve Care

In the case study on research in practice, Joel experienced some of the typical barriers nurses face in applying research to practice. An initial barrier is the confusion between "doing" research and "utilizing knowledge" from research studies. Haller and others (1979) found that when nurses were asked how they might use research in practice, they most frequently referred to replicating research studies. Since nursing education programs provide students with very little exposure to research utilization, such confusion is understandable.

The organizational climate of clinical practice settings is likely to support rather than challenge skeptical views about research utilization. Most practice settings are very action-oriented, and nurses' workloads allow little time for systematic planning and evaluation of client care. In addition, little funding is available for extensive literature searches or studies to evaluate practice innovations. These problems are accentuated in chronic care institutions, where financial constraints are more severe and caseloads are heavier; thus, nurses may be discouraged from implementing innovative approaches.

Slow Dissemination of Findings. Another problem that discourages nurses from utilizing research findings is the difficulty of gaining timely access to relevant research information (Barnard 1980; Lelean 1982). This problem is due in part to the time required for publication of research findings. Publication of an article in a journal such as *Nursing Research* can take as long as two years. If the investigator also wishes to publish in a practitioner journal, the article must be revised and resubmitted, which takes even longer (Barnard 1980).

Furthermore, nurses have little time to search for studies relevant to their clinical practices. Although research journals are beginning to be more available in practice settings, resources for facilitating computer searches or other rapid retrieval methods may be very limited. Many nursing administrators are aware of nurses' problems in acquiring research information and are attempting to develop better mechanisms for disseminating research findings. However, there is still a wide discrepancy between the ideal and the reality. In a study by Hefferin, Horsley, and Ventura (1982), hospital administrators and researchers identified ten very effective methods for communicating research findings to practicing nurses, but only two of these methods were actually being used in more than 50% of the hospital settings.

Recent advances in communication technology suggest solutions to this problem. Communication by space satellites will eventually enable nurse-investigators to disseminate research findings to practitioners with very little time delay. Teleconferencing between investigators and nurses also will facilitate the communication of clinical problems and research needs. As computer systems develop, they can store books and periodicals as well as research data, all of which can be retrieved on clinically based video monitors. These advances should greatly facilitate the utilization of research findings in practice (Barnard 1980).

Limited Skills in Using Research. Nurses attempting to use research findings in practice often have difficulty evaluating reports and determining how the findings apply to their specific practice situations (Downs 1984; Hefferin, Horsley, & Ventura 1982; Krueger, Nelson, & Wolanin 1978; Lelean 1982). Problems in evaluation are due largely to the practitioners' lack of experience in evaluating studies, specifically in regard to the limitations of various research designs. Nurse-investigators may contribute to these problems by failing to point out the strengths and weaknesses of their research studies or by presenting findings in terms that would not be understood by practitioners (Downs 1984; Hefferin, Horsley, & Ventura 1982). Barnard (1980) suggests that researchers need to bring their research findings to the individual case level so that nurses can more readily recognize the practice implications.

In assessing the applicability of research findings, practitioners must consider not only the quality of the research study but whether the findings actually apply to the clients in their practice setting. This consideration is especially important, since many nursing studies have been conducted with small groups of clients and never replicated in other settings (Lelean 1982). Haller, Reynolds, and Horsley (1979) advise nurses to be aware of the differences between research goals and clinical goals when assessing the usability of a study. Innovations based on research findings must be systematically evaluated in the clinical setting in order to assure their overall benefits to clients. The desired effect of a new nursing practice, as well as unexpected outcomes, should be compared against those of the traditional practice, using well-defined outcome measures (Haller, Reynolds, & Horsley 1979).

The above discussion makes it obvious that utilization of research requires nurses to make many judgments that directly affect patient care. While nurses certainly are capable of making such judgments, they may lack sufficient knowledge and experience to safely apply research findings in practice. Studies suggest that while nurses make many practice innovations, they usually implement new practices on a basis of trial and error rather than systematically evaluating the outcome of new innovations (Hefferin, Horsley, & Ventura 1982). More organized utilization of research findings in clinical settings is needed in order to assure the safe introduction of practice innovations.

Interventions:
Problem-Solving Strategies

Nurses can use several strategies to overcome the problems associated with nursing research. First of all, individual nurses can increase their competence in handling research through education. The ANA guidelines on research (ANA 1980) specify that "all" nurses should be involved in the research process "in a manner that is consistent with their educational preparations, practice roles, personal interests and capabilities." In interpreting these guidelines to rehabilitation nurses, Bondy (1983) states:

> This does not mean that every nurse must "do research." It does mean, first, that nurses must maintain enquiring minds and continue to search for those questions and answers that will improve practice. Second, nurses must be prepared to integrate their practice appropriately with the research process; and third, nurses must be accountable for the reading, use, and evaluation of nursing research in their areas of practice.

If these basic guidelines are followed, practicing nurses should be capable of participating responsibly in research.

It is not necessary to receive an advanced degree in order to obtain adequate knowledge and skills in nursing research. Much knowledge can be gained in self-directed study, in continuing education courses, and in research seminars sponsored by universities, hospitals, and professional organizations. Nurses who actively participate in state nursing association activities and in clinical specialty organizations should have good access to information on educational programs related to research. Nursing research interest groups also have been organized in many geographic locations, and these groups welcome new members.

In addition to improving their own knowledge and skills, practicing nurses ultimately will benefit from encouraging more research courses in nursing schools. Textbooks in nursing need to be more research-based (Lelean 1982), and curriculums need to provide greater opportunities for nurses to learn about research applications in clinical settings. Nursing faculty might also be urged to teach a broader range of research methods (Davis 1981), which would increase options for investigating practice-relevant problems and assist nurses to better evaluate the applicability of other investigators' findings.

Developing a Research Climate in the Practice Setting

The existence of a supportive research environment in the practice setting is crucial to nurses' involvement in the research process (Batra 1983; Hunt et al. 1983; Todd & Gortner 1982). In commenting on the nurse administrators' role in research, Hunt and others (1983) state:

> Nursing administration within a service setting must articulate the value of research to clinical practice by creating a climate conducive to research. This is done by incorporating research goals into departmental philosophies, beliefs, and by-laws, by including research objectives in position descriptions, and by raising the level of research awareness and skills through nursing research committee activities and program offerings.

Staff nurses can help to create a positive research climate in the practice setting by supporting the development of nursing research policies and partici-

pating in research programs. Research policies should include (1) guidelines for assuring ethical and safety standards; (2) performance expectations for participation by head nurses, assistant head nurses, and staff nurses; (3) criteria for evaluating and rewarding nurse-investigators; and (4) procedures for facilitating research development, such as granting of clinical release time for investigative activities (ANA 1975; Davis 1981).

Organizational Structures. A formal nursing research committee is one of the most effective organizational structures for stimulating nursing research activity in the practice setting. Research committees have been instituted successfully in a variety of settings, including Veterans Administration hospitals (Batra 1983), private hospitals (Spross et al. 1981), and university medical centers (Fuhs & Mohr 1981; Hunt et al. 1983; Todd & Gortner 1982). The research committee may be primarily responsible for educational activities and consultation (Batra 1983), or it may have a wide range of functions, such as the development of research policies and procedures, planning of educational programs, development of research resources and communication networks, and review and monitoring of nursing research projects (Fuhs & Mohr 1981).

In some hospital settings, an individual from the nursing research committee also serves on the hospitalwide Institutional Review Board or Human Subjects Committee (Spross, Kilpack, & Marchewka 1981). The presence of a nurse on this committee helps to ensure nurses' participation in decisions concerning patients' rights and other ethical issues. Nurse representation on Institutional Review Boards also may enhance other professionals' awareness of the value of nursing and behavioral science research in health care (Robb 1981).

Creating a position in the practice setting for a doctorally prepared nurse researcher should greatly facilitate the development of nursing research. The nurse-researcher can serve as a teacher and role model for other nurses and can assume a major responsibility for developing organizational structures for conduct and utilization of research.

Educational Programs. An active research education program in the practice setting can help nurses gain the necessary skills and self-confidence to participate effectively in nursing research. Educational activities may include formal research seminars, courses, and workshops, as well as informal luncheon forums, group discussions, and journal clubs. If possible, research programs should be instituted on an ongoing basis. All nurses should attend orientation sessions and structured in-service programs on the conduct and utilization of research. Nurses who expect to be more involved in research activities can also have more focused work sessions with colleagues in their clinical areas to identify specific practice problems and to discuss research applications (Davis 1981).

It may be advantageous for research education to be integrated into the quality assurance program (Batra 1983). Using research methods to obtain quality assurance data can help nurses gain skill in conducting evaluation studies as well as in applying research findings to validate practice standards. A nursing research newsletter also can be very supportive to nurses actively participating in research activities. This type of publication can reward nurses for their efforts, as well as facilitate communication about research activities both within the clinical setting and throughout the larger community (Fuhs & Mohr 1981).

Nurses who work in long-term care institutions or other settings where no research is performed may have difficulty obtaining research training or access to current research literature. In such situations, it will be necessary to initiate contact with libraries and resource centers and to participate actively in professional nursing organizations. It is possible to develop an active research education program in the practice setting, even when no nurses with advanced research training are on the staff. Interested nurses should review the nursing literature to locate articles on developing research programs in clinical settings. Some authors on this topic include Batra (1983), Davis (1981), Fuhs and Mohr (1981), and Spross, Kilpack, and Marchewka (1981). If the clinical agency is near a university, the nursing

faculty might be willing to assist in program development.

Support Services. Support services such as library assistance, clerical and reproduction services, computer terminals, and funding for literature searches also help to create a positive research climate in the practice setting. Nurses can become quite knowledgeable about research and its applications without such services, but they provide needed information and enable completion of nursing research projects in a reasonable time period. A very useful resource, which is becoming more available in clinical settings, is the computer-assisted literature search. Computer searches can save much time, as well as helping nurses to complete more comprehensive literature reviews.

Batra (1983) also describes a LATCH (Literature Attached to Charts) service that is implemented in some health care institutions. In this system, the library staff retrieves resource materials pertinent to specific patients' health problems and sends the materials to clinicians on the individual treatment units. The rapid availability of resource materials reinforces a learning attitude and helps to assure the utilization of recent research findings

Nurses in clinical settings will benefit from having adequate space for their research planning activities, away from the direct patient-care area. This is especially important for developing less action-oriented work habits (Davis 1981). Nurse-investigators' lack of immediate availability during clinical release time for research also may assist other staff members to recognize the value and high priority of research activities.

Utilizing Educational Resource Materials

Information on research and research utilization is becoming much more accessible to practicing nurses. Textbooks on nursing research methods, nursing research journals, and other health care journals and resource materials are now available in many clinical settings. Articles and columns on research applications are also appearing more regularly in nursing specialty journals (Kirchhoff 1983). An article by Bondy (1983) in *Rehabilitation Nursing,* for example, provides practical guidelines that nurses in chronic care institutions can use to determine the applicability of new research findings.

Morse and Conrad (1983) detail an eight-step procedure for applying research findings in practice. The suggested procedure includes

1. Defining the clinical problem or need
2. Locating information or studies relevant to the problem
3. Determining the "soundness" or reliability of the reviewed research findings
4. Assessing whether findings from the reviewed studies are applicable to the present problem
5. Preparing a written plan for application of the research
6. Obtaining cooperation and permission
7. Implementing the plan
8. Evaluating the entire process.

After evaluating the application of research to practice, nurses are encouraged to publish their results and to communicate with the original researchers so that new information can be made available to other practitioners.

A variety of learning materials for critiquing research reports is available. *A Sourcebook of Nursing Research* (Downs 1984) provides excellent case examples of both experimental intervention studies and observational studies to guide the nurse through the critiquing process. Nurses also may find suggestions offered by Morse and Conrad (1983), Jacox and Prescott (1978), and Norbeck (1979) very useful.

Use of Innovation Protocols

Two groups of nurse-researchers have developed models for systematically introducing research findings into clinical practice. In a project sponsored by the Western Council of Higher Education in Nursing (WCHEN) in the mid-1970s, dyads of nurse-researchers and clinicians worked on retrieving and applying relevant research reports. This project was very successful in increasing the individual nurse-clinician's

use of research in practice, although the clinicians assessed the overall impact of the project on their service agencies to be minimal (Krueger, Nelson, & Wolanin 1978).

The other utilization project, "Conduct and Utilization of Research in Nursing" (CURN), was initiated by faculty at the University of Michigan School of Nursing in the late 1970s. In this project, nurse-researchers and clinicians collaborated in developing problem-specific innovation protocols to guide practitioners in applying research findings. Each CURN protocol begins with a discussion of the clinical problem being addressed. The innovation under consideration then is described, including information on the types of clients most likely to benefit. The protocol next provides a summary of research studies (called the *research base*), which support the innovation. The protocol then details specific procedures to be followed to implement the practice innovation systematically and evaluate its impact (CURN 1983; Haller, Reynolds, & Horsley 1979).

At the present time, CURN protocols for the implementation of ten nursing practice innovations have been published. Protocols most relevant to long-term or chronic care include those on catheterization procedures, distress reduction, decubiti treatment, pain reduction, and mutual goal setting (CURN 1983). Nurses are encouraged to review these protocols, both for their substantive content and to learn the methodology of research utilization. The procedure manual, *Using Research to Improve Nursing Practice: A Guide* (CURN 1983), is a very useful addition to the research protocols. This manual should help nurses better understand the process of building a scientific research base for practice and stimulate ideas about practice innovations.

Developing Support Networks and Collaborative Relationships

Collaboration with other clinical nurses and nurse-investigators is very important for the practicing nurse who desires active involvement in research. Research collaboration can both be personally very rewarding and provide opportunities for the sharing of expertise, physical resources and facilities, and financial obligations (Hunt et al. 1983; Todd & Gortner 1982).

Various structures for research collaboration have been described in the nursing research literature. Hunt and others (1983) describe a nursing research network organized by nurses in three teaching hospitals in Boston. Each of the participating hospitals had its own resources and program for nursing research, and the network was created to facilitate sharing ideas, developing mutual practice standards, and planning joint educational activities and research projects. Organized research networks are especially useful for nurses whose practice is isolated from research settings. Interaction with professional colleagues is essential for personal growth as well as for planning strategies to effect organizational change. Hunt and others (1983) give suggestions for how to develop successful research networks and effectively manage group process problems.

Collaboration between Clinicians and Researchers. Collaboration between clinicians and researchers also is essential for the development of a research-based nursing practice. *Traditional models* of research do not adequately foster such collaboration, however. In the typical research model, university faculty members conduct research investigations and report their findings in research journals. In this model, clinicians are consumers of research and do not actually participate in the research. In the *agency research model,* clinicians identify problems in their practice settings, and the agency hires a researcher to investigate the problems and offer solutions. Findings from this type of study may be more relevant to practice but often cannot be generalized beyond the specific practice setting (Loomis & Krone 1980).

Collaborative research, as defined by the CURN project staff, is "research in which university-based researchers and agency-based clinicians, as equal contributors, collaborate at each stage of the research process" (Loomis & Krone 1980). This type of collaboration helps to assure that problems studied are

relevant to clinical practice and increases the potential for utilization, since findings from a study can be readily converted into practice innovations. The innovations can be retested (replicated) in a variety of settings.

Most nurses who work in clinical settings will find that faculty-clinician collaboration provides the most effective means of implementing clinical research studies. To avoid falling into traditional student-instructor roles, it becomes important to clarify such roles and responsibilities in planning sessions. Circulating the minutes of each planning session to all those on the research project enhances communications and promotes a collegial atmosphere.

Consortium Model of Collaboration. Nurse-investigators living in different geographic locations can form consortiums to work on collaborative research projects. The model for this type of nursing research collaboration was initiated when WCHEN was awarded its grant for regional nursing research development (Krueger, Nelson, & Wolanin 1978). Several consortiums of nurse investigators were organized through regional workshops sponsored by WCHEN, and they subsequently planned and conducted a series of multisite clinical investigations, including the previously discussed studies on research utilization (Bergstrom et al. 1984).

The consortium model of collaboration has many advantages. A major advantage to investigators is the benefit of each other's expertise and assistance. The WCHEN-sponsored consortium for "Nursing Interventions in Problems of Tube Feeding" had seven coinvestigators. Eight other nurses collaborated on the project, contributing expertise from a variety of areas (Bergstrom et al. 1984).

Another advantage of the consortium model is the large number of clients who can be included in a research study. Large samples allow for more complete data analysis, since subjects can be studied as a total group and also categorized into subgroups according to specific characteristics, such as diagnosis, severity of illness, ethnicity, or geographic residence. The findings from multisite investigations are open to wider generalization, since clients represent a wide range of possible subjects. Finally, research conducted through consortium groups tends to be more cost-effective because project management activities, such as computer services and staff assistance, can be centralized (Bergstrom et al. 1984).

Although consortiums are very beneficial, there are difficulties inherent to conducting research with a group of investigators. In comparison with individual research, consortium participation is very demanding. Many joint decisions need to be made concerning project management, and frequent meetings and telephone conferences may be required to resolve misunderstandings among consortium members. Because of the necessary coordination involved in multisite studies, consortium projects also may progress very slowly. Strong leadership, attitudes of give and take, and mutual trust and support are very necessary to maintain motivation and morale (Bergstrom et al. 1984).

Overall, collaborative research projects can be very personally rewarding experiences, and the findings from these projects can have wide-ranging clinical implications. As in any other type of collaboration, mutually agreed-upon goals and expectations among participants are necessary for assuring successful working relationships. At the beginning of any collaborative endeavor, it is very helpful to have open discussions about expectations, research goals, and working arrangements. In addition, decisions regarding publication rights and ownership of the research data should be made (Todd & Gortner 1982). Collaboration can become very difficult if disagreements over these issues surface during conduct of the research investigation.

Financing Nursing Research

Financing nursing research can pose problems, but nurses should not let those problems discourage them from pursuing their research goals. It is important to remember that research projects in clinical settings often can be carried out with very limited funding (Leininger 1983; Martinson 1983). Many descriptive and exploratory studies, as well as small pilot studies of nursing intervention projects, may

require funds only for literature searches, supplies used in the project, and support services such as secretarial or computer assistance. Although it is very desirable for nurse-investigators to be paid for the time they spend on research activities, many studies actually do not necessitate such coverage.

Leininger (1983) provides several suggestions for how nurses can economize to limit the costs of research. She suggests

1. Use phase-in research plans, based on funding availability
2. Borrow or rent, rather than buy, expensive equipment
3. Use data banks for study when possible
4. Conduct multidisciplinary studies or collaborate with other investigators to share expenses
5. Use standardized instruments and less costly data collection methods
6. Reduce photocopying and use of office supplies
7. Reexamine policies and procedures that are expensive or outdated.

Leininger also encourages nurses to develop good grantsmanship skills, so that their research studies can be funded. Critiques from peers should be sought to improve chances of competing successfully for research grants.

Federal Sources of Funding. Financial support for health research is available from a variety of sources. Most health research funds are administered through agencies of the federal government, and investigators obtain these funds by successfully competing in the grant program of the U.S. Public Health Service. The National Institutes of Health (NIH), in the Department of Health and Human Services (DHHS), are the primary funding agencies for health research. Each of the institutes determines its own priorities for research and administers its own research programs.

The NIH institutes most likely to have programs matching nurses' interests in research on chronic illness are the National Institute on Aging (NIA), the National Institute of Arthritis, Diabetes, and Digestive and Kidney Diseases (NIADDK), the National Institute of Neurological, Communicative Disorders and Stroke (NINCDS), the National Cancer Institute (NCI), and the National Heart, Lung and Blood Institute (NHLBI). Although much of the grant money awarded through these institutes is for biomedical research, a number of programs solicit grants for studies on sociocultural and behavioral factors related to disease progression, coping with aging and specific illness conditions, and long-term care and rehabilitation (Martinson 1983).

Two other agencies in DHHS that may be of particular interest to nurses are the Health Resources and Services Administration (HRSA) and the Alcohol, Drug Abuse, and Mental Health Administration (ADAMHA). The HRSA, whose primary concern is the health care delivery process, funds studies on the cost-effectiveness of alternative health care delivery systems, such as home health care, as well as studies that focus on improving health services for underserved population groups. The HRSA programs are interdisciplinary, and collaborative research studies are encouraged. ADAMHA funds studies on mental health and mental illness, dependency states, and drug and alcohol abuse (Martinson 1983). Nurses interested in research in these areas are encouraged to contact the agency for information on specific program announcements. ADAMHA also provides an excellent clearinghouse for educational information on mental health issues. Brochures and other printed materials are available upon request.

The Division of Nursing in the Health Resources Administration, DHHS, funds a major portion of nursing research studies. The nursing research grants program is part of the greater Public Health Service grant system, and investigators compete for funding as they do in the NIH institute programs. The Division of Nursing funds studies on a wide variety of health care issues, although studies with direct implications for clinical nursing practice are given the highest priority. Block, Gortner, and Sturdivant (1978) provide an excellent overview of the Division of Nursing grants programs, and nurses interested in applying for grants are encouraged to review this publication.

Staff in the Nursing Research Branch suggest that prospective applicants initiate contacts with the branch officers early in their proposal development to obtain specific guidance. Beginning nurse-researchers may be more successful in obtaining funding for their studies if they ally themselves with more experienced investigators. Grant reviewers carefully evaluate the capabilities of the principal investigator of a study, as well as the total research team, in determining whether the necessary expertise is available to complete the proposed study successfully (Block, Gortner, & Sturdivant 1978).

Nurses may be reluctant to apply for federal research grant monies because of the tough competition for funds; however, Gortner (1983a) strongly urges nurses to compete for grants. She emphasizes that "for nursing research, health services research, and social and behavioral sciences research, the proportion of proposals approved in any given round (one-quarter to one-third of all reviewed) is comparable to the proportion approved in the biomedical science review rounds." Gortner (1983a) also emphasizes the importance of nurses' being prepared for setbacks as well as success in the grant world. When a proposal is rejected, the nurse-investigator has an excellent opportunity to learn from the reviewers' critiques. The proposal then can be improved and resubmitted for funding.

Other Sources of Funding. A growing number of private foundations, corporations, and other agencies are funding nursing research studies. The National Directory of Research Foundations lists nearly 3,000 foundations that provide grants for research (Leininger 1983). The Kellogg Foundation and the Robert Wood Johnson Foundation have funded several extensive health research projects, including a number of nursing demonstration studies on long-term care.

Recent corporate donors to the American Nurses Foundation research fund include the Pfizer Foundation, the Burroughs Wellcome Fund, the Bristol-Myers Fund, and the American Hospital Corporation (ANF 1984). Organizations such as the state chapters of the American Lung Association and the American Association of Retired Persons also provide seed monies for projects specific to their interests. Nurses often neglect to request funding from these sources, although their research interests may be compatible with those of the funding agencies.

From 1955 to 1983, the American Nurses Foundation (ANF) provided financial assistance to 172 nurse-investigators for clinical research studies (ANF 1984). The foundation grants are primarily for new investigators, although experienced investigators initiating new areas of research are also eligible. Grants from the foundation are quite competitive, but the successful nurse-scholars are well rewarded for their efforts. Sigma Theta Tau also has a small grants program for new nurse-investigators. Funds from this program can be used for exploratory research purposes or for pilot studies of more extensive intervention projects.

A number of health care institutions are beginning to develop their own internal sources of funding to stimulate the development of nursing research. Whether the funds are derived from developmental grants, fund-raising drives, or charitable contributions, they can be very supportive to nurses' research activities. Nurses interested in developing strong research programs in their practice settings are encouraged to discuss their financial needs with the development staff of their respective institutions. The aggressive pursuit of funding to research goals eventually will be rewarded.

Regional and National Level Strategies

Nurses can be encouraged by efforts currently being made at the regional levels to support nursing research. Conferences and seminars that focus on substantive and methodological research issues, as well as on strategic planning for research development, now are frequent occurrences. These conferences help to strengthen networks between nurse-clinicians, researchers, and educators and provide forums that address problems related to research utilization, resource development, and practice standards.

Since the early 1970s, there has been extensive lobbying at the national level to increase the visibility of nursing in the scientific community and to strengthen the federal government's commitment to nursing research. These efforts have begun to be successful. In 1983, the Institute of Medicine issued a report on nursing and nursing education that acknowledged the critical role of nursing and the need for federal support of nursing research:

> A substantial share of the health care dollar is expended on direct nursing care, yet the professionals who deliver this care work without the benefit of a strong organizational base to stimulate and support scientific investigations in their field. This committee believes that a center for nursing research is needed at a high level of the federal government to be a focal point for promoting the growth of quality nursing research (Institute of Medicine 1983).

Legislation for establishment of an Institute for Nursing within the NIH was introduced to Congress in late 1983 by Republican Senator Madigan of Illinois. The legislation was approved by Congress but subsequently vetoed by President Reagan. At the time of this writing, the ANA continues to press for such legislation. An NIH task force has outlined recommendations for the strengthening of nursing involvement and nursing research within the existing NIH structure. These recommendations include the establishment of a postdoctoral research training program for nurse-scientists and appointment of more nurses to advisory and review boards. As an alternative to the NIH Institute for Nursing, a Center for Nursing Research within the Division of Nursing also is being planned.

Summary and Conclusions

Research is a growing component of the professional nurse's role, since research contributes to the understanding of clients' health problems, assists practitioners in identifying effective strategies for promoting clients' successful adaptation, and documents the cost-effectiveness of nursing practice. Research can be carried out by the nurse or findings from studies can effectively be utilized to benefit client outcomes. Yet, for a variety of reasons, a great majority of practicing nurses neither carry out nor utilize research.

At the turn of the century, health research focused on infectious diseases. As these diseases were brought under control, the focus turned to the biomedical aspects of chronic conditions. The concurrent increase in federal funding led to the establishment of a number of institutes and broadened the research base to a multidisciplinary endeavor. Nursing research focusing on client care is relatively recent and looks promising, even though obtaining adequate funding continues to be difficult.

Several areas of research can add to the knowledge base needed for chronic care nursing practice: studies on the environmental, psychosocial, and behavioral factors of illness; studies on impact of chronic illnesses on clients and their families; and studies on the effectiveness of nursing interventions on both illness and client adaptation. Nursing investigations take the form of either observational studies to gain information or interventional studies to test the effectiveness of nursing practice. Methodology can be quantitative or qualitative, and both methods can be used to cross-validate research findings. Quantitative methods are useful for hypothesis testing and program evaluation, and qualitative methods help formulate hypotheses.

In spite of the inherent benefits of research on chronic illness, few studies are being performed. This is due to a number of problems. The difficulties involved in doing research in the practice setting include limited support from colleagues, limited resources available for research development, and conflicts and competing demands of the workplace. Problems also exist in the utilization of research to improve client care, including the slow dissemination of research findings, limited skills in critiquing studies, and insufficient knowledge and experience to safely apply research findings to practice.

There are a number of strategies for overcoming problems. Skill in handling research and knowledge of research activities can be gained through some kind of educational program or course and developing a research climate in the clinical practice setting. Utilizing research can be improved by systematically determining how to integrate findings into practice, learning how to critique studies, using innovative protocols, and making findings more available to the practitioner.

The nurse interested in doing research must develop support networks and collaborative relationships through, for example, collaboration between clinicians and researchers or among researchers living in different geographic areas. Research also requires funding, which can come from federal or private sources. Funding agencies require the submission of a study proposal, and even rejection of the proposal can be used to strengthen it for resubmission.

Although real obstacles must be overcome in integrating research in practice settings, nurses in many institutions have successfully organized strong support networks to foster their research interests. Nursing research has greater visibility at the national level, and nurse-researchers are beginning to be better integrated into the scientific community, as well as the political community. More active political involvement by nurses can greatly help the profession obtain the funding and support it needs for rapid research development.

STUDY QUESTIONS

1. According to the 1980 ANA guidelines, what level of educational preparation does an R.N. need to participate in nursing research?
2. What three strategies can staff nurses use to promote nursing research development in the practice setting?
3. What is the nursing administrator's role in fostering a positive research climate in the practice setting? Discuss this role.
4. What are the major deterrents to utilizing nursing research findings in clinical practice?
5. What are some good sources of information on nursing research methods and research utilization?
6. What are some of the major features of qualitative and quantitative research methods? How can a nurse-investigator combine the two methodologies to cross-validate a study?

References

American Nurses Association, (1975) *Human Rights Guidelines for Nurses in Clinical and Other Research,* Kansas City: American Nurses Association

American Nurses Association, (1980) *Guidelines for the Investigative Functions of Nurses,* Kansas City: American Nurses Association

American Nurses Association, (1984) *Nursing Research: Directions for the Twenty-first Century,* Kansas City: ANA Cabinet on Nursing Research

American Nurses Foundation, (1984) *1983 Abstracts of ANF Funded Research,* Kansas City: American Nurses Foundation

Barnard, K. E., (1980) Knowledge for practice: directions for the future, *Nursing Research, 29*(4):208–212

Batra, C., (1983) Motivating nurses to do nursing research, *Nursing and Health Care, 4*(1):18–22

Bergstrom, N., Hansen, B., Grant, M., Hanson, R., Kubo, W., Padilla, G., and Wong, H., (1984) Collaborative nursing research: Anatomy of a successful consortium, *Nursing Research, 33*(1):20–25

Block, D., Gortner, S., and Sturdivant, L. W., (1978) The nursing research grants program of the Division of Nursing, U.S. Public Health Service, *Journal of Nursing Administration, 8*(3):40–45

Bondy, K. N., (1983) Developing a research base for practice, *Rehabilitation Nursing, 8*(4):9–11

Chenitz, W. C., (1981) Adjusting to institutional life: A special status passage of elders, Paper presented at the 12th International Congress of Gerontology, Hamburg, Germany, July 12–17, 1981

Conduct and Utilization of Research in Nursing Project, (1983) *Using Research to Improve Nursing Practice: A Guide,* New York: Grune & Stratton

Corbin, J. M., and Strauss, A. L., (1984) Collaboration: Couples working together to manage chronic illness, *Image, 16*(4):109–115

Davis, M. Z., (1981) Promoting nursing research in the clinical setting, *Journal of Nursing Administration, 11*(3):22–27

Department of Health, Education and Welfare, (1979) Healthy People: The Surgeon General's Report on Health Promotion and Disease Prevention, 1979, DHEW Publication No. (PHS) 79-55071, Public Health Service, Washington, D.C.: U.S. Government Printing Office

DeVon, H., and Powers, M., (1984) Health beliefs, adjustment to illness, and control of hypertension, *Research in Nursing and Health, 7*:10–16

Dimond, M., (1979) Social support and adaptation to chronic illness: The use of maintenance hemodialysis, *Research in Nursing and Health, 2*:101–108

Dimond, M., and Jones, S. L., (1983) *Chronic Illness Throughout the Life Span,* Norwalk, Conn.: Appleton-Century-Crofts

Downs, F., (1984) *A Sourcebook of Nursing Research,* Philadelphia: Davis

Fagin, C. M., (1982) The economic value of nursing research, *American Journal of Nursing, 82*(12):1844–1847

Fuhs, M. F., and Mohr, K., (1981) Research program development in a tertiary care setting, *Nursing Research, 30*(1):24–27

Goodwin, L. D., and Goodwin, W. L., (1984) Qualitative vs. quantitative research or qualitative and quantitative research? *Nursing Research, 33*(6):378–380

Gorenberg, B., (1983) The research tradition of nursing: An emerging issue, *Nursing Research, 32*:347–349

Gortner, S. R., (1980) Nursing research: Out of the past and into the future, *Nursing Research, 29*(4):204–207

Gortner, S. R., (1982) Reflections from research participants, *AORN Journal, 36*(5):842–846

Gortner, S. R., (1983a) Researchmanship: Maintaining the momentum, *Western Journal of Nursing Research, 5*(1):104–106

Gortner, S. R., (1983b) The history and philosophy of nursing science and research, *Advances in Nursing Science, 2*(1):1–8

Haller, K. B., Reynolds, M. A., and Horsley, J., (1979) Development of research-based innovative protocols: Process, criteria and issues, *Research in Nursing & Health, 2*:45–51

Hammond, J., (1979) Home health care cost effectiveness: An overview of the literature, *Public Health Reports, 94*:305–311

Hefferin, E. A., Horsley, J., and Ventura, M. R., (1982) Promoting research-based nursing: The nurse administrator's role, *Journal of Nursing Administration, 12*(5):34–41

Heinrich, J., and Block, D., (1980) Summary of "knowledge for practice" conference group sessions, *Nursing Research, 29*(4):218

Hoeffer, B., and Archbold, P. G., (1983) Problems in doing research: Interfacing quantitative and qualitative methods, *Western Journal of Nursing Research, 5*(3):254–257

Hunt, V., Stark, J. L., Fisher, K. H., Joy, L., and Woldum, K., (1983) Networking: A managerial strategy for research development in a service setting, *Journal of Nursing Administration, 13*(7):27–32

Institute of Medicine, (1983) *Nursing and Nursing Education: Public Policies and Private Actions,* Washington, D.C.: National Academic Press

Jacox, A., (1980) Strategies to promote nursing research, *Nursing Research, 29*(4):213–217

Jacox, A., and Prescott, P., (1978) Determining a study's relevance for clinical practice, *American Journal of Nursing, 78*(11):1882–1889

Kirchhoff, K. T., (1983) Using research in practice: Should staff nurses be expected to use research? *Western Journal of Nursing Research, 4*(3):245–247

Knafl, K. A., and Howard, M. J., (1984) Interpreting and reporting qualitative research, *Research in Nursing & Health, 7*:17–24

Krueger, J. C., Nelson, A. H., and Wolanin, M. O., (1978) *Nursing Research: Development, Collaboration and Utilization,* Germantown, Md.: Aspen Systems

Larson, E., (1984) Health policy and NIH: Implications for nursing research, *Nursing Research, 33*(6):352–356

Leininger, M. M., (1983) Creativity and challenge for nurse researchers in the economic recession, *Journal of Nursing Administration, 13*(3):21–22

Lelean, S. R., (1982) The implementation of research findings into nursing practice, *International Journal of Nursing Studies, 19*(4):223–230

Lindemann, C. A., (1984) Nursing research: The key to excellence, in *Issues in Professional Nursing Practice: Theory and Research as Basic to Nursing Practice,* Kansas City: American Nurses Association, pp. 1–5

Loomis, M. E., and Krone, K. P., (1980) Collaborative research development, *Journal of Nursing Administration, 10*(12):32–35

Martinson, I., (1978) Home care for children dying of cancer, *Pediatrics, 62*:106–113

Martinson, I., (1983) Funding for research, *Journal of Gerontological Nursing, 9*(7):378–383

Morse, J. A., and Conrad, A., (1983) Putting research into practice, *Canadian Nurse, 79*(8):40–43

National Center for Health Statistics: Health, United States and Prevention Profile, (1983) DHHS Publication No. (PHS) 84-1232, Public Health Service, Washington, D.C.: U.S. Government Printing Office, December 1983

Norbeck, J. S., (1979) The research critique: A theoretical approach to skill development and consolidation, *Western Journal of Nursing Research, 1*(3):298–305

Robb, S., (1981) Nurse involvement in institutional review boards: The service setting perspective, *Nursing Research, 30*(1):27–38

Schwartz, D. R., (1981) *Faculty Research Development Grants: A Follow-up Report,* publication number 14-1835, New York: National League for Nursing

Spross, J. A., Kilpack, V., and Marchewka, A. E., (1981) Committee evolution in a medical setting, *Nursing Research, 30*(1):30–31

Swanson, J. M., and Chenitz, W. C., (1982) Why qualitative research in nursing? *Nursing Outlook, 30*(4):241–254

Todd, A. H., and Gortner, S. R., (1982) Researchmanship: Removing obstacles to research in the clinical setting, *Western Journal of Nursing Research, 4*(3):329–333

Ventura, M. R., Young, D. E., Feldman, M. J., Pastores, P., Pikula, S., and Yates, M. A., (1985) Cost savings as an indicator of successful nursing intervention, *Nursing Research, 34*(1):50–53

CHAPTER FIFTEEN
Alternative Modalities

Introduction

Clients and their families often seek help outside traditional medicine. That action is not necessarily a reflection of noncompliance. When people have symptoms (such as pain) or illnesses (such as terminal cancer) that do not respond to traditional medical treatment, alternative treatment may provide them with a sense of more control and greater choice in the direction and emphasis of treatment. When the alternative option can be used in conjunction with traditional treatment it may become even more desirable.

Dealing with chronic pain or terminal conditions is only one of many reasons given for selecting nontraditional forms of health care. Some people find that nontraditional practitioners provide the care and support they find lacking in their dealings with traditional medical care. Others select nontraditional treatment because of their cultural beliefs. Some individuals in good health seek alternate health care for preventive purposes or to maximize their well-being in the expectation that such practices will enhance their lives.

In the Western world, state licensure laws have long regulated the practice of physicians, nurses, pharmacists, and other health providers identified as the traditional practitioners. Now many other providers, such as chiropractors and acupuncturists, are being regulated through licensure. At one time, physicians were the only licensed diagnosticians and prescribers of health care. Other health professionals

now diagnose and prescribe within the areas of their expertise and qualifications. Some of them, such as nurses, are still considered to be within the traditional health care realm; others are not.

Unfortunately, many traditional providers, including nurses, view *all* alternatives as less valid or less acceptable than more traditional practices. Such attitudes deny clients a maximum range of choices to fill their needs. In addition, alternative practitioners are frequently classed together, as if they were a single entity, and labeled as quacks by many orthodox health care professionals, often without any prior investigation of the effectiveness of or basis for the treatment provided. This labeling occurs even when an alternative is actually quite effective.

This chapter explores reasons why individuals seek alternative treatments, looks at some of the problems related to their use, and discusses some common or popular approaches.

What Are Alternative Modalities?

An alternative treatment modality can be defined as a health intervention not "approved" by the community of orthodox medicine. Individuals may seek such treatment without orders or permission from their physicians. This does not imply that all physicians object to the use of all alternative approaches, but rather that they tend not to be prescribed or recommended.

The use of alternative treatment is not new in this country. The survival of early American colonists was due, in part, to their ability to use home remedies. In 1721, the city of Boston had only one doctor and treatment was primitive, including such practices as bloodletting. For about 200 years after the arrival of the first colonists, there were no hospitals or medical schools. Choking, broken bones, hemorrhage, poisoning, gangrene, snakebite, fever, gunshot or arrow wounds, and so on had to be treated at once by the best means known at that time (Meyer 1973).

A great number of alternative practices stem from folk tradition, although many alternatives have other sources. Every cultural, ethnic, and religious group has as part of its heritage the development of a system of treatment of sickness. One of the authors can remember watching her maternal grandmother make a poultice of fried onions placed between sheets of flannel cloth, to be applied to the chest for upper respiratory congestion. Treatments like this are passed down through tradition from one generation to the next and can be numbered among choices available to an individual when sickness occurs.

From an historical viewpoint, folk medicine has provided many useful drugs and treatments. For example, lithium is a natural substance found in the water of mineral springs; the ancient Greeks used water containing lithium salts to treat "mania and melancholy" (Kruger 1974). In the 1970s lithium was rediscovered as a valuable treatment for manic depression.

Another drug has a similar history. An 18th century doctor was asked to examine a man suffering from heart failure and dropsy but could offer no effective treatment. After his return from a short trip, the doctor found the man up and about with all the swelling gone. The man told the doctor he had been cured by a local charwoman who had given him an herb—foxglove. The doctor had the herb analyzed, and medicine gained a new drug, digitalis (Kruger 1974).

Why Individuals Seek Alternative Treatment

Individuals with chronic diseases will look for health care outside the traditional realm for a number of reasons: frustration with how their health and illness problems are being handled, feelings that ordered treatment is inadequate in alleviating symptoms or in correcting disease process, preference for cultural or ethnic practices, or a desire to enhance wellness. The client may feel, "What do I have to lose?"

Pain commonly motivates people to seek relief elsewhere. If you have ever been in pain during a long, lonely night, waiting for the dawn to come, you have had a glimpse into the world of a person who experiences chronic or intractable pain. When the pain that accompanies disorders such as arthritis and late-stage cancer no longer responds adequately to medical treatment, afflicted persons may try anything they feel holds a promise of relief.

Impaired mobility, which occurs with chronic conditions such as multiple sclerosis, amyotrophic lateral sclerosis, and arthritis, is frequently given as a reason for seeking alternative treatment. Mobility limitations can create a change in one's self-concept, ability to function, and roles; financial security may even be threatened. The failure of traditional medical treatment to improve mobility may lead these people on a search for other means to greater functioning.

Negative experiences with traditional health care can create a climate of distrust. Consequently, the individual may be more likely to reject treatment provided by orthodox practitioners. In addition, family members or others who have lost confidence in traditional treatment may encourage or influence the client to look elsewhere. Those families who consider traditional treatment ineffective may seek alternative ways to achieve improvement, regardless of cost.

The devastation and helplessness of a terminal illness are factors that make people feel there is nothing to lose and everything to gain from looking elsewhere for health care. Often, alternative practitioners offer these people hope that in turn improves their mental status. Belief in the efficacy of a treatment is an extremely important factor in recovery or improvement. These treatments have been known to delay progression of symptoms or improve the client's health status.

Because increased technology and other factors have sent health care costs soaring so dramatically

(Somers & Somers 1977), the government has found it necessary to monitor cost as well as quality of health care services (see Chapter 17). Furthermore, the diseases that plague our urbanized and aging population (for instance, vascular disease, cancer, respiratory disorders, and mental illness) are not only costly to treat but not very amenable to conventional medical treatments or cures. Cost can influence a client's choice of treatment and can motivate client or family to look for more reasonably priced, and more effective, care.

Some people do not want the discomfort, inconvenience, or frequency involved in traditional medical treatment. This aversion can make a "simple" treatment or "cure" seem more attractive and acceptable. Furthermore, when unhealthy life-styles underlie illness, people who cannot confront the need to change may search for unorthodox, simplistic, magical remedies.

Clients' desire for autonomy and control over their own bodies in a system that seems increasingly impersonal, fragmented, and incomprehensible has also contributed to the growth of alternative methods. In fact, over the past few decades self-care has become a trend in our society—a trend involving individuals who increasingly feel they can make decisions about their health, prevention of illness, and treatment of disease. In fact, many American households now have self-care reference books, and household members check out and initially treat their own symptoms rather than seeing a physician. A trip to the local pharmacy, where you can find machines to take your own blood pressure, do-it-yourself pregnancy detection kits, blood glucose monitoring devices, and a growing array of vitamins and minerals, confirms this trend.

Problems and Issues Related to Alternative Modalities

Numerous difficulties plague the client seeking relief or cure when traditional medicine has failed to improve health status or ameliorate symptoms. Quacks abound, treatment can conflict with sociocultural values, methods used may conflict with accepted health practices or may have no scientific basis, insurance companies may be unwilling to cover costs that are incurred, and competency of practitioners may be difficult to determine. In addition to clients, both orthodox and alternative practitioners find that their practices are sometimes negatively affected by these same problems. A brief discussion of each of these issues is therefore in order.

Quackery

Quackery is something to be avoided. Both clients and health professionals are faced with the perplexing problem of differentiating quackery from effective, worthwhile alternative treatment modalities. Miracle cures are often sought by people in need—people who are willing to believe anything that is presented as effective. In fact, Americans spend billions of dollars each year on frauds, hoaxes, and false cures (Vickery & Fries 1981). It is quackery that often leads people to label all alternatives as ineffective or dangerous.

A quack is "one who pretends to cure a disease" (Woolf 1980), which implies that the provider is aware that the proffered treatment is a hoax. Historically, quacks have promoted their treatments for their own profit (Martin et al. 1983). The Food and Drug Administration estimates that at least two billion dollars are spent each year on worthless tests and treatment (Holland 1981). Furthermore, to complicate the issue, quackery can occur within, as well as outside, orthodox medicine.

Johnson (1984) reported the following guidelines for recognizing fraudulent treatment, presented originally in the October 1984 issue of the *Harvard Medical School Health Letter:*

1. Words such as *miracle, cure,* and *breakthrough* are often used.
2. Ingredients are not identified.
3. Support of experts who are not named or fully identified is asserted.
4. Claims of effectiveness for a wide variety of conditions are made.

5. The product is declared as *all natural.*
6. There are vague allusions to "public research," sometimes with an offer to supply references.

To avoid fraudulent practices, the client should define treatment goals as clearly and realistically as possible before accepting proffered treatment. Questions should be asked regarding what changes or benefits are expected from the chosen treatment. Decisions should be made in advance about how to measure the effect of the treatment in terms of expected improvement, activity tolerance, pain intensity, weight change, or dollars and time expended. When openness and trust exist between client and health care professional, the professional may be particularly helpful in identifying goals, alternatives, and methods of evaluating results of treatment.

Substitution for Known Effective Treatments

People move from traditional to other modalities when traditional treatment is no longer effective or when the individual rejects effective treatment in hope of finding some miracle cure. Unfortunately, desperate people are often willing to try anything. This is especially tragic when traditional treatment for a disorder might lead to control or cure. Time spent on ineffective choices, regardless of the reason, delays treatment and may result in a poor outcome for the client.

But many non-traditional approaches do not have negative outcomes. If value is determined by results, there are many alternatives to medical practice that are effective and lead to improvement. When this happens, the client and family feel that the treatment was worthwhile.

Rejection of traditional treatment can create feelings of frustration among many health care professionals, which may surface as anger directed at the client. Some health care providers may demand that the client choose between traditional and nontraditional treatment rather than encouraging the individual to consider both, even when the latter does not conflict with the former.

Cultural Conflict

Although folklore serves as the basis of many different kinds of health care, including traditional medicine, different cultural groups often do not agree with the methods and treatment offered by orthodox medicine. Many individuals see diseases as having different bases from those generally accepted in Western culture. There is also a difference in what symptoms constitute illness among different groups and what degree of impairment is necessary before one is even considered ill (Murray & Zentner 1979). Given these factors, it is not surprising that individuals often choose familiar, and frequently effective, treatment before turning to Western methods.

As we have noted, folk treatments are common to every culture and are handed down from generation to generation. Even though some of these treatments have gained acceptance, other treatments have not. A client may feel torn between the use of orthodox medical treatment and the use of familiar folk medicine that he or she sees as a viable alternative. Traditional health care professionals, unfamiliar with the treatment basis of the folk medicine or the individual's reason for selecting such treatment may assume that the alternative is ineffective and therefore object to its use.

Costs

Because of the rising cost of health care, it is not surprising that individuals may try to find more cost-effective treatment. Mastering relaxation or biofeedback may be a less expensive, yet effective, treatment for migraine headaches when compared with the ongoing cost and potential dangers of chronic use of a prescription drug. The use of transcutaneous electrical nerve stimulation (TENS) to control low back pain may be less expensive then prescription drugs, a back brace, and repeated hospitalization for pelvic traction.

Although some alternative treatment modalities are effective and less expensive than traditional treatment, not all are. When traditional treatment is considered the best, regardless of cost, the health professional should share this information with the client. Optimally, the choice of care should be based on the client's informed decision. Although the health professional may not agree with the client's selection, the provider should continue to be supportive and work cooperatively with client and alternative health care provider.

Clients must realize that not all alternatives are cheaper; some are more costly than traditional medical treatments. The "Mexico Cure" for arthritis may cost $300 for a miracle medicine that, when analyzed, is a few dollars' worth of cortisone and phenylbutazone. Such treatment is effective only for limited periods of time, and prolonged use of these medications can be extremely expensive, as well as causing serious side effects.

Lack of Payment

Tied to costs, another problem of alternative treatment is that the client's insurance company may not pay for nontraditional treatment. Insurance companies justify refusal on the grounds that the modality is not accepted by the medical community. This stance often forces the client to use traditional methods even though he or she feels that an alternative would be more effective. For example, an insurance company may pay for a prescription medication to curb the appetite of an obese client but not pay for a class in relaxation techniques to reduce the stress that may be causing the overeating, in spite of possible medical problems, such as diabetes mellitus and hypertension, that are related to obesity. There are times when an insurance company will consider reimbursement, especially if a primary provider makes appropriate referrals or provides data to support the benefit of an alternative modality. However, payment usually requires that a review board (often of physicians) approve the treatment.

Failure of the insurance company to pay for treatments may intensify the financial burden on the entire family. Adding financial stress to the other stresses imposed by the chronic illness on the client and family can lead to family discord and disruption of family functioning.

Separating Fact from Fiction

Both nonprofessionals and professionals face the problem of differentiating fact from fallacy with respect to cause and effectiveness of treatment. It is very difficult when reading books, magazines, and the daily newspaper to discriminate proven fact from hypothesis or conjecture. Some people believe that what is printed is true, since they lack the knowledge or resources to evaluate critically what they read. In addition, when medical treatment has "failed" them, they tend to believe in anything that seems to offer promise. It is this need to find help that makes people gullible.

Titles used by individuals also influence potential clients. Many books that promote various treatments or cures are written by Dr. So-and-so, yet the kind of doctorate the author holds is not listed, nor where the special expertise was obtained. The title *doctor* denotes authority, special knowledge, and prestige in American society. When a suggested treatment is potentially harmful, people can be fooled into trying it because the author uses a title. This does a disservice to all legitimate health care providers, especially those outside the mainstream, because poor outcomes raise the suspicion that all alternative treatment is quackery.

Scientific versus Empirical Treatment

Scientific investigation in medicine uses the experimental model for determining if a treatment truly makes a difference. The best experimental models use a double-blind approach, in which neither client nor physician knows which subjects are receiving the treatment. The treatment group is then compared to a control group that did not receive the treatment. An excellent example of this method is the Veterans Administration Cooperative Study Group study that provided convincing evidence for a step approach to hypertension management (VACSG 1967, 1970). Good studies should also control for other variables that could affect the outcome, such as age, sex, and occupation.

The Hawthorne and placebo effects, which can be strong and dramatic, can influence study outcomes. The *Hawthorne effect* occurs when subjects in the experimental group perform or respond better simply because they are aware that they are the "experimental" group. This happens merely because of the attention and expectations they feel and not because of the independent, or treatment, variable being tested.

The *placebo effect* occurs when a subject feels better just because he or she took a pill, received a special bath or massage, or the like, not because the treatment actually had any pharmacologic or physiologic effect (Brody 1982). The client's belief in the treatment influences intrinsic neurochemical changes that have a significant physiological impact (Levine, Gordon, & Fields 1978). It is the body's response, but not necessarily to the specific treatment used. The placebo effect has withstood scientific investigation and is a well accepted fact in the clinical practice of medicine. As an example, it is acknowledged that the action of a drug can be enhanced or hindered by the social context in which it is given (Berblinger 1963).

One of the most important ingredients that enhances the placebo effect is a positive attitude toward the placebo's effectiveness. This phenomenon has been well demonstrated by faith healers. Expectations about the effects of the treatment, the extent of fear or pain, the confidence and trust placed in the practitioner, and the choice of treatment all strongly influence the client's response to any therapy. Positive placebo responses are much more likely in chronic remittant diseases or when the central nervous system is being treated (LaPatra 1978).

Not all traditional treatment is based on science and not all alternatives on word of mouth. Much of medical treatment is really empirical; that is, things were tried, found effective, and used without any experimental design at all. However, more valid scientific research is done in traditional medicine than is done by practitioners of alternative treatments. This is in part the result of funding provided by the federal government for such research.

Finding Competent Practitioners

An individual may decide, with or without medical approval, to try an alternative treatment modality.

Once that decision is made, where does one find someone who is competent? Although many practitioners of alternative modalities are licensed, there is no licensing or certification procedure for many others. In other words, inconsistencies and gaps in standards for licensure and certification make it difficult to decide who is competent. Acupuncture is a case in point. It is considered acceptable (and even reimbursable) when acupuncture is practiced by physicians (very few of whom have had adequate training in that modality). Yet in many states, no mechanism exists to license Oriental practitioners who have extensive specialized training and legitimate credentials.

Similar quandaries exist among other health disciplines. Relaxation techniques and biofeedback are being offered by many levels of health professionals. Some are well trained, some are not. If the treatment is ordered by a primary provider, insurance payment is generally made without investigation of qualifications. One can ask if there should be some kind of regulatory system that would control who can provide certain treatments. If so, who should establish and control this system? And how do you control for the many quacks or frauds who go unregulated?

At present, control seems unlikely. Therefore, each individual should take responsibility for seeking information to make an informed decision. However, becoming informed on competency and qualifications is a difficult task for client and professional alike.

Common or Popular Treatment Modalities

The health care professional has a responsibility to help clients make the informed treatment decisions that will be most therapeutic or meaningful to them. This requires a climate conducive to open communication about any treatment under consideration. If the health professional is not familiar with the alternative drug or treatment, efforts should be made to find unbiased or impartial information.

Clients also need a supportive environment and a sense that the professional is their advocate, who will focus on helping them live life to the fullest despite chronic illness. This may entail that the client learn to live with some pain, some immobility, or the reality of his or her own mortality. It may require learning ways to monitor symptoms and make appropriate adjustments in medications, activities, and so forth, in order to avoid potential problems. Or it may require that professionals give clients support and show a willingness to help them make intelligent decisions on alternative treatments. Above all, clients need to feel a sense of dignity, and such feelings come largely from having control over oneself and one's environment (Prescott & Flexer 1982).

The remaining sections of this chapter describe some alternative modalities currently in use in this country. The list is not all-inclusive, nor will these modalities be presented in depth. No judgment of their validity as treatment is intended, although pros and cons are included.

Diets

The use of diet—low-sodium diets for cardiac problems and calorie-controlled diets for diabetes, for example—as part of medical management of many diseases is well known to health professionals. Diets are also commonly used for weight control, as evidenced by the multitude of books offering diets to achieve a slim and youthful self. Diets are frequently used as preventive treatment, to achieve maximum health, or to reverse effects of some pathologies, such as arthritis or cancer. Frequently, individuals having diseases such as cancer, obesity, senility, and arthritis have been promised (and believe in) "cures" effected by adherence to a certain diet. However, since food is the primary source of nutrients, the misuse of diets can create health problems.

The content, frequency, and ritual that comprise dietary intake are greatly influenced by an individual's culture. Such influences against certain foods are so strong that, even in famine situations, recipients of food packages have starved rather than eat forbidden food. Belief in the magical power of certain foods to prolong life, increase vitality, and cure illness is also widespread (Miller 1981).

Diets can be prescribed or self-instituted. They can focus on eliminating certain foods that are considered harmful, combining certain foods for a given effect, or avoiding additives. Diets are used to control various symptoms such as the pain of arthritis, to manage weight, to effect preventive treatment, and so forth. Each diet claims different values, emphasizes different approaches, and works for different people. Because diets are so widely used for so many different reasons, only a few are described here. It is not our intent to condone or condemn any of them.

Arthritis Diets.[1] A number of the diets used by arthritics are basically sound from a nutritional standpoint, but they restrict the intake of certain foods that seem to increase symptoms. Individuals who use these diets find that they are very helpful, even though the medical community as a whole does not support diet as a basis for treating arthritis. Clients who find relief through these diets should not be discouraged from their use, but rather, allowed to integrate their food preferences into the medical regimen.

One such diet is presented by C. Dong, a physician who suffered from crippling arthritis as a young adult (Dong & Banks 1975). Based on the concept that rheumatic diseases have a food allergy component, this diet emulates simple Chinese food intake and consists primarily of any kind of rice, all seafoods and vegetables, vegetable oils (particularly safflower and corn), egg whites, honey, nuts (not processed) and seeds, tea or coffee, and herbs and spices. Restricted foods include meats (except occasional white meat of chicken), fruit, dairy products, whole eggs, alcohol, and all additives, preservatives, and chemicals. Dr. Dong has found that people who consume this diet have decreased symptoms and maintain normal lab values.

Zen Macrobiotic Diet. The word *macrobiotic* is derived from the Greek *macros* ("great" or "long") and *bios* ("life"). Popular among only a few people in metropolitan centers such as New York and Los

---

[1]Information on arthritis diets courtesy of Ilene Lubkin.

Angeles, the diet is professed to have curative powers for such illnesses as cancer. Developed by Ohsawa, after being told that he was dying of an incurable disease, the diet consists of decreasing food intake over ten levels until only brown rice remains. Nutritionally unsound, the diet is condemned by the Council on Foods and Nutrition of the American Medical Association. Numerous deaths have resulted from it, as have cases of scurvy, severe anemia, hypocalcemia, and hypoproteinemia (Kuske 1983; "Unproven" 1983a). It is mentioned not because it is recommended by the authors but because it is used by people often desperate for some help.

Pritikin Diet. Developed in 1974, the Pritikin diet advocates an intake high in carbohydrates, high in fiber, and extremely low in fat (less than 10% of total calories), low in cholesterol (less than 100 milligrams per day), and free of sugars and processed foods (Kuske 1983). An individual who consumes approximately 1,400 calories per day meets the requirements for essential nutrients, except some of the recommended iron (Taylor & Anthony 1983). Although balanced, this diet is considered less palatable to Americans who are accustomed to the flavor of a higher fat intake. Those who adhere to this diet feel it is effective in reversing atherosclerotic changes.

Scarsdale Diet. Designed by Dr. Herman Tarnower for weight loss, the Scarsdale diet consists of foods high in protein, low in carbohydrates, and low in fat. Specific menus are provided, and the strict regimen is to be followed for two week periods with a modified regimen in between. Initially, no more than 1,000 calories are recommended (Kuske 1983). Some authors state that the quantity of foods to be eaten is not clearly described. The diet is also low in milk, bread, cereals, iron, vitamin A, calcium, and riboflavin, and it is recommended for use only under medical supervision (Taylor & Anthony 1983).

Dr. Atkins's Revolution. The Atkins diet, also intended for weight loss, recommends zero carbohydrates, high fat, and moderate protein intake. Because of the high fat content, the diet produces a state of ketosis. The diet also induces fatigue and hypoten-

sion and has the danger of potential vascular damage, fetal brain damage, and accelerated atherosclerosis (Kuske 1983).

Megavitamin Therapy. Although not truly a dietary modification, megavitamin therapy involves the use of massive doses of vitamins to effect nutritional and health goals. Between 1900 and 1950, knowledge in the field of nutrition reached a major height with the discovery of vitamins, minerals, and essential amino acids. Many vitamins are known to be "essential nutrients"; that is, they cannot be synthesized by the body, must be supplied from foods, and are essential for normal body function or growth. Clearly, many disorders such as rickets (vitamin D), pellagra (B_{12}), beriberi (B_1), and chilosis (B_2) are due to vitamin insufficiency.

Many Americans are consuming high doses of vitamin C, vitamin A, and vitamin E in the belief that such action can enhance their health. For example, Linus Pauling recommends regular use of large doses of ascorbic acid to help prevent common colds. One text listed 28 disorders that can be alleviated or cured by taking vitamin E (Kruger 1974). Whether these improvements result from a placebo effect or from actual physiologic changes has not been fully studied. Generally, orthodox medicine discounts the effectiveness of megavitamin therapy.

Care should be taken in suggesting the use of megavitamins, since excessive dosages of some vitamins can cause adverse effects in the body. Vitamins in large doses may act as drugs and not as nutrients. Using vitamin C as an example, it is known that large doses of ascorbic acid can lead to the formation of oxalate stones. Ascorbic acid can destroy a high percentage of vitamin B_{12} in a given meal. For diabetics, glycosuria tests (Testtape and Clinitest) are invalidated by consumption of large doses of ascorbic acid (Feldman 1983). The public must be aware that massive doses of vitamins may not be harmless and that toxic effects can occur.

Drugs Not Approved by the FDA

The first Pure Food and Drug Act in the United States was passed in 1906. Since that time, the federal Food and Drug Administration (FDA) has been a watchdog to protect Americans from drugs not fully tested. For example, when the drug thalidomide was used in Europe, thousands of infants were born with missing extremities. Most Americans were spared this tragedy due to our strict drug regulations (Miller 1981). A number of drugs used to treat some chronic diseases are illegal in this country but available in Europe and other countries where regulations are not as strict. DMSO, laetrile, and iscador are examples of drugs considered effective by many people but not approved for use in the United States.

Dimethyl Sulfoxide (DMSO). Dimethyl sulfoxide is a byproduct of the paper-making industry and has been used as an industrial solvent since the 1940s. DMSO has been claimed as an effective treatment for arthritis, mental illness, emphysema, and cancer. For cancer, the drug is usually given intravenously. The rationale is that DMSO penetrates the shell around the cancer cell and becomes a vehicle for any other medication that is concurrently administered. The period of treatment for cancer at the Degenerative Disease Medical Center in Las Vegas is four weeks. The cost of the treatment, which includes laetrile and procaine hydrochloride as well as DMSO, is $4,000. Aetna Life Insurance Company has refused to pay for treatments involving the administration of DMSO for cancer. DMSO causes damage to the skin and eyes. In 1978, the FDA approved a 5% sterile aqueous solution of DMSO for symptomatic relief of interstitial cystitis. A 90% solution of DMSO is approved for use in veterinary medicine for horses and dogs. No other usage of the drug has been approved by the FDA ("Unproven" 1983b), although many of those who use the veterinary solution topically feel it is quite helpful.

Laetrile. Laetrile has been promoted as an anticancer vitamin, and many individuals suffering from that disease have turned to this product. Yet every American nutritional society of scientific repute has said laetrile is not a vitamin. The promoters of laetrile made enormous profit from its sale, according to *The New York Times* (June 26, 1977). One promoter was estimated to take in $150,000 to $200,000 a month in laetrile sales (Martin 1977). In 1976, Mexico canceled its approval of laetrile, stating that "no positive results were obtained in clinical research." Nevertheless, terminally ill people use and claim some relief from this drug.

Iscador. Iscador is a preparation made from various kinds of mistletoe. It was first proposed for the treatment of cancer in 1920 by a man in Switzerland. The drug received a great deal of visibility from 1920 through 1979 in articles in the annual reports of the Society for Cancer Research in Ashuheim, Switzerland. Its proponents recommend iscador for the treatment of inoperable tumors, for preoperative treatment of tumors, as adjuvant therapy for solid tumors, and for precancerous conditions when indicated. The drug has been approved for use in Austria, Switzerland, and West Germany. However, no attempt has been made to conform to standards of the FDA in the United States. Manufacturers of the drug in Switzerland stated in 1981 that "the FDA regulations are devised for chemically definable substances and as such are not compatible with a drug like iscador that represents a whole plant extract" ("Unproven" 1983c).

Alternative Systems of Medical Care

A number of health practitioners provide alternative or complementary approaches to health care management. Many of these practitioners undergo extensive training to reach a level of competency and pass rigorous national and state licensing board examinations. These fields of practice have many devoted clients. Only a few are discussed here.

Chiropractic.[2] Considered by many people to be part of orthodox health care, chiropractic is still seen by others as an alternative modality. Chiropractic manipulation was introduced in the late 1800s by Daniel D. Palmer, on the premise that illness is essentially

---

[2]The authors wish to thank Hugh J. Lubkin, D.C. for content on chiropractic.

functional and becomes organic only as an end process (Haldeman 1980). Palmer's first client, a deaf employee, had an amazing portion of his hearing restored within 24 hours after being adjusted. Another of Palmer's clients, Samuel Weed, named this manipulative process *chiropractic,* which means "with hands."

The basis of chiropractic practice is correction of vertebral subluxation and improvement of nerve function. Normally, as nerve roots exit from the intervertebral foramen, fatty connective tissue protects the nerves from compression (Haldeman 1980). In subluxation, the soft tissue around the nerve becomes compressed or irritated. Compression and local edema can ensue, resulting in diminished blood supply to the nerve, nerve root, and spinal cord. If not corrected, vertebral subluxation can result in ischemia and decreased function of the nerve, tissue, or organ (Pansky & Allen 1980). Eventually, ischemia can culminate in nerve death, which becomes more serious than the original problem.

A criticism of chiropractic is that once manipulative therapy is started, regular treatments are necessary to maintain optimum health. However, in most cases, clients must realize and accept that no treatment can miraculously reverse or cure their problems in just weeks. These people often have serious, chronic conditions that, at best, can be effectively managed to reduce symptomology and pain. Many of these clients have tried a multitude of other approaches before turning to chiropractic care. As effective chiropractic management provides welcome relief, these individuals often enjoy a reduction or elimination of pain, musculoskeletal symptoms, and any associated drug consumption. Often, chiropractic manipulations can be so effective that clients can reduce their treatments to occasional visits as needed.

Today, modern chiropractors are licensed primary health care providers with a wide scope of practice. Clinically, chiropractic health care is effective with many disorders related to the autonomic, peripheral, somatic, and central nervous systems (Haldeman 1980). Chiropractic also focuses on preventive health care and correction of athletic injury.

In addition, chiropractic research is currently exploring the effects of improved nerve innervation on various disease states, including internal organ dysfunction and improved postsurgical recovery.

Chiropractic philosophy still supports the concept that body tissues and organs function best with optimal neural and hormonal innervation and that disease is often the result of a lack of nerve innervation or function. Chiropractors strive, through carefully calculated manipulations of spinal misalignment, to restore maximum nerve innervation, which allows the body either to resist disease and illness or to heal quickly from disease or insult.

Homeopathy. This system of medicine was originated in the early 19th century by Samuel Hahneman. It is often successful in treating various infectious diseases. Homeopathy is largely responsible for the development of the use of nitroglycerine for angina pectoris and some other present day medications. The basic principle is as follows:

> The remedy for any case of disease or illness is the substance that, when administered systematically to a healthy person, yields precisely the symptomatology of this case.... Homeopathy holds that when the patient receives the one remedy whose symptomatology most perfectly matches his or her own symptoms, the whole disease is removed, root and branch (Coulter 1978).

Once a drug is selected it is then administered in the minimum effective dose, usually much less than the ordinary allopathic medication doses. Proponents cite the advantages of small dosages: rare sensitivity or toxic reactions, minimal expenses, and a holistic approach (Baker 1978). The precise matching of client symptoms with one of thousands of homeopathic remedies demands considerable time and individual attention, perhaps also contributing to the satisfaction some clients feel.

Naturopathy. Claiming roots in ancient practices, naturopathic medicine purports to be a separate and distinct healing art employing a holistic approach that supports physiologic and natural processes. Health maintenance and promotion and disease prevention through education, nutrition, mental hygiene, and physical fitness are emphasized. Practitioners describe naturopathy as treating all types of illnesses, referring to and cooperating with licensed physicians, and as an alternative complementary to other healing arts (Boucher 1978).

Modalities Involving Mind Control

Relaxation/imagery, biofeedback, yoga, and transcendental meditation are addressed under this category.

Relaxation/Imagery. Hans Selye, an endrocrinologist and director of the Institute on Experimental Medicine and Surgery at the University of Montreal, is well known for his work related to stress response in humans. According to Selye, chronic stress can lead to hormonal imbalance, increased blood pressure (which can lead in turn to kidney damage), and suppression of the immune system (which could lead to cancer) (Selye 1956; Simonton, Matthews-Simonton, & Creighton 1978). Both relaxation and imagery are utilized to help reduce stress and related problems.

A technique for progressive systemic muscle relaxation was developed in the 1930s by Dr. Edward Jacobson, inventor of electromyography. In the 1970s, a renewed trend toward holistic medicine led to an increased interest in his technique. Progressive relaxation involves the purposeful tensing and then relaxing of specific muscle groups (Agrar 1983). Characteristics common to all types of relaxation techniques include rhythmic breathing, decreased muscle tension, and, occasionally, an altered state of consciousness (Dimotto 1984).

Relaxation techniques can decrease heart rate, blood pressure, respiration, oxygen consumption, carbon dioxide production, muscle tension, and metabolic rate, as well as increase peripheral vasodilation and modify peripheral temperatures (Graves & Thompson 1978).

Simonton and Matthews-Simonton recommend the use of guided imagery along with a relaxation program. Simonton, a physician, believes that stress

increases a person's susceptibility to illness and that, when compounded by an attitude of hopelessness or helplessness, can contribute to, not cause, cancer (Simonton, Matthews-Simonton, & Creighton 1978). Simonton and Matthews-Simonton combine relaxation with imagery as a tool to communicate with the unconscious, to decrease tension and stress, and to comfort and alter feelings of hopelessness and helplessness. Simonton does not recommend his program in lieu of medical treatment; rather, he recommends it in conjunction with the usual traditional medical treatment (Simonton, Matthews-Simonton, & Creighton 1978).

Biofeedback.

The presentation to a person of on-going biological information, such as heart rate, usually by means of meters, lights, or auditory signals, so that he or she can become aware of inside-the-skin behaviors. Biofeedback training means using the information in learning how to self-regulate the biological process being displayed (Green 1978).

Currently biofeedback research is being conducted toward efforts to achieve control of the autonomic nervous system, to relieve hypertension, cardiac dysrhythmias, migraines, asthma, epilepsy, back pain, and muscle tension.

Sensitive instruments such as electroencephalography (EEG), electromyelography (EMG), thermometers, and so on, convert minute amounts of electrical energy, reflecting somatic and autonomic processes, to audible or visible signals. With training and practice, many individuals learn to omit the electronic instrumentation (external feedback). These individuals develop a conscious "feedback loop" and are trained to perceive directly and to react or adjust to their bodies in response to inside-the-skin events (Green 1978): "Biofeedback practice, acting in the opposite way to drugs, increases the person's sensitivity to inside-the-skin events."

Biofeedback has been effectively used to help relieve many types of pain. "Dr. Ronald Melzack, an authority on pain, has found that it is not biofeedback alone that prevails over pain. Rather, pain is relieved by distraction, suggestion, relaxation and sense of control that are all part of the biofeedback procedure" (LaPatra 1978). Holroyd stated:

> In some instances, biofeedback training may be effective because it indirectly induces the patients to alter their interactions with the environment, not because it enables them to directly control problematic physiological responses. It is therefore crucial that treatment procedures be developed that focus on altering cognitive and behavioral responses to stress, in addition to physiological responses (Holroyd 1979).

Biofeedback is a proven and valuable adjunct to many treatments, especially when combined with other approaches.

Yoga. Yoga is a complex system of beliefs and practices to integrate the mind and body. It developed in India out of Hindu philosophy before the second century B.C. Like many other religions and philosophies, yoga extols the virtues of meditation in clearing the mind of thoughts, easing tensions, releasing energy, and increasing self-awareness (Kruger 1974). The awakening of Kundalini, the powerful reservoir coiled like a snake at the base of the spine, results in the sensation of tremendous heat and energy. This energy is awakened and released by ascetic practices including chanting, breathing, exercises, positions, and meditation (Grisell 1979).

The most popular and best known system of yoga is Hatha Yoga, exercises and positions (asanas and mudras) to prevent and cure disease by strengthening muscles and nerves, keeping the spine flexible, and maintaining function of the glands. Yoga also includes breathing techniques (pranayamas) during which the body is purified and universal energy and knowledge are drawn in.

Another variation of yogic healing is ayurvedic medicine, involving diet, herbs, and natural and Indian folk remedies. There is much similarity to traditional Chinese medicine, as both are based on the Taoist philosophy that humanity is one with the universe. Ayurvedic medicine endorses diet based on fruits and vegetables, seeds and nuts, milk, buttermilk, and honey and avoidance of meat, eggs, fish,

sweets, and conventional medicine and surgery (Kruger 1974).

Relaxation and reduction of tension are demonstrable benefits of meditation and exercise for some practitioners of yoga, and dietary recommendations offer benefits for some. However, individual limitations and requirements, such as avoidance of spinal hyperextension or inclusion of ample dietary iron, must not be overlooked.

Transcendental Meditation (TM). In the 1970s, the Maharishi Mahesh Yogi founded TM, a more secular movement that gained wide popularity in the United States. Reputable medical research has documented the following physiologic effects during meditation: decreased blood pressure, heart and respiratory rates, oxygen consumption and carbon dioxide elimination, accompanied by a rise in electrical skin resistance and alpha brain waves. Advantages are that TM requires meditation for only 20 minutes twice daily, with no religious commitment, and it is easily learned (Kruger 1974).

Stimulation/Manipulation of the Body

Another group of alternative modalities involves body stimulation. Acupuncture/Chinese medicine, transcutaneous electrical nerve stimulation (TENS), massage, and therapeutic touch are discussed under this heading.

Acupuncture/Chinese Medicine. In 1971, acupuncture burst into the American public's awareness following the U.S. ping pong team's trip to China. When President Richard Nixon toured China a year later, his Air Force physician witnessed, and journalist James Reston experienced, the use of acupuncture as an anesthetic. To the Chinese, acupuncture is but one part of a complex system of traditional Chinese medicine that has been practiced for 5,000 years. After the Communist Revolution (1949), doctors practicing Chinese medicine were encouraged, and they outnumbered those trained in the West by three to one by the 1960s. During the Cultural Revolution of 1966–1976, medical and nursing schools closed and traditional Chinese methods received further emphasis. Today, traditional Chinese medicine (including acupuncture) is practiced in conjunction with Western medicine by doctors both in rural areas and in clinics and hospitals (Kruger 1974; Dimond 1984).

Traditional Chinese medicine is based on the view that all things in humanity and nature are related. A human being is seen as a microcosm of the universe, which encompasses the five elements of wood, fire, earth, metal/air, and water—all governed by the opposing but complementary forces of *yang* and *yin,* which must be in harmony. The objective of traditional Chinese medicine is to maintain or restore equilibrium, to treat the cause rather than the symptoms (Bresler, Kroening & Volen 1978).

Energy or life force, *ch'i,* circulates through fourteen meridians (channels or pathways) that pass through the body; illness is a result of an interruption or imbalance of this energy flow. Hundreds of vital points have been identified along the meridians, and each point has a specific function and action.

Needles made of stainless steel, precious metal, porcelain, or other materials, varying in diameter and length, are inserted at these points. Stimulation of some points results in tonification, and of others, sedation of the related organ. The results are also affected by the way the needles are inserted (angle and depth) and manipulated (rotated, twirled, left in place) (Kruger 1974).

Acupuncture is frequently practiced in conjunction with other elements such as moxibustion, herbal treatments, and massage. Described as painless, acupuncture sometimes causes sensations ranging from a dull ache to a brief sharp pain. Commonly, the presence of warmth, itching, numbness, tingling, and prickling are viewed as evidence that the treatment is working.

How acupuncture works is a tantalizing mystery. There may be multiple mechanisms, represented by a variety of theories, including the placebo effect, hypnosis, and even Melzack and Wall's gate control theory (1965), which proposes that an area within the spinal cord acts as a gate in response to electrical input from both peripheral and central nerves. Some

feel that acupuncture may effect complex mobilization of the immune and inflammatory system, and others believe that it sets off subtle psychologic responses (Kruger 1974).

It is said that the most important diagnostic tool of the Chinese physician is the complicated art of pulse reading. Each of the 28 qualities of the 12 pulses (6 on each wrist) relates information from every organ and system. In addition, detailed histories are taken and complex evaluations of body, tongue, and facial tone examination are done (LaPatra 1978).

Transcutaneous Electrical Nerve Stimulation (TENS). Electrical stimulation through the skin is a form of therapy that began as an alternative modality and is increasingly being accepted by traditional medical practitioners. TENS evolved in 1967 as a clinical application of Melzack and Wall's gate control theory (Moore & Blacker 1983). Though the mechanism of action is still unclear, the stimulation of larger peripheral nerves apparently blocks transmission of pain impulses. Another possibility is release of the body's own analgesic, endorphins, as a result of nerve stimulation (Taylor et al. 1983).

TENS has been used to relieve chronic pain states as well as to reduce pain associated with surgery, childbirth, and chronic disease. Studies of its application indicate that TENS is more successful for some types of chronic pain, such as back pain, than for others. Proper selection of clients and thorough instruction and preparation are essential for best results. Advantages to clients include avoidance of the hazards of analgesic medication and the ability to control their own therapy (Meyer 1982). In recent years, electrical stimulation has also been used to enhance bone growth and to maintain some of the size and function of paralyzed muscles.

Massage. In recent years, the trend to self-awareness and getting in touch with and healing one's own body and emotions has led to incorporating massage independently or with alternative therapies. It has been pointed out that hands were the first instruments of healing. As early as the seventh century A.D., massage was taught in China, and certain acupuncture points are still used in this way as acupressure massage to equalize the life forces of *yang* and *yin,* thereby achieving balance and equilibrium of the body (Kruger 1974).

Japanese massage, like Chinese massage, may be based on manipulation of vital spots, called *tsubo,* on the meridians for the treatment of many diseases. There are other types of Japanese massage. One, *shiatsu,* which originated about 50 years ago, includes prolonged finger pressure and spiritual concentration. Shiatsu is thought to stimulate the parasympathetic nervous system and produce relaxation (Masunaga 1978). Japanese specialists have combined oriental (amma) massage with techniques to evolve a "distinctive Japanese massage system unlike any other in the world" (Serizawa 1978, p. 207).

A number of modern massage methods are suggestive of acupressure massage, but the "points" and techniques vary. The principle behind *zone therapy* is that every organ muscle in the body has a corresponding area in one or both feet; *reflex therapy* is similar. *Polarity therapy* employs (along with exercise, diet, and "right thinking") heavy pressure by thumbs, knuckles, and elbows to special points (Pannetier 1978). There are Swedish, Turkish, Italian, and Austrian styles of massage and many variations of psychotherapy interwoven with different types of massage.

Rolfing, invented in the 1950s by Ida Rolf, a biochemist, is a form of very deep, intensive massage that purports to use the force of gravity and manipulation by the rolfer as tools in permanently restructuring the whole body and, as the founder said, to improve functioning and competence (Rolf 1978). The client is encouraged to cry out, express pain, and relieve tensions (Kruger 1974).

William Reich, a psychoanalyst, was innovative and highly influential in combining massage with psychotherapy. He is recognized for his thesis that neurotics build up "compensatory muscular armor" as a defense against their repressed anxieties. Bioenergetics, founded by Alexander Lowen and based on Reichian therapy, incorporates massage and its associated release of tension and anger (Kruger 1974).

Many healing capabilities are attributed to various forms of massage, including relief of pain, stimulation of blood and lymph circulation, speeding up of waste elimination, reduction of swelling, lowering of blood pressure, and foremost, of course, relaxation of muscles (LaPatra 1978).

Therapeutic Touch. The touch of a healer is intended to be a channel for the flow of healing energy from the healer to the afflicted. Many clients describe sensations of heat and tingling during contact healing. Many healers often have a unique awareness of their own bodily energy; some healers feel that this energy comes not from themselves but from the environment or a higher source. Since earliest times, helping and healing have been accomplished by the laying on of hands. The modern term for this modality is *therapeutic touch* (Grad 1979; Krieger 1979a).

Delores Krieger, a nurse clinician and researcher, has studied and written extensively about healing. She describes it in terms of *prana,* an Eastern concept meaning both the spiritual life force or energy and physical inhalation and exhalation (Krieger 1978). In the mid-1970s, Krieger carried out studies measuring changes in hemoglobin values as indicators of responses by clients to therapeutic touch by nurses. She later described two implications of her studies: (1) therapeutic touch can be taught, and (2) "touch affects the healee's [client's] blood components and brain waves and . . . elicits a generalized relaxation response" (Krieger 1979b). Krieger states, "The practice of therapeutic touch is a natural potential in physically healthy persons who are strongly motivated to help ill people" (Krieger 1975).

Recently, Quinn (1984) tested the thesis that "If an energy exchange is the means by which therapeutic touch has an effect, contact should not be required to achieve the effect." Subjects tested with noncontact therapeutic touch demonstrated a decrease in anxiety significantly greater than the control group. Quinn concludes that "At a time when an estimated

50 to 80% of all human illness is attributed to psychosomatic, stress related origins, a noninvasive, natural intervention that can help to decrease anxiety would appear to have an important contribution to make" (Quinn 1984).

Of that there is no doubt, but exploration of this alternative treatment modality, though increasing, is still in its infancy. In a recent careful review of the research literature, Clark and Clark (1984) concluded that the current research supporting the nursing practice of therapeutic touch is, at best, weak and requires replication and expansion with clear, objective evidence before this treatment can gain professional credibility.

Summary and Conclusions

Once health practitioners accept the right of the chronically ill client to determine what treatment modalities are most effective and meaningful, support should be given to the client's choices. Only through a willingness to accept that there are alternatives to orthodox medical practice and that all health care providers need to be informed about them can health professionals provide the assistance clients seek.

In the Western world, most individuals seek orthodox medical care when ill. However, this care is not always effective in controlling symptoms or prolonging life. People in need will seek ways of resolving their difficulties, and this often means alternative approaches to health care. In addition, many people follow other health practices, either because such practices are culturally correct or because they feel that their health will be enhanced. Although these modalities are not frequently prescribed or often approved by the medical community, many are effective, legitimate routes to health care. Problems that make it difficult to choose among valid alternatives include quackery, costs, insurance payment for treatment, determining the best treatment for the given client or situation, separating fact from fiction, and determining competency of practitioners.

In spite of these problems, clients will and do seek alternatives. Some of these alternatives have been presented. The list is only partial and meant to stimulate health care providers to explore their clients' needs in view of the ever-growing availability of beneficial and effective alternative modalities.

STUDY QUESTIONS

1. What is an alternative modality?
2. Why do clients/families seek alternative treatments?
3. What is the danger of quackery, and about how much money is spent on such treatment?
4. How do the problems of effectiveness of health care, cultural conflict, false claims, and finding competent practitioners adversely affect clients and practitioners, both traditional and alternative?
5. How do costs of treatment and insurance payments influence choice of treatment?
6. Why is it important for health care practitioners to be familiar with alternative treatment modalities?
7. What are the advantages and disadvantages of diets used by clients with or without the approval of their primary provider?
8. What can chiropractors, homeopaths, and naturopaths do to help clients?
9. How can relaxation/imagery, TENS, TM, or therapeutic touch be used to enhance health or improve chronic illnesses?
10. How would you counsel a client who is interested in acupuncture, massage, yoga, or biofeedback as a treatment choice?

References

Agrar, W. S., (1983) Relaxation therapy in hypertension, *Hospital Practice, 18*(50):129–137

Baker, W. P., (1978) Homeotherapeutics, in Kasloff, L. J. (ed.), *Wholistic Dimensions in Healing: Resource Guide,* Garden City, N.Y.: Doubleday, pp. 49–50

Berblinger, K. W., (1963) The physician, patient and pill, *Psychosomatics, 4*(9):265–269

Boucher, J. A., (1978) Naturopathic medicine: A separate and distinct healing profession, in Kasloff, L. J. (ed.), *Wholistic Dimensions in Healing: Resource Guide,* Garden City, N.Y.: Doubleday, pp. 80–81

Bresler, D. E., Kroening, R. J., and Volen, M. P., (1978) Acupuncture in America, in Kasloff, L. J. (ed.), *Wholistic Dimensions in Healing: Resource Guide,* Garden City, N.Y.: Doubleday, pp. 132–134

Brody, H., (1982) The lie that heals: The ethics of giving placebos, *Annals of Internal Medicine, 97:*112–118

Clark, P., and Clark, M. J., (1984) Therapeutic touch: Is there a scientific basic for practice? *Nursing Research, 33:*37–41

Coulter, H. J., (1978) Homeopathy, in Kasloff, L. J. (ed.), *Wholistic Dimensions in Healing: Resource Guide,* Garden City, N.Y.: Doubleday, pp. 47–48

Dimond, E. G., (1984) The breaking of a profession, *The Journal of the American Medical Association, 252:*3160–3164

Dimotto, J. W., (1984) Relaxation, *American Journal of Nursing, 84*(6):745–758

Dong, C. H., and Banks, J., (1975) *The Arthritic's Cookbook,* New York: Bantam

Feldman, E. B., (1983) *Nutrition in the Middle and Later Years,* Boston: John Wright

Grad, H. A., (1979) Some biological effects of the laying on of hands and their implications, in Otto, H. A., and Knight, J. W. (eds.), *Dimensions in Holistic Healing: New Frontiers in the Treatment of the Whole Person,* Chicago: Nelson-Hall, pp. 199–209

Graves, H. H., and Thompson, E. A., (1978) Anxiety: A mental health vital sign, in Long, D. C., and Williams, R. A. (eds.), *Clinical Practice in Psychosocial Nursing: Assessment and Intervention,* New York: Appleton-Century-Crofts

Green, E., (1978) Biofeedback, in Kasloff, L. J. (ed.), *Wholistic Dimensions in Healing: Resource Guide,* Garden City, N.Y.: Doubleday, pp. 169–171

Grisell, R. D., (1979) Kundalini yoga as healing agent, in

Otto, H. A., and Knight, J. W. (eds.), *Dimensions in Holistic Healing: New Frontiers in the Treatment of the Whole Person,* Chicago: Nelson-Hall

Haldeman, S., (1980) *Modern Developments in the Principles and Practice of Chiropractic,* New York: Appleton-Century-Crofts

Holland, J. C., (1981) Patients who seek unproven cancer remedies: A psychological perspective, *Clinical Bulletin, 11*(3):102–105

Holroyd, K., (1979) Stress, coping, and the treatment of stress-related illness, in McNamara, J. R. (ed.), *Behavioral Approaches to Medicine: Application and Analysis,* New York: Plenum, pp. 191–217

Johnson, G. T., (1984) Studies help spot fraud in medicine, *Kansas City Star,* November 29, 1983, p. 3B

Krieger, D., (1975) Therapeutic touch: The imprimatur of nursing, *American Journal of Nursing, 75:*786

Krieger, D., (1978) The potential use of therapeutic touch in healing, in Kasloff, L. J. (ed.), *Wholistic Dimensions in Healing: Resource Guide,* Garden City, N.Y.: Doubleday, pp. 182–183

Krieger, D., (1979a) Therapeutic touch and contemporary applications, in Otto, H. A., and Knight, J. W. (eds.), *Dimensions in Holistic Healing: New Frontiers in the Treatment of the Whole Person,* Chicago: Nelson-Hall, pp. 297–303

Krieger, D., (1979b) *The Therapeutic Touch,* Englewood Cliffs, N.J.: Prentice-Hall

Kruger, H., (1974) *Other Healers, Other Cures: A Guide to Alternative Medicine,* New York: Bobbs-Merrill

Kuske, T., (1983) Quackery and fad diets, in Feldman, E. (ed.), *Nurtition in the Middle and Late Years,* Boston: John Wright

LaPatra, J., (1978) *Healing,* St. Louis: McGraw-Hill

Levine, J. D., Gordon, N. C., and Fields, H. L., (1978) The mechanism of placebo analgesia, *Lancet, 2:*654–657

Martin, D. S., (1977) Laetrile—a dangerous drug, *Cancer Journal for Nurse Clinicians, 27*(5):301–304

Martin, D. S., Allen, C. N., Cohen, R. J., Lerner, I. J., Lewis, J. P., and Pinsky, C. M., (1983) Ineffective cancer therapy: A guide for the layperson, *Journal of Clinical Oncology, 1*(2):154–163

Masunaga, S., (1978) Shiatsu, in Kasloff, L. J. (ed.), *Wholistic Dimensions in Healing: Resource Guide,* Garden City, New York: Doubleday, pp. 212–214

Melzack, R., and Wall, P. D., (1965) Pain mechanisms: A new theory, *Science, 150:*971

Meyer, C., (1973) *American Folk Medicine,* New York: Crowell

Meyer, T. M., (1982) TENS: Relieving pain through electricity, *Nursing 82, 12*(9):57–59

Miller, S. A., (1981) *Nutrition and Behavior,* Philadelphia: Franklin Institute Press

Moore, D. E., and Blacker, H. M., (1983) How effective is TENS for chronic pain? *American Journal of Nursing, 83*:1175–1177

Murray, R., and Zentner, J., (1979) *Nursing Assessment and Health Promotion through the Life Span* (2d ed.), Englewood Cliffs, N.J.: Prentice-Hall

Pannetier, P., (1978) Polarity therapy, in Kasloff, L. J. (ed.), *Wholistic Dimensions in Healing: Resource Guide,* Garden City, New York: Doubleday, pp. 216–217

Pansky, B., and Allen, D. J., (1980) *Review of Neuroscience,* New York: Macmillan

Prescott, D. M., and Flexer, A. S., (1982) *Cancer: The Misguided Cell,* New York: Scribner's

Quinn, F., (1984) Therapeutic touch as energy exchange: Testing the theory, *Advances in Nursing Science, 6*(2):42–49

Rolf, I. P., (1978) Rolfing, in Kasloff, L. J. (ed.), *Wholistic Dimensions in Healing: Resource Guide,* Garden City, N.Y.: Doubleday, pp. 225–227

Selye, H., (1956) *The Stress of Life,* New York: McGraw-Hill

Serizawa, K., (1978) Massage, in Kasloff, L. J. (ed.), *Wholistic Dimensions in Healing: Resource Guide,* Garden City, N.Y.: Doubleday, pp. 206–208

Simonton, O. C., Matthews-Simonton, S., and Creighton, J. L., (1978) *Getting Well Again,* New York: J.D. Tarcher

Somers, A. R., and Somers, A. M., (1977) *Health and Health Care,* Germantown, Md.: Aspen Systems

Taylor, A. G., West, B. A., Simon, B., Skelton, J., and Rowlington, J. C., (1983) How effective is TENS for acute pain? *American Journal of Nursing, 83*:1171–1174

Taylor, K. B., and Anthony, L. E., (1983) *Clinical Nutrition,* St. Louis: McGraw-Hill

Unproven methods of cancer management: Macrobiotic diets, (1983a) *Cancer Journal for Clinicians, 33*(1):60–63

Unproven methods of cancer management: DMSO, (1983b) *Cancer Journal for Clinicians, 33*(2):122–124

Unproven methods of cancer management: Iscador, (1983c) *Cancer Journal for Clinicians, 33*(3):186–188

Veterans Administration Cooperative Study on Antihypertensive Agents, (1967) Effects of treatment on morbidity in hypertension: 1. Results in patients with diastolic blood pressure averaging 115 through 129 mm Hg., *Journal of the American Medical Association, 202*:1028

Veterans Administration Cooperative Study on Antihypertensive Agents, (1970) Effects of treatment on morbidity in hypertension: 2. Results in patients with diastolic blood pressures averaging 90 through 114 mm Hg., *Journal of the American Medical Association, 213*:1143

Vickery, D., and Fries, J., (1981) *Take Care of Yourself,* Reading, Mass.: Addison-Wesley

Woolf, H. B. (ed.), (1980) *Webster's New Collegiate Dictionary,* Springfield, Mass.: G.T.C. Merriam

Bibliography

Charney, E., (1967) How well do patients take oral penicillin: A collaborative in private practice, *Pediatrics, 40*(2):188–195

DeJarnette, M. B., (1978) Cranial technique, in Kasloff, L. J. (ed.), *Wholistic Dimensions in Healing: Resource Guide,* Garden City, N.Y.: Doubleday, pp. 84–85

Fanslow, C. A., (1983) Therapeutic touch: A healing modality throughout life, *Topics in Clinical Nursing, 5*(2):72–79

Gottlieb, R., (1978) Developmental vision therapy, in Kasloff, L. J. (ed.), *Wholistic Dimensions in Healing: Resource Guide,* Garden City, N.Y.: Doubleday, pp. 90–91

Kroening, R. J., Volen, M. P., and Bresler, D., (1979) Acupuncture: Healing the whole person, in Otto, H. A., and Knight, J. W. (eds.), *Dimensions in Holistic Healing: New Frontiers in the Treatment of the Whole Person,* Chicago: Nelson-Hall, pp. 427–438

May, W. B., (1978) The position of the mandible (lower jaw) as it relates to stress in the human system, in Kasloff, L. J. (ed.), *Wholistic Dimensions in Healing: Resource Guide,* Garden City, N.Y.: Doubleday, pp. 85–87

Perry, H. T., (1978) Temperomandibular joint technique, in Kasloff, L. J. (ed.), *Wholistic Dimensions in Healing: Resource Guide,* Garden City, N.Y.: Doubleday, pp. 88–89

Rubenfeld, I., (1978) Alexander: The use of self, in Kasloff, L. J. (ed.), *Wholistic Dimensions in Healing: Resource Guide,* Garden City, N.Y.: Doubleday, pp. 222–224

P A R T   F O U R

Impact of the System

◇

CHAPTER SIXTEEN
The Agency Maze

Introduction

The chronically ill frequently need to use health care resources beyond those their families can provide. This is a result of the long-term, multifaceted nature of their illnesses. In the past, an ill person had few options for care. The family, physician, and hospital were the most common resources. Today, the network of medical, social, and support agencies has become extremely complex and confusing for both the professional caregiver and the consumer. Coordinating this complex health care requires special skills and sometimes a little luck.

Medical technology has brought about extensive demographic changes. Many people who survive acute disease now live with chronic illness. Neonatal intensive care units, for example, have decreased infant mortality in this country, resulting in a higher incidence of congenital abnormalities and physically and emotionally handicapped individuals (Harding, Heller, & Kesler 1979). Medical technology has also prolonged the lives of others, leading to longer life expectancy and increases in the proportion of the elderly. These changes present new challenges for the health care system since the "dependent population" increases while "able-bodied workers shrink in number" (Morris 1983).

The rise in chronic illness has influenced political trends. Equal access to health care was the political issue of the 1960s and 1970s. The health care system responded by increasing services. As a result, mental health centers, neighborhood medical clinics, and regional medical programs, such as heart, cancer, and stroke programs, were established. The cost was absorbed by a healthy economy (Lewis 1983).

In the 1980s, however, the political trend was reversed. Federal health planning fell short on cost containment and medical expenses had become exorbitant (see Chapter 17). Not only has Medicare spending increased tremendously (Feder 1983) but the federal budget is plagued by an economic recession that can no longer absorb such costs. As a result, medical cost control has become today's major political issue (Lewis 1983). The federal government has imposed constraints through numerous control measures. This has meant a loss of 25% of federal health care funding in 1982 (Brown 1983), and about half of these cuts affected Medicare and Medicaid (Friedman 1982).

Cuts have eroded public health and mental health services and present a serious threat to community-based programs still in action (Callahan 1983). While high technology services supported by the private sector are expanding and competing in the medical market place, supportive care for the chronically ill and needy has been curtailed. Thus, the original federal aim of equal access to health care has been defeated (Yordy 1983).

Client Needs and Community Resources

The deinstitutionalization of the chronically mentally ill from state hospitals to the community began in the 1960s (Caton 1981). Underlying the movement was the premise of offering rehabilitation and resocialization of the mentally ill to the community, as well as saving costs of care. Because of poor planning, however, communities were not ready to handle this influx. Confusion and much needless suffering ensued. The movement did survive, and community residential care of the long-term mentally ill is likely to last.

New developments affecting the physically afflicted chronically ill appear to have taken a similar course. Hospital cost containment is leading to early discharges. Consequently, extended care facilities and families are expected to take over the care of the chronically ill and aged. Clear sign of a response to this phenomenon is the present home care boom (Home care today 1984). The National Home Care Association reports a 241% increase in home health care agencies (Dunphy 1984). As was the early deinstitutionalization movement, this new trend is poorly organized. The mushrooming of home care agencies can be attributed to a desperate attempt to meet the needs of clients quickly and to an opportunity to make money.

Needs of the Chronically Ill

The community-based health care system is faced with the challenge of providing and organizing presently available resources to meet the needs of the partially dependent chronically ill. For this chapter, needs are categorized into four groups: medical, psychological/spiritual, rehabilitation, and optimal functioning in activities of daily living (ADL) (see Table 16-1).

Medical needs include assistance in obtaining proper medical diagnosis, treatment, and supervision. Psychological/spiritual needs ask for help in adjusting emotionally and spiritually to the situation and coping with the on-going illness. Rehabilitation needs require specialized assistance to restore and maintain body functions or life-style. ADL needs ask for creative problem solving to provide the client with as much independence and autonomy as possible.

Several points need to be addressed when discussing client needs. First, education is one of the most important needs. Research has shown that 28% of clients discharged from hospitals do not adhere to their prescribed treatment (Marcus et al. 1980). In addition, the Food and Drug Administration (FDA) reports that a number of studies indicate "that as many as half of the people taking medicines aren't taking them properly" (FDA 1983). Ineffective communication between the physician, the pharmacist, and the client was the reason cited. Poor compliance with medication regimens may, therefore, mean that clients need more careful instructions and interpretation of their medical treatment (see Chapter 12).

Second, in some categories listed in Table 16-1, the needs of the physically ill and mentally ill are similar. However, the rehabilitation needs of the chronically impaired mentally ill are markedly different, specifically in the areas of self-sufficiency and productivity. The deinstitutionalization movement was a disappointment in terms of rehabilitation and resocialization of the long-term hospitalized client. Goals for the chronically mentally ill were to relearn community living, become achievement and success oriented, and maintain a job. Such goals were rarely reached, since the typical level of functioning in this group is incongruent with such goals. After years of living in institutions, clients develop a dependent lifestyle. They feel little pressure to perform and their motivation to achieve is minimal (Spivack et al. 1982). As a result, rehabilitation aims had to be adjusted over time. These adjustments have turned to a maintenance rather than a curative focus, which is more appropriate for the client and keeps the health provider in touch with realistic planning.

Finally, the professional caregiver must remember that physical rehabilitation is always coupled with psychological rehabilitation. A stroke client will not regain the ability to walk if the will to get better is lacking. The client's psychological needs have to be met before rehabilitation can become truly effective. On the other hand, good progress in physical functioning will give a client courage to go on.

Available Community Resources

Two trends are presently influencing the availability of community resources: cost control, which results

TABLE 16-1. Needs of the Chronically Ill

Medical Needs	
Physical Illness	Supervision of treatment regimen
	Maintenance of physical care
	Understanding purpose of treatment
	Skillful administration of treatment
	Obtaining necessary equipment and supplies for treatment
Mental/Emotional Illness	Ongoing monitoring of medication
	Monitoring of behavior changes
	Assistance with administration of medication

Psychological/Spiritual Needs	
Physical and Mental/Emotional Illness	Emotional support from family and friends
	Help with acceptance of limitations
	Help to feel like a productive member of the family and community
	Assistance to gain positive self-concept and body image
	Avoidance of unduly restrictive and overprotective parenting (children)
	Maximizing independence
	Encouragement to express feelings
	Consistency and continuity of care to provide a sense of security
	Opportunity to participate in religious activities and counseling
	Help with acceptance of chronicity of illness

Rehabilitation Needs	
Physical Illness	Rehabilitation training: exercises, vocational training
	Supervision of prescribed rehabilitation program
	Long-term follow-up and evaluation of rehabilitation program
Mental/Emotional Illness	Assistance in coping with life stressors
	Help with locating support systems
	Learning social and job skills

Needs for Optimal Functioning in Activities of Daily Living	
Physical and Mental/Emotional Illness	Evaluation of client's total functioning level in the environment
	Help in utilization of strengths for self-care
	Assistance with daily self-care as necessary

in shrinking public funds, and the home health care boom. The first trend has influenced various federal and state agencies. Overall, expenditures of public funds have not grown concomitantly with expanded needs for services. Medicare and Medicaid, which provide coverage for periodic hospitalization and limited coverage for extended care or home care, are still the most important funding sources for the poor and the elderly. Presently, both systems are struggling for survival ("DRGs" 1984). State psychiatric hospitals, which still are the only available temporary resource for intermittent flare-ups of many mental disorders, are confronted with serious difficulties as well; services have been cut back to minimal standards (Andrulis & Mazade 1983). In addition, daily newspapers report that other agencies dependent on

TABLE 16-2. Creative Community Responses

Problem	Community Responses
Scarcity of Funds	Development of new methods to procure private and corporate funds; for example, increase proportion of private funds via fund raising to compensate for loss of public funds (Lewis 1983)
	Use of volunteer services, such as crisis counseling, friendly visitors, sitters
	Involvement of churches in providing community services
	Physicians' donation of time to treat the needy and elderly
	Rise in self-help and support groups that provide mutual support and help with coping, such as ostomy, diabetes, drug abuse, and mastectomy groups (Cole, O'Connor, & Bennett 1979)
Need for Home Care	Private enterprise taking root in health care business; for example, home health agencies, extended care facilities (Home care today 1984)
	Rise of voluntary and nonprofit agencies to deliver supportive care, such as housekeeping, shopping, transportation (Lee & Stein 1980)
Lack of Resources to Meet Psychological Needs	Rise of self-help groups Summer camps for children and families that provide education and counseling, such as diabetes, leukemia, epilepsy camps (Rose 1981)

government funding, such as community mental health centers, state and county health departments, the Department of Public Health, schools, courts, and prisons, have had to cut various services and have serious financial difficulties.

The second trend, the home health care boom, is closely related to the first. Cuts in Medicare and Medicaid require hospital cost savings and the most obvious method is to discharge clients earlier. This leads to a great need for home care agencies.

In addition to providing more home care agencies, communities have responded in many ways to fill the gaps created by the two trends. Some community actions taken are listed in Table 16-2.

All types of agencies (government, private, self-help, and voluntary) are frequently associated with a national organization that oversees and regulates state and local activities. As indicated in the *Encyclopedia of Associations,* these national organizations (such as the American Cancer Society, the Heart and Lung Association, or the National Association of Home Care) provide the consumer with information about local services. Their focus is coordination, re-

search, and consumer education rather than direct care to clients (Akey 1984).

Local agencies and local constituents of national agencies that provide more direct services are located primarily in metropolitan areas. Prior to 1980, the National Health Planning Commission, in an effort to provide equal access to health care, provided services for rural areas and low-income urban areas. Now, many of these agencies have run out of funds and have had to close their doors (Friedman 1982). Even the survival of low-cost self-help groups is assured only if enough committed participants volunteer their time and energy. This dependency on funds and volunteers explains the distinct advantage that wealthy urban communities have over others with respect to the availability of services.

Positive Effects on the Client and the Professional

Much of the chapter's content, so far, has a negative or ominous ring. But agencies have positive influences on both clients and professionals. The client benefits from trends involving an increased focus on the humaneness of care, innovations in health maintenance, health promotion, rehabilitation, and the inclusion of support services in health care arrangements. The expansion of home health services and the multitude of new programs provide the professional with increased resources for matching client needs with available services and have led to the creation of many new professional roles. In addition, increased public awareness of the needs of the chronically ill and the willingness of the consumer to support creative programs have been helpful to the client and the professional alike.

Humane Care

Increased awareness of more than physical needs of the chronically ill person has positively affected the health care system. This is evidenced by the recent trends within nursing education and other human service professions to increase the focus on psychosocial needs of clients (Lancaster 1980; Erikson 1981). Nurses have demonstrated their concern with maintaining the client's health in all areas of life by establishing goals of care that transcend the execution of physicians' orders.

These changes are apparent in hospitals that employ increasing numbers of baccalaureate-prepared nurses who not only allow clients to express their worries but help them adapt to new treatment regimens, daily living activities, or socialization. Most large hospitals also employ clinical nurse-specialists for specific health conditions, such as diabetes. These specialists educate clients, work closely with physicians and other professionals, serve as liaison persons or client advocates, and, above all, try to bridge the gap between hospital and home care by planning ongoing care and supervision for the client. Some clinicians make home visits and others work closely with the visiting nurse agencies and refer clients to necessary support services (Home care today 1984).

Psychiatric liaison nurses have further humanized care for many clients suffering from chronic illness through providing better understanding of their psychological needs and coping behaviors, especially for those who are terminally ill and for their families. These nurse-specialists help nurses to accept clients' reactions better through facilitating open communication, allowing clients to vent their feelings and express anger, sadness, and grief. Such acceptance leads to the giving of care in a more understanding manner. Group counseling sessions for staff or client/families are also provided and have been effective (Lewis & Levy 1982).

Humanness of care is not restricted to hospital settings. Many professional nurses and social workers are involved in outpatient and home care services, where their roles as liaison and client advocates have had positive effects on clients and their families (Lang & Mitrowski 1981).

Health Maintenance, Health Promotion, and Rehabilitation

The rise in the number of chronically ill and the scarcity of financial resources have resulted in the evolution of new organizations, such as health maintenance organizations (HMOs), that provide regular supervision and health promotion. In spite of resistance from private physicians and the American Hospital Association, many health planners agree that HMOs hold promise for future health care (Callahan 1983). HMOs provide prevention and health education as well as acute and long-term care. Services are prepaid and participating clients are entitled to regularly scheduled health visits as well as hospitalization. The chronically ill benefit from the inclusion of services by physical therapists, dieticians, social workers, and counselors, some of which might be hard for individual clients to locate.

Some medical centers have also responded to changing health care needs by reorganizing their ambulatory services to more comprehensive programs, establishing their own home care programs, helping clients gain access to services, or educating clients to cope with illness. Clients benefit by easy access (Rucklin, Norris, & Eggert 1982) and programs such as social support systems of similarly afflicted people (Cole, O'Connor, & Bennett 1979). The oncology service of Detroit's Harper-Grace Hospital, in partnership with Wayne State University, is an example of a program that combines inpatient and out-patient services, including educational programs, discussion groups, and a yearly "We Can Cope" weekend retreat. Educational sessions, which are taped, can be borrowed in order to reinforce learning. Transportation is provided for radiation treatment. Preventive services include classes on breast examination, how to stop smoking, and how to improve one's life-style (Conway 1984).

Support Services and Increased Quality of Life

Home health agencies have increased in number, expanded their range of services, and in fact become more comprehensive. Home health aides, trained to give basic care such as baths, linen changes, and simple medical procedures, are now available. Homemaker services, which include housekeeping, shopping, meal provision, and transportation, are now provided by many agencies so the chronically ill can be maintained at home. Although not proven to be cost-effective, homemaker services have an influence on reducing the mortality rate among the elderly (Weissert et al. 1980). A Milwaukee study found that special services, such as transportation and nutrition, shortened the length of stay during rehospitalization (Applebaum, Seidl, & Austin 1980).

Transportation, which seems to have special importance to the client's psychological well-being, is often provided by churches or public agencies in metropolitan areas; these services are sometimes limited in rural communities. Transportation enhances participation in social activities, church services, and community functions. Such participation provides mental stimulation, a sense of belonging, the satisfaction of contributing to worthwhile activities, and a sense of being less dependent.

Effects on the Professional

The trend toward increasing numbers of agencies has also expanded the role of professionals who are responsible for locating or providing services. For example, home care nurses are now becoming administrators, planners, and organizers. Other health care providers, including social workers and psychologists, also have expanded their roles to include serv-

ing as liaison or referral people or by facilitating community support groups (Lang & Mitrowski 1981). Pharmacists are increasingly involved in client education rather than just dispensing medications (Hahn, Barkin, & Oestreich 1982). The novice caregiver, planning extended care for clients, finds experienced and well-educated professionals willing to share their knowledge for the sake of clients.

An even newer trend is comprehensive case management projects such as On Lok and ACCESS. On Lok is a San Francisco–based agency that draws funds from block grants and the private sector and serves as a model that may work elsewhere. Its outreach programs are locally controlled by a community board to provide consumer input (Rucklin, Norris, & Eggert 1982). On Lok provides a service package of medical, rehabilitation, maintenance, and custodial care for clients with functional deficits. An innovative, cost-saving idea that is incorporated in the project is monetary compensation for participating caretaking family members, which reduces the need for hospitalization and provides a means by which the family can care for loved ones at home. ACCESS (Assessment for Community Care Services) is a comparable project in the state of New York that manages to keep the daily cost for care at 52% of the institutional rate allowed by Medicaid (Eggert, Bowlyow, & Nichole 1980).

Comprehensive health care has advantages for both client and professional. Clients are spared anxiety and frustration in finding their way through the agency maze; caregivers are provided help in handling referrals more effectively. Comprehensive service packages are often more effective in meeting clients' needs than referrals to dispersed individual agencies. In addition, the caregiver's time is saved in locating resources. The case study on innovative resources demonstrates the way one family benefited from health care innovations.

Problems, Unresolved Issues, and Negative Effects

In spite of many exciting innovations in health care, progress is stalled by several unresolved issues: frag-

---

◇ CASE STUDY ◇
Innovative Resources

Bobby, the only son of Eva and Robert F., suffers from severe cerebral palsy and is wheelchair bound. He cannot speak because of poor muscle control, although he has always been able to make his wants known by signs and sounds. When Bobby was very young, a visiting nurse taught Eva how to provide basic physical care and alerted the family to their right to have Bobby evaluated by the public school system for special preschool training. As a result, Bobby became part of a program staffed by special education professionals. The family was taught how to work with Bobby in improving daily living skills, bowel and bladder control, and discipline.

When Bobby reached school age, the preschool staff helped the family adjust to a new program administered by the local university. This program had not only special education faculty and students but physical therapists, speech therapists, and other allied health professionals. Team functions were designed to maximize the child's potential, work cooperatively with the parents, and provide liaison between parents and the staffs of

the neurology and orthopedic clinics that treated Bobby. The family was fortunate to have a special education student work with them for several months. She taught Eva and Robert many ways to make physical care for Bobby easier. She helped find funding for a patient lift and a specially equipped transport van.

Bobby was also provided with a small electronic communication device, and he learned to activate special meaningful sounds in order to communicate. His ability to operate the device at age 11 was a major turning point for the family. Now that he could communicate, frustration was reduced, and his potential for further development was greatly enhanced. Eva and Robert are extremely grateful for the care and concern of these health caregivers. Eva feels obliged to contribute service to other families. She has established a cerebral palsy support group and has become involved in community-wide fund raising for the university program, so that more children can have a new way of living.

---

mentation of the health care system, lack of communication between agencies and caregivers, high cost for services, and politics. These unresolved issues have a negative effect on clients and professionals alike. Each of these issues is discussed separately.

Fragmentation

The need for certain types of health care has changed rapidly. The response by health planners has been rushed, erratic, and disorganized. This response was an attempt to find solutions to local health needs by well-meaning professionals and consumers. In addition, the federal government has encouraged profit-making businesses to enter the scene. It is ironic that while the government has imposed rules and regulations in order for agencies to obtain funding, it has also redistributed or cut back funds. Today's health care system consists of thousands of federal, state, and local agencies offering various services that compete with each other for funding from the private and public sectors and fight for survival (Waitzkin 1983).

In such a situation, fragmentation is unavoidable. This has led to duplication and unequal distribution of services.

Without either a centralized organization to oversee these developments or guidelines to monitor developments, confusion is unavoidable. In the 1970s, the aim of the National Health Planning and Resource Development Act (PL 93–641) was to organize health care. Nationwide, 200 health system agencies (HSAs) were established. Many HSAs were effective in curtailing overbedding and improving health care planning in their communities. One of their tasks was to collect health statistics that were to be used in a national survey. Yet 22 of these agencies collected inadequate statistics (Marcus et al. 1980). Since then, many attempts at unification and joint organization have been dismissed and are now discouraged by the Reagan administration, which believes in free, competitive enterprise (Yordy 1983).

In spite of trends toward consolidation of services to render health care comprehensive, many towns and cities have an abundance of small subspecialty clinics that lack resources for complex care. In other geographic locations, families in need have few community alternatives. Harding, Heller, and Kesler (1979) describe the frustrations of families with chronically ill children who go "doctor-shopping" because physicians neither meet their psychological needs nor refer them to an effective agency. Physicians are not adequately trained to deal with psychological or social problems, and they often neglect to refer clients to available social and health agencies.

Lack of Communication

Communication between agencies and health professionals is difficult in a complex and fragmented health care system. Many agencies operate with a self-centered attitude and an individual budget. Their caregivers have knowledge of few other agencies that could complement their services. Consequently, referrals are made according to a fixed routing system to a few widely used resources. Such referral techniques are quicker to make and less bothersome but neglect to consider community services and resources that would better meet individual clients' needs (Friedemann 1983).

Of particular importance is the insufficient communication between hospitals and home care teams. Some needed referrals are never made or are made too late to be helpful even when critical to clients. Discharging clients on weekends, when they cannot be seen by a public health nurse until Monday, may be dangerous. Clients may need rehospitalization because family members are not sufficiently skilled in taking care of them and encounter unexpected difficulties at home (Wheeler-Lachowycz 1983). In addition, frustrations and anxiety arise because of lack of communication among health professionals, double messages given to families, disruption of care, and insufficient education of the caretakers (Wheeler-Lachowycz 1983; Home care today 1984).

Cost for Service

Fragmentation and duplication of services, as well as the need for technical advances and complex meth-ods of care, have driven up costs (Waitzkin 1983). Cuts in government funding have not reduced the actual cost of health care; instead, cost cutting has eroded the public services used mainly by the disadvantaged. For example, the 40% payment by Medicaid for nursing-home care is insufficient to assure survival of such institutions. As a result, nursing homes select those clients who cost less and pay more, while closing the doors to others (Feder 1983).

Over the years, medical costs paid through Medicare and Medicaid have increased and health care institutions have charged the government increasing amounts. Today, government cost containment measures have resulted in the loss to Medicare and Medicaid of billions of dollars in federal funds through budget cuts (Friedman 1982). In 1965, Medicare covered roughly 50% of all medical expenses of the elderly; in 1981, only 38% (Brown 1983). In addition, these clients pay coinsurance of 29% (Friedman 1982), and cost-sharing of up to $2,500 is presently under discussion (Feder 1983). Many clients no longer qualify for coverage because of more restrictive regulations, and those who do qualify are discharged from hospitals sooner than in the past, increasing their need for extended care and home services (see Chapter 17).

Politics and Power

The competition between government and private health care planners concerns money and power. The lobbying power of the medical profession and hospital administrations has been considerable in the past. Lobbyists have convinced the federal government of the need for advanced medical technology and expanded services and have justified rising costs (Waitzkin 1983). Recently, however, their influence has diminished while government cost-saving measures have gained importance. Today's health care institutions are forced to initiate care in less expensive settings and to consolidate services.

As a result of scarce public funding, institutions have turned to private funding sources. Competition is stiff and, on account of the lack of systematic evaluations of services, choices are often made at random rather than on the basis of sound knowledge and reason. Many agencies and services continue to be short lived and local health care systems are in a constant state of flux. Experimental services are discontinued after the federal funding period has ended, old and established agencies often find it difficult to survive, and new services are often an effort to cover financial losses in other service areas (Waitzkin 1983). Such strategies are successful only if they are well planned and managed. Private enterprise is equally vulnerable to competition, and a high turnover may be expected in health care services that depend on capital gains.

Effects on the Client

The effect on clients lost in a fragmented maze of agencies is confusion. Clients may have difficulty perceiving their complex needs. Frustration results when they find out that they do not qualify for a service, that no such service is available in the area, that they cannot obtain satisfactory services, or that they cannot afford services. Often, clients get false or contradictory information about services and later discover that the agency cannot meet their needs. When assistance in locating agencies is not forthcoming, clients may give up trying to establish contact. In addition, without adequate information to make knowledgeable choices, clients are likely to become confused or discouraged by the large selection of agencies that offer similar services.

Once a client has decided to accept a service, satisfaction is not guaranteed. For example, because of a lack of adequate funds for private care, a family may have sent its mentally ill family member to a state hospital. Treatment may include heavy sedation, which results in a marked reduction in activity participation. The family members become distressed because they have no power to influence care and no alternative services from which to choose. Disadvantaged clients often find services inadequate. Community mental health centers may have long waiting lists for counseling service, or medical clinics may be staffed with doctors and nurses who are too busy to listen to a client's problem.

In many instances, lack of communication among health professionals and agencies can leave clients with either no referral or one that is useless, such as to an agency that no longer exists. Referrals are sometimes done hastily, without exploring what services the client actually needs or wants. For clients with psychological needs, inadequate counseling often causes difficulty accepting extended treatment plans or failure to follow through due to anxiety about treatment and/or ambivalent feelings about the need to change their behavior.

Clients in need of prolonged services can find their savings depleted over time. Although those with medical insurance find part or all of their hospitalization expenses covered, outpatient and home care is inadequately covered under private insurance plans, Medicare, or Medicaid (Dunphy 1984). When Medicare or Medicaid clients cannot afford coinsurance and deductibles, they may not seek health care except in an emergency. The elderly are particularly affected by this problem, and some areas have set up special clinics or have private physicians who volunteer their services to meet the medical needs of the elderly (Friedman 1982). Many senior citizens, however, do not have access to such care or do not know about it.

Many of the chronically ill fall through loopholes in the system and go without care or supportive help. Some people no longer qualify for Medicaid or Medicare, others do not have private insurance coverage because they are self-employed or unemployed, and many run out of insurance benefits if they need long-term rehabilitation or support services (Friedman 1982). For example, clients having no need for skilled nursing care do not quality for Visiting Nurse Association services and therefore pay 81% more for support services from private companies (Callahan 1983). Although there is more health care provided now than there was 20 or 30 years ago, good health care is becoming more of a privilege of the wealthy than a right for all.

People who are satisfied with or benefit from comprehensive health care still remain threatened by the political power play previously described. Chronically ill clients need consistency and a sense of security, which are hard to find in a system submerged in constant changes in rules and regulations. Agencies fighting for survival reduce the number of staff personnel or cut services. This influences the quality of care all clients receive. The ultimate threat to clients is the closing of an entire agency on which they depend. Many clients who lose their support system in this manner feel betrayed and angry, depressed and disillusioned. They may not have the energy to establish contact with other agencies, especially if they see their future as equally uncertain.

A last problem worth mentioning is the client's frustration about repeated data collection. Clients in need of several services are forced to have a lengthy interview with each agency they contact and give the same information many times. Sharing data among agencies has become difficult due to legal restrictions to maintain client confidentiality. Agencies are required to get a written consent from the client before they can pass on treatment information. Hospitals and the Visiting Nurses Association in Michigan have a relatively free information exchange and use release-of-information forms, but most other agencies contacted by the authors prefer to collect their own data base on each client. Much valuable information is necessarily lost in the archives of agencies and much time of the client and professionals goes to waste. Often, only the clients and their families know all the historical facts of the illness and treatments and sometimes report overlapping services, useless treatments, and resulting frustration and anger.

Effects on the Professional

Well-meaning and hard-working caregivers often get equally disheartened in their attempts to connect clients with services. Often, there are no services of the kind a client needs; at other times, waiting lists are discouragingly long. In addition, agencies chosen for a service do not always perform at the level promised. As acting liaison persons, the authors frequently have felt the clients' anger directed at them even though they were in no position to change the situation. Over time, professionals in this situation may become angry and suffer burn-out. Professional dis-

appointment is especially acute if a great deal of energy was spent getting a client ready to accept a referral for service. For example, a nurse or social worker may counsel a depressed client repeatedly over an extended period of time until psychological barriers against accepting help from a mental health agency are overcome. If the client walks out angrily after just one or two counseling sessions because the psychologist seemed insensitive to her or his problems, the referring caregiver may feel demoralized and give up trying.

The intake process required by most agencies often involves filling out lengthy forms as well as collecting statements from other professionals that verify the client's condition. This may discourage the caregiver from making referrals. In addition, the complex referral system in many metropolitan areas requires skills or time that some caregivers lack.

Professionals may lack information about available services, about whether agencies perform efficiently, or about the level of education of their staff. Communication about emerging agencies is poor, and a community's services can change so fast that it is difficult for even the most skilled health care worker to keep up to date. Making referrals, for most professionals, is only a small portion of their daily work, which may account for the limited time and energy allocated to keeping informed.

All these problems can lead professionals to feel as frustrated and confused as their clients. The development of specialized referral agencies is much needed. However, such agencies are not likely to appear in great numbers in the very near future. The next section of this chapter attempts to give caregivers guidelines for organizing their efforts to match the client's needs with community resources.

Dealing with the Agency Maze

The last section briefly introduced a multitude of problems and unresolved issues facing the chronically ill and professionals who must deal with agencies. Solutions for the problems of fragmentation, interagency communication difficulties, rising costs, and power politics can not be addressed satisfactorily within the limitations of just a few pages. The reader is encouraged to refer to Chapters 13 and 17 and to more advanced sources for additional information and suggested solutions to these serious problems. The rest of this chapter is devoted to providing a practical "how to" approach to finding one's way into, around, and through the agency maze. The authors' model, Dealing with the Agency Maze, is designed to help the client and professional caregiver minimize the confusion, frustration, and discouragement that come from inadequate interaction with the agency maze. Before discussing this model, it is helpful to visualize the need-resource linking relationship. The following diagram illustrates the relationship among client, caregiver, and community resources:

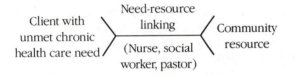

Agency maze appropriately describes the complex of community resources for the chronically ill. Chronic illnesses frequently require more assistance than the family can provide. Thus, the health provider's help in locating, matching, and using outside resources can be critical. This role requires skill in linking the client's needs with community resources. Caregivers who enter this maze without experience or knowledge can easily get frustrated or give up. The inexperienced who persist may eventually find their way through the maze. Practice is important if caregiving professionals are to function effectively in this role.

Although the diagram indicates that any helping professional can link client and resource, generally the hospital-based nurse refers clients in need of agency services to the discharge planner, social worker, home care coordinator, or community health nurse. However, understanding the process of obtaining the correct agency can help the staff nurse who initially advises clients or can lead to obtaining orders for referral early on during hospitalization. Knowing the process will also be helpful during those times

or situations when the hospital-based nurse may need to make agency referrals without the aid of those who are more experienced.

Experienced caregivers have gained their understanding of community resources and the linking process with the help of others as well as by trial and error. Inexperienced caregivers, just entering the maze, often are faced with immediate problems and little time to experiment with the system. How can they deal most effectively with the agency maze? The path presented in this chapter leads the caregiver and client through the maze of resource procurement and results in meeting the client's needs (see Figure 16-1). Following this path also allows the caregiver to leave the maze with increased knowledge and experience. Each step taken by the caregiver is described individually and in detail.

Identify Client Needs

The process of identifying needs corresponds directly to the first step in any problem-solving approach, the assessment of the problem. A comprehensive data base should be collected from a variety of sources: clients, significant others, the physician, the hospital, medical records, service agencies, agency referral forms, and so on. Assessment comprises the accurate collection of information and determination of which information is crucial. For example, a critical factor in assessment is determining the client's financial status, since ability to pay affects eligibility for services. Unfortunately, questions about income can be perceived by caregiver and client as prying into private matters. Justifying the need for asking such questions requires recognizing the value of financial data for agency selection. Practicing with a friend or colleague to find words that are comfortable to use is often helpful. The client can be prepared for such questioning by explaining the purpose and need for such questions. For example,

> "Mr. Green, there is one more area of information I need to ask about. It is sometimes difficult for people to talk about money matters, but the information is needed in our planning. It will help us to determine what agency to select: a public one, a tax-sup-

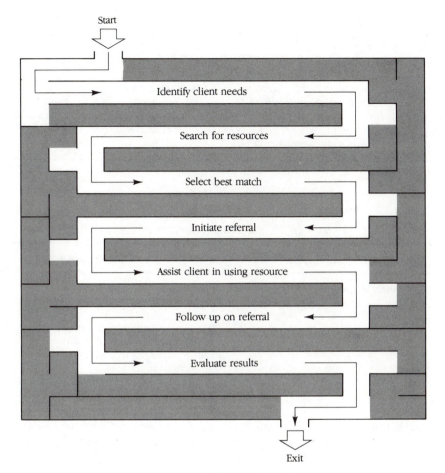

Start

Identify client needs

Search for resources

Select best match

Initiate referral

Assist client in using resource

Follow up on referral

Evaluate results

Exit

FIGURE 16-1. Dealing with the Agency Maze

ported one without fees, or one that charges for services or has a sliding fee scale. We want the agency that can do the job best."

Once assessment is complete, the caregiver and client list all needs in the four categories: medical, psychological/spiritual, rehabilitation, and optimal functioning in ADL. The assessment process and determination of needs are illustrated by the case study of Mrs. Kim.

Search for Resources

Although knowledge about community services and functions is extremely helpful to clients and families, many beginning caregivers do not have this knowledge. Thus the caregiver needs a systematic approach to find information about the numbers of agencies and services offered in many communities. Consequently, the second step is locating agencies that offer services to meet the client's listed needs. In order to limit the number of possible agencies, an initial choice needs to be made regarding the type of agency the client wants and needs.

Determining the Type of Agency. The client's financial situation and means of transportation will influence whether a public or private agency is preferred and where it needs to be located. These factors

◇ C A S E S T U D Y ◇

Mrs. Kim: Assessment and Categorizing Needs

Mrs. Kim, a 45-year-old former schoolteacher, has multiple sclerosis (MS), which was diagnosed eight years ago. She is married, has two children ages 12 and 8, and lives in a suburban community with a large selection of service agencies. Mrs. Kim has to be hospitalized periodically for treatment but, with the support of her family and community resources, is able to remain at home. The community health nurse collected data and determined corresponding needs (see Table 16-3).

TABLE 16-3. Mrs. Kim's Categories of Need

Data	Need Category
Medical Diagnosis: multiple sclerosis	*Medical* Requires ongoing medical supervision, outpatient clinic visits Needs hospitalization during exacerbations Needs to understand purpose of treatment Family needs information about disease, prognosis, treatment Needs consistency between hospital and home care
Disease process has depleted her strength and stamina for extended activities. Can ambulate short distances with leg braces and assistance of one person. Longer distances require use of wheelchair.	*Rehabilitation* Needs daily walking with assistance Needs periodic supervision and encouragement of daily exercise program Needs assessment of living facility for wheelchair access (planning for future)
Spends much time watching television. Complains of having nothing useful to do.	Needs occupational therapy assessment
Physical limitations prevent some self-care activities of personal hygiene, dressing, and meal preparation. Family cannot provide help with bath or noon meal preparation.	*Optimal functioning in ADL* Needs service agency to provide assistance with bathing, shampoo, and dressing Needs noon meal preparation
Family does most of cooking, all cleaning, laundry, and shopping.	Teach family to give Mrs. Kim opportunities for self-care and help with daily tasks within her capability
Uses religion as a significant support system but because of physical and financial limitations has been unable to attend services.	*Psychological/spiritual needs* Needs a church that is wheelchair accessible and provides transportation Needs financial support toward handicapped vehicle (discuss with family)
States that she is very lonely being at home all day alone.	Needs friendship, companionship, and mental stimulation during day (assess community resources for visiting companions, social support groups)

TABLE 16-4. Examples of Local Resources Nationwide*

- Telephone book, Yellow Pages
  (Explore the categories "Social Service Organizations," "Nurses," "Health Maintenance Organizations," etc. Also consult the Index to the Yellow Pages. Letter *I,* for example, lists "Ileostomy Supplies," "Infant and Toddler Programs," "Information Bureaus," and "Invalid Supplies."
- Chamber of Commerce directories
- Social service directories from the United Fund and others
- Advertisements in newspapers
- Television and radio announcements and commercials
- Computer data bases and information systems

*See Appendix A for a listing of selected national agencies that focus on chronic illnesses.

must be discussed in depth with the client, since this information may automatically limit choices. For example, the caregiver need not inquire about services of agencies that are too expensive or too distant from home if the client has no transportation.

Locating Suitable Agencies. Even after the elimination process, locating agencies may seem overwhelming if the caregiver has no plan to follow. Most organizations have a resource file or more experienced team members who can help. Such information is useful even though it may need updating.

Let us assume, however, that no resource file exists. The first step we suggest here is to consult major information sources on either a national or local level and begin your own file. There are two valuable sources on the national level. First, *The National Health Information Clearing House* in Washington, D.C., assists consumers and health professionals in locating health resources (their toll-free number is 800-336-4797). Second, *The Encyclopedia of Associations* is available in the reference section of most community and university libraries. The two most useful sections for caregivers are labeled "Social Welfare" and "Health"; both sections list many agencies for the blind, the handicapped, drug abuse, alcohol abuse, and so forth.

On a local level one can contact local health departments; local, state, and federal government offices; local referral centers; neighborhood informa-

tion centers; crisis centers; or hospital social workers or discharge planners, such as home care coordinators. Other printed materials, television, and radio could also be explored. Table 16-4 lists examples of resources available in all areas of the country. Appendix A lists selected national and common local agencies that focus on chronic illnesses. It is also a good idea to stay alert to announcements of new agencies at all times and add them to your file.

Once information on agencies is obtained, it needs to be stored for future reference. For frequently used agencies, one's memory may well suffice. In some agencies, computers, which make information updating easy, are available to store material for future reference. But most professionals still use written cards in their resource file. These cards should include not only the agency name, address, and phone number, but information about type of agency, funding source, and contact person. In addition, seven areas of assessment need to be explored and noted on this card. These areas are discussed in the next step of our model. Some agencies provide a brochure or pamphlet that describes their services. These should be filed together with the resource card.

Integral to locating resources is establishing professional relationships with other health care providers. Called *networking,* this is accomplished by contacting key resource individuals. Networking skills are a most valuable asset to caregivers. The saying

◇ C A S E   S T U D Y ◇
Mr. Mitchell, R.N., B.S.: Networking

March, 1984. While attending a workshop on third-party reimbursement of health services, Mr. Mitchell meets Mrs. James from the Department of Social Services (DSS), Ms. Kelly from Community Mental Health (CMH), Ms. Stabb from the community hospice program, and Mr. Hadley from the local chapter of the American Diabetes Association. Mr. Mitchell introduces himself to all four agency representatives and writes down their names.

April, 1984. Mr. Mitchell receives a new client, Mrs. Jewel, who is a 50-year-old widow. She has diet-controlled diabetes and progressive blindness and lives on a pension and Social Security. She complains of loneliness because she cannot go out of the house. Assessment also indicates that she needs help with meal preparation. The VNA's resource file contains a resource for meal preparation, Meals on Wheels, whose contact person is Mrs. Hoover. Mr. Mitchell calls her and initiates a referral for Mrs. Jewel. He also remembers the people he met at the workshop. He calls Mr. Hadley (Diabetes Association) and reminds him of their meeting the pre-

vious month. Then he explains his client's needs. Mr. Hadley recommends that he call three people: Mr. Jackson at the Leader Dogs for the Blind; Mr. Hunrich from the Senior Citizens' Visitors Group; and Miss Fuller, who is in charge of "Talking Books" at the library. Figure 16-2 shows the networking system developed by Mr. Mitchell as he goes through the process of linking this client to suitable resources.

May, 1984. Another new referral, Mr. Crane, is blind and wants to obtain a leader dog. Mr. Mitchell calls Mr. Jackson (Leader Dogs for the Blind), reminds Mr. Jackson of their last contact, provides updated information on Mrs. Jewel, and explains Mr. Crane's needs. Since Mr. Crane sounds like a good candidate, arrangements are initiated for a direct contact between this client and this agency. The following diagram illustrates the use of Mr. Mitchell's previously developed network for another client.

Mr. Crane ⟩   Mr. Mitchell   ⟨ Mr. Jackson
(Client) ⟩———————————⟨ (Leader Dogs)
          (Nurse)

"It's who you know, not what you know, that counts" illustrates the importance of personal contacts. Let us follow Mr. Mitchell, a new nurse working with the Visiting Nurse Association (VNA), and see the way he uses networking.

This case study illustrates the way in which professional relationships become basic components of networks: new resource persons are added to the file and the relationships of old contacts are reinforced by providing feedback on a client's progress, acknowledging previous help, or helping other agency professionals and their clients in a similar manner.

Finding Specific Information about Agencies.
Locating resources is only the beginning. In order to determine if the client's needs and agency resources are compatible, the caregiver also needs specific information about what services are provided. The name usually gives a clue to the agency's function:

Vocational Rehabilitation, Heart Association, Department of Community Mental Health. However, to compare agency services to client needs requires a seven-area agency assessment (see Table 16-5). The first three areas should be assessed in the order indicated; the priority of the others depends on the situation. A brief description of each assessment area follows.

Eligibility Requirements. Some agencies screen clients according to medical diagnosis, type of disability, age (child or adult), and financial status. Eligibility questions *must* be asked first in order to save time. A client on Medicaid will not be seen by an agency that does not accept Medicaid recipients. Such information needs to be noted for further reference with other clients.

Geographic Location/Accessibility. Physical location affects usefulness of services. Clients may have

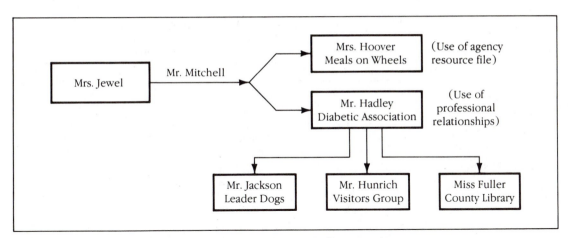

FIGURE 16-2. Mr. Mitchell's Networking

TABLE 16-5. Areas of Assessment

- Eligibility requirements
- Geographic location and accessibility
- Types of services required
- Comprehensiveness of service
- Credentials of the agency and its staff
- Direct cost to the client
- Referral process and contact person

transportation problems, be unwilling to travel long distances, or fear the neighborhood where the agency is located. Screening agencies by location saves time and unnecessary work.

Types of Service Provided. Services can generally be categorized as research, education, or direct-care service (Akey 1984). Most chronic illness problems require direct-care services. Each of our needs areas has various types of agencies (see Table 16-6). Caregivers have to inquire carefully about these services in detail. This can be done by contacting key persons of each agency, past consumers (clients), or professionals who have previously used such agencies.

Comprehensiveness of Service. The chronically ill generally need care in more than one area. It would be easier and more efficient if the client and family could deal with one person or agency to meet three needs, rather than dealing with three different agencies. For example, a hospice nurse can meet the client's personal care needs and psychosocial needs and the family's need to deal with grieving. Comprehensiveness of service does not mean superiority of services. The caregiver arranging services needs to evaluate, individually, the quality of each service against comprehensiveness before reaching a decision.

Credentials of the Agency and Its Staff. Credentials imply some level of quality based on standards. The area of credentials is a highly relevant issue in home care. Certain terms need to be understood by the caregiver and the client in selecting a quality home care agency (see Table 16-7).

Once credentials of the agency have been determined, credentials of the staff need to be considered. Usually, formal educational preparation of professionals is considered a measure of their ability; however, educational credentials do not always represent quality of care. The alcohol therapist who has only a high school education but was an abuser and now

TABLE 16-6. Agencies That Meet Need Categories
(Partial Listing)

Need	Agency
Medical	Hospital
	Medical clinic
	Physician's office
	Nursing home
	VNA
Psychological/Spiritual	Counseling agency
	Alcoholics Anonymous
	Pastoral care services
	Crisis center
Rehabilitation	Department of Vocational Rehabilitation
	Association for Retarded Citizens
	Hospital physical therapy
Optimal level of ADL	Housing commission
	Meals on Wheels
	Home health care
	Homemakers

has 15 years of alcohol counseling experience may be more effective than an inexperienced counselor with a master's degree in psychology. Networking and personal contacts greatly enhance decisions about what agencies and which professionals have accomplished the best results for clients.

Direct Costs to the Client.   Some agencies charge no client fees, being supported by tax revenues or donations. Other agencies accept total or partial payment from third-party payers, such as Medicare, Medicaid, or private insurance. Certain agencies have a sliding fee scale based on the client's ability to pay, and still other agencies, usually privately owned, will charge the client the entire fee for services rendered (Clark 1984). It is useful to weigh cost carefully against quality of service, even if the client has no financial difficulties and is willing to pay the fee.

Referral Process and Contact Person.   In order to prepare the client, the caregiver needs to inquire from the agency what paper work will be needed and who the intake worker is. This will be discussed

in detail as a major step in progressing through the maze.

By going through the steps in the maze up to this point, the caregiver has assessed the client's needs and identified one or more resources to help solve the client's problem. If only one agency is available, it is obviously the one to contact. But what if there is more than one? What criteria can help the caregiver and the client make the best selection?

Select the Best Match

This step requires cooperation between caregiver and client. It is very easy for a busy caregiver to assume that professional judgment is enough and therefore make decisions *for* instead of *with* the client. This can result in making choices too quickly. The client and family should make the ultimate choice. Participating in the decision says two important things to the client: the decision is his or hers and the caregiver will help with the referral.

Often, caregivers know from experience that one agency gives better care than another. This knowl-

TABLE 16-7. Terms Used for Accrediting Agencies*

Bonded agency: The agency has obtained a bond that acts as an insurance policy. The agency pays a fixed amount of money, similar to a premium for insurance, for the bond. The bond serves simply as a security in case the agency is sued by a client and loses the court case. It does not ensure quality of service.

Certified agency: These agencies are eligible to be reimbursed for Medicaid and Medicare service. To qualify, the agency must meet basic federal and state requirements for financial management and standards for patient care. Certification implies some quality.

Accredited agency: Accreditation is granted by special nonprofit groups whose goal is excellence of care. The agency must pass a detailed and careful review of its services, policies, practice, patient records, and management procedures. Accreditation is voluntary and is the best predictor of quality available.

*National groups most commonly involved in accrediting for home care: National Homecaring Council, National League for Nursing, American Public Health Association, Joint Commission on the Accreditation of Hospitals.

edge should be shared with the client so that, ultimately, a more informed choice can be made. When possible, it is useful to share written agency information, such as what is noted on the resource card or a copy of the agency's brochure. There are effective and ineffective ways of sharing unwritten knowledge about an agency's quality, as shown in the following example:

Ineffective: "They are doing a terrible job."

Effective: "I've talked with several people who have used this agency before and were not satisfied. They complained of long waiting time and constant staff turnover. This means that you may not see the same person each week."

Information and explanations should be given about all possible agencies and resources. Then the family or client is ready to decide which would work best.

Decision making can sometimes be difficult. When a client is undecided or refuses to make any decision, the caregiver may be asked to assume this responsibility. Depending on the situation, the caregiver might act or refrain from acting for the client. Care must be taken not to push a client into using a resource on the basis of the caregiver's value system. If the client lacks motivation—for example, showing reluctance to start needed mental health counseling—decisions should be delayed until feelings of resistance have been worked through so that the

client can accept help. It can be hard for caregivers who want immediate action or solutions to adjust their own pace to that of the client. It is useful to look at the treatment goals and be sure they are truly set by the client.

Initiate the Referral

Let's assume that the client has selected an appropriate agency and is ready to proceed. This fourth step is achieved by answering four questions: Whom do I contact? How do I contact? What do I ask? What should the client expect?

Whom Do I Contact? The correct contact person's name can often be learned while collecting information about the agency. But, in many situations, the first person the client will see is not the regular contact person but an intake worker who is to collect preliminary information. It can be helpful if the referring caregiver can share some client data on the telephone to start the referral process.

How Do I Contact? How to make contact may be listed under "referral process" on agency brochures. If the information is not available, a telephone call is needed to find out if the process should be initiated by client or caregiver, if it needs to be done in person, or if it requires that the client be accompanied by the caregiver. When talking to an agency about the needs of a client, the caregiver must respect confidentiality. Either of two measures should be used to assure confidentiality: (1) avoid using the client's name or other identifying characteristics when explaining the client's needs; (2) obtain the client's written permission to communicate personal information.

What Do I Ask? The situation determines what should be asked. The client's eligibility must be confirmed. The agency's ability to provide the required service and its clear understanding of the client's needs should be determined. It is appropriate to ask when the client can be seen, since time is a prime factor: Is there walk-in service? What is the appointment procedure? Is there a waiting list or waiting period, and if so, how long is it? What is the cancellation policy, if any? If the waiting list is very long, say 3 to 6 months, then even a perfect match of client need and agency may be of no help to the client.

What Should the Client Expect? The client should be told that often the first visit may be simply to collect information. Preparing the client for the intake process ahead of time decreases frustration for both client and agency. Intake can include forms to fill out, documents that need to be seen regarding medical status or finances, and so forth. The client should be informed as to how long the first interview will probably last and whether or not service will be provided during that first contact.

The first four steps in this model can be carried out by most health professionals without much difficulty. But the next three steps require more sophisticated need-resource linking. These remaining steps will be noted briefly here so that the clinical practitioner or novice community worker has a greater understanding of the process taken by community health nurses and social workers with more experience. The experienced professional thus proceeds to assist the client in dealing with the remaining three steps: using the resource, taking necessary follow-up steps, and evaluating the results.

TABLE 16-8. Checklist for Smooth Referrals

1. Does the client have in writing:

   Name and address of the agency?
   Name of the person to contact?
   Date and time of the appointment?
   Directions to get to the agency?

2. Does the client have transportation?

3. Does the client have child or adult care, if needed?

4. Does the client know how and whom to contact if the appointment must be canceled?

5. Can the client effectively explain his or her needs?

6. Is the client comfortable in making this contact?

Assist the Client in Using the Resource

Facilitation is the key work for this step. To help the client make the initial contact successful, the experienced caregiver cannot take the process for granted (see Table 16-8). Any written material the client receives should take into account the client's literacy and visual acuity. If transportation is a stumbling block, and private or public transportation is not readily available, resourcefulness is needed. Acceptable options include local church, volunteer groups, or special agencies offering transportation services.

If child or adult care is needed, this can prevent the client or family member from leaving the home. Joint problem solving with the client, done in advance of the actual appointment, will usually lead to a solution. Again, church groups or adult day care organizations may be of assistance. Should cancellation be necessary, knowing how to cancel an appointment enhances the client's acceptance to the agency, since it shows a degree of responsibility. Some clients do not operate under such a value system and do not realize the negative impression they may leave if they fail to cancel (Murray & Zentner 1979). Educating the client to agency expectations is an important caregiver task.

When a client is insecure or unable to explain his or her needs, providing an opportunity for role playing can be helpful. If role playing reflects a deficiency in the client's communication skills, roles can be reversed. This allows the caregiver to model skills that enhance communication. Then, by again reversing roles, the client can try out the approach presented by the caregiver. Basic principles in learning as well as experience support the value of this technique. The client may also feel insecure about initiating contact with the agency. This can usually be handled, in advance, by encouraging verbalization of fears followed by problem solving, such as identifying what is needed to increase comfort level. It can sometimes be as simple as bringing a book to read while waiting or asking a friend or relative to come along on the intake visit.

Follow Up on the Referral

This step is based on the principle of continuity of care. Even if all the preceding steps were executed properly, something could still go wrong. Talking to the client shortly after the first contact with the new agency allows the caregiver to ask if the appointment was kept, what happened during the visit, if the visit was satisfactory, and what the client wants to do next. If the appointment was missed, the reasons need to be explored and solutions suggested before another appointment is made. If the client did not understand what happened during the first visit, it needs to be clarified. For example, a rheumatoid arthritis patient may be unclear as to why blood samples are necessary before receiving colloidal gold injections. Knowing the importance of baseline blood values and the need for regular evaluation to assure that gold was not causing harmful side effects can lead to continued cooperation.

Satisfaction with the outcome of the visit can range from high to low. Dissatisfaction can be the result of overly high expectations or of the agency's not meeting the client's needs. What the client wants to do next will depend on the degree of satisfaction. In reality, few agency services are perfect matches for all needs. Those services that prove ineffective should be quickly terminated. Good and fair services, however, require evaluation of how well the client be-

lieves his or her needs were met. If using this resource is to be continued, the caregiver continues the role of liaison person by enhancing communication between client and agency staff in order to develop a trusting relationship between them. As trust grows, the need for a liaison decreases and eventually disappears. Closure is frequently accompanied by a final statement of support such as, "Here are my name and phone number. Call me if you need help in the future."

Evaluate the Results

Much of the evaluation has been done throughout the referral process. A final evaluation allows for the examination of each step of the process and resultant outcomes. For unsuccessful referrals, evaluation allows the caregiver to determine where things went astray. It is important to know if client needs were accurately identified, if the agency was screened effectively, if the best match was made between client and agency. Also evaluate if the referral was initiated appropriately, if the client received the necessary assistance in making contact with the agency, and if follow-up was complete. A negative response to any of these points allows the caregiver and client to focus on the origin of the problem so a solution can be sought.

Record evaluation information on the resource card for future reference. Sharing such information, which can take weeks or months to collect, saves time and speeds up the process of future referrals. The case study of Paul S. illustrates the entire process of traveling through the agency maze and illustrates that more than one person may be involved in the need-resource linking process. Yet, in this situation, the office nurse assumed primary responsiblity for following the process through to completion.

Summary and Conclusions

The first section of this chapter focused on many of the health care issues that have affected resources for the chronically ill. Not only has the health care deliv-

◇ CASE STUDY ◇
Paul S.: Dealing with the Agency Maze

Paul S., a 50-year-old, was a happily married man with three grown children when his wife, Edna, had a radical mastectomy for breast cancer. Now, a year later, Edna was undergoing chemotherapy because of metastasis. Edna was experiencing some pain and her stamina and activity level were significantly decreased.

Paul was irritable at work, since he was sleeping poorly as a result of a great deal of stress. His secretary, Mary, who was also a family friend, knew that Edna's health problems had been emotionally upsetting to her husband. Although Mary had no experience in using community resources, she decided to seek professional assistance for her employer when her support as a friend was no longer sufficient. With the S.s' permission, she called the office of their family physician and described the problem to Ms. Reis, the office nurse.

Identify Client Needs. Ms. Reis collected the following information about Paul S.:

- He had been sleeping only 3 to 4 hours a night during the past two weeks.
- He was short tempered and irritable with his subordinates at work.
- He was confused about his wife's condition and how to help her.
- He feared his wife's imminent death.
- He was receptive to professional help.
- He had insurance covering professional mental health counseling and could also afford to pay for counseling service.

Ms. Reis realized that Paul's psychological/spiritual needs were approaching a crisis situation requiring rapid intervention.

Search for Resources. In addition to several agencies that might be helpful, Ms. Reis checked the office resource file and found a new agency, Counseling for Coping. The brochure describing their services indicated that the agency might be appropriate to Paul's needs. Even though she had never used this agency, she knew that new agencies frequently had shorter waiting time.

Select the Best Match. Over the telephone, Ms. Reis shared information about all the identified resources with Mary so they could discuss which would best meet Paul's needs. The new resource, a partnership of independent nurse-practitioners, seemed most appropriate. Although the agency did not allow third-party reimbursement, it was chosen because it not only offered the type of service that was needed but could take Paul shortly. Ms. Reis suggested that Mary share their thinking with the S. family. She provided photocopies of the file cards on all the resources and made a note to herself to call within a couple of days in order to follow up on the situation.

Initiate the Referral. Mary shared this information with Paul and Edna, who were agreeable to whatever she could arrange. Mary called Counseling for Coping and talked directly to Mrs. Davis, the nurse counselor, who not only described the agency services in detail but indicated that she was also the intake worker. An appointment for an intake interview and problem assessment was made for the next day. Mary obtained directions to the agency and instructions for parking.

Assist the Client in Using the Resource. Mary gave Paul the information on the agency's name, address, and phone number, Mrs. Davis' name, and information on the intake procedure and agency services. She offered him a ride, but he preferred to take his own car. He kept his appointment. Paul had no problems with expressing his needs and seemed comfortable in seeking help.

Follow Up on the Referral. Ms. Reis called Mary the next morning and asked if the agency had been contacted and if Paul had been seen. Mary gave her a progress report.

Evaluate the Results. One week later, Ms. Reis called the S. family. She found out that Paul was feeling better, that he was sleeping better and was consequently more rested. Three weeks later, during an office visit, Ms. Reis took the opportunity to talk to Paul about the service he obtained at Counseling for Coping. He reported that he was very well satisfied with the way they had helped him express his concerns and had helped him understand what to expect in the future. He stated that Mrs. Davis was now seeing him and his wife together and was helping them communicate more effectively. A summary of Paul's comments were recorded on her office file card, and this information was shared with other nursing and medical personnel.

ery system experienced major changes over the last few decades, but advances in medical technology have drastically increased the incidence of chronic illness. Although political support for access to health care was on the rise during the 1960s and 1970s, it has since decreased, largely as a result of national efforts toward cost containment. Funding for health care needs of the chronically ill has been particularly affected by these federal budget cuts. These national economic trends have led to more privately run agencies and a mushrooming of home care agencies.

The next section described the needs of the chronically ill and many of the community resources required to meet these needs. Resources and agencies can be public or private, official or voluntary, and these classifications provide a clue as to the type of service they offer and their source of funds.

The rapid changes in the health care delivery system have had several positive effects on client and professional alike. Increased awareness of the needs of the chronically ill has encouraged better educational preparation of the caregiver and has increased coordination of health services by way of interdisciplinary health teams. New delivery systems have been developed, such as HMOs and combined service agencies providing both support and basic services. As a result, clients have more choices with respect to kinds of services. This enhances both the quality of life and the client's autonomy.

Unfortunately, there are also negative effects. The unresolved issues discussed included fragmentation of services, duplication of service, lack of communication among agencies, and political changes that have resulted in closure of some agencies and the infringement of competition and profit making on quality of service. Any of these can result in the client's not receiving the necessary service and feeling overwhelmed by the system. The professional can also be overwhelmed by the system.

To help the caregiver restore a sense of control, a model for dealing with the agency maze was recommended. This seven-step model can be used with the chronically ill and generalized to other populations that need community resources.

In the future, ongoing research in chronic illness will help document and validate the health care needs of these clients. Advocacy organizations will increase public awareness and provide political pressure to ensure recognition of the needs of special groups such as the elderly. The referral process will also continue to change. As more agencies like On Lok and ACCESS develop, health care for the chronically ill will become more coordinated and comprehensive.

In addition, computer technology will make information collection and resource retrieval a much more manageable task. Computerized locating services are becoming available locally, regionally, nationally, and internationally. For example, the International Association of Gerontology hopes to begin an International Resource Center on Aging under the guidance of the United Nations. Its goals include the collection, storage, and exchange of information among member agencies (Gerontology 1982). Even with the existing gaps in health care, that same kind of center could be forthcoming for the chronically ill. However, no matter how sophisticated computer searching or system reorganization becomes, the chronically ill will still require the assistance of skilled professionals. Understanding the model presented here and gaining experience in using it will be a valuable asset for the caregiver in any setting.

STUDY QUESTIONS

1. Explain how demographic changes within the population are related to chronic illness.
2. Give three examples of needs a chronically ill person may have in each category:
   • medical
   • psychological/spiritual
   • rehabilitation
   • optimal functioning
   Use as examples the following individuals:
   • a young child having epilepsy
   • a woman who has leukemia
   • an elderly man having leg ulcers

References

Akey, D. S. (ed.), (1984) *Encyclopedia of Associations* (18th ed.), Vols. I and II, Detroit: Gale Research Company, Book Tower

Andrulis, D. P., and Mazade, N. A., (1983) American mental health policy: Changing directions in the 80's, *Hospital and Community Psychiatry, 34*(7):601–606

Applebaum, R., Seidl, F. W., and Austin, C. C., (1980) Wisconsin Community Care Organization: Preliminary findings from the Milwaukee experiment, *Gerontologist, 20*(3):350–355

Brown, L. D., (1983) Health policy in the Reagan administration: A critical appraisal, *Bulletin of the New York Academy of Medicine, 59*(1):31–40

Callahan, J. J., (1983) Long-term care and home health services, *Bulletin of the New York Academy of Medicine, 59*(1):69–74

Caton, C. L., (1981) The new chronic patient and the system of community care, *Hospital and Community Psychiatry, 32*(7):475–478

Clark, M. D., (1984) *Community Nursing: Health Care for Today and Tomorrow,* Reston, Va.: Reston

Cole, S. A., O'Connor, S., and Bennett, L., (1979) Self-help groups for clinic patients with chronic illness, *Primary Care, 6*(2):325–340

Conway, K., (1984) Cancer patients find they're not alone, *Detroit Free Press,* March 15, 1984, pp. B1–B2

DRGs: New prescription for Medicare's ills, (1984) *Gray Panther Network,* 3, Spring

Dunphy, J., (1984) For the elderly, no place like home, *Detroit Free Press,* May 15, 1984, pp. 1B and 3B

Eggert, G. M., Bowlyow, J. E., and Nichole, C. W., (1980) Gaining control of the long-term care system: First returns from the ACCESS experiment, *Gerontologist, 20*(3):356–363

Erikson, K., (1981) *Human Services Today* (2d ed.), Reston, Va.: Reston

Feder, J., (1983) Effects of changing federal health policies on the general public, the aged and the disabled, *Bulletin of the New York Academy of Medicine, 59*(1):41–49

Food and Drug Administration, (1983) Patient education fliers mailed to Social Security recipients, *FDA Drug Bulletin, 13*(2):17

Friedemann, M. L., (1983) *Manual for Effective Community Health Nursing Practice,* Monterey, Calif.: Wadsworth Health Science Division, Brooks/Cole

Friedman, E., (1982) Access to care: Serving the poor and elderly in tough times, *Hospitals, 56*(23):83–90

Gerontology, foundations of a policy for the aged in the 80s and beyond, (1982) *Gerontology, 28*(4):271–280

Hahn, A. B., Barkin, R. L., and Oestreich, S. J., (1982) *Pharmacology in Nursing* (15th ed.), St. Louis: Mosby

Harding, R. K., Heller, J. R., and Kesler, R. W., (1979) The critically ill child in the primary care setting, *Primary Care, 6*(2):311–324

Home care today, (1984) *American Journal of Nursing, 84*(3):341–342

Lancaster, J., (1980) *Community Mental Health Nursing: An Ecological Perspective,* St. Louis: Mosby

Lang, P. A., and Mitrowski, C. A., (1981) Supportive and concrete services for teenage oncology patients, *Health and Social Work, 6*(4):42–45

Lewis, A., and Levy, J. S., (1982) *Psychiatric Liaison Nursing: The Theory and Clinical Practice,* Reston, Va.: Reston

Lewis, I. J., (1983) Evolution of federal policy on access of health care: 1965–1980, *Bulletin of the New York Academy of Medicine, 59*(1):9–20

Marcus, A. C., Reeder, L. G., Jordan, L. A., and Seeman, T. E., (1980) Monitoring health status, access to health care, and compliance behavior in a large urban community: A report from the Los Angeles health survey, *Medical Care, 18*(3):253–265

Morris, R., (1983) Will the growth of health and welfare services be resumed? *American Journal of Public Health, 73*(7):732–733

Murray, R., and Zentner, J., (1979) *Nursing Assessment and Health Promotion through the Life Span* (2d ed.), Englewood Cliffs, N.J.: Prentice-Hall

Rucklin, H. S., Norris, J. N., and Eggert, G. M., (1982) Management and financing of long-term care services: A new approach to a chronic problem, *New England Journal of Medicine, 306*(2):101–105

Spivack, G., Siegel, J., Sklaver, C., Deuschle, L., and Garrett, L., (1982) The long-term patient in the community: Life style patterns and treatment implications, *Hospitals and Community Psychiatry, 33*(4):291–295

Waitzkin, H., (1983) Community based health care: Contradictions and challenges, *Annals of Internal Medicine, 98*(2):235–242

Weissert, W. G., Won, T. T., Livieratos, B. B., and Pellegrino, J., (1980) Cost-effectiveness of homemaker services for the chronically ill, *Inquiry, 17*(3):230–243

Wheeler-Lachowycz, J., (1983) How to use your VNA, *American Journal of Nursing, 83*(8):1164–1167

Yordy, K. D., (1983) New directions in federal policies for health care: A critique, *Bulletin of the New York Academy of Medicine, 59*(1):21–30

Bibliography

Alleyne, S. I., Vassall-Hurd, A. V., and Morgan, A. G., (1982) End-stage renal disease in Jamaica: How patients cope in a developing society, *Health and Social Work,* 7(2):130–133

Barey, P. T., and Lewis, L., (1980) Extending home care services: An experiment that failed, *Nursing Outlook,* 28(11):680–684

Cohodes, D. R., (1983) Evolution of health planning, *New England Journal of Medicine, 308*(17):1037–1038

Csank, J. Z., and Zweig, J. P., (1980) Relative mortality of chronically ill geriatric patients with organic brain damage, before and after relocation, *Journal of the American Geriatric Society, 28*(2):76–83

DeChristopher, J., (1981) Children with cancer: Their perceptions of the health care experience, *Topics of Clinical Nursing, 2*(4):9–19

Dimond, M., (1979) Social support and adaptation to chronic illness: The case of maintenance hemodialysis, *Research in Nursing and Health, 2*(3):101–108

Donaldson, K., (1979) Advocacy program for the elderly, *Advocacy Now, 1*(2):60–63

Lee, J. T., and Stein, M. A., (1980) Eliminating duplication in home care for the elderly, *Health and Social Work,* 5(3):29–36

Muller, E. M., and Taylor, I. A., (1980) Effective functioning of chronic psychiatric patients in aftercare settings, *Journal of Psychiatry, 25*(8):651–658

Murray, R. B., and Zentner, J. P., (1979) *Nursing Concepts for Health Promotion* (2d ed.), Englewood Cliffs, N.J.: Prentice Hall

Neufeld, G. R., (1977) *Advocacy and the Human Service Delivery System,* Washington, D.C.: Office of Human Development Services Publication SHR–0006389 (Available from Themes and Issues, DD/TAS, Suite 300, NCNB Plaza, Chapel Hill, N.C., 27514)

Rose, V., (1981) Juvenile diabetes, *Midwife-Health Visit-Community Nurse, 17*(9):372–374

Stern, R., and Minkoff, K., (1979) Paradoxes in programming for chronic patients in a community clinic, *Hospital and Community Psychiatry, 30*(9):613–617

C H A P T E R   S E V E N T E E N

Financial Impact

◇

Introduction

Health care costs in the United States have risen 20% faster than other consumer price indexes (CPIs). Health care spending in the United States has more than tripled between 1971 and 1981 (Freeland & Schendler 1983). Expenditures for medical care and other health-related activities increased an astronomical 1500% between 1950 and 1978 (Herrell 1980). Considering these astounding figures, it is no wonder that health care and health care delivery have emerged as national political issues.

What has caused this dramatic spiraling of health care costs, making it an issue upon which economists, health care providers, legislators, and the public have debated and speculated? Two causes for this growth are under consideration. First, the actual increase in population in the United States provides more people who funnel more money into the health care budget. Second, the increase in actual income within the general population releases more financial resources into health care (Freeland & Schendler 1983). But even when health care cost figures are controlled for inflation, income, and population growth, a conspicuous rise in these expenditures still exists. Obviously, other reasons are contributing to much of the rise in health care costs.

The public has communicated to its political leaders that medical care is a right, not simply a privilege. As a nation, we expect and demand much from the medical profession, and this automatic assumption of access to medical care carries with it a heavy financial burden and a corresponding increase in health care costs. And this financial crisis in health care will continue to grow as health care costs escalate faster than any other price index.

The U.S. government is spending an increasingly larger portion of our Gross National Product on health care. In 1950, 4.4% of the GNP was spent on health care. By 1960, that figure had risen to 5.3%, and in 1970 the costs had reached 7.5%. By 1981 we were spending 9.8% of our GNP on health care with this upward trend projected to increase to 12% by 1990 (Freeland & Schendler 1983).

Aging also influences health care costs. In 1983, 12% of the U.S. population was over 65 years of age. In the year 2025, it is estimated that the number of elderly will increase to 19%. As our population ages, we will most certainly witness a proportional increase in health care spending, since statistics demonstrate that chronic illness increases with age and that the chronically ill are the largest users of the health care dollar. The current estimate of the percentage of health care resources consumed by the chronically ill is 80%, with this estimate including most of the medical facilities, services, and biomedical research (Evans 1983a). Simply stated, the longer a person lives, the more susceptible that person becomes to functionally limiting chronic illnesses and thus to greater utilization of health care.

◇ C A S E S T U D Y ◇
Cycle of Impoverishment

Mr. C., a middle-class father of two, had been an electrician all his adult life. At age 42, he began experiencing some pain and stiffness in his joints, making the execution of his job duties very difficult. He visited his doctor, who diagnosed his condition as rheumatoid arthritis. His disease progressed rapidly, affecting his hips, hands, knees, and neck. Hospitalization, treatment, and medication resulted in mounting medical bills. His insurance covered most of these costs. His illness forced him to use all his allotted sick time, which severely affected his income.

Within nine months, he was entirely unable to work. He was subsequently laid off. Losing his job meant losing his medical insurance, even though his medical bills continued to mount. Costly gold salt injections were prescribed. His wife was forced to work, but her salary was only a fraction of what he had been earning. Medical and hospital bills consumed the "nest egg" of $100,000 within two years after he lost his job. The family had to apply for Medicaid to meet medical expenses. This meant that they had to deplete their real property so that they would be eligible.

Problems and Issues of Financial Impact

Except possibly for the very wealthy, the financial frustration and burden borne by the chronically ill cross nearly every socioeconomic level. For many of the chronically ill, the onslaught of their disease exhausts their finances and forces them to search continually for new ways to help pay for their many and mounting medical bills. An individual who is sick and weary must deal with the insurance company's paper work, interpret benefits, and decipher the company's detailed billing procedures. Most insurance companies are geared to helping the acutely ill, not the chronically ill, as is witnessed in clauses excluding preexisting conditions (Katz & Capron 1975). When chronic illnesses are covered, the coverage is usually limited to exacerbations of symptoms, instead of the ongoing management of the disease.

The chronically ill commonly find themselves in a cycle of impoverishment: the individual suffers an onslaught of a chronic illness, medical bills mount rapidly, income is lost, as is social position, which ultimately can lead to loss of job and associated health insurance benefits. Chronic illness frequently leaves the individual with no means to pay for health care. The case study of Mr. C. demonstrates this cycle of impoverishment.

Unfortunately for Mr. C., and others pauperized by chronic illness, once they reach this welfare level, it is highly unlikely that they will ever regain their financial independence. Medicaid laws, by necessity, have been developed to discourage abuse, but they markedly discriminate against the chronically ill who, before becoming eligible for public funds, must deplete their resources to the poverty level. With those who are already poor, chronic illness sustains them at the poverty level, transforming them into indigents. The majority of Americans cannot afford the economic burden imposed by chronic illnesses.

Increasing Health Care Costs

The reasons for the dramatic increase in our health care expenditures are many and complex. One question asked is: Who is absorbing these dramatic increases in health care expenditures? Over the last 30 to 40 years, the United States government has absorbed the major portion of this growth, while private spending declined markedly. Prior to that time, private sources covered most health care costs, but now spending on national health care is experiencing a reversing trend, which becomes obvious from a look at the figures for the last 30 years. Private spending has declined from 72.8% in 1950 to 59.4% in 1978, while public spending has increased from

TABLE 17-1. Aggregate and Per Capita National Health Expenditures, by Source of Funds, and Percentage of Gross National Product, Selected Calendar Years, 1929-1978

Calendar Year	Gross National Product (in Billions)	Health Expenditures								
		Total			Private			Public		
		Amount (in Billions)	Per Capita	Percentage of GNP	Amount (in Billions)	Per Capita	Percentage of Total	Amount (in Billions)	Per Capita	Percentage of Total
1929	$103.1	$3.6	$29.49	3.5	$3.2	$25.49	86.4	$0.5	$4.00	13.6
1935	72.2	2.9	22.65	4.0	2.4	18.30	80.8	.6	4.34	19.2
1940	99.7	4.0	29.62	4.0	3.2	23.61	79.7	.8	6.03	20.3
1950	284.8	12.7	81.86	4.5	9.2	59.62	72.8	3.4	22.24	27.2
1955	398.0	17.7	105.38	4.4	13.2	78.33	74.3	4.6	27.05	25.7
1960	503.7	26.9	146.30	5.3	20.3	110.20	75.3	6.6	36.10	24.7
1965	688.1	43.0	217.42	6.2	32.3	163.29	75.1	10.7	54.13	24.9
1966	753.0	47.3	236.51	6.3	34.0	169.81	71.8	13.3	66.71	28.2
1967	796.3	52.7	260.35	6.6	33.9	167.61	64.4	18.8	92.74	35.6
1968	868.5	58.9	288.17	6.8	37.1	181.40	63.0	21.8	106.76	37.0
1969	935.5	66.2	320.70	7.1	41.6	201.83	62.9	24.5	118.87	37.1
1970	982.4	74.7	358.63	7.6	47.5	227.71	63.5	27.3	130.93	36.5
1971	1,063.4	82.8	393.09	7.8	51.4	244.12	62.1	31.4	148.97	37.9
1972	1,171.1	92.7	436.47	7.9	57.7	271.78	62.3	35.0	164.69	37.7
1973	1,306.6	102.3	478.38	7.8	63.6	297.17	62.1	38.8	181.22	37.9
1974	1,412.9	115.6	535.99	8.2	69.0	319.99	59.7	46.6	216.00	40.3
1975	1,528.8	131.5	604.57	8.6	75.8	348.61	57.7	55.7	255.96	42.3
1976	1,700.1	148.9	678.79	8.8	86.6	394.73	58.2	62.3	284.06	41.8
1977	1,887.2	170.0	768.77	9.0	100.7	455.27	59.2	69.3	313.50	40.8
1978[1]	2,107.6	192.4	863.01	9.1	114.3	512.62	59.4	78.1	350.40	40.6

[1]Preliminary estimates.

Source: U.S. Social Security Administration, (1980) Social Security Bulletin, Annual Statistical Supplement 1977-1979, Washington, D.C.: U.S. Government Printing Office.

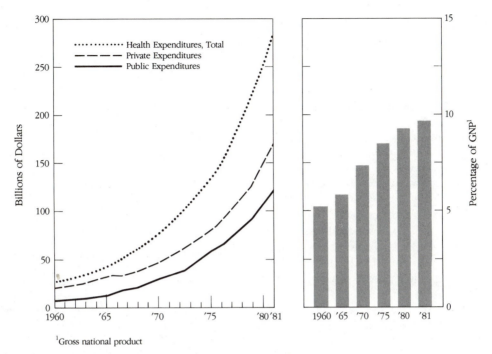

Gross national product

Source: Chart prepared by U.S. Bureau of the Census. For data, see Table 17-1.

FIGURE 17-1. National Health Expenditures: 1960–1981

27.2% in 1950 to 40.6% in 1978 (Cost of Disease and Illness in the U.S. 1978). Table 17-1, containing data provided by the Social Security Bulletin, describes this course. Figure 17-1 graphically depicts changes in spending patterns. Continuing this trend of increased public spending will have an impact on how Congress allocates our tax dollars.

One principal reason for the increase in public spending for health care is the demands and expected "right" to high-quality medical care that all Americans feel they deserve. Public expenditures on health care merely mirror society's expectations. This right or expectation translates into legislation for more extensive Medicare and Medicaid coverage, which in turn expands public spending. Additionally, each newly created government program and regulation dictates more subsidized government jobs, further enlarging our public spending (Caldwell 1982). Simultaneously, private spending has decreased as

employers and employees assume more of their own medical care costs through prepayment plans. The plans relieve employer and employee of potentially significant expenses.

Where do these federal dollars go? End stage renal disease (ESRD) is a particularly catastrophic, costly illness covered by Medicare, and renal dialysis clients are commonly singled out as the major consumers of the federal health care dollar. But statistics clearly show that *all* the chronically ill spend tremendous amounts of money and should be included as major spenders of the federal dollar. Vital statistics put out by the United States government in 1980–1981 show that 14.6% of noninstitutionalized Americans have chronic activity limitations and that this group uses 58% of all short-term hospital stay days. In another study of medical care resource utilization, 13% of the chronically ill were found to exhaust 87% of hospital costs (Zook & Moore 1980). Studies repeatedly demonstrate that the chronically ill are high consumers of medical care, especially expensive hospital care (Schroeder, Showstack, & Roberts 1979).

But is this appropriate utilization of hospital and other health care resources? Most services received by a client are ordered by the physician, with between 50% and 80% estimated to be controlled by the physician (Eisenberg & Rosoff 1978). Kurylo (1976), in reviewing the literature on misutilization of health care resources, documents how inpatient care is repeatedly overutilized. She cites one study asserting that one-fourth of patients in a general hospital had "no diagnostic or therapeutic requirements at hospital level" (p. 77). From another study, she notes that 11.8% of clients in chronic hospitals had insufficient medical grounds for admission. Quite obviously, the chronically ill place a considerable strain on the health care budget.

One must ask why the chronically ill are so frequently overhospitalized. A number of reasons have been proposed:

1. *Financial incentives:* Hospitalization is revenue-generating for both the physician and the hospital (Schroeder & Showstack 1978).
2. *Social reasons:* The client is unable to manage at home any longer (Glass et al. 1977).
3. *Malpractice scare:* The fear of lawsuits fosters "defensive medicine" (Curran 1975).
4. *Government reimbursement:* The present reimbursement system encourages hospitalization in order to receive payment (Kleczkowski & Mach 1979).
5. *Inefficiency:* Delays and inefficient use of diagnostic and treatment facilities unnecessarily prolong hospitalization (Zimmer 1967).

Increased Cost of Medical Advances. Advances in medical technology, treatments, and diagnostic tests are frequently singled out as being integral factors in the appreciation of health care costs. When new cancer drugs emerge on the market, frequently no less expensive generic equivalent exists. The client has no choice but to use the expensive medication if ordered by the physician. In one recent study, antineoplastic drug costs rose from 5.74% to 16.74% of a total hospital's drug budget (Nyman, Dorr, & Hall 1981). Computed tomography (CT) scanners, organ transplants, renal dialysis, and other costly procedures increase the health care budget. And each hospital in each community seems to feel the need to have every improved piece of equipment.

Representative Paul G. Rodgers, Democrat, of Florida, described this problem when addressing the National Leadership Conference on America's Health Policy in 1976. He noted that

> Now we're going through this business with the scanner. What's it cost? $300,000 to purchase and install. And the Society of Neuroradiologists, a group that probably would not necessarily err on the side of too little, has estimated that there ought to be six or seven scanners in the Washington area.... We already have three and a dozen more on order right here in the nation's capital. This cost will run from about $4 to $7 million. That's at today's prices. And in England, do you know how many they have? Two, and I think that's where they invented it (quoted in Iglehart 1982).

If hospitals and clinics did not insist on having their own expensive pieces of equipment, major savings could be realized (Devey 1981). One can question if it is worth spending $600 on diagnostic tests to gain 97% accuracy, when $75 would offer 95% accuracy. When further expense only produces markedly diminishing returns, there is need to evaluate the efficacy of the tests involved. Medical specializations also add to the health care budget. We see not only internists, obstetricians, pediatricians, surgeons, and so on, performing tests previously done by less expensive general practitioners, but multiple subspecialists within each of these groups.

Estimates of the financial effect of technology on cost per diem in hospitals range from 33% to 75%, with 50% being the average (Evans 1983a). Technology can also be fingered as the culprit in rising health care costs in relation to the trend toward shorter but more care-intensive hospital stays. In other words, clients spend fewer days during each hospitalization but receive more diagnostic tests, laboratory evaluations, and X rays, which have actually increased the general cost of each day in the hospital (Evans 1983a). The costs associated with renal dialysis units, medical intensive care units (MICUs), and other high-technology medical practices is only a part of a more pervasive problem. The very effectiveness of this technology results in a growing number of people who survive formerly fatal disorders and need to be maintained by this same expensive technological medicine. This guarantees that health care costs will continue to escalate.

There is some question as to whether all this "high-tech" medicine is improving our nation's health. Many researchers have questioned whether there is a positive, direct correlation between health and the amount of medical care provided (Fuchs 1974; Turnbull et al. 1979; Rice & Wilson 1976). Coronary by-pass surgery is a case in point, since it is a very costly surgical procedure with questionable efficacy. Results for clients who have three artery involvement are clearly not impressive and their rate of return to work is insignificant (Evans 1983b). If social and economic factors are considered, not simply medical services, then altered personal behavior has the greatest potential for reducing coronary disease, cancer, and other major killers (Fuchs 1974).

Other researchers feel that health care spending has had a positive effect, especially for the elderly. Drake (1978) cites a 9.6% increase in life expectancy from 1965 to 1975 and a decrease in death rates from heart disease and cerebral vascular accidents of 14.9% and 19%, respectively, during the same ten years.

Continued controversy can be expected over the cost of high technology and its value to the nation's health. The renal dialysis program is a prime example of the soaring costs of our technology. Sixty thousand renal dialysis patients consume nearly $2 billion annually in Medicare funds. Without this critical treatment, these people would die. Can society deny them this life-saving treatment? And yet providing just this one treatment modality creates a mind-boggling health expenditure.

Physician Fees. The debate continues over whether physician fees contribute significantly to spiraling costs. Some reports state that physicians' incomes are rising faster than those of any other occupation (Culliton 1978), whereas others claim that a 25% reduction in physician incomes would decrease national health expenditures by only 2.7% (Ayres 1977). Physician fees are not rising as rapidly as medical care in general; hospital room rates have risen more rapidly than any other form of medical care (Statistical Abstract of the U.S. 1982–83, p. 98). See Figure 17-2.

Some physicians claim they have had to raise their fees because of high malpractice insurance premiums. It was in 1975 that the medical profession first coined the phrase *the crisis in medical malpractice*. That year, insurance companies increased their premiums, on a national scale, between 100% and 750% (Curran 1975). This massive increase had some effect on physician behavior. Although the actual amount (1% in 1975) paid in medical malpractice premiums may be a small percentage of the total health care expenditures (Somers 1977), there is consensus that it leads to costly physician behavior, commonly referred to as *defensive medicine*. Fear of malpractice litigation has led the physician to be overly cautious and order additional, and frequently unnecessary, X rays, laboratory tests, and hospital days (Zucker 1980). The actual effect on the health care budget is unknown, but one can speculate that all this additional testing to assure maximum accuracy in diagnosis adds to rising costs.

The Focus on Acute Care. The focus on acute hospital care over ambulatory and home care adds to the crisis in health care. Acute hospital care provides necessary but expensive service for short-term illnesses, but most diseases are of a chronic nature and they need management on a long-term, out-of-hospital basis. Both ambulatory care and home care are highly appropriate most of the time for managing chronic illnesses. Excessive and unnecessary hospitalizations are major offenders of the overburdened health budget.

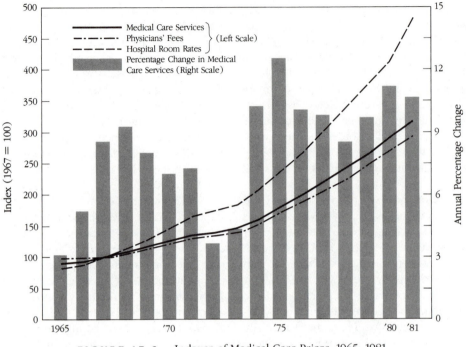

FIGURE 17-2. Indexes of Medical Care Prices: 1965–1981

Frequently, hospitalization is not necessary to accomplish health goals. In a study of Hodgkins lymphoma staging (Corder et al. 1981), unnecessary hospitalizations accounted for 68% of the "perceived excess charges." Inversely, home care and ambulatory care have proven less costly than acute care for similar treatment and procedures, and in some studies, have been demonstrated to be the superior form of treating the chronically ill. Zwaag and others (1980) studied a group of chronically ill individuals who needed ongoing evaluation and discovered that when care was shifted from major medical centers to neighborhood clinics, attention focused on client education, follow-up, and support rather than medical work-up. In addition, health care became more accessible, which contributed to the significant drop in missed appointments and proved to be a major factor encouraging a large portion of clients to remain in the medical system many years after referral.

Reimbursement. Our current system of reimbursement provides few incentives to keep health care costs down. In fact, our present system of reimbursement is commonly viewed to be a major contributor to the escalating health care budget (Eisenberg & Rosoff 1978; Roemer & Shonick 1973; Zucker 1980). With present forms of insurance reimbursement, the incentive is to hospitalize the client for therapies that could be administered at home, because hospital admissions and diagnostic tests generate revenue for the physician and the hospital. In addition, payment for many procedures is not reimbursed when performed on an outpatient basis.

Most people (76% in 1980) have some form of hospital insurance (Evans 1983a). When there is no outpatient coverage, the physician will hospitalize the client for procedures that can be administered less expensively on an outpatient basis in an attempt to save the client money. Since third-party reimbursement facilitates the detached attitude that "the money doesn't come out of the patient's pocket anyway," it is no wonder that physicians engage in this revenue-generating behavior. This common practice is mistakenly seen as benign, when actually we all absorb these "hidden costs" in increased insurance premiums and decreased insurance benefits.

Lack of both continuity and coordination of care also adds to medical expenses. In our complex medical care delivery system, a chronically ill individual can easily be receiving care from many different specialists in several different health care facilities. This commonly leads to fragmentation and duplication of care and tests. For instance, a diabetic with renal failure would be under the care of several specialists—nephrologist, endocrinologist, ophthalmologist, and cardiologist—all for complications from diabetes! The coordination of this client's care in an effort to minimize duplication of tests and increase sharing of medical information is no easy task.

Direct versus Indirect Costs

Illness expenditures can be measured by a combination of both direct and indirect costs. Direct costs include all medical and hospital-related expenses, drugs, laboratory charges, X rays, and so on. Indirect costs are related to morbidity and mortality rates. Included in indirect costs are vocational rehabilitation and social services, special diets, and special equipment, as well as loss of productivity and of income.

One common method to measure costs is the economic theory of human capital. This theory measures the value of a life saved in terms of the goods and services produced over a sustained working lifetime after recovery. Cost of economic contribution can then be approximated against this output (Cromwell & Gertman 1979). Some factors that contribute to the measurement of both direct and indirect costs of any illness are age at death, duration of illness, incidence rate of the illness, and disability caused by that illness. When these factors are all taken into consideration, a more accurate estimate of the true cost

of illness can be established. The relationship between direct and indirect costs for the client is important information needed for the formation of health care policies.

Direct Costs. Fortunately, as mentioned, the great majority of the American population is covered by some form of health insurance, which defrays a good portion of direct costs. Of the respondents in a 1978 Gallup survey, 90% had some sort of health insurance; however, only 59% had extended or catastrophic coverage (Schroeder 1981). Good insurance coverage is not always adequate for the chronically ill, since they have much higher direct medical costs than the average population. Meenan and others (1978) found that rheumatoid arthritics have direct medical costs three times higher than most Americans, and that rheumatic diseases are among the most prevalent chronic illnesses.

In one study, cancer patients, most of whom had both outpatient and inpatient insurance coverage, still had to pay just under 20% of their direct-care costs out of pocket (Cromwell & Gertman 1979). The expenses incurred, but not covered, included equipment such as wheelchairs, cancer-related home nursing, and uncovered drug costs. Items such as these, which are frequently not covered by insurance, can quickly multiply an individual's overall medical bill. Even with catastrophic coverage usually covering 80% of the bill, the remaining 20% of expenses for a chronic illness like cancer or cardiovascular disease can quickly place an extraordinary strain on personal finances.

Indirect Costs. Indirect costs are the heaviest financial burden for any client, since these costs are rarely covered by insurance (McNaull 1981). Rheumatoid arthritics have been shown to have indirect costs that are three to five times higher than their direct costs (Meenan et al. 1978). Cardiac disease clients have indirect costs as much as 4.5 times the direct costs involved in their treatment (Hartunian, Smart, & Thompson 1980). Indirect costs are also incurred by the family and friends of the chronically ill, as they provide unpaid nursing and other services and experience income loss as a result of the family member's illness (see Chapter 8).

The middle class, dependent on salaries for financial solvency, is especially susceptible to the crippling medical costs of chronic illnesses. There exist today a good number of chronic illnesses with treatment costs far exceeding any individual's financial means. McClure summarizes this critical situation well:

> The U.S. remains one of the few industrialized countries where an individual can be bankrupted by medical expense. Presently, approximately 10% of U.S. households spend directly (excluding employer or other contributions) in excess of 15% of their income annually for health insurance premiums and out-of-pocket medical bills. Almost 4% spend more than 25% of their income on such expenses (McClure 1976).

Given McClure's statistics and the U.S. position, alone among industrialized nations in allowing medical expenses to bankrupt families, an evaluation of our health care spending and budget is in order.

Loss of income is by far the greatest privation and plays a tremendous role in the psychosocial impact of chronic illness. If a middle-class breadwinning man suffers significant loss of wages, this may necessitate his wife's entering the job market or the illness may mitigate his changing jobs. The same would be true if a working woman is forced to leave her employment or change jobs to accommodate her illness. In either case, the change is often to a lower salary level. One study showed that 76% of working rheumatic arthritics experienced major changes in their employment (Meenan et al. 1978). Marked changes in income can also place stress on marriage, roles, and how time is spent, and can bring up previously unaddressed issues of power between husband and wife. Meenan and associates' study (1978) of rheumatoid arthritics showed that 18% of the married respondents were divorced or separated, compared to a national average of 11%.

Who Is Most Impacted?

Both the poor and the elderly, primarily women, are severely affected by chronic illness. Given the profile of these two groups, the implication is that chronic illness afflicts those who can least afford it. These findings should also have bearing on health care policy formation.

The Poor. Unfortunately, the poor (commonly considered those whose income is in the lowest 20% in the U.S.) are affected most by chronic illness, even though they can least afford the financial impact and monetary burden. Chronic illness most severely affects the life-style and income of this group. The high prevalence and severity of chronic illness among the poor are due to the economic dynamics of chronic disease and the cycle of impoverishment discussed earlier in the chapter. Chronic illness limits the job opportunities, mobility, and financial resources of the poor, in turn cutting off the opportunity to rise above limited monetary means.

Although both poor and nonpoor are affected by the same types of chronic diseases, the prevalence, severity, and activity limitation of illness are overly represented among the poor. In one government study (Health Characteristics of Persons with Chronic Activity Limitation 1978), the difference between activity limitation due to chronic conditions of poor and higher-income groups was represented by a 26.6% to 10.4% ratio. The difference increases even more dramatically for people between ages 45 and 64, considered to be peak income-earning years. In this age group, 46.8% of the poor reported some degree of limitation compared to 19.1% of the more affluent (see Table 17-2). These figures demonstrate how chronic illness not only sustains poor people at poverty level but maintains the "health gap" between those who are poor and those who are not (Health Characteristics 1978).

Currently, the government is spending more money on medical care and less on human service programs. This is a devastating policy for the chronically ill since chronic illness is, by nature, neither curable nor preventable. Even though chronically ill people need more medical treatment than the general public, they have an even greater need for health-related and support services, including assistance with ambulation, bathing, housekeeping, and shop-

TABLE 17-2. Percentage of Persons Limited in Activity through Chronic Conditions, by Age and Family Income: United States, 1977

| | Percentage Limited in Activity | | |
Age	Family Income Less than $6,000	Family Income $6,000+	Percentage Difference between Income Categories
All ages	26.6	10.4	156
Under 17 years	4.5	3.2	41
17–44 years	14.2	7.1	100
45–64 years	46.8	19.1	145
65 years and over	50.3	37.8	33

Source: Unpublished data from the Health Interview Survey, National Center for Health Statistics. Data are based on household interviews of the civilian, noninstitutionalized population. Excludes unknown income.

ping. Greatest benefit could be derived if these services were provided and complemented with periodic professional monitoring of illness and treatment (Ricker-Smith 1982).

Is spending more and more money on treatment of chronic illness efficacious when one witnesses the significant economic and psychosocial problems that result? Meenan and Yelin (1981) note that we are probably at the point of diminishing returns with most chronic diseases, since additional technological therapy produces progressively less improvement in health status. Spending less on actual medical care and more on physical and vocational rehabilitation, as well as social and human services, would better serve the chronically ill by improving their plight. Spending money in this way presents a provocatively different approach from spending more on new technology.

The Elderly. The second largest group of people overly represented among the chronically ill are elderly White women. These women are especially susceptible to the cycle of impoverishment as, statistically, they outlive their husbands by 7.7 years (*World Almanac and Book of Facts* 1983), have had meager

earning power, have limited knowledge of financial management, and suffer tremendous loss in income after their husbands die. Women are more likely to have a higher prevalence of chronic diseases, such as congestive heart failure or arthritis, that are *not* among the leading causes of death. The disability and limitations of activity that result from these chronic conditions further limit these women from improving their economic and social situation.

Elderly White women far exceed any other group of nursing home residents (see Figure 17-3). It is estimated that 99% of nursing home residents have some kind of chronic illness, with an average of 3.9 chronic conditions per resident (*U.S. Vital Health Statistics* 13 1981, p. 12).

Almost one-third of the clients who enter nursing homes as private patients eventually become Medicaid clients (Kane & Kane 1981), which is further evidence of the pauperization of chronic illness. Medicaid is the largest single payer of nursing home care for elderly persons. Private insurance and Medicare pay for negligible amounts of this long-term care (U.S. General Accounting Office 1983). An elderly person on a fixed income is hard pressed to afford nursing home charges of $1,200 to $3,000 a

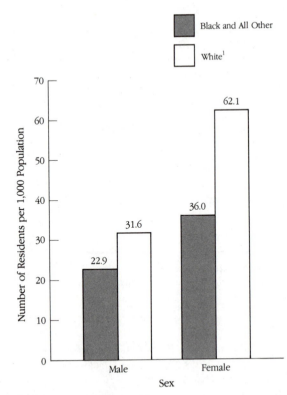

¹Includes persons of Hispanic origin.

Source: U.S. Vital Health Statistics, (1981) Series 13, 59, p. 26.

FIGURE 17-3. Number of Nursing Home Residents per 1,000 Population 65 Years of Age and Over, by Race and Sex: United States, 1977

month for a semiprivate room in a facility that provides decent quality care. A handsome life savings of $100,000 would easily be consumed in a few short years.

Inadequate Assistance from Federal Programs

The federal government has five main programs meant to assist the chronically ill financially and medically: Medicare (Part A and Part B), Medicaid, Social Security Disability, SSI, and Title XX. These federal programs are jointly operated with state, and occasionally county, governments, except Medicare, which is operated entirely at the federal level. Since the mandates of most of these programs are directed

partially from either state or county governments, their services and eligibility requirements vary.

Medicare and Medicaid. Medicare and Medicaid were passed in 1965 as part of the Social Security Act to provide basic health care to the elderly and disabled. They provide services in different ways. Medicare is a national health insurance program for the elderly and for those with some specified chronic conditions, and Medicaid is a program for the poor.

Medicare. This program is administered entirely on a federal level and benefits are uniform throughout the country. The program contains two parts. Part A is a hospital insurance program that includes acute care hospitalization for an allowable number of days per benefit period for all people over age 65 and for some disabled people, such as individuals with ESRD. People who are covered pay an initial deductible fee, after which 80% of "reasonable" charges are covered. Skilled nursing facilities are also covered for a maximum number of days if such care is needed, but only after acute hospitalization (*Your Medicare Handbook* 1984).

Part B is a voluntary medical insurance supplement for those interested individuals who can afford the monthly premiums. In 1984, part B premiums were $14.60 a month. As in Part A, 80% of "reasonable" charges for outpatient care are covered. These include physician services, medical supplies and services, diagnostic tests and X rays, ambulance, some outpatient services, physical and speech therapy, home health visits if ordered by a physician, and chiropractic care. Because the charges covered as "reasonable" are not always the same as actual charges, physician and other outpatient services frequently expect clients to pay the difference (Stevens & Stevens 1974).

Medicaid. Legislated under Title XIX of the Social Security Act, this program is meant to provide medical care to the eligible poor and indigent. All Supplemental Security Income (SSI) recipients are offered automatic eligibility. Every state now participates in the Medicaid program, which is both state and federally funded. However, the amount and kind of coverage vary by state; some cover only mandatory services for the categorically needy and others provide additional services. Services covered include inpatient and outpatient hospital care, physician office visits, skilled nursing home and intermediate care, periodic screening, diagnostic and X ray tests, and family planning. Optional services include dental and mental health care in some states (Kane & Kane 1981).

Recipients of this program must meet strict financial eligibility requirements. Individuals may have no more than $1,500 in any liquid asset (cash, stocks, bonds) to be eligible for Medicaid. Fees paid are usually much lower than usual charges made by providers, and reimbursement is generally slow and cumbersome.

Inadequacies of Medicare and Medicaid. Both these programs are geared to help the acutely ill (Newacheck et al. 1980). Coverage favors acute inpatient hospital stays, which are generally not optimal for the treatment of long-term chronic illness in which symptoms flare up only periodically. Monitoring and ongoing treatment are better received in ambulatory or decentralized clinics, physicians' offices, or home nursing services (Garfield et al. 1976; Zwagg et al. 1980). In many instances, services included under these programs can be covered only after an admission to an acute care hospital.

Analysis of what Medicare does not cover shows that the chronically ill are the big losers. Routine physical exams, custodial care at home, extended care facilities, eyeglasses, hearing aids, and drugs outside the acute hospital setting are all services needed by the chronically ill but not covered by Medicare (*Your Medicare Handbook* 1984).

As noted, Medicaid is not administered equally in all states. Although states that provide extended services do have fairly comprehensive medical coverage, many providers refuse to take clients in these programs because of the low reimbursement rates, the slowness of payments, and the potential for rejected claims. Where only minimum services are covered, health care can be inadequate except for acute flare-ups.

The natural outcome of favoring inpatient care is that the chronically ill receive financial and medical support primarily when they end up in an acute care institution rather than on an ongoing basis. Covering acute phases of chronic illness is less efficacious because many social and psychological facets are not considered. It would be more advantageous for both the client and our staggering health care budget if these people were treated as outpatients.

Social Security Disability. Part of the Social Security Administration (SSD) is financed by taxes paid by employees, employers, and some self-employed people. Eligibility requirements are strict. It is mandatory that the insured have a work history and have contributed to the system. To receive benefits, the worker-recipient must have a disability preventing gainful employment that is projected to last at least one year. Dependents become eligible in the event of disability or death of the insured. Those who are eligible for SSD benefits include workers disabled before age 65, widows and widowers who are disabled or caring for dependent children, unmarried dependent children under age 18 (22 if in high school or college full time), or disabled individuals under age 22 (U.S. Department of Health and Human Services 1983).

Processing applications takes at least four months, which means that a disabled worker may be without income for that period. This can place the uninsured and unemployed chronically ill individual and family in dire straits for what can seem an interminable length of time. SSD provides income, not health insurance. Eligibility for Medicare comes only after recipients have been receiving SSD benefits for 24 months (U.S. Department of Health and Human Services 1983). Only ESRD clients receive immediate Medicare benefits upon diagnosis of their disease.

Supplemental Security Income. SSI became effective in 1974 in an effort to reorganize and revamp the array of state-operated welfare programs. SSI provides a uniform, federal minimum-level income payment standard for poor aged, blind, or disabled people. Organized under the nationally operated Social

◇ CASE STUDY ◇
Falling through the Cracks

Mrs. T., a mother of three, was 47 years old when she was diagnosed as having breast cancer with bone metastasis. Her husband's income was $24,000 per year. His covered health benefits offered only hospital insurance, so they were forced to pay for all her outpatient services out of pocket. The progression of her disease necessitated pinning a pathologically broken hip, radiation, and chemotherapy treatments. When these treatments were done in the hospital, they were covered. But often these treatments were done on an outpatient basis. Mrs. T. was ineligible for Social Security Disability because she hadn't been disabled for at least two years. She was also ineligible for SSI and Medicaid because the family had too many liquid assets, some property they had purchased as an investment but that was currently unsalable. In other words, their income and situation exempted them from any financial assistance.

Although this was a middle-income family, they could not begin to pay for the treatments that were averaging $500–600 monthly. After only one year, this family was deeply in debt to the teaching hospital where Mrs. T. was receiving treatment. Since they were not able to make the smallest dent in her enormous medical bill, Mrs. T. was transferred to the nearest county facility, where she could receive treatment for a reduced fee. This facility was much farther from her home than the medical center, requiring that she travel great distances for treatment. All this proved to be traumatic to the entire family. Had they been very poor, or very rich, many of their problems would not have existed.

Security Administration, SSI is financed by the U.S. Treasury rather than by Social Security taxes; thus no work history is required for these benefits (*A Guide to Supplemental Security Income* 1984).

Financial eligibility requirements are very similar to those for Medicaid. An individual may have no more than $1500 in any liquid assets (that is, checking or savings accounts, cash, stocks, or bonds); a couple may have no more than $2250. In 1984, the payment schedule was $314 per month for an individual living alone and $472 per month per couple (*A Guide to SSI* 1984). This amount of money is frequently inadequate to provide food, shelter, clothing, and medical care for these individuals.

Title XX. Also part of the Social Security Act passed in 1974, Title XX is operated at both state and federal levels. The federal Title XX goals (Nelson 1982) are

1. To prevent, reduce or eliminate dependency by achieving or maintaining economic self-support.
2. To achieve or maintain self-sufficiency while reducing or preventing dependency.
3. To prevent or remedy neglect, abuse or exploitation of children and adults unable to protect their own interests. Included here is the preserving, rehabilitating or reuniting of families.

4. To avoid or reduce inappropriate institutional care through forms of less intensive care such as community-based or home-based care.
5. When other forms of care are inappropriate, to secure admission or referral for institutional care. Included here is the provision of services to individuals in institutions.

Eligibility is determined by a financial means test, but SSI, Medicaid, and Aid to Families with Dependent Children (AFDC) recipients are automatically eligible. Services provided under this act for eligible recipients include legal and transportation services, day care, family counseling, protective services, information and referral, at-home services, education, and training.

Although all these programs are designed to aid the medically and financially needy, many clients "fall through the cracks" and, because of rigid eligibility requirements, may not receive assistance. Such a situation is illustrated by the case study discussing "falling through the cracks."

Mrs. T.'s case is not unique. In a number of chronic illnesses, treatment costs far exceed any individual's financial means. Unfortunately, these programs are structured in such a way that those who are from the middle classes can, and do, become bankrupt.

Solutions to Rising Health Care Costs

As we have seen, the chronically ill are burdened with multiple financial problems, persistently leading to impoverishment. Society also pays a heavy price in maintaining the present system of health care costs. We will now look at suggestions and possible solutions aimed at reducing this rapidly growing and increasingly overwhelming problem. Although these suggestions are noted in the literature, they are not presented in depth, nor are they all inclusive. Rather, considering the limitations and constraints of a single chapter, the authors hope primarily to stimulate the reader into investigating additional solutions to the problems of rising medical costs for the chronically ill.

Ambulatory Care

Given that hospital costs have risen faster than other medical care indexes, and that the chronically ill are hospitalized excessively, a change of focus from acute to ambulatory care would help ease this financial problem. Serious consideration and efforts are being made to dialyze ESRD clients at home rather than at centers. In 1980, Roberts, Maxwell, and Gross found that a shift from dialysis center to home could save $7,000 to $8,000 per person per year of life. These figures are in all likelihood conservative, considering the recent increase in center dialysis costs. In yet another detailed study of the chronically ill and physically disabled, no significant differences in improvement were found between those receiving treatments at home versus at the clinic. Yet clinic costs were 21% higher than home care (Gersten, Cenkovich, & Dinken 1968).

Rehabilitation

Improving the rehabilitation of the chronically ill decreases the frequency and need for acute hospitalization and thus cuts medical expenses (Johnson & Keith 1983). With rehabilitative measures, everyone profits. The client's dignity and self-determination are restored and the client is returned to a higher functional level (see Chapter 18), and the public's

financial obligation is diminished through decreased cost of long-term maintenance. Unfortunately, we are not employing rehabilitation to its fullest today. Only 6.6% of impaired applicants to Social Security Disability ever received physical or occupational therapy (Smith & Lilienfeld 1971).

Choice of Setting for Treatment

Challenging the rationale for physicians' choices is always treading in dangerous waters, but there is room for question. Physicians tend to select hospitals for diagnosis and treatment, since payment by insurance companies is more complete in these settings. As noted earlier, clients generally have more comprehensive inpatient than outpatient coverage, so part of the physician's decision is an attempt to save clients out-of-pocket money. Unfortunately, this practice is not cost-effective because many diagnostic tests and treatments can be less expensively administered on an outpatient basis.

One Hodgkin's lymphoma staging study (Corder et al. 1981) showed that physicians unnecessarily hospitalized clients for this procedure. The authors recommend that the expenses of Hodgkin's lymphoma staging could be appreciably reduced by decreasing hospitalization. This is only one example of how decision making influences cost. Undoubtedly physicians can modify diagnostic and treatment formats to save client, as well as public, expense in numerous other ways. This single change will demand involvement of and responsibility by private physicians.

Prevention

Focusing on preventive health care through health education and teaching everyone healthier life-styles will also lower medical costs by decreasing the number of chronically ill and the severity of chronic illnesses. Weight and stress reduction, smoking cessation, and prenatal classes are just some of the methods now available that contribute to this effort. Even the simple gesture of buckling a seat belt saves lives and money.

How effective can these preventive programs be? Cooper and Rice (1976) estimated that in 1972 the *annual* savings of preventable illness, based on costs of broad categories of illnesses in the U.S., would include approximately 400,000 lives and $5 billion in medical costs. These are very meaningful and significant figures. Of equal importance is the fact that when antihypertensive programs prevent diseases such as cerebral vascular accidents (CVA), we not only prevent a disability with large medical costs to the individual and society but also maintain that individual as a healthy, contributing member of the community with less likelihood of future mental and physical disability.

There seems to be a great consensus regarding improving health by changing some of our negative behaviors. More illnesses would be prevented and lives saved, especially between the ages of 40 and 64, by significant reductions in sedentary living, alcoholism, overnutrition, hypertension, and excessive cigarette smoking than can be saved by the best current medical practice (Kristein, Arnold, & Wynder 1977).

Is Treatment Always Cost-Effective?

This is a most provocative question. Some researchers, using cost-benefit analysis outcomes, reviewed programs geared to prevent recurrence of chronic disorders such as heart disease and cancer (Luginbuhl et al. 1980). Cost-benefit analysis compares earned income over time against cost to the individual and society. They note a much higher recurrence rate in individuals who have already suffered one such episode of these diseases. Although CCU care has reduced mortality rates, the cost of trying to prevent death from cardiac disease, once the disease has occurred, may be far costlier than the individual's future earnings. These authors question if preventing deaths from these diseases is an efficacious method of spending our public health care dollars. Although many individuals surviving catastrophic illnesses produce additional income that would have been lost had they not survived, many others do not. The combination of health care costs, disability, and retirement payments produces a loss of net earnings of $3.9 billion (Luginbuhl et al. 1980).

Their analysis produces a rather harsh conclusion for health care policy formation by reducing benefits of health care expenditures solely to the financial level. They propose encouraging medical interventions that will increase the population's net income while discouraging interventions that decrease net income. This, they note, could be a better way of maximizing health care expenditures than limiting financial investment in institutional health care. Unfortunately, they have not taken into consideration other goals in medicine and society, such as the reduction of pain and suffering and increasing the length and quality of life.

Expanded Nursing and Other Health Provider Roles

Health care practitioners other than physicians can provide effective ways of trimming health care costs. Registered nurses, who primarily staff hospitals and physicians' offices, could be used more extensively in many of their newer roles to perform more functions and, in this way, keep health care costs lower than those of using more expensive physicians. Nurses can also play a major role in screening hospital admissions, thereby preventing or lowering unnecessary and costly admissions. Clinical nurse-specialists can help formulate nursing care plans that would lead to more effective care, which could lead to earlier discharge.

Nurse-practitioners, who once were used primarily in rural areas suffering from the physician shortage, now provide primary care in clinics, homes, and hospitals at reduced costs and with high client satisfaction (Garfield et al. 1976). New health practitioners (NHP), consisting of both nurse-practitioners and physician assistants, were studied in a prepaid primary care practice, where they used protocols to provide patient care. The protocol system was compared with the physicians-only nonprotocol system. Costs of average visits under the protocol system, including NHP time and charges, lab tests, and medications were 20% less than those from physicians (Garfield et al. 1978). The protocol system lowered costs by minimizing physician time while maximizing physician output. The doctor's time per patient was reduced by 92%.

Costs are saved largely because of the large salary differential between NHPs and physicians. Not only is money saved but clients are more satisfied. Another study (Thompson, Basden, & Howell 1982) using family nurse practitioners (FNPs) in a health maintenance organization (HMO) found that

1. Waiting time at the clinic was reduced.
2. The quality of examinations did not diminish when performed by the FNPs.
3. Unit cost per client decreased.
4. Clients examined by the FNPs voiced greater satisfaction.
5. Counseling and education were emphasized.

National Approaches to Reducing Health Care Costs

Many endeavors to change the system of health care delivery have been proposed. All are intended to provide high-quality care at reduced costs to the consumer and the public. With the growing financial crisis in health care, economists, health care providers, and elected officials are all looking for new and more cost-effective ways to deliver medical care while simultaneously assuring access to high-quality care. Considering the current public sentiment regarding inflationary health care costs, the climate is ripe for change. Some of these proposals geared to changing our health care delivery system are described.

Health Maintenance Organizations. HMOs, such as Kaiser-Permanente Health Plan, Inc. (primarily in California but with facilities in ten other states), provide medical care for subscribers with costs coming only from their monthly premiums. These premiums are charged for a total care package including hospitalization. Since no additional money is provided, there is a strong incentive to use preventive and maintenance care, which keeps costs down (Roemer & Shonick 1973; Rabkin 1983).

HMOs function by making contracts with consumers (or employers on their behalf) to assure the delivery of stated health services of measured quality. These consumers are offered a broad range of personal health service benefits, including, at a minimum, physician services and hospital care. Subscribers must be preenrolled, usually through some group, and fees are paid in advance (Roemer & Shonick 1973). An HMO coordinates its members' entire care.

Preferred Provider Organizations. Another means for health providers to help keep costs down is the use of PPOs. By banding together, an organized group of physicians, dentists, clinics, or other health care providers can contract with an insurance company or large employer to provide services at a reduced fee (Kodner 1982).

PPOs are often compared to HMOs but differ on two significant accounts. PPOs are not entities like HMOs, nor do they coordinate their participants' care. Rather, the PPO is designed around contractual relationships among all participating parties. The hospital and physician are guaranteed a client load with prompt payment. Employers receive reduced fees and better health care coverage for their employees. Employees/clients receive reduced medical care costs. In addition, the client can retain the freedom of choosing his or her own physician or hospital as long as he or she pays the additional fee required for that choice (Kodner 1982).

National Health Insurance. Proposed periodically in Congress, NHI would provide guaranteed health care for all U.S. citizens (Falk 1977). The United States is the only major Western nation without a comprehensive health insurance program for its citizens (Schroeder 1981). Such a program might include a regulatory body that would set rates for hospital costs similar to a public utility. England, Sweden, and the Netherlands all have health care systems that serve as examples of NHI programs.

In the last few years, legislative activity regarding NHI has decreased (Schroeder 1981), which could be due to the public's growing awareness of rapidly escalating medical costs. Probably because of the dramatic increase in our health care budget, the focus of proposed health legislation has changed from reimbursing the costs accrued for health care and related social programs to containing medical costs (Starr 1982).

Catastrophic Health Insurance. Different from NHI, this type of insurance would prevent people from becoming indigent because of major illness (Zucker 1980). This form of insurance is based on an economic, rather than the customary medical, definition of catastrophe. For instance, once an individual's medical bills rose above $5,000 or 15% of one's income, this insurance would begin picking up all medical expenses. In an atmosphere where politicians and the public are crying to cut health care costs, CHI is less costly than NHI and probably would be more acceptable.

Diagnosis-Related Groups (DRGs). This recently instituted Medicare payment system places a limit on the amount paid in hospital bills for specific diagnoses regardless of the length of hospitalization. The DRG system is a way of measuring the hospital's resource utilization performance and costs (Simborg 1981). The plan, first tried in New Jersey's acute care hospitals, was designed to provide incentives to decrease costs to the government. New Jersey set payment rates for all private and public payers on the basis of what type of patient case mix was being treated, rather than on the number of hospital days. The program was effective in reducing costs.

The United States government adopted this approach for its Medicare payment system. Under DRGs, the client is classified by one of 383 mutually exclusive categories (Fetter et al. 1980). These are either principal diagnoses, secondary diagnoses, or special procedures (diagnostic or surgical).

Speculation exists regarding problems that may sabotage the cost-effectiveness of the DRG system.

First, marginal admissions might be encouraged to maximize reimbursement. Second, a system could be devised whereby the more costly diagnoses were always listed as primary diagnoses, enabling higher reimbursement rates. Third, less costly diagnoses could possibly be changed to more costly "rule out" diagnoses, such as admitting a "probably transient ischemic attack" as a "rule-out CVA," which has a larger reimbursement rate (Fetter et al. 1980).

Summary and Conclusions

Health care costs have increased progressively and continuously. One reason is that the public feels that each member of society has a right to medical care, yet many questions and problems result from this escalation. Not only have health care costs increased for many reasons, but each person is affected by indirect costs as well as direct costs, the latter usually being picked up by insurance companies or the government. The poor, the elderly, and others who fall between the cracks suffer severe consequences from the financial impact of health care. Available solutions in dealing with rising health care costs need to be seriously considered if we are to arrive at a workable answer.

Like the certainty of death and taxes, illness is part of our daily existence. Chronic illness is costly and its prevalence will surely increase as the American population ages. It is an economic sign of the times when the first question asked of us upon entering our physician's office is "Do you have any insurance?" rather than "What ails you?" With health care expenditures projected to be 12% of the Gross National Product by 1990, careful planning and discussion are needed to curb this escalation. Ideally, we will not witness a reversal of the public's edict of health care for all, as this would make health care a privilege of the financially secure few rather than a right of all. The challenge of the future is: How do we continue delivering high-quality care and make advances in medical technology and research while simultaneously limiting spending?

Considering the state of medical science, a re-evaluation of our budget may prove that spending 12% of the GNP on health care *is* appropriate. Nevertheless, more than dollars are at issue; ethics, values, and human rights are involved. How do we equitably and rationally divide limited financial resources to meet individual, national, and international needs? The $2 billion spent annually by the Medicare program on 60,000 renal dialysis clients could provide a great deal of care for thousands of others who are chronically ill. But do we risk the lives of these individuals to offer more routine treatment to a far greater number of people? The public, legislators, and health care providers grossly underestimated the cost of renal dialysis when they included this treatment under Medicare. Yet, considering our belief in the sanctity of life, the same decision would probably have been made had an accurate cost been known.

We now find ourselves in a similar situation with the emergence of costly heart and liver transplants. In the future, new and even more exorbitantly costly life-saving measures will be discovered and those who could benefit from these measures will clamor for them. How do we decide who should receive what treatment? Who should pay? There are no blueprints for this type of decision-making process.

Inasmuch as vast public funds are being spent, the public, medical professionals, other health care providers, courts, and legislatures all need to be involved in the allocation of health care resources. However, as we plan our complex health care system, we need to focus on the objectives, priorities, and human rights involved. Where could we, or should we, draw the line on costs versus needs? Rationality, creativity, intelligence, and sensitivity are required when analyzing this complicated issue. Judgments made for or against increased spending require that consequences of those decisions be fully considered.

STUDY QUESTIONS

1. Why have health care and its associated costs become a national political issue?
2. In what ways has federal and private payment of health care expenditures changed over the last 20 years? How does this influence costs?
3. What factors influence overutilization of hospitals for care of the chronically ill?
4. How do technology, malpractice rates, and the reimbursement system affect cost of health care?
5. How do direct and indirect costs affect the health care consumer?
6. Who are the most adversely affected by the present system of payment for health care? How are these people affected?
7. What are the advantages and disadvantages of assistance provided by federal programs?
8. How can ambulatory care and rehabilitation programs better serve the chronically ill while limiting health care costs?
9. What part does prevention play in decreasing health care costs?
10. What are the advantages and disadvantages of trying to make health care cost-effective? of using paramedics?
11. In what ways can high-quality care be attained while reducing costs through changes in the health care system itself?

References

A Guide to Supplemental Security Income, (1984) United States Department of Health and Human Services, January

Ayres, J., (1977) Decelerating skyrocketing health-care cost, *New England Journal of Medicine, 296*:391–392

Caldwell, J., (1982) Home care: Utilizing resources to develop home care, *Hospitals, 21*:68–72

Cooper, B. S., and Rice, D. P., (1976) The economic cost of illness revisited, *Social Security Bulletin 39,* pp. 21–36

Corder, M., Lachenbruch, P., Lindle, S., Sisson, J., Johnson, P., and Kosier, J., (1981) *American Journal of Public Health, 71*(4):376–380

Cost of Disease and Illness in the U.S. in the Year 2000, (1978) *Public Health Reports Supplement, 93*(5):497–506

Cromwell, J., and Gertman, P., (1979) The cost of cancer, *Laryngoscope, 89*:393–409

Culliton, B., (1978) The high cost of getting well, *Science, 200*(26):883–885

Curran, W., (1975) Malpractice insurance: A genuine national crisis, *New England Journal of Medicine, 292*(23):1233–1234

Devey, G., (1981) Technology: Focus on management grows in face of high costs, *Hospitals, 7*:169–173

Drake, D., (1978) Does money spent on health care really improve U.S. health status?, *Hospitals, 52*:63–65

Eisenberg, J., and Rosoff, A., (1978) Physician responsibility for the cost of unnecessary medical services, *New England Journal of Medicine, 299*(2):76–80

Evans, R., (1983a) Health care technology and the inevitability of resource allocation and rationing decisions (part I), *Journal of the American Medical Association, 249*:2047–2053

Evans, R., (1983b) Health care technology and the inevitability of resource allocation and rationing decisions (part II), *Journal of the American Medical Association, 249*:2208–2217

Falk, I. S., (1977) Proposals for national health insurance in the U.S.: Origins and evolutions and some perceptions for the future, *Millbank Memorial Fund Quarterly, 55*:161–191

Fetter, R. B., Shin, Y., Freeman, J. L., Averill, R. F., and Thompson, J. D., (1980) Case mix definition by diagnosis-related groups, *Medical Care, 18*(Suppl.):1–53

Freeland, M., and Schendler, C., (1983) National health expenditure growth in the 1980's: An aging population, new technologies, and increasing competition, *Health Care Financing Review, 4*(3):1–7, 12–18

Fuchs, V., (1974) *Who Shall Live?* New York: Basic Books

Galblum, T., and Trieger, S., (1982) Demonstrations of alternative delivery systems under Medicare and Medicaid, *Health Care Financing Review, 3*(3):37–38

Garfield, S., Collen, M., Feldman, R., Soghikian, K., Richart, R., and Duncan, J., (1976) Evaluation of an ambulatory medical-care delivery system, *New England Journal of Medicine, 294*(8):426–431

Garfield, S., Komaroff, A., Pass, T., Anderson, H., and Nessim, S., (1978) Efficiency and cost of primary care by nurse and physician assistants, *New England Journal of Medicine, 298*(6):305–309

Gersten, J., Cenkovich, F., and Dinken, H., (1968) Comparison of home and clinic rehabilitation for chronically ill and physically disabled persons, *Archives of Physical Medicine and Rehabilitation, 49*:615–640

Glass, R., Mulvihill, M., Smith, H., Peto, R., Bucheister, D., and Stoll, B., (1977) The four score: An index for predicting a patient's non-medical hospital days, *American Journal of Public Health, 67*:751–755

Hartunian, N., Smart, C., and Thompson, M., (1980) Economic costs of cancer, motor vehicle injuries, coronary heart disease and stroke: A comparative analysis, *American Journal of Public Health, 70*(12):1249–1257

Health Characteristics of Persons with Chronic Activity Limitation, (1979) *U.S. Vital Health Statistics,* Series 10, No. 137, pp. 133–139

Herrell, J., (1980) Health care expenditures: The approaching crisis, *Mayo Clinic Proceedings, 55*:705–710

Iglehart, J., (1982) New Jersey's experiment with DRG-based hospital reimbursement, *New England Journal of Medicine, 307*(26):1655–1660

Johnson, M., and Keith, R., (1983) Cost-benefits of medical rehabilitation: Review and critique, *Archives of Physical Medicine and Rehabilitation, 64*:147–152

Kane, R., and Kane, R., (1981) A guide through the maze of long-term care, *Western Journal of Medicine, 135*(6):503–510

Katz, J., and Capron, A. M., (1975) *Catastrophic Diseases: Who Decides What?* New York: Russell Sage Foundation

Kleczkowski, B., and Mach, E., (1979) Some reflections on containing the rising cost of medical care under social security, *Social Science and Medicine, 13*(1):21–32

Kobrinski, E., and Matteson, A., (1981) Characteristics of high-cost treatment in acute care facilities, *Inquiry, 18*:179–184

Kodner, K., (1982) Getting a fix on PPO's, *Hospitals, 56*:59–63

Kristein, M., Arnold, C., and Wynder, E., (1977) Health economics and preventive care, *Science, 195*:457–461

Kurylo, L., (1976) Measuring inappropriate utilization, *Hospital Health Service Administration, 21*(1):73ff

Luginbuhl, W., Forsyth, B., Hirsch, G., and Goodman, M., (1980) Prevention and rehabilitation as a means of cost containment, *Journal of Public Health Policy, 2*:103–115

McClure, W., (1976) The medical care system under national health insurance, *Journal of Health Politics, Policy, and Law, 1*:22–28

McNaull, F., (1981) The costs of cancer: A challenge to health care providers, *Cancer Nursing, 4*:207–212

Meenan, R., and Yelin, E., (1981) The impact of chronic

disease: A sociomedical profile of rheumatoid arthritics, *Arthritis and Rheumatism, 24*(3):544–549

Meenan, R., Yelin, E., Henke, C., Curtis, D., and Epstein, W., (1978) The cost of rheumatoid arthritis, *Arthritis and Rheumatism, 21*(7):827–833

Nelson, G., (1982) A role for Title XX in the aging network, *Gerontologist, 21*(1):18–25

Newacheck, P., Butler, L., Harper, A., Piontkowski, D., and Franks, P., (1980) Income and illness, *Medical Care, XVIII*(12):1165–1176

Nyman, J., Dorr, R., and Hall, G., (1981) Escalating costs of cancer chemotherapy, *American Journal of Hospital Pharmacy, 38*:1151–1154

Rabkin, M., (1983) Control of health care costs, *New England Journal of Medicine, 309*(16):982–984

Rice, D., and Wilson, D., (1976) The American medical economy: Problems and perspectives, *Journal of Health Politics, Policy and Law, 1*:151–174

Ricker-Smith, K., (1982) A challenge for public policy: The chronically ill elderly and nursing homes, *Medical Care, XX*(11):1071–1078

Roberts, S., Maxwell, D., and Gross, T., (1980) Cost-effective care of end-stage renal disease: A billion dollar question (part 1), *Annals of Internal Medicine, 92*:243–248

Roemer, M., and Shonick, W., (1973) HMO performance: The recent evidence, *Millbank Memorial Fund Quarterly, 51*(3):271–272

Schroeder, S., (1981) National health insurance: Always just around the corner? *American Journal of Public Health, 71*(11):1101

Schroeder, S., and Showstack, J., (1978) Financial incentives to perform medical procedures and laboratory tests, *Medical Care, XVI*(4):289–291

Schroeder, S., Showstack, J., and Roberts, E., (1979) Frequency and clinical description of high-cost patients in 17 acute care hospitals, *New England Journal of Medicine, 300*(23):1306–1309

Sex differences in health and use of medical care, (1979) *Vital Health Statistics,* Series 3, No. 24, Washington, D.C.: U.S. Government Printing Office

Simborg, D., (1981) DRG creep, *New England Journal of Medicine, 304*(26):1602–1604

Smith, R. T., and Lilienfeld, A. M., (1971) Social Security Disability program: Evaluation study, United States Department of Health, Education and Welfare, *Publication No. 55A 72-11801, Washington, D.C.: USDHEW, U.S. Social Security Administration, Office of Research & Statistics*

Somers, H., (1977) The malpractice controversy and the quality of patient care, *Millbank Memorial Fund Quarterly, 55*:200–230

Starr, P., (1982) Transformation in defeat: The changing objectives of national health insurance 1915–1980, *American Journal of Public Health, 72*(1):78–86

Statistical Abstract of the United States, Washington, D.C.: United States Department of Commerce, Bureau of the Census, 1982–1983, p. 98

Stevens, P., and Stevens, R., (1974) *Welfare Medicine in America,* New York: The Free Press

Terris, M., (1980) The costs and benefits of prevention, editorial, *Journal of Public Health Policy, 1*:285–291

Thompson, R., Basden, P., and Howell, L., (1982) Evaluation of initial implementation of an organized adult health program employing family nurse practitioners, *Medical Care, XX*(11):1109–1127

Turnbull, A., Graziano, C., Baron, R., Sichell, W., Young, C., and Howland, W., (1979) The inverse relationship between cost and survival in the critically ill cancer patient, *Critical Care Medicine, 7*(1):20–23

United States Department of Health and Human Services, (1983) *If You Become Disabled,* April

United States General Accounting Office, (1983) Report to the Subcommittee on Health and the Environment, Committee on Energy and Commerce, House of Representatives, Medicaid and nursing home care: Cost increases and the need for services are creating problems for the states and the elderly, October, p. i

United States Vital Health Statistics, (1981) Series 13, No. 59, p. 26

What You Have to Know about SSI, (1983) United States Department of Health and Human Services, July

World Almanac and Book of Facts, (1983) New York: Newspaper Enterprise Association, p. 958

Your Medicare Handbook, (1984) United States Department of Health and Human Services, January

Zimmer, J., (1967) An evaluation of observer variability in a hospital bed utilization study, *Medical Care, V*(4):221–222, 230–234

Zook, C., and Moore, F., (1980) High cost users of medical care, *New England Journal of Medicine, 302*(18):996–1002

Zucker, J., (1980) Catastrophic health insurance and cost containment: Restructuring the current health insurance system, *American Journal of Law and Medicine, 6*(1):83–103

Zwagg, R., Mason, W., Joyners, B., and Runyan, J., (1980) Cost of chronic disease care, *Journal of Chronic Diseases, 33*:713–720

Bibliography

Berk, A., Phil, M., and Chalmers, T., (1981) Cost and efficacy of the substitution of ambulatory for inpatient care, *New England Journal of Medicine, 304*(7):393–397

Birnbaum, H., (1978) *Cost of Catastrophic Illness,* Lexington, Mass.: Heath

Blagg, C., (1983) After ten years of the Medicare End-Stage Renal Disease Program, *American Journal of Kidney Disease, 111*(1):1–3

Carey, L., (1982) Health costs, competition and the physician, *American Journal of Surgery, 143*:2–5

Cluff, L., (1981) Chronic disease function and the quality of care, *Journal of Chronic Diseases, 34*:299–304

Cunningham, R., (1981) Rise in malpractice scare forces look at previous scare, *Hospitals, 6*:85–90

Curran, W., (1983) Medical malpractice claims since the crisis of 1975: Some good news and some bad, *New England Journal of Medicine, 309*(18):1107–1108

Dirks, J., Schraa, J., Brown, E., and Kinsman, R., (1980) Psychomaintenance in asthma: Hospitalization rates and financial impact, *British Journal of Medical Psychiatry, 53*:349–354

Eisenburg, J., and Williams, S., (1981) Cost containment and changing physicians practice behavior, *Journal of the American Medical Association, 246*:2195–2201

Gibson, R., and Waldo, D., (1981) National health expenditures, 1980, *Health Care Financing Review, 3*:1–54

Ginsberg, E., (1982) More care is not always better care, *Inquiry, 19*:187–189

Goodman, L., and Steiber, S., (1981) Public support for national health insurance, *American Journal of Public Health, 71*(10):1105–1107

Haggerty, R. J., (1977) Changing lifestyles to improve health, *Preventive Medicine, 6*:274–289

Komaroff, A., Flatley, M., Browne, C., Sherman, H., Fineberg, E., and Knopp, R., (1976) Quality efficiency and cost of a physician-assistant protocol system for management of diabetes and hypertension, *Diabetes, 25*:297–306

Kramer, J., Yelin, E., and Epstein, W., (1983) Social and economic impacts of four musculoskeletal conditions, *Arthritis and Rheumatism, 26*(7):901–907

Lansky, S., Black, J., and Cairns, N., (1983) Childhood cancer, *Cancer, 52*:762–766

Mechanic, D., (1978) Approaches to controlling the costs of medical care: Short range and long range alternatives, *New England Journal of Medicine, 298*(5):249–254

Medsger, A., and Robinson, H., (1972) A comparative study of divorce in rheumatoid arthritis and other rheumatic diseases, *Journal of Chronic Diseases, 25*:269–275

Porter, G., (1983) After ten years of the Medicare End-Stage Renal Disease program, *American Journal of Kidney Diseases, 111*(1):1–4

Schechter, E., (1981) Commitment to work and the self-perception of disability, *Social Security Bulletin,* Vol. 44, Part 1

Stein, R., Jessop, D., and Reissman, C., (1983) Health care services received by children with chronic illness, *American Journal of Diseases of Children, 137*:225–230

Strauss, A., (1975) *Chronic Illness and the Quality of Life,* New York: Mosby

Walsh, J. H., (1978) Federal health spending passes the $50-billion mark, *Science, 200*:886–887

Wilson, R., and White, E., (1977) Changes in morbidity, disability and utilization differentials between the poor and the non-poor, *Medical Care, XV*(8):633–646

Yelin, E., Feshbach, D., Meenan, R., and Epstein, W., (1979) Social problems, services, and policy for persons with chronic disease: The case for rheumatoid arthritis, *Social Science and Medicine, 13C*:13–20

CHAPTER EIGHTEEN

Rehabilitation

◇

Introduction

One wonders, as one cares for clients in some stage of chronic illness, what would be the impact of an organized rehabilitation program on the trajectory of their illnesses or on the quality of their lives (see Chapters 2 and 6). The purpose of this chapter is to explore why such programs are not readily available; why public laws do not support rehabilitation, specifically for chronic illness; and what could make such programs possible.

In general, rehabilitation programs deal with individuals whose disabilities are secondary to mobility problems (see Chapter 5). Yet there are many chronically ill persons who are physically mobile but could benefit in other ways from the many techniques and methods involved in the field of rehabilitation. For example, a systematic program teaching how to breathe properly (to increase O_2 uptake and decrease fatigue) would help an individual with chronic obstructive pulmonary disease (COPD). This person could also be taught ways to spare energy by using rehabilitation skills for such purposes as dressing efficiently and managing daily hygiene. The individual could then function as a more productive member of society.

In separate interviews, a number of personnel in two fairly large local rehabilitation centers concurred that rehabilitation would improve the quality of life for those with chronic illnesses, including COPD, congestive heart failure (CHF), and arthritis. They identified economics as the major reason for the lack

of availability of such programs, although all acknowledged that even before the economic crunch clients with chronic illnesses were rarely referred to those centers.

Definitions

Defining some of the concepts developed in this chapter accentuates the physiological, psychological, economic, and vocational factors contributing to the most meaningful life possible for those who have chronic illnesses. A definition of *chronic illness* is provided in Chapter 1. The words *rehabilitation, disability,* and *handicap* need explanation before their relationship to chronic illness can be fully understood.

Rehabilitation. Most health personnel give only lip service to the need for restorative services for individuals with chronic diseases. Moreover, many chronic illnesses are rarely indexed in the rehabilitation literature, despite exceptions such as cerebral vascular accidents (CVA), which would qualify as both a mobility problem and a chronic disease. Nevertheless, an awareness of how rehabilitation is viewed in rehabilitation literature is important if one is to appreciate its value for the chronically ill.

The literature on rehabilitation does contain many definitions pertinent to rehabilitation, but chronic illness is mentioned only in passing, even though the ideas of disability and handicap are implicit. Table 18-1 presents definitions pertaining to

TABLE 18-1. Definitions of Rehabilitation

Source	Definition
Kottke 1980	"Restoration of the functional capacity of the patient with chronic disease or physical disability is the goal of rehabilitation medicine."
Stryker 1977	"Rehabilitation is a creative process that begins with immediate preventive care in the first stage of an accident or illness. It is continued throughout the restorative phase of care and involves adaptation of the whole being to a new life." [This definition comes from a nursing viewpoint.]
Verville 1979	"All items of services and equipment which might be necessary to restore the full function of a disabled person including medical care, psychological services, social services and economic support through a job or otherwise."
National Council on Rehabilitation Education 1961	"The restoration of the individual to the fullest physical, mental, social, vocational, economical capacity of which he is capable."
Krusen et al. 1971	"A creative procedure which includes the cooperative efforts of various medical specialists and their associates in other health fields to improve the mental, physical, social and vocational aptitudes of persons who are handicapped, with the objective of preserving their ability to live happily and productively on the same level and with the same opportunities as their neighbors."
Yesner 1971	"Treatment process designed to help physically handicapped individuals make maximal use of residual capacities and to enable them to obtain optimal satisfaction and usefulness in terms of themselves, their families, and their community."
Rusk 1977	Ultimate restoration of a disabled person to his maximum capacity—physical, emotional, and vocational.
Cole and Cole 1982	Process that promotes a stabilization of lost function and institutes adaptive mechanisms that allow resumption of responsibilities for part or all of one's life.

rehabilitation. Inherent in all these definitions is the concept of maximizing the potential of the individual physically, psychologically, socially, and vocationally. The difficulty is not whether the chronically ill may be considered eligible for rehabilitation services *by definition*. The fact of the matter is that individuals with mobility problems seem to receive priority. These clients are usually young, the exceptions being those older individuals who have had a CVA.

Disability/Handicap. Rehabilitation definitions all speak to the problems of disability, and many relate to the handicapped or use words such as "impairment" to indicate some decrease in function. Ab-

sence of clear differentiation among these terms causes confusion: which indicates decreased function without incapacitating the individual, and which refers to being incapacitated (see Table 18-2)? There are times when the words are used interchangeably.

Whether an impairment constitutes a disability or handicap is not exclusively a medical judgment, since such judgment needs to encompass consideration of the whole person, including such factors as abilities, skills, and possibilities of adaptation. Unfortunately the distinction between impairment and disability is not always recognized, and the existence of impairment is sometimes taken as prima facie evidence of disability. This confusion leads to problems in the

TABLE 18-2. Definitions of Disability/Handicap

Source	Definitions of Disability
The Social Security Act	Disability (except for certain cases of blindness): "Inability to engage in substantial gainful activity by reason of any medically determinable physical or mental impairment which can be expected to result in death or which has lasted or can be expected to last for a continuous period of not less than 12 months" [section 223 (d) (1)]. This act goes on to define a physical or mental impairment as: "An impairment that results from anatomical, physiological, or psychological abnormalities which are demonstrable by medically acceptable clinical and laboratory diagnostic techniques" [section 223 (d) (3)].
Bowe 1978	*Disability* is an impairment that results from disease, accident, or a defective gene. "If the impairment persists for 6 months or longer and interferes with a person's ability to do something—walk, talk, dress, lift—they have a disability." He believes the "problem of disability" has become one of our most urgent national concerns and states that by the year 2000 there will be one chronically ill, over 65, or disabled citizen for every able-bodied person in this country.
Albrecht 1976	"Disability refers to limitations in the kind and amount of individual physical and mental function" and "Disability affects not only socialization of the individual with an injury or disease, but all of the persons of importance in their lives and those with whom he interacts socially."
Athelston 1982	"A disability exists when an impairment causes an inability to perform some major life function such as self care, mobility, communication, or employment."

Source	Definitions of Handicap
Bowe 1978	When a "disability, in interaction with a specific set of environmental conditions, makes one unable to perform certain activities, they are handicapped."
Athelston 1982	"Handicap results when a disability interacts with the environment to impede individual's functioning in some area of life such as work, travel, or fulfilling family or other social roles."
Roberts and Roberts 1979	Handicap "is a collective result of all the hindrances that a disability places between an individual and optimum functional potential."

medical-legal system in connection with disability determination and compensation proceedings and in self-definitions of people with impairments who may be motivated to identify themselves as disabled (Athelston 1982).

Chronic Illness. Reif (1975) identified three general features of chronic illness:

1. The disease symptoms interfere with many normal activities and routines.

2. The medical regimen is limited in its effectiveness.

3. Treatment, although intended to alter the symptoms and long-range effects of the disease, often disrupts the usual patterns of living.

Looking at these characteristics, one can see that chronic illness, like disability or handicap, can in many ways alter an individual's ability to function. The goals of rehabilitation are such that the chronically ill could benefit, whether disabled or not, in the same way that the disabled can benefit.

Historical Perspective

To give context to our concern for the inadequacy of rehabilitation for the chronically ill, we must place the entire field of rehabilitation in its historical perspective. Rehabilitation history reflects people's persistent apathy and insensitivity toward the young, old, poor, mentally impaired, and physically disabled, all of whom are at a disadvantage in comparison with the general population. Primitive peoples, using the philosophy that only the fit should survive, abandoned the disabled and old. Even after such practices had stopped, it was many centuries before people in disadvantageous positions received more than alms. Our current enlightened standards for the care of the disadvantaged still contain an element of apathy and insensitivity toward these individuals (Stryker 1977).

The evolution of rehabilitation for the physically disabled and aged is tied to the growth of social consciousness, with its component sense of responsibility. Marine hospitals, where the disabled could receive care for illnesses, were established in England as early as 1588, at a time when extremely punitive measures were directed toward dependency and disability in the general population. In England in 1601, efforts were made to help the disabled through the passage of the Poor Relief Act. This law outlawed begging (which had previously been sanctioned as legitimate), classified dependent people, and attempted to assist both the poor and the disabled. Our present welfare system, a legacy of that law, still wrestles with some of the same issues that were addressed at that time. In 1842, England launched massive attacks against poverty; later the United States followed suit. Both the Poor Relief Act and the establishment of marine hospitals were efforts to make the poor and disabled self-sufficient by improving their health and thus lessening their dependence on public welfare (Stryker 1977).

The groundwork for modern rehabilitation was laid at the turn of the 19th century. According to Stryker, the nursing literature of that time showed evidence of convalescent nursing care and the need for occupational therapy, which then referred to the constructive use of idle time. The first medical social service department was started at Bellevue Hospital in New York City. Two other dimensions were added at that time—home care and education. Lillian Wald began the first visiting nursing service, and the first professorship of physical therapy was established at the University of Pennsylvania (Stryker 1977).

War influenced the field of rehabilitation. Modern warfare produced new kinds of injuries, which required a new medical approach. For the first time, large numbers of people were maimed and disabled from a cause other than an accident of birth. The term *rehabilitation* came into being during World War I even though the high death rate from spinal cord injuries minimized the importance of rehabilitation. The first inclusive textbook on rehabilitation treatment methods was written in 1941. However, it was not until World War II that rehabilitation demonstrated its restorative power by making it possible for soldiers to return to active duty. Rehabilitation was also used with men who had been hospitalized since World War I, leading in some instances to discharge after 20 years of hospitalization (Stryker 1977).

After World War II, much interest in all phases of rehabilitation continued. Along with industrial growth came an increasing number of industrial injuries. More automobiles brought still more injuries, which in turn led to further need for rehabilitation. Legislation during the postwar period included the Vocational Rehabilitation Act of 1943 and its 1954 amendments. This legislation broadened the scope of both vocational and medical rehabilitation services to disabled citizens and made funds available for professional training and research. As an outgrowth of rehabilitation efforts of World War II, early ambulation was initiated in civilian hospitals in 1944 (Kottke 1980).

Both medicine and nursing rehabilitation organizations now exist. The American Academy of Physical Medicine and Rehabilitation, founded in 1938, set the standards and requirements for the practice of rehabilitation medicine. In 1947 rehabilitation medicine became a board-certified specialty and the American Board of Physical Medicine and Rehabilitation was established. For many years, nurses concerned with the quality of rehabilitation nursing met informally all over the United States. Feeling an increasing need to share their knowledge and experience, they formed the Association of Rehabilitation Nurses (ARN) in 1974 and now have a journal, *The ARN Journal,* related to their specialty.

Public Policy Concerning the Disabled

"Public policy" refers here to the basic philosophy of federal and state governments as reflected in laws dealing with the needs of the disabled, including their rehabilitation (Verville 1979a). There are many policies affecting programs for the disabled, which can include the chronically ill, yet the care provided is still disappointing. Attention to this issue may be lacking because solutions are difficult or approaches do not fit neatly into single categories of health care such as vocational services or education (Verville 1979b). Also, the political impact of the rehabilitation movement is slight compared to efforts put out for acute health care and general education.

Krause (1976) notes that neither poverty nor industrial work has a positive impact on one's health and that occupational health hazards have been well documented. These factors and others have led to enormous changes in the enactment of laws dealing with occupational needs. Every state has Workers' Compensation programs initiated to supply a form of health insurance; the burden of proof of industrial injury falls on the worker, but the law requires the employer to provide coverage. Most states now require vocational rehabilitation to avert the necessity of adding so many workers to the welfare rolls. Costs of these programs are passed on to consumers either directly, through welfare (when workers exhaust their disability benefits), or indirectly, through payments from injury funds in Social Security (Krause 1976). Since corporations pay the bill, they fight to keep amounts down, and their lobbies have often been successful in defeating or weakening occupational health and safety legislation (Krause 1976). Focus is on mobility, and attempts to rehabilitate dis-

abled workers are not usually mandatory. The worker is paid a subsidy for a limited period and then ends up on welfare rolls (Krause 1976). Chronic illnesses are not covered.

Two issues related to income support or disability insurance have seriously affected rehabilitation. First, the definition of disability is definitely linked to earning capacity. A person who earns more than the allowed amount each month loses eligibility for income support and health coverage. This stipulation is a work disincentive and undercuts the effect of rehabilitation. In addition, reports indicate serious discrepancies between myth and reality of rehabilitation effectiveness for the disabled on disability insurance or Supplemental Security Income (SSI). It is also believed that disability insurance rolls have increased because of abuse (Verville 1979a).

Second, disability is essentially an impairment or ailment that presumably prevents one from working and that continues for a long time. This view can become a self-fulfilling prophecy. If benefits are provided only to people whose impairments prevent them from working, then those who are disabled and need income and health coverage will not easily be vocationally rehabilitated (Verville 1979a).

Health Care for the Disabled

The disabled get short shrift from both Medicare and Medicaid, which require being on SSI or having disability insurance. Medicaid does not supply enough coverage to deal with rehabilitation since nearly 50% of Medicaid money goes to either acute care or convalescent and custodial care. Medicare's long waiting period, currently 29 months, delays coverage for the disabled. Two other policies affecting the disabled under Medicare and Medicaid are (1) that support is provided only when one is so disabled for so long that rehabilitation may not be appropriate, and (2) that support is provided primarily for institutionalized care. Such policies could encourage incapacity rather than restoration and productivity (Verville 1979b).

National health insurance could achieve equity of access to health services and provide quality care and cost-effectiveness for the disabled and chronically ill people (Roemer 1980). Rusk (1978) notes that rehabilitation services would be the most effective way to make national health insurance work until corrective treatment for diabetes, cancer, demyelinating diseases, atherosclerosis, and other chronic diseases are found. Rusk goes on to say that rehabilitation personnel have the expertise to teach people to live with residual capacities and return to the community rather than remaining in institutions.

Vocational Rehabilitation

The Rehabilitation Act of 1973 mandated only that physicians recognize the need for rehabilitation services and that they refer patients to professionals who could provide such services. This act was amended in 1978 with encouraging changes that broadened the federal rehabilitation program to include improvement of physical, psychological, social, or vocational functions for the handicapped of any age. The act now creates a public or community service jobs program for the disabled, as well as programs for on-the-job training and employment in industry. It focuses on comprehensive rehabilitation services for the disabled (who may have no immediate vocational potential), the handicapped, the aged, and children (Verville 1979b). However, there is difficulty obtaining money for implementation of necessary new programs (Verville 1979b).

Two elements in this act are not directly vocational. The first is an independent living program that makes it possible for the handicapped to live and work within the community. The second establishes a National Institute for Research for the Handicapped, which stresses developing research to deal with the needs of all the handicapped (Verville 1979b). These elements allow for some focus on the chronicity aspects of disabilities and handicaps.

Verville (1979a) summarizes current government policy regarding the disabled and their rehabilitation:

1. To guarantee equal treatment and opportunity to the disabled who are competent to participate in benefits offered by those institutions receiving federal aid, including education, transportation, jobs, and health and social services.
2. To provide income protection through disability insurance to the above disabled workers and their families and to the poverty-stricken disabled through SSI if they have no ability to work regularly.
3. To provide hospitalization and medical services to disabled workers when sufficient time has passed to assure that they have a real disability (29 months) and when those individuals have no regular work capacity; and to stress convalescent and custodial institutional care.
4. To provide vocational rehabilitation to a limited number of disabled in order to restore their vocational capacity, if feasible, and to provide jobs for a limited number, particularly through public service jobs.
5. To assist the few who cannot work to live independently.

Since the majority of those having chronic illnesses are elderly, it is important to look also at legislation that can specifically affect rehabilitation for their age group (see Table 18-3). It must be noted, however, that there is no central coordinating agency, and variable definitions of *disabled, elderly,* and *elderly disabled* further complicate matters for personnel seeking services for their older clients.

Problems and Issues of Rehabilitation

Laws do not specifically address rehabilitation of the chronically ill; rather, they speak to disability and handicap. Full enforcement or voluntary adoption of these laws becomes the crux of the matter. Verville (1979a) notes that insufficient expenditures for care and services, as well as modest numbers of qualified professionals and educational, social, and vocational institutions and facilities, reflect our limited expectations of disabled persons. The problems described by Verville (1979b) can be summed up as follows:

1. The disabled are not encouraged to become rehabilitated and work.
2. Financing of rehabilitative care for disabled adults is inadequate at the times when most

TABLE 18-3. Legislation Affecting Older Americans*

Legislation	Purpose
Pratt-Smoot Act, 1931	Makes the Library of Congress materials and services accessible to those who cannot read conventionally printed materials. Braille books, talking book machines, cassette players, and so on, are provided at no cost.
Civil Rights Act, 1957	Included in this act is the stipulation that programs receiving federal funds may not deny services because of age.
The Urban Mass Transportation Act, 1964	The aim of this act is to provide mass transportation that is planned and designed to meet special needs of the elderly and handicapped. Cooperative transportation arrangements between Area Agencies on Aging and agencies that provide transportation services are provided. Independent functioning that is prerequisite to rehabilitation success requires access to mass transportation.
Older Americans Act, 1965	To be eligible for the OAA, a person must be over 60. There is no economic means test. A major objective is to keep older persons independent and to postpone or prevent institutionalization. Various social services, such as transportation, escort, shopping assistance, legal aid, homemaker chore service, and counseling, are provided. The act also funds training in gerontology.
The Adult Education Act, 1966 Higher Education Act, 1965	These acts aim at providing lifelong learning, including job training for older retired people. Both these acts expand educational opportunities for adults who are not adequately served by current community educational services. AEA provides basic skills to increase levels of employability, productivity, and income. HEA provides postsecondary education.
The Domestic Volunteer Service Act, 1973	Makes available programs in which older persons may donate their time and talents to service activities. Volunteers are usually paid for meals and transportation and sometimes receive a small stipend. Some programs are Retired Senior Volunteer Programs (RSVP), Foster Grandparents, and Volunteers in Service to America (VISTA).
The Age Discrimination in Employment Act, 1975 (amended 1978)	ADEA prohibits discrimination in hiring practices for persons between the ages of 40 and 70. It also addresses the topic of mandatory retirement based solely on age. Enforcement is the responsibility of the Department of Human Development, and there is a provision for the Secretary of Labor to investigate the feasibility of raising the age limit even higher.

*For additional information on legislation affecting older people, contact the National Senior Citizens Law Center in Washington, D.C.

needed. (Vocational Rehabilitation, Medicaid, and Title XX provide for some comprehensive rehabilitation programs. These programs produce positive results only when the client obtains a job with substantial compensation, including health insurance.)

3. Demands on medical care increase without the financial capacity to deliver such care. In addition, limited numbers of professionals and facilities are available to deliver services, and few professionals have the ability to work with other systems of service.

Impact of Economics

Rehabilitation workers frequently are oblivious to the economic, policy, and political realities surrounding a social reform they appear to support (Krusen et al. 1971). Adequate financing for rehabilitative care is not generally provided when most needed—that is, before disabilities become permanent. Financing for health care and rehabilitation is very limited. The severely disabled person is encouraged to retain government-provided income and health coverage rather than becoming rehabilitated to work. Clients are often told they have a lifelong grant of benefits (Krusen et al. 1971). A more complete discussion of economic issues is presented in Chapter 17. However, it needs to be emphasized that Medicare limits hospitalization payments for chronic illness and health maintenance services, which would be an important aspect of care of the chronically ill. Private insurance companies also restrict and limit their coverage and can assign physicians who may or may not be rehabilitation oriented.

The policy of paying hospitals according to diagnosis-related groups (DRGs) is the latest in a series of legislative attempts to contain costs and will have an impact on rehabilitation for the chronically ill. Since DRGs allow only specific payment for specific illnesses, any additional time needed for the care of the client must be paid for by the hospital. There is concern that clients will be released too soon, particularly the elderly, who constitute the majority of the chronically ill. It is well known that the elderly take longer to recover from acute illnesses or flare-ups of their chronic conditions. The DRG system, phased in completely by 1986, could result in premature release of the elderly as well as others who have not fully recovered. With inadequate recovery and inadequate rehabilitation, these individuals will have to pay more money out of pocket for prolonged health care or therapy. If the elderly do not eat because they are saving for a possible medical crisis, why would they spend money for rehabilitation?

Most government-financed payment programs seek to correct the "fee for service" arrangements, which gave health workers an incentive to run up costs. Some systems, such as Medicaid, rely on contracts that set daily costs and fees in advance. The reimbursement of doctors under one system and hospitals under another creates confusion. Hospitals might make money discharging the client as early as possible, whereas the doctor, on the other hand, may want to keep the client in the hospital for treatment because fees for hospital visits are higher than those for office visits. And the client gets lost in the shuffle.

When hospitalizations for acute illness are limited by a time frame, how can there be an opportunity to evaluate and teach clients how to maximize their potential? Dealing with the loss of function takes time in the same way that initial recovery of physiological homeostasis does. Mastering new methods or skills is not a quick process, especially for those with decreased function and limitation of energy resources.

Impact on Income. Salary loss is expected when an individual cannot work or work activity is curtailed because of illness. Frequent absenteeism can also result in job loss. The cost of illness in terms of medications, treatment, medical visits, and other expenses also cuts into income. With such limitations on income, individuals are not likely to consider rehabilitation as an answer to their difficulties, especially if it means further expenses, delays in returning to work, or cuts in benefits (Krause 1976).

Workers' Compensation, when available, often provides funding at a poverty level and for a limited time. In addition, payments for the occupational diseases that develop slowly, such as black lung disease and radiation poisoning, are lower than those for traumatic and more socially visible damage (Krause 1976). The largest cost of disability is the cost of maintaining an individual as a dependent. Social Security disability insurance is projected to cost $70 billion in 1986 unless a significant number of recipients can be rehabilitated so they do not become permanently dependent upon the program (Kottke 1980).

Costs of Chronic Illnesses. Dr. Kottke, in his comments on economics given to the Academy of

Physical Medicine and Rehabilitation, noted that the major costs of chronic disability pertain to maintaining dependent individuals and their families when there is a loss of functional capacity. These costs are also reflected in loss of productivity, either by client or by family members who quit work to provide home care (Kottke 1980).

We still calculate only the direct costs of necessary health services as the cost of illness. If we do not establish effective rehabilitative management of chronic disease, we will experience increasing cost of welfare services. Even the government, which has to pay both health and welfare costs, makes no attempt to compare total cost of illness *with* rehabilitation to costs of medical care and maintenance *without* rehabilitation. It is not surprising that the rehabilitation of the handicapped does not appear to provide great savings when three-fourths of the cost of nonrehabilitation is ignored (Kottke 1980). A fixed delay from the onset of disability until eligibility for services begins has been a major way to reduce costs of certain federal rehabilitation programs so that the cost of direct rehabilitation services appears to be reduced. Ironically, welfare costs are subsequently greatly increased, leading to more government expenditures because of deterioration secondary to neglect (Kottke 1980).

Health insurance has only slowly begun to cover the cost of chronic diseases. Often insurance premiums are increased when coverage includes outpatient or long-term care, making the policy less attractive—except to the 10% who need this type of coverage. It is difficult for the health care consumer who has no chronic illness to see any advantage to paying for protection against the accumulating costs of chronic disability (Kottke 1980).

Any exotic disease that catches the imagination or frightens the general public and legislators gets funding. Witness the AIDS (acquired immune deficiency syndrome) scare of the 1980s. When enough clamor was heard, the Secretary of Health and Human Services "found" $40 million for AIDS research in the back of her vast empire (Weissman 1983). This is equivalent to the government's spending $10,000 in research per affected person. That sum, if spent

in similar proportions on cancer or heart disease, would swamp the federal budget. Using this ratio, research into Alzheimer's disease, which incapacitates so many older Americans, should be financed to the tune of $20 billion per year and arthritis for $320 billion (Weissman 1983). Yet only a fraction of that amount is spent for research on those diseases, which are less dramatic but affect millions.

Lack of Professional Interest in Rehabilitation

The average medical doctor seems to lose interest in the chronically ill and those with residual disability after the acute phase of illness has passed. Many nurses do not have a rehabilitation focus, and this problem is compounded by physicians who do not recognize the need for rehabilitation. When there is an insensitivity to the need for rehabilitation, referral is made to a clinical subspecialty rather than a physiatrist. Those referrals that are made for rehabilitation are usually unstructured or incomplete. Thus, clients lose the opportunity to improve the quality of their lives.

But lack of referral for the chronically ill is not the only manifestation of limited professional interest. Only half of the medical schools teach rehabilitation medicine to their students, and few physicians have had any training to prepare them for handling rehabilitation problems (Kottke 1980; Anderson, Fenderson, & Kottke 1983). Only 0.5% of physicians in practice have specialized in rehabilitation. The 900 board-certified physiatrists practicing in the United States today represent less than one-fourth the number needed—a disparity between availability and demand that is the major obstacle impeding rehabilitation for the handicapped (Kottke 1980). Physical medicine and rehabilitation (PM&R) has not gained acceptance in medical school curriculums because physiatrists emphasize care of the long-term disabled client rather than the client with an acute disease. As a result, clinical management, as well as research and teaching of chronic disease and rehabilitation, takes second place (Fowler 1982).

Fowler (1982) feels that the long-term viability of this specialty in clinical practice will depend on both a better-defined teaching and research foundation of academic physiatrists and the establishment of a credible presence in the centers of medical education. As of 1980, there were no established qualifications of training and experience for the physician who is going to prescribe and supervise rehabilitation medicine. Kottke feels that the establishment of such criteria would encourage physicians who do not have such knowledge and experience to refer clients to the physiatrist. When the nonspecialist decides which clients would benefit from rehabilitation, a number of individuals remain untreated. The decision not to treat practically guarantees permanent disability and dependency for many who have a potential for improvement. Clients consigned to dependency in institutions attest to the need for an adequate evaluation of their potential for rehabilitation.

Interestingly, there seems to be little concern for the lack of nurses or allied professionals gravitating to rehabilitation (Fordyce 1981). Many nursing schools still do not have well-defined rehabilitation or aging content in their curriculums. The acute illness model continues to be the primary emphasis in these schools. The nursing literature has a minimal content on rehabilitation nursing, and what is available is principally skills oriented. Personal observation indicates that many nurses do not seem to be interested in the care of the chronically ill and do not identify the need for rehabilitation techniques to improve function and quality of life. Some physical and occupational therapy personnel also note that their schools are reducing the number of candidates entering these programs. This change, of course, will influence availability of rehabilitation services to both the disabled and the chronically ill.

For those clients in extended care facilities rather than acute hospital beds, there is even greater limitation on rehabilitation services that would restore them to more independent living (Kottke 1980). Institutional rehabilitation in these facilities is poor or nonexistent. Even though the same standards of eligibility for rehabilitation exist in nursing homes as on the "outside," the availability of services is worse. Usually a rehabilitation program is conducted for an hour or so twice a week, and in most instances attendance is not required or encouraged.

Problems with Rehabilitation Teams

Among members of rehabilitation teams, there seems to be considerable dissatisfaction with how the team functions. Inadequacy of functioning may be the result of some people's difficulty in sharing team responsibility, which could be secondary to a lack of understanding of or commitment to the concept of a team. Health care providers are often task oriented and focus on "doing their own thing." Personal experience with teams indicates that most time is spent on case preparation and little, if any, on learning how to work together. Various disciplines represented on the team do not always acknowledge the value of the educational preparation and knowledge base of their colleagues; there can be a myopic view of the contribution of each member. Physical and occupational therapists sometimes push to practice and prescribe independently of the physician-leader (Fordyce 1981). The nurse coming onto the team as a rehabilitation specialist is probably the newest member and may not have had special training for the role (Rothberg 1981).

To assure future success of rehabilitation practice, we need to change our focus from multidisciplinary to interdisciplinary teams (Rothberg 1981). The multidisciplinary approach occurs when an individual's allegiance is to his or her respective profession; we look to our peers for approval and more often than not are reluctant to accept guidance from other professionals. If this system survives, the problems of chronic illness will continue to be neglected (Fordyce 1981). Not only do the interdisciplinary team members understand their discipline-oriented activities but each team member takes on the responsibility of group effort on behalf of the client (Rothberg 1981).

Rehabilitation teams tend not to work with the chronically ill. Apparently the rehabilitation team does not fully recognize the need of the chronically ill for its services, even though rehabilitation directors do acknowledge that restorative services for the chronically ill would improve quality of life. Rehabilitation is denied when a physician does not identify the need, although, as mentioned earlier, economics is considered the major cause for lack of referral.

◇ CASE STUDY ◇
Distancing of the Chronically Ill

M.J. has been wheelchair bound for several years because of a spinal injury—an obvious physical handicap. She has undergone extensive rehabilitation and drives a specially fitted car and runs a small business. One day, she could not find a "handicapped" parking space near her store. Her first instinct was to verify that the handicapped spaces were being used legitimately. She said that when she looked around inside the store she "didn't see anyone in a wheelchair or anything." What M.J. didn't notice was the shopper who was quite incapacitated with emphysema. Later questioning of this woman brought out the information that she felt guilty using a "handicapped" parking place because she felt, "People look at me funny." She thought that others didn't feel she had the right to use such a space because her impairment was not openly visible.

Restorative programs place greater emphasis on motor goals than on assisting the client to master manageable activities of daily living (ADLs). In addition, the staff and perhaps the family often deny the client a decision-making role (Fordyce 1981).

All of this is unfortunate, since the clientele of America's health care system consists predominantly and increasingly of people with problems of chronicity: chronic illness, chronic disability, chronic impairment. The health care system continues to function and to allocate priorities as if it were still dealing only with acute illness or disability. Most people with chronic illness need the interdisciplinary and comprehensive contribution of rehabilitation and are usually not getting it (Fordyce 1981). The name of the game continues to be acute illness.

Social Invisibility

Zola (1981), who is himself physically handicapped, feels that people who are chronically ill or physically handicapped are made socially invisible (see Chapter 4). He notes that in the eyes of the "able bodied" the physically handicapped become "look-alikes." This distancing of those who are different is attributed to the nature of society and the nature of people. "The . . . discomfiting confrontation of the 'able bodied' with the 'disabled' is not just a symbolic one" (Zola 1981). Zola feels there is an unspoken truth in the sentiment "I'm glad it's not me," commonly felt in the presence of the aged, the suffering, or the dying. In the United States we never tire of denying that we grow old and die, not of "natural causes" and old age but of some chronic disease. Zola feels that this avoidance of reality is a burden carried by the chronically ill in general and the physically handicapped in particular. With many chronic illnesses, however, distancing is not as obvious, since there is rarely an observable handicap, as illustrated in the case study of M.J.

Zola comments further on the experience of having to live according to someone else's definition of physical independence. He talks about people who have to overcome much reluctance, fear, and even pain as they exert considerable efforts to reach former capabilities (Zola 1982). Few seem to consider making the most of what functioning remains, particularly as it relates to the client's life-style. For example, someone with COPD needs help to make a decision about whether to dress or to eat when energy and oxygen capacity allow for only one activity or the other. If some sort of rehabilitation service were offered, chronically ill clients such as this individual would regain more of their social and psychological independence.

Impact on Family

Disability can have a catastrophic impact, not only on clients but on those others who are important to their lives. For example, financial resources are seriously diminished (see Chapter 17). One study showed a decrease in income of more than 40% (Albrecht 1976). Such loss adversely affects families who did not have high predisability incomes. These families are now faced with endless medical and drug expenditures in addition to their expenses of everyday living. Even if they have insurance coverage, most insurance policies have deductible clauses or have upper limits of payments. The family that has to support a severely and/or chronically disabled member is often financially ruined (Albrecht 1976).

Although families do help clients adjust, they can also impede mastery of necessary skills by refusing to become involved or by their "ambiguous or unrealistic expectations" (Albrecht 1976). Health personnel, especially nurses, are in a strategic spot to identify the areas in which families are at risk. Some families already have difficulties before the diagnosis is made. Family members may suffer from feelings of powerlessness and fears about the client's fate. They may be unsure of their ability to handle the needs of the client as a family member, of economics (especially if the client is the breadwinner), or of decisions that must be made. There are many questions: Can they manage at home? Can home be adapted for the patient? Is there agreement on the role of the family in the rehabilitation plan? Can they carry through even if there is agreement? Even the best-adjusted families may transfer their frustration to health personnel, particularly the rehabilitation team. Frustration may be manifested by critical comments even though the client may be making progress.

There is a lot of stress for clients, families, and staff in a rehabilitation setting. The professional needs to know if the family members recognize the significance of rehabilitation teaching when the client is not obviously disabled. The client needs to realize the importance of teaching at a time when he or she does not feel too bad. A chronically ill individual often rules the family, but the family may become reluctant to cooperate. Unless institutionalized clients receive rehabilitation, their status will not improve, but the high cost of dependency will increase nevertheless.

Arthritis sufferers, who constitute the greatest proportion of clients with musculoskeletal diseases, exemplify the impact of a neglected chronic disorder. Arthritis increases directly with age and inversely

with education and income (Kottke 1980). The client, the family, and the health care system tend to neglect necessary maintenance care, thus precipitating a progressively downhill course for the client. Long-term preventive maintenance such as a planned exercise program to help retain function for ADLs would reduce disability for millions of arthritics. The problems of management are compounded by the need for continuing medical, supportive, and environmental services, which must be maintained for years. There is never a dramatic improvement or cure as a psychological reward for the participants. Under these circumstances, it is difficult to persist in efforts and expenditures needed to maintain ADLs when there is so little immediate response (Kottke 1980).

Rehabilitation of stroke victims demonstrates how highly cost-effective such programs can be, in addition to improving the quality of life. Many unrehabilitated stroke clients still occupy an excessively large proportion of beds in institutions because they were not referred for rehabilitation consultation. Referral often depends on the age of the client, the old and old-old being referred less frequently than others (Kottke 1980).

Transportation

Transportation of clients for outpatient rehabilitation is usually erratic and often dependent on transportation programs. Yet even in England, where such rehabilitation is stressed, transportation is undependable. In both the United States and England, this problem is due to unavailability of vehicles, lack of money to support such programs, lack of family support for program objectives, and lack of client interest (Bowe 1978). In addition, some families are not concerned enough to have the client ready for pick-up, and some do not encourage participation. For the client, the need to be transported for therapy can mean a long ride for a short visit and an exhausting, perhaps painful experience.

Role

It was noted earlier that there can be financial advantages to remaining ill. Whether clients would identify the need for rehabilitation in order to improve the quality of their lives might be a problem. Many individuals enjoy the sick role to the extent that they would not participate in any program that would alter that status. Other clients find that they are forced into a sick role by their families. Families and even some health personnel do not always encourage a person, especially an older person, to adapt to the disability to the fullest extent possible. Doctors tell arthritics not to walk, daughters tell their mothers with congestive heart failure (CHF) to rest "because it's time to take it easy." Bowe (1978) notes that recently disabled people end up with perceptions of diminished worth as human beings because of the impact of problems of daily living that come from disability, reduced social status, and decreased income. As self-concepts become damaged, aspirations are lowered and isolation increases, further handicapping the individual.

In his discussion of socialization and the disability process, Albrecht (1976) identifies the following difficulties:

1. Clients, families, and medical staffs are not prepared to handle long-term consequences of injury and disease conditions. People used to die sooner from heart and respiratory diseases and serious accidents.
2. Modern medical practice can prolong life but cannot seem to adjust to the ramifications of that change.
3. Clients and those around them are not socially and psychologically ready to deal with chronic medical conditions. "Physical disability has a major impact on all components of the socialization process."
4. Clients have to redefine their roles, a difficult process because their disability affects their interactions with others and they cannot rely on old patterns and role expectations.

Taking on the impaired role is a difficult process for some because it contradicts many cherished values. Some individuals are uncertain about assuming the role; others may prefer to retain the sick role for the secondary gain of continued dependence on others (Fordyce 1976) (see Chapter 3). When role

change is needed, it might be handled better if the individual had an idea of how long the disability would last. If clients think the disability is permanent, then the adoption of the impaired role could facilitate their rehabilitation. On the other hand, if the disability is seen as being of short duration, then the client might prefer to remain in the sick role and refuse to learn adaptive behaviors such as breathing exercises (Fordyce 1976).

The total impact of disability on values and norms is beyond the realm of this chapter. Albrecht (1976) discusses the complexity of the shocks to the disabled person and those around him or her. His examples include the need for the reconstruction of roles and social interaction patterns, as well as sexuality and physical independence. In particular, behavior required of sick persons is antithetical to behavior valued by the larger society. Persons are also judged by society to be in some way responsible for what has happened and to have earned their present status. This attitude often produces guilt and embarrassment in client and family (Kübler-Ross 1969).

Interventions and Solutions

If the client's status cannot be improved, care must be directed toward preventing further disability. Changes in the client who is chronically ill are often subtle. Being able to do independent daily care (ADLs) should be as important as vocational rehabilitation, which has been the emphasis of public policy. The nurse is in an ideal position to intervene appropriately with clients and family in relation to ADL limitations.

For the chronically ill and their families, quality of life and usefulness to society can be improved if the system will recognize the necessity for teaching and rehabilitation as a means to utilizing or enhancing remaining functions. Health care workers, particularly nurses, should begin to collect data to demonstrate that institutionalization can be avoided or delayed with structured rehabilitation, teaching, and counseling. There is also the possibility of reducing hospitalizations for the chronically ill when both client and family are adequately prepared for living in the community.

Many of the suggestions made here are currently not possible but dependent on changes in public policy and funding. It must be remembered that when all costs (medical as well as financial, personal, and social) are considered, providing rehabilitation services is really more feasible than neglecting them. It behooves all health professionals to become active in working for such policy changes.

Kottke (1980) presents a proposal not only to increase the quality of life but to reduce the total cost of disability. He advocates that programs should be established on the basis of ability to restore the individual to "optimal potential for functioning in society." He suggests that the process of implementing such programs should focus not on avoiding immediate costs but on providing services to restore optimal levels of performance for the individual. Such programs would meet client needs by not only requiring medical and surgical care at the onset of disability but incorporating rehabilitation immediately and continuously. He also feels that necessary equipment (braces, prostheses, wheelchairs, and so forth), assistive home modifications, and necessary transportation should be included.

There are many settings for care of the disabled and handicapped, but home is usually best. To enhance the quality of life for the client with chronic illness and to provide respite for the caregiver, we must consider increasing the use of such options as neighborhood ambulatory and day care centers, extended or intermediate care facilities, foster homes, and regional rehabilitation centers such as the Veteran's Administration Medical Centers. Dependable and inexpensive transportation is a prerequisite to the provision of such services.

Interdisciplinary Health Teams

Typically, hospitals view the discharged client as cured and no longer of concern. Although the health professions are effective in preventing deaths, their interventions are leaving increasing numbers of clients who have chronic disabilities without restoration to optimal levels of function within limits of remaining abilities. The result is increases in cost for maintenance plus costs of medical care because of continued disability. One of the major solutions to the problems that affect the quality of life for the chronically ill is rehabilitation through the creation of an interdisciplinary team of health care givers.

Rothberg, the only nurse yet to be president of the American Academy of Physical Medicine and Rehabilitation, reexamined "health teams" because of her belief that the future of successful rehabilitation practice depends on directing our efforts toward the establishment of truly interdisciplinary teams. Her conclusion is that team members must understand and accept the content description of each other's roles and come to some agreements regarding practice boundaries. She goes on to describe some of the tasks the team must undertake in order to be genuinely interdisciplinary and to produce improved services to clients (Rothberg 1981).

Roemer also sees the further development of the team approach in rehabilitation as a means of cost containment in conjunction with high-quality care. Such an approach will result in greater organization of ambulatory services in health maintenance organizations and health centers that are "conducive to rich use of allied health personnel and to team provision of services" (Roemer 1980).

In view of economic cutbacks, health workers could benefit by acting as advocates for the interdisciplinary team as a whole. As individuals, members of the team could schedule follow-up visits periodically to assess the client's changing needs throughout the course of the disease. Members of the health and rehabilitation team would be able to focus on the aspects of the client's program to which they could make their greatest contribution without spending time reviewing and repeating actions of other team members.

Roles for Professional Nurses. Professional nurses are ideally suited to be coordinators for interdisciplinary teams because only they have a truly holistic picture of the client. One could say that a sole nurse with a "rehab conscience," not necessarily a specialist, would be a godsend in such a situation. At one physical therapy unit the department head agreed that a well-educated rehabilitation nurse would make an ideal team leader for an interdisciplinary team. Writing about Lydia Bailey, who founded the famous Loeb Center for Rehabilitation in New York, Bowar-Ferres provided a definition of nursing based on a helping model:

> What nurses at Loeb strive for and achieve most of the time is to help the patient determine what his goal is, perhaps help him to bring it into clearer perspective and then, with him, work out ways to get there, with the patient's pace consistent with his medical treatment plan and congruent with the patient's sense of who he is (Bowar-Ferres 1975).

In order to perform this role maximally, nurses need the inclusion of rehabilitation as a distinct part of their undergraduate curriculum. Rehabilitation should also be encouraged as an area of specialization in graduate school. In addition, concepts relating to this field should be developed for continuing education requirements and required for those who care for the disabled or clients with chronic illnesses. One study involving individuals with spinal cord injury demonstrated that across professional disciplines, nursing showed the highest proportion of chart entries focused on client teaching (Bleiberg & Merbitz 1983).

Nurse-practitioners with rehabilitation expertise, in addition to their other knowledge, could develop another variation on interdisciplinary teams. They could contract to serve several extended or intermediate care facilities and work with a physical therapist, an occupational therapist, and a nutritionist to see that *all* clients receive rehabilitation training. If a physiatrist is available, he or she could be used for consultation. Such a program would allow for maintenance of primary care, directed nursing care, and all rehabilitation services.

Independence in Practice.   In many countries rehabilitation therapists tend to work with greater autonomy than they do in the United States. It is customary for the physician to write an order for "phys-

ical therapy" that gives the therapist full freedom to evaluate the client and determine treatment (Roemer 1980). Considering the paucity of physiatrists in this country and the inexperience of many physicians prescribing rehabilitation, granting more independence to therapists seems in order. Greater independence would permit therapists to provide service to industry, schools, health maintenance organizations (HMOs), community health centers, and regional rehabilitation centers.

Forming coalitions with other professionals who serve on rehabilitation teams not only could improve the quality of health care for the chronically ill but would promote mutual support. Coalitions could work for policies that would allow all residence facilities for chronically ill or disabled people to be considered rehabilitation centers. Such action would restore the morale of those who work in both intermediate and extended care facilities by emphasizing that they are employed in something other than warehouses for the old. Coalitions could also provide support for therapists pushing for independence from physician members of their discipline, many of whom are not trained physiatrists (Fordyce 1981).

Neighborhood Centers

Centers that would serve chronically ill and disabled individuals and their families could be established in intermediate or extended care settings—an intervention that would require a change in funding policy. Ideally, any chronically ill or disabled individual, regardless of age, who is cared for at home would be eligible to attend. Such centers would give respite to the caregiver, and further, would greatly improve the quality of life for many homebound clients. People who are not yet incapacitated would benefit from a well-planned program that could serve as a great morale booster, as well as preventing further functional disabilities. In addition, classes dealing with the aged and aging could be provided in the neighborhood centers, which would be open to the general public. Rehabilitation professionals might consider an advocacy stance for the establishment of such centers.

◇ CASE STUDY ◇
Making Decisions: The Client's Choice

A.B. is a quadriplegic who has been in intensive rehabilitation to teach him to perform his own ADLs. He is now capable of dressing, transferring, and feeding himself but still needs assistance to bathe. These activities fatigue him tremendously, leaving little energy for anything else. He and his wife have discussed these limitations frequently and he has decided that to retain some quality to his life, it is more crucial for him to go to work every day rather than feed or dress himself. His wife concurs. Consequently, A.B.'s wife performs these ADLs for her husband, drives him to his office, and in this way, allows him to share in the role of providing for the family.

This behavior caused much distress to his therapists who feel that independence is an essential goal. Yet, this decision is based on rational thought to best meet the needs identified by the client and his family.

Research

Not enough research is done in the field of rehabilitation. More research needs to be directed toward validating that hospital stays could be shortened by rehabilitation and that readmissions would be reduced. Research might well indicate that earlier referral to a formal rehabilitation program would improve the client's medical status. Such findings could positively influence legislation and public funding for the chronically ill.

Schuman (1980) did a study in a skilled nursing facility using a team of therapists and ward personnel. The study demonstrated an increase in permanent discharges, increase in home discharges, and decrease in mean length of stay. This study warrants replication using an interdisciplinary team.

Evaluating the Client

We need to be concerned with assisting clients to make the most of remaining abilities, rather than trying to return them to their prior level of functioning. This approach is especially applicable to chronically ill clients, who probably were not evaluated for their functional disabilities in the first place. Evaluating remaining abilities provides the health professional with a means of assisting clients to make choices. As an example, clients who have congestive heart failure (CHF) need to learn how to monitor their energy levels and select activities that they feel are most important. Making choices requires clients to understand that some activities must be left until a later time or omitted entirely.

Involving the Family. Family input is essential when assessing a client's residual functional abilities and deciding what activities are of major importance. When options are available, the team is responsible for educating the client and family about the consequences of decisions. Once a decision is made, as in the case study of A.B., the professional should support it, not condemn it, and should assist client and family to succeed.

Using an Evaluation Tool. Functional assessment is an important step in the treatment of the client with chronic illness. It is vital to know whether the client has the ability to perform tasks independently or with assistance and whether such performance is easy or difficult. Assessment must include vocational activities, ADLs, and related skills such as bending, stooping, and lifting. Rehabilitation philosophy begins with fundamental behavioral issues and considers that the *actual* environment where these behaviors take place is important.

The best indicator of value for service is outcome, measured by the degree of improvement of function and quality of life. Outcome needs to be measured by parameters of client performance throughout the life span, rather than by length of survival (Kottke et al. 1982). To identify these parameters accurately requires the use of a scale that recognizes small changes in function so that a precise evaluation can be done throughout the entire range of performance.

Table 18-4 is an example of a tool that might be used by a nurse to evaluate ADLs and to define benefits of therapy. Such tools provide information for

TABLE 18-4. Functional Assessment Screening Questionnaire

Rate answers to the following questions along the line from:

<u>5</u> Excellent   <u>4</u> Good   <u>3</u> Average   <u>2</u> Poor   <u>1</u> Very Poor

1) Compared to other persons your age, would you say your health is   _____

2) Your ability to be as active as others your age is   _____

3) Your physical ability to do things you *need* to do is   _____

4) Your physical ability to do things you *want* to do is   _____

Please answer yes or no to the following questions:

Do you have any difficulty at all with:

Personal Care Tasks:

Shampooing your hair
Fastening buttons, zippers or snaps
Putting on shoes or tying shoe laces
Cutting your toenails
Getting up from a low seat

Household Tasks:

Cooking on stove
Washing windows or walls
Cleaning the floor when something is spilled
Taking care of your laundry
Doing grocery shopping
Doing gardening
Performing child care

Vocational Tasks:

Concentrating on one task for at least 15 minutes
Reaching, grasping or pinching
Sitting for long periods
Standing for long periods
Climbing ladders
Manipulating foot pedals

Transportation Tasks:

Operating an automobile
Boarding and exiting from a bus

Leisure Tasks:

Playing your favorite sports
Seeing the TV set
Listening to music
Carrying on a conversation

With permission of Gary B. Seltzer et al., (1982) Functional assessment: Bridge between family and rehabilitation medicine within an ambulatory practice, Archives of Physical Medicine and Rehabilitation, 63(10):453–457 the interdisciplinary team dealing with the client. More important, nurses can absorb the role of evaluating the client when settings provide only contract rehabilitation services rather than ongoing formal rehabilitation services. This more limited service is included at many extended care and intermediate care facilities.

Education

Once evaluation has been made, a plan of action needs to be developed and undertaken. Anderson (1978) states that even though rehabilitation is both *treatment* and *training,* it is the training that makes rehabilitation unique. He proposes that if professionals in the rehabilitation setting were more aware of the educational frame of reference, client compliance rates would be greater (see Chapter 12). Most nurses are well prepared in the concepts of teaching and could educate client and family about the goals and objectives of the program. Anderson notes that the medical model of care reinforces the playing of the sick role (see Chapter 3). Under the educational model, clients learn to assume the role of the partially disabled, one that is not too familiar in our society, particularly for men who see no gray area between being totally disabled and fully able bodied.

Beginning with diagnosis, the responsibility for educating the client and family lies with health care providers. Education includes not only management of the disease but prevention of further incapacity. Essentially, nurses should assume their preventive role early in the acute stage of disability. Continuous effort should be made to guard against focusing only on the physiological demands of the acute condition, which tends to obliterate equally valuable preventive and restorative roles. The failure to give suitable emphasis to responsibilities for prevention can lead to increased risk of greatly prolonging the client's hospitalization and ultimately reducing the quality of life (Christopherson et al. 1974). In addition, clients and health workers need to learn that rehabilitation does not have to take place in special buildings with special equipment. In a home environment, for example,

soup cans could be used for weights to build muscles that would otherwise atrophy.

Education of the general public to preventive aspects of chronic illness has also been neglected. Recent studies have clarified the roles of nutrition, exercise, and the intelligent utilization of medical care in acute heart disease. Habits of daily living are difficult to correct because they are so intimately integrated with people's life-styles. Each member of the health team needs to be responsible for reorienting the general public toward better health practices. The educated consumer will in turn make demands on the health care system for better care. We see this effect already in the successes of the severely handicapped in having architectural barriers removed and in obtaining more money for independent living.

Home Visits

Home visits by health workers would enhance the client's and family's ability to live with chronic disease. Such visits help keep the client as active and independent as possible throughout the course of the disease by evaluating strengths and weaknesses, by focusing on assets and strengths, and by evaluating dependency on family. Through home visits, health workers are able to continue their interest in the client and family, which serves to decrease depression and hopelessness by "enhancing self-image and quality of life" (Coe 1976).

National Health Insurance

A national health insurance plan of some sort is in order so that rehabilitation needs of all chronically ill clients can be met from the day of diagnosis. Great gains have been made with respect to public policy through the efforts of aging and disabled people, but often money is not allocated to follow through. Nurses, because of their numbers, could be a great political force to agitate for an adequate health insurance plan. Nurses need also to pursue changes in reimbursement policies for themselves as well as their colleagues, the physical and occupational therapists.

The government, in many instances, will pay more to keep a person in an institution than to subsidize transportation so the client can either receive therapy while remaining at home or have a means of going to work. When there is inadequate funding to pay for needed health services that can keep a family member active and involved, families and friends may be forced to expend tremendous amounts of money, even to the point of bankruptcy. If one accepts limits on available monies, an alternative to the current system would be to provide some sort of voucher system whereby clients and families could decide what services they would buy.

Society could benefit if the disabled had some form of health insurance that has no waiting period and that provides coverage for comprehensive rehabilitation services. Benefits would also be derived if there were provisions for work incentives under SSI and disability insurance that included increased earning limits and allowances for work-related expenses. In addition, our capacity to deliver effective rehabilitation services could be expanded through a major government-wide research effort spearheaded by the New Institute created under PL 94-602 (Verville 1979a). Until comprehensive health insurance is available, we need private insurance companies to make provisions of the same kind for their clients. We need a fairer Workers' Compensation package that will cover the economic, physiological, and psychological needs of workers who are highly prone to environmental risks leading to chronic illness. In spite of the legal commitments that were added to the Rehabilitation Act of 1978, it does not appear that financial commitment is forthcoming for the total implementation of the concept set forth in this act.

Summary and Conclusions

The laws noting that rehabilitation is a right of the disabled and handicapped could be interpreted to include the rights of chronically ill people. Some of these laws strongly imply that money is to be spent for necessary services. However, these laws have not been fully implemented. One major reason is the manner in which money and health care are distributed: the health care system has not demonstrated to those who control health care dollars that rehabilitation is a way of decreasing the waste of millions of dollars and person-hours. Other problem areas that impede the implementation of rehabilitation programs, in addition to legislation and finances, include the lack of adequate numbers of trained personnel; the inability to recognize the need for referrals for many deserving clients and the resultant lack of such referrals; and the lack of interdisciplinary teams to provide quality care.

With sufficient economic support for rehabilitation, health care personnel could improve the quality of life for the chronically ill in many ways. Such support is dependent on changes in public policy and attitudes regarding chronic illness and the disabled. Not only do we need more qualified personnel to provide rehabilitation services, but professionals, the public, and legislators must be educated in the advantages of such change. Creative and innovative health personnel and interdisciplinary teams could improve the status of the chronically ill with resources presently available in most health care settings.

One can focus on changing the health delivery system to increase the effectiveness of rehabilitation (Fordyce 1981) or on encouraging the individual to focus on maximizing remaining functions rather than belaboring lost ones (Zola 1981), or both.

Health professionals must realize that rehabilitation needs to deal with the concept of chronic illness as a disability and, depending on the circumstances, as a handicap. Chronic illness thus becomes amenable to all the precepts of rehabilitation. If we are to enhance the feelings of self-worth of all our clients, then we must change the emphasis of our care to deal primarily not with the acutely ill but with the large and growing population of chronically ill individuals who could benefit from our abilities to maximize their remaining function.

STUDY QUESTIONS

1. Provide at least two reasons why there are not more rehabilitation programs available to the chronically ill.

2. Does the difference in meaning of the words *disability, handicap,* and *impairment* influence current legislation? How does chronic illness fit into these definitions?

3. What is the historic development of rehabilitation? How does this relate to attitudes held by people and to current policy and legislation?

4. What five problem areas affect the provision of rehabilitation to the chronically ill? How do these areas influence rehabilitation services?

5. What interventions should be available if we, as health professionals, are to increase the quality of life and usefulness of clients who are chronically ill? Discuss five such solutions.

6. Identify someone you know who is chronically ill and could benefit from rehabilitation. How would you help this individual and family?

References

Albrecht, G. L. (ed.), (1976) *The Sociology of Physical Disability and Rehabilitation,* Pittsburgh: University of Pittsburgh Press, pp. 257–285

Anderson, T. P., (1978) Educational frame of reference: An additional model for rehabilitation medicine, *Archives of Physical Medicine and Rehabilitation, 59*(5):203–206

Anderson, T. P., (1983) An alternative frame of reference for rehabilitation: The helping process versus the medical model, *Archives of Physical Medicine and Rehabilitation, 64*(2):85–87

Anderson, T. P., Fenderson, D. A., and Kottke, F. J., (1983) Strategies for recruiting medical students, *Archives of Physical Medicine and Rehabilitation, 64*(2):85–87

Athelston, G. T., (1982) Vocational assessment and management, in Kottke, F. J., et al. (eds.), *Krusen's Handbook of Physical Medicine and Rehabilitation* (3d ed.), Philadelphia: W.B. Saunders, pp. 163–189

Bleiberg, J., and Merbitz, C., (1983) Learning goals during initial rehabilitation hospitalization, *Archives of Physical Medicine and Rehabilitation, 64*(10):448–450

Bowar-Ferres, S., (1975) Loeb Center and its philosophy of nursing, *American Journal of Nursing, 75*(5):810–815

Bowe, F., (1978) *Handicapping America,* New York: Harper & Row

Bowe, F., (1980) *Rehabilitating America,* New York: Harper & Row

Christopherson, V. A., et al., (1974) *Rehabilitation Nursing Perspectives and Applications,* New York: McGraw-Hill

Coe, R. M., (1976) Some notes on rehabilitation and models for interdisciplinary collaboration, in Albrecht, G. L. (ed.), *The Sociology of Physical Disability and Rehabilitation,* Pittsburgh: University of Pittsburgh Press, pp. 247–256

Cole, T. M., and Cole, S. D., (1982) Rehabilitation of problems of sexuality in physical disability, in Kottke, F. J., et al. (eds.), *Krusen's Handbook of Physical Medicine and Rehabilitation* (3d ed.), Philadelphia: W.B. Saunders, pp. 889–905

Fordyce, W. E., (1976) A behavioral perspective in rehabilitation, in Albrecht, G. L. (ed.), *The Sociology of Physical Disability and Rehabilitation,* Pittsburgh: University of Pittsburgh Press, pp. 73–95

Fordyce, W. E., (1981) On interdisciplinary peers, *Archives of Physical Medicine and Rehabilitation, 62*(2):51–53

Fowler, W. M., Jr., (1982) Viability of physical medicine and rehabilitation in the 1980's, *Archives of Physical Medicine and Rehabilitation, 63*(1):1–5

Kottke, F. J., (1980) Future focus of rehabilitation medicine, *Archives of Physical Medicine and Rehabilitation, 61*(1):1–6

Kottke, F. J., Stillwell, K., and Lehmann, J. F., (1982) *Krusen's Handbook of Physical Medicine and Rehabilitation* (3d ed.), Philadelphia: W.B. Saunders, pp. xi–xix

Krause, E. A., (1976) The political sociology of rehabilitation, in Albrecht, G. L. (ed.), *The Sociology of Physical Disability and Rehabilitation,* Pittsburgh: University of Pittsburgh Press, pp. 201–221

Krusen, F. H., et al. (eds.), (1971) *Handbook of Physical Medicine and Rehabilitation* (2d ed.), Philadelphia: W.B. Saunders

Kübler-Ross, E., (1969) *On Death and Dying,* London: Tavistock

Reif, L., (1975) Beyond medical intervention: Strategies for managing life in face of chronic illness, in Davis, M., et al. (eds.), *Nurses in Practice: A Perspective in Work Environments,* St. Louis: C.V. Mosby

Roberts, M., and Roberts, A., (1979) Psychological rehabilitation of the handicapped, in Leon, A. S., and Amundson, G. T. (eds.), *Proceeds of the First International Conference on Lifestyle and Health,* Minneapolis Department of Conferences, University of Minnesota

Roemer, R., (1980) Health service developments: Their impact on regulation and functions of rehabilitation personnel, *Archives of Physical Medicine and Rehabilitation, 61*(4):182–187

Rothberg, J. S., (1981) The rehabilitation team: Future direction, *Archives of Physical Medicine and Rehabilitation, 62*(8):407–410

Rusk, H. A., (1964) Preventive medicine, curative medicine—the rehabilitation, *New Physician, 13*:165–167

Rusk, H. A., (1978) Rehabilitation medicine: Knowledge in search of understanding, *Archives of Physical Medicine and Rehabilitation, 59*(4):156–160

Schuman, J. E., (1980) Rehabilitative and geriatric teaching programs: Clinical efficacy in a skilled nursing facility, *Archives of Physical Medicine and Rehabilitation, 61*(7):310–315

Seltzer, G. B., et al., (1982) Functional assessment: Bridge between family and rehabilitation medicine within an ambulatory practice, *Archives of Physical Medicine and Rehabilitation, 63*(10):453–457

Sink, J. M., and Craft, D., (1982) Legislation affecting rehabilitation of older people, *Journal of Rehabilitation,* 85–89

Stryker, R., (1977) *Rehabilitative Aspects of Acute and Chronic Nursing Care,* Philadelphia: W.B. Saunders

Verville, R. E., (1979a) The disabled, rehabilitation and current public policy, *Journal of Rehabilitation,* 48–51

Verville, R. E., (1979b) The rehabilitation amendments of 1978: What do they mean for comprehensive rehabilitation? *Archives of Physical Medicine and Rehabilitation, 60*(4):141–144

Weissman, G., (1983) Research on AIDS gets big dollars, *San Francisco Chronicle,* October 1

Yesner, H. J., (1971) Psychosocial diagnosis and social services—one aspect of the rehabilitation process, in Krusen, F. H., et al. (eds.), *Handbook of Physical Medicine and Rehabilitation* (2d ed.), Philadelphia: W.B. Saunders

Zola, I. K., (1981) Communication barriers between "the able bodied" and "the handicapped," *Archives of Physical Medicine and Rehabilitation, 62*(8):355–359

Zola, I. K., (1982) Social and cultural disincentives to independent living, *Archives of Physical Medicine and Rehabilitation, 63*(8):394–397

Bibliography

Archives of Physical Medicine and Rehabilitation, (1979) *60*(1), entire issue dedicated to independent living

Gans, J. S., (1983) Hate in the rehabilitation setting, *Archives of Physical Medicine and Rehabilitation, 64*(4):176–179

Granger, C. V., (1982) Health accounting—functional assessment in the long term patient, in Kottke, F. L., et al. (eds.), *Krusen's Handbook of Physical Medicine and Rehabilitation* (3d ed.), Philadelphia: W.B. Saunders

Rusk, H. A., (1977) *Rehabilitation Medicine* (4th ed.), St. Louis: C.V. Mosby

Wallace, S. G., and Anderson, A. D., (1978) Imprisonment of patients in the course of rehabilitation, *Archives of Physical Medicine and Rehabilitation, 59*(9):424–429

A P P E N D I X A

Selection of National Organizations Related to Chronic Illness*

Name and Address	Type of Service/Comments
AGING	
American Association of Homes for the Aging 1050 17th St., N.W., Suite 770 Washington, D.C. 20036	Education, service
American Association of Retired Persons (AARP) 1909 K St. N.W. Washington, D.C. 20049	Service, newsletter
Children of Aging Parents (CAPS) 2761 Trenton Rd. Levittown, PA 19056	Education, self-help groups, newsletter
Divorce After 67 c/o Turner Geriatric Clinic 1010 Wall St. University of Michigan Ann Arbor, Michigan 48109	Support; research; counseling; legal, medical, and financial information
Elder Craftsmen 135 E. 65th St. New York, N.Y. 10021	Provides a nonprofit outlet for elders' crafts on consignment
Fifty Upward Network (FUN) P.O. Box 4714 Cleveland, OH 44126	Education; support for middle-aged women who are single, divorced, or widowed
Gray Panthers 3635 Chestnut St. Philadelphia, PA 19104	Education, research, service, referral, newsletter
Legal Services for the Elderly 132 W. 43rd St., 3rd Fl. New York, N.Y. 10036	Service, funded by grants and Legal Services Corporation

*Source: Akey, D. S. (ed.), (1984) *Encyclopedia of Associations* (18th ed.), Detroit: Gale (Vol. I, parts 1 and 2; vol. III, issues 1 and 2). The organizations selected for the Appendix are only a small sample of many thousands listed.

Name and Address	Type of Service/Comments
National Association of Older Worker Employment Services c/o National Council on Aging West Wing 100 Suite 208 600 Maryland Ave. S.W. Washington, D.C. 20024	Education, service, newsletter

CANCER

Corporate Angel Network (CAN) Hangar F, Westchester Airport White Plains, N.Y. 10604	Service, air transportation on U.S. corporation aircraft for cancer patients to treatment centers
Lost Chord Clubs c/o American Cancer Society International Association of Laryngectomies 777 Third Ave. New York, N.Y. 10017	Support groups, newsletter

Forty-two additional organizations are listed under *Cancer.*

HANDICAPPED

Accent on Information P.O. Box 700 Bloomington, IL 61701	Computerized retrieval system to help the disabled live more effective lives by providing them information
Amputee Shoe and Glove Exchange 1635 Warwickshire Dr. Houston, TX 77077	Service
Handicapped Introductions P.O. Box 48 636 W. Oxford St. Coopersburg, PA 18036	Education, workshops, counseling, introductions

Fifty-four additional organizations are listed under *Handicapped.*

HEARING AND VISION

American Council of the Blind Parents	Support Outreach
Independent Visually Impaired Enterprisers	Education Newsletter
Visually Impaired Data Processors International	

The above three organizations are in care of
American Council of the Blind
1211 Connecticut Ave., N.W., Suite 506
Washington, D.C. 20036

Seventy-three additional organizations are listed under *Blind.*

Dogs for the Deaf 13260 Hwy. 238 Jacksonville, OR 97539	Service, newsletter

Thirty-one additional organizations are listed under *Deaf.*

Name and Address	Type of Service/Comments

MENTAL ILLNESS

American Anorexia Nervosa Association
133 Cedar Lane
Teaneck, NJ 07666

Information and referral, counseling, self-help, newsletter

National Alliance for the Mentally Ill
1234 Massachusetts Ave., N.W., No. 721
Washington, D.C. 20005

Self-help, education, advocacy, research, newsletter

National Society for Children and Adults with Autism
1234 Massachusetts Ave., N.W. Suite 1017
Washington, D.C. 20005

Education, referral, placement, newsletter

Phobia Society of America
6191 Executive Blvd.
Rockville, MD 20852

Service, self-help, clearinghouse for resources, newsletter

MENTAL RETARDATION

Mental Retardation Association of America
211 E. 300 South St. Suite 212
Salt Lake City, UT 84111

Support, research, education, legislation

PKU Parents
518 Paco Dr.
Los Altos, CA 94027

Support, education, newsletter

Nineteen additional organizations are listed under *Mental Retardation*.

NEUROLOGIC AND/OR MUSCULAR DISORDERS

Alzheimer's Disease and Related Disorders Association
360 N. Michigan Ave. Suite 601
Chicago, IL 60601

Education, research, support, newsletter

American Paralysis Association
4100 Spring Valley Rd. Suite 104 L.B. 3
Dallas, TX 75234

Research, fund raising, speakers bureau, newsletter

Association of Sleep Disorders Center
P.O. Box YY
East Setauket, NY 11733

Diagnosis, treatment, education, research, newsletter

Lupus Foundation of America
11673 Holly Springs Dr.
St. Louis, MO 63141

Education, support, research, newsletter

National ALS Foundation (Amyotrophic Lateral Sclerosis)
185 Madison Ave.
New York, NY 10016

Education, service, research, newsletter

National Committee on the Treatment of Intractable Pain
P.O. Box 9553 Friendship Station
Washington, D.C. 20016

Education, research, speakers bureau, legislation, newsletter

National Migraine Foundation
5252 N. Western Ave.
Chicago, IL 60625

Education, research, newsletter

Name and Address	Type of Service/Comments
Paget's Disease Foundation P.O. Box 2772 Brooklyn, NY 11202	Education, help to locate financing of service, newsletter
Parkinson Support Groups of America 11376 Cherry Hill Rd. No. 204 Beltsville, MD 20705	Education, self-help, legislation, clearinghouse, newsletter

Thirty-one additional organizations are listed under *Neurologic Disorders.*

REHABILITATION

National Association of Rehabilitation Professionals in the Private Sector 1133 15th St. N.W. Suite 1000 Washington, D.C. 20005	Information exchange
National Rehabilitation Information Center 4407 Eighth St. N.E. Washington, D.C. 20017	Clearinghouse, international on-line computer, research, education, newsletter in braille and printed editions
National Wheelchair Athletic Association 2107 Templeton Gap Rd. Suite C Colorado Springs, CO 80907	Amateur sports events, newsletter

Twenty-three additional organizations are listed uner *Rehabilitation.*

SUBSTANCE ABUSE

Alcoholics Anonymous World Services P.O. Box 459 Grand Central Station New York, NY 10163	Service
American Atheist Addiction Recovery Groups P.O. Box 6120 Denver, CO 80206	Self-help for nonreligious persons, speakers bureau, pamphlets
BACCHUS (Boost Alcohol Consciousness Concerning the Health of University Students) 124 Tigert Hall University of Florida Gainesville, FL 32611	Self-help, support, newsletter
Straight, Inc. P.O. Box 40052 St. Petersburg, FL 33743	Service to adolescent substance abusers, newsletter

Twenty-five additional organizations are listed under *Drug Abuse.*

Thirty-one additional organizations are listed under *Alcohol Abuse.*

OTHER ORGANIZATIONS

Self Help Center 1600 Dodge Ave. Suite S-122 Evanston, IL 60201	Clearinghouse for information on all types of self-help groups: alcohol, drugs, batterers, depression, emphysema, epilepsy, chronic mental illness, gambling, impotence, overeating, child abuse, burn victims, mistresses, and so on

Name and Address	Type of Service/Comments
American Allergy Association P.O. Box 7273 Menlo Park, CA 94025	Service, education, newsletter
American Cleft Palate Association Administrative Office 331 Salk Hall University of Pittsburgh Pittsburgh, PA 15261	Education, research; referral, newsletter
American Federation of Home Health Agencies 429 N St. S.W. Suite S-605 Washington, D.C. 20024	Education, legislation
Coronary Club 3659 Green Rd. Cleveland, OH 44122	Education, rehabilitation
Herpes Resource Center Box 100 Palo Alto, CA 94302	Support, education, research, newsletter
Know Problems of Hydrocephalus Rt. 1 Box 210A River Road Joliet, IL 60434	Education, public policy, referral, newsletter
National Association for Sickle Cell Disease 3460 Wilshire Blvd. Suite 1012 Los Angeles, CA 90010	Education, service, legislation, newsletter
National Burn Victim Foundation 308 Main St. Orange, NJ 07050	Education, referrals, counseling, self-help groups, newsletter
National Foundation for Ileitis and Colitis 295 Madison Ave. New York, NY 10017	Education, research, newsletter
National Ichthyosis Foundation P.O. Box 252 Belmont, CA 94002	Education, research, support, newsletter
Premenstrual Syndrome Action P.O. Box 9326 Madison, WI 53715	Education, counseling, newsletter
Resolve, Inc. P.O. Box 474 Belmont, MA 02178	Counseling, referral and support related to infertility, newsletter
Step-Up Foundation (Society to Educate Persons with Urinary Problems) Box 8 Dunbridge, OH 43414	Education, research, support
TOPS Club P.O. Box 07489 4575 S. Fifth St. Milwaukee, WI 53207	Self-help weight control, newsletter

Author Index

Subject Index